## The American Civil War Surgery Series

### Edited by Ira M. Rutkow, M.D., Dr.P.H.

1. S.D. Gross: *A Manual of Military Surgery* (Philadelphia, 1861)

2. S.P. Moore: *A Manual of Military Surgery, Prepared for the Use of the Confederate States Army*. (Richmond, 1863)

3. S.W. Mitchell, G.R. Morehouse and W.W. Keen: *Gunshot Wounds and Other Injuries of Nerves* (Philadelphia, 1864)

4. J.J. Chisolm: *A Manual of Military Surgery* (Richmond, 1861)

5. F.H. Hamilton: *A Practical Treatise on Military Surgery* (New York, 1861)

6. E. Warren: *An Epitome of Practical Surgery for Field and Hospital* (Richmond, 1863)

7. C.S. Tripler and G.C. Blackman: *Hand-book for the Military Surgeon* (Cincinnati, 1861)

8. S. Smith: *Hand-book of Surgical Operations* (New York, 1862)

9. F. Formento: *Notes and Observations on Army Surgery* (New Orleans, 1863), bound with:

   M. Schuppert: *A Treatise on Gun-shot Wounds: Written for and Dedicated to the Surgeons of the Confederate States Army* (New Orleans, 1861)

10. J.H. Packard: *A Manual of Minor Surgery* (Philadelphia, 1863)

11. Adjutant-General and the Surgeon-General: *List of Battles and Roster of Regimental Surgeons and Assistant Surgeons During the War of the Rebellion* (Washington, D.C., 1883)

# List of Battles and Roster of Regimental Surgeons

# An Alphabetical List of THE BATTLES OF THE WAR OF THE REBELLION,

Compiled from the
Official Records of the office
of the Adjutant-General and
the Surgeon-General, U.S.A. and

# A Roster of all THE REGIMENTAL SURGEONS AND ASSISTANT SURGEONS

in the Late War
and Hospital Service

Reprinted with a New Index to Names and Introduction

by Ira M. Rutkow, M.D., Dr.P.H.

Norman Publishing
San Francisco
1990

Published by Norman Publishing
Division of Jeremy Norman & Co., Inc.
442 Post Street
San Francisco, California 94102-1579



Library of Congress Cataloging-in-Publication Data

Wells, J. W. (John Wesley)
An alphabetical list of the battles of the War of the Rebellion / compiled from the official records of the Adjutant-General and the Surgeon-General, U.S.A. and a roster of all the regimental surgeons and assistant surgeons in the late war and hospital service; reprinted with a new index to names and a new introduction by Ira M. Rutkow.
p. cm. — (The American Civil War Surgery Series ; 11)
"By J.E. Wells and N.A. Strait, revised by Newton A. Strait"—Added t.p.
Reprint. Originally pub.: Rev. ed. Washington, D.C. : G.M. Van Buren, 1883.
ISBN 0–930405–10–2 (alk. paper)
1. United States—History—Civil War, 1861-1865—Campaigns. 2. United States—History—Civil War, 1861-1865—Registers. 3. United States. Army—Surgeons—Registers. I. Strait, N. A. (Newton Allen), d. 1922. II. Title. III. Series: American Civil War surgery series ; no. 11.
E470.1.W48 1990
973.7'3—dc19
The American Civil War Surgery Series, no. 11.

This book is printed on acid-free paper, and its binding materials have been chosen for strength and durability.

Manufactured in the United States of America.

# PREFACE

The beginnning of the Civil War found the United States Army Medical Department unprepared to cope with the rapidly intensifying crisis. Its resources in supplies and personnel were pitifully inadequate and did not provide any overall medical plan to care for the wounded soldiers. In 1860, the Army's medical staff consisted of the Surgeon-General, thirty surgeons, and eighty-three assistant surgeons. Three surgeons and twenty-one assistant surgeons were from the South and eventually resigned their commissions. Only five surgeons and eight assistant surgeons whose homes were in the South remained on the medical staff. Three other assistant surgeons were dismissed for disloyalty. The medical corps thus began its wartime service with approximately ninety officers.

Although termed "surgeons," most of these men in fact had little or no operative experience and were really capable of only general medical practice. During the war more than 12,000 physicians were called into service in either the field or hospital. These doctors were also called surgeons, but only a few had received training in surgery. This unfortunate practice of referring to all physicians in Army service as surgeons has complicated efforts to understand the problems of the Civil War soldier in obtaining medical and surgical care.

The problems of providing medical care in the Union Army have been documented in George W. Adams's *Doctors in Blue*. Much of the following information is derived from his admirable monograph. The Northern medical services were organized into seven distinct categories:

1. Surgeons and Assistant Surgeons of the United States Army. This was the regular Medical Corps and consisted of men in service when the war began and additional personnel authorized by Congress. They were used primarily for staff duty.

2. Surgeons and Assistant Surgeons of Volunteers. These were the former "brigade surgeons" created by Congress to supplement the work of the regular staff surgeons. A total of 547 commissions were issued.

3. Regimental Surgeons and Assistant Surgeons, commissioned by state governors rather than by the Congress or the President. There were 2,109 Surgeons and 3,882 Assistant Surgeons, the largest category within the entire medical hierarchy.

4. Acting Assistant Surgeons, United States Army. These physicians were known as the "contract" surgeons. They held no commission but received the pay of first lieutenants. There were a total of 5,532 Acting Assistant Surgeons; most worked in the general hospitals in the North. They also continued their civilian practice.

5. Medical officers of the Veterans Corps.

6. Acting Staff Surgeons.

7. Surgeons and Assistant Surgeons of Colored Troops. These physicians received presidential commissions, but were ineligible for staff positions. They were mainly assigned to various Black troops.

Most of the Regimental Surgeons and Assistant Surgeons noted in the reprinted roster are found in categories 3 and 7. Many received pensions and therefore the federal and state government maintained post-office addresses.

The Medical Service of the Confederate States Army has been ably described by H. H. Cunningham in his *Doctors in Gray*. In 1916, at the 19th Annual Meeting of the Association of Medical Officers of the Army and Navy of the Confederacy, it was reported that 3,237 surgeons or assistant surgeons had been nominated by Jefferson Davis (1808–1889) and confirmed by the Senate for duty in the Army's Medical Service. In addition, another 107 had served in the Navy. It is important to realize that these figures exclude contract physicians. Like the North, the South paid contract surgeons on a part-time basis while they continued their civilian practice.

Unfortunately, almost all the important papers of the Medical Department of the Confederate States Army were burned when the buildings in Richmond that housed the Surgeon General's office were destroyed by fire during the evacuation of that city (April 2, 1865). As a consequence, there are no detailed lists outlining who the Confederate surgeons were and what unit they served with.

It is known that the Confederate Medical Department was arranged quite similarly to that of the Union Army. This was a deliberate act on the part of the Confederate Surgeon-General Samuel Preston Moore (1813–1889), who had previously served in the United States Army. Each army corps, of which there were eighteen in September 1864, had a medical director. The medical director was immediately responsible to one of five medical directors of the army. Immediately below the corp medical director came the chief surgeons of the various army divisions. These physicians were recommended for appointment by the medical director and were free from all regimental tasks. Below the division level was the brigade, each of which had a senior surgeon, who was not relieved from regimental service. Within each brigade were numerous regiments and they generally had one surgeon and one assistant surgeon. Supporting these physicians were the countless contract doctors.

The overall effectiveness of the Union and Confederate medical services should be judged in the context of mid nineteenth-century military medicine. In spite of disorganization, shortages of supplies, and overwhelming difficulties in taking basic measures to protect public health, the overall care rendered to both the Union and Confederate soldier must be considered more than adequate when compared with the care received by soldiers in the European wars of that era.

ADOPTED BY THE PENSION BUREAU, SECOND AUDITOR, THIRD AUDITOR, AND SECOND COMPTROLLER, TREASURY DEPARTMENT.

---

# AN ALPHABETICAL LIST

OF THE

# Battles of the War of the Rebellion,

WITH DATES,

From Ft. Sumter, S. C., April 12 and 13, 1861, to Kirby Smith's Surrender, May 26, 1865,

COMPILED FROM THE OFFICIAL RECORDS

OF THE OFFICE OF THE

## Adjutant-General and the Surgeon-General, U. S. A.,

BY J. W. WELLS AND N. A. STRAIT,

REVISED BY NEWTON A. STRAIT,

WITH THE ADDITION OF MANY INCIDENTS OF THE WAR,

Giving the number killed, wounded, and missing in each of the important Battles, Union troops engaged, names of the Generals killed and wounded in both armies; also the *total* number of enlistments, number discharged, number wounded, number missing, number of deaths, number killed in battle, number of graves, and

## A CHRONOLOGICAL HISTORY OF THE WAR OF THE REBELLION,

AND A LIST OF THE PRESIDENTS AND VICE-PRESIDENTS OF THE UNITED STATES FROM WASHINGTON TO ARTHUR,

AND A

ROSTER OF ALL THE

## REGIMENTAL SURGEONS AND ASSISTANT SURGEONS

IN THE LATE WAR AND HOSPITAL SERVICE,

With their last known post-office address, with date of muster out of each regiment and organization, and number of regiments, batteries, and independent companies from each State.

---

WASHINGTON, D. C.
G. M. VAN BUREN, PUBLISHER.
1883.

E. W. Oyster, Printer,
339 Penna. Ave., Washington, D. C.

# AN ALPHABETICAL LIST OF BATTLES

OF THE

## WAR OF THE REBELLION,

### WITH DATES.

---

| | | |
|---|---|---|
| Abbeville | Miss | Aug. 12, 23, 25, 1864. |
| Abb's Valley | Va | May 8, 1864. |
| Aberdeen | Ala | Nov. 17, 1864. |
| Aberdeen | Ark | July 9, 1862. |
| Abingdon | Va | Dec. 15, 1864. |
| Abo Pass | N. Mex. | July 3, 1865. |
| Ackworth | Ga | June 3, 4, 1864. |
| Acton | Minn | Sept. 2, 3, 1862. |
| Adairsville | Ga | May 17, 18, 1864. |
| Adamsville | Tenn | April 4, 1862. |
| Aetna | Mo | July 22, 1861. |
| Aiken | S. C | Feb. 11, 1865. |
| Albuquerque | N. Mex. | April 9, 1862. |
| Aldie | Va | Oct. 9, 31, 1862, June 17, 1863. |
| Alexandria | La | April 26, 1864, May 2–8, 1864. |
| Alimosa | N Mex. | Oct. 4, 1861. |
| Allatoona | Ga | Oct. 5, 1864. |
| Allen's Farm | Va | June 29, 1862. |
| Alliance Steamer | Fla | March 8, 1865. |
| Alpine Gap | Ga | Sept. 11, 1863. |
| Alpine Station | Va | Jan. 4, 1862. |
| Altoona Hills | Ga | May 25–June 4, 1864. |
| Amelia Springs, or Jettersville | Va | April 5, 1865. |
| Amitie River | La | March 28, 1863, March 18, 1865. |
| Anandale | Va | Dec. 4, 1861. |
| Anderson's Crossroads | Tenn | Oct. 2, 1863. |
| Anderson's Gap | Tenn | Oct. 1, 1863. |
| Anthony's Hill | Tenn | Dec. 25, 1864. |
| Antietam, or Sharpsburg | Md | Sept 16, 17, 1862. |
| Antioch Station | Tenn | April 10, 1863. |
| Antoine | Ark | April 2, 1864. |
| Anxvois River | Tenn | Oct. 20, 1862. |
| Apache Cañon, or Glorietta | N. Mex. | March 26–28, 1862. |
| Apache Pass | Ariz | July 15, 1862. |
| Appomattox Court-House, or Clover Hill, (Lee surrendered) | Va | April 9, 1865. |
| Arivapo Cañon | | June 8, 1864. |
| Arkadelphia | Ark | Feb. 15, 1863, March 28, 1864. |
| Arkansas Post | Ark | Jan. 11, 1863. |
| Arkansas River | Ark | Dec. 18, 1864. |
| Armstrong Ferry | Tenn | Jan. 22, 1864. |
| Arrowfield Church | Va | May 9, 10, 1864. |
| Arrow Rock | Mo | July 29, 1862. |
| Arthur's Swamp | Va | Aug. 29, 30, Sept. 30, Oct. 1, 1864. |
| Ash Bayou | La | Nov. 19, 1864. |
| Ashby's Gap | Va | Sept. 22, 1862, July 12, 1863, July 18, 1864, Feb. 18, 1865. |
| Ashepoo River | S. C | May 16, 1864. |
| Ashland | La | June 6–8, 1863. |
| Ashland | Va | May 11, 30, 1864, March 15, 1865. |
| Ashley's Mills | Ark | Sept 7, 1863. |
| Ashley's Station | Ark | Aug. 24, 1864. |
| Ashton | La | May 1, 1864. |

| | | |
|---|---|---|
| Ashwood | Miss | June 25, 1864. |
| Ashwood Landing | La | May 1-4, 1864. |
| Assault on Fort Wagner | S. C. | July 10, 11, 1863. |
| Atchafalaya | La | Sept. 9, 10, 1863. |
| Atchafalaya River | La | Sept. 7, 1863, July 28, 1864. |
| Athens | Ala | Jan. 25, Sept. 23, Oct. 1, 2, 1864. |
| Athens | Ky | Feb. 23, 1863. |
| Athens | Mo | Aug. 5, 1861. |
| Athens Ranch | Col | Aug. 22, 1864. |
| Atlanta. (See also siege of) | Ga | July 21–Aug. 25, Nov. 9, 1864. |
| Atlee's | Va | March 1, 1864. |
| Attack on transport Crescent City | | May 18, 1863. |
| Attempt on rebel ram Arkansas | | July 15, 1862. |
| Auburn | Ga | July 18, 1864. |
| Auburn | Va | Oct. 14, 1863. |
| Augusta | Ark | April 1, Sept. 2, 1864. |
| Augusta | Ky | Sept. 27, 1862. |
| Austin | Ark | Aug. 31, 1863. |
| Austin | Miss | Aug. 2, 1862. |
| Averill's raid in West Virginia | | Aug. 25–30, 1863. |
| Averill's raid in Southwest Virginia | | Dec. 8–21, 1863. |
| Averysboro, or Smith's Farm | N. C | March 15, 16, 1865. |
| Avoyelle's Prairie | La | May 14, 16, 1864. |
| Bachelor's Creek | N. C. | Nov. 11, 1862, May 23, 1863, Feb. 1–3, 1864. |
| Bacon Creek | Ky | Dec. 26, 1862. |
| Bad Lands | D. T. | Aug. 8, 1864. |
| Bagdad | Ky | Dec. 12, 1861. |
| Baker's Creek | Miss | May 16, 1863, Feb. 5, 1864. |
| Baker's Springs | Ark | Jan. 24, 25, 1864. |
| Baldwin | Miss | June 9, Oct. 2, 1862. |
| Baldwin's Ferry | Miss | May 13, 1863. |
| Ball's Bluff, or Edward's Ferry, Harrison's Island, and Leesburg | Va | Oct. 21, 1861. |
| Ball's Crossroads | Va | Aug. 27, 28, 1861. |
| Ball's Ferry | Ga | Nov. 24, 25, 1864. |
| Ball's Mills | Mo | Aug. 28, 29, 1861. |
| Baltimore, streets of | Md | April 19, 1861. |
| Baltimore Crossroads | Va | June 26, 1863, July 2, 1863. |
| Barber's Crossroads | Va | Nov. 5, 1862, Sept. 1, 1863. |
| Barber's Place | Fla | Feb. 9, 10, 1864. |
| Barboursville, also Red House | W. Va. | July 12, Sept. 18, 1861. |
| Bardstown | Ky | Oct. 4, 1862. |
| Barnett's Ford | Va | Feb. 7, 1864. |
| Barnwell's Island | S. C | Nov. 24, 1863. |
| Barrancas | Fla | July 22, 1864. |
| Barren Fork | I. T | Dec. 19, 1863. |
| Bartlett's Mills | Va | Nov. 27, 1863. |
| Barton Station | Miss | April 16, Oct. 20, 1863. |
| Bastin Mountain | Mo | Nov. 9, 1862. |
| Batesville | Ark | July 14, 1862, Feb. 4, 1863. |
| Bath | Va | Jan. 4, 1862, Sept. 8, 1863. |
| Baton Rouge | La | Aug. 5, 1862, Sept. 8, 1863, March 8, May 3, and June 16, 1864. |
| Battery Huger | Va | April 18, 1863. |
| Battle Creek | Tenn | June 21, 1862. |
| Baxter's Springs | Ark | Oct. 6, 1863. |
| Bayle's Crossroads | La | Oct. 12, 1861. |
| Baylor's Farm | Va | June 15, 1864. |
| Bayou Barnard | I. T | July 28, 1862. |
| Bayou Biddell | La | Oct. 15, 1864. |
| Bayou Boeuff | La | Dec. 13, 1863, May 7, 1864. |
| Bayou Bontecom | La | Nov. 21, 1862. |

| | | |
|---|---|---|
| Bayou Bordeaux | La | Nov. 3, 1863. |
| Bayou Cache, or Cotton Plant, Round Hill, Bayou De Vieu, and Hill's Plantation | Ark | July 7, 1862. |
| Bayou De Glaize, or Old Oaks, Simmsport, Yellow Bayou, and Calhoun Station | La | May 18, 1864. |
| Bayou De Mora | La | May 12, 1864. |
| Bayou De View | Ark | July 7, 1862. |
| Bayou La Fourche, or Ash Bayou | La | Nov. 19, 1864. |
| Bayou La Mourie | La | May 7, 1864. |
| Bayou Macon | La | May 10, 1863. |
| Bayou Mason | Miss | July —, 1864. |
| Bayou Metoe | Ark | Aug. 27, Sept 1, 1863. |
| Bayou Pierre | Miss | May 2, 1863. |
| Bayou Rapids | La | March 21, 1864. |
| Bayou Roberts | La | May 8, 1864. |
| Bayou Sara | Miss | Nov. 9, 1863. |
| Bayou Saint Louis | Miss | Nov. 17, 1863. |
| Bayou Teche | La | Nov. 3, 1862, Jan. 14, 1863. |
| Bayou Tensas | La | June 30, Aug. 10, 1863, July 30, Aug. 26, 1864. |
| Bayou Tunica | La | Nov. 9, 1863. |
| Bay Springs | Miss | Oct. 26, 1863. |
| Beachtown | Ga | July 22, 1864. |
| Bealington | W. Va | July 8, 1861. |
| Bealton | Va | Oct. 24, 1863, Jan. 14, 1864. |
| Bean's Station | Tenn | December 9, 1862, Dec. 10, 14, 1863. |
| Bear Creek | Ala | April 17, Oct. 26, 1863. |
| Bear Creek | Mo | Feb. 5, 1863. |
| Bear Creek | Miss | Oct. 27, 1863. |
| Bear Creek Station | Ga | Nov. 16, 1864. |
| Bear River | W. T | Jan. 29, 1863. |
| Bear-Skin Lake | Mo | Sept. 7, 1863. |
| Bear Wallow | Ky | Dec. 25, 1862. |
| Beaver Creek | Ky | June 27, 1863. |
| Beaver Creek | Mo | Nov. 24, 1862. |
| Beaver-Dam Lake | Miss | May 24, 1863. |
| Beaver-Dam Station | Va | May 9, 1864. |
| Beckwith Farm | Mo | Oct 13, 1861. |
| Beech Creek | W. Va | Aug. 6, 1862. |
| Beech Grove | Ky | Jan. 19, 20, 1862. |
| Beech Grove | Tenn | June 25, 1863. |
| Beersheba Springs | Tenn | Nov. 26, 1863, March 20, 1864. |
| Beher's Mills | Va | Sept. 2, 1861. |
| Belcher's Mills | Va | May 16, Sept. 17, 1864. |
| Bellefield | Va. | Dec. 9, 1864. |
| Belmont | Mo | Nov. 7, 1861. |
| Bennett's Mills | Mo | Sept. 1, 1861. |
| Benton | Miss | May 7, 1864. |
| Bentonville | Ark | March 6, 1862, Feb. 20, Aug. 15, 1863. |
| Bentonville | Mo | Feb. 19, 1862, May 22, 1863. |
| Bentonsville | N. C | March 18-21, 1865. |
| Bent's Old Fort | Tex | Nov. 24, 1864. |
| Bermuda Hundred | Va | May 4, 16–30, June 2, Aug. 24, 25, Nov. 30–Dec 13, 1864. |
| Berry's Ferry | Va | May 16, 1863. |
| Berryville | Va | Dec. 1, 1862, June 6, 12, Oct. 18, 1863, Aug. 21, Sept. 3, 4, 1864, April 17, 1865. |
| Berryville Pike | Va | Aug. 10, 1864. |
| Bertrand | Mo | Dec. 11, 1861. |
| Berwick | La | April 26, 1864. |
| Berwick City | La | March 13, 1863. |
| Bethesda Church | Va | May 30–June 6, 1864. |
| Bett's Farm | Mo | July 24, 1862. |

| | | |
|---|---|---|
| Beverly | W. Va. | July 12, 1861, April 24, July 2, 1863, Oct. 29, 1864, Jan. 11, 1865. |
| Beverly Ford | Va. | June 9, Oct. 22, 1863. |
| Bidnella Crossroads | Va. | March 1, 1864. |
| Big Beaver Creek | Mo. | Nov. 7, 1862. |
| Big Bethel, or Great Bethel | Va. | June 10, 1861, April 4, 1862. |
| Big Black River | Miss. | May 3, 17, July 4, 5, Oct. 13, 1863, Feb. 4, 1864. |
| Big Black River Bridge | Miss. | Aug. 12, Sept. 11, 1863, Nov. 27, 1864. |
| Big Blue | Mo. | Oct. 23, 31, 1864. |
| Big Creek | Ark | July 10, 1863, July 26, 1864. |
| Big Creek | Mo. | Sept. 9, 1862. |
| Big Creek Gap | Tenn. | Sept. 4, 1862. |
| Big Hatchie River, or Metamora | Miss. | Oct. 5, 1862. |
| Big Hill | Ky. | Aug. 23, 1862. |
| Big Hill Road | Ky. | Oct. 23, 1862. |
| Big Hurricane Creek | Mo. | Oct. 19, 1861. |
| Big Indian Creek | Ark | May 27, 1862. |
| Big Indian Creek | Mo. | May 26, 1862. |
| Big Mound | D. T. | July 24, 1863. |
| Big North Fork Creek | Mo. | June 16, 1864. |
| Big Pigeon River | Tenn. | Nov. 5, 6, 1864. |
| Big Pine Creek | Cal. | April 10, 1863. |
| Big Piney | Mo. | July 25, 26, 1862. |
| Big River Bridge | Mo. | Oct. 15, 1861. |
| Big Sandy | Col. | Nov. 29, 1864. |
| Big Sewell | W. Va. | Dec. 12, 1863. |
| Big Shanty | Ga. | June 6, Sept. 2, Oct. 3, 1864. |
| Big Springs | Ky. | Jan.—, 1865. |
| Binniker's Bridge | S. C. | Feb. 9, 1865. |
| Birch Coolie, or Acton | Minn. | Sept. 2, 3, 1862. |
| Bird Song Ferry | Miss. | June 18, July 4, 5, 1863. |
| Bird's Point | Mo. | Aug. 19, 1861. |
| Birmingham | Miss. | April 24, 1863. |
| Bisland | La. | April 12–14, 1863. |
| Black Bayou | Miss. | April 10, 1863, March 19, 1864. |
| Blackburn's Ford | Va. | July 18, 1881, Sept. 19, 1862, Oct. 15, 1863. |
| Black Cañon | A. T. | May 6. 1865. |
| Black Creek | Fla. | July 27, 1864. |
| Blackford's Ford | Va. | Sept. 20, 1862. |
| Black-Jack Forest | Tenn. | March 16, 1862. |
| Blackland | Miss. | June 4, 1862. |
| Black River | La. | Nov. 1, 1864. |
| Black River | Miss. | July 1, 2, 1863. |
| Black River | Mo. | Sept. 12, 1861, July 8, 1862, Sept. 17–20, 1864. |
| Black Run | Mo. | July 8, 1862. |
| Blackville | S. C. | Feb. 11, 1865. |
| Black Walnut Creek | Mo. | Nov. 29, 1861. |
| Black Warrior Creek | Ala. | May 1, 1863. |
| Black Water | Mo. | Dec 19, 1861, Oct. 12, 1863, Sept. 23, 1864. |
| Blackwater | Va. | Sept. 28, Oct. 24, 1862, March 17, 1863. |
| Blain's Crossroads | Tenn. | Dec. 16, 1863. |
| Block House, No. 4 | Tenn. | Aug.—, 1864. |
| Block House, No. 5 | Tenn. | Aug. 31, 1864. |
| Block House, No. 2 | Tenn. | Dec. 2, 3, 1864. |
| Block House, No. 7 | Tenn. | Dec. 4, 1864. |
| Bloomfield | Mo. | May 11, July 19, Aug. 25, 29, Sept. 11–13, 1862, March 1, April 29, 30, May 12, 1863. |
| Bloomfield | Va. | Nov. 2, 1862. |

| Place | State | Date |
|---|---|---|
| Blooming Gap | Va | Feb. 13, 1862. |
| Blount's Farm | Ala | May 2, 1863. |
| Blount's Mills | N. C. | April 9. 1863. |
| Blountsville | Tenn | Sept. 22, Oct. 13, 1863. |
| Blue Gap | Va | Jan. 7, 1862. |
| Blue Island | Ind | June 19, 1863. |
| Blue Mills | Mo | July 24, 1861. |
| Blue Mills Landing | Mo | Sept. 17, 1861. |
| Blue River | Mo | June 18, 1863. |
| Blue Springs | Mo | March 22, 1863. |
| Blue Springs | Tenn | Oct. 10, 1863. |
| Blue Springs | Ala | March 25, 1865. |
| Bluffton | S. C | June 4, 1863 |
| Bob's Creek | Mo | March 7, 1862. |
| Bogg's Mills | Ark | Jan. 24, 1865. |
| Bogler's Creek, or Ebenezer Church and Maplesville | Ala | April 1, 1865. |
| Bole's Farm | Mo | July 23, 1862. |
| Bollinger County | Mo | Jan. 14, 1864. |
| Bolivar | Miss | Aug. 25, Sept. 19, 1862, May 3, 1864. |
| Bolivar | Tenn | Aug. 30, Sept. 21, 1862, Feb. 13, March 9, Dec. 24, 25, 1863, Feb. 6, March 29, May 3, 1864. |
| Bolivar | Va | July 4–7, 1864. |
| Bolivar Heights | Va | Oct. 16, 1861. |
| Bollinger's Mills | Mo | July 29, 1862. |
| Bolton | Miss | July 4, 5, 1863. |
| Bolton's Depot | Miss | July 16, 1863, Feb. 4, 1864. |
| Bone Yard | Tenn | Feb. 10, 1863. |
| Bonfonca | La | Nov. 26, 1863. |
| Boone | N. C. | April 1, 1865. |
| Boone Court-House | W. Va | Sept. 1, 1861. |
| Booneville | Mo | June 17, Sept. 13, 1861, Oct. 12, 13, 1863, Oct. 9–11, 1864. |
| Boonsboro | Ark | Nov. 7, 28, 1862. |
| Boonsboro | Md | Sept. 15, 1862, July 7–9, 1863. |
| Boonville | Miss | May 30, July 1, 1862. |
| Boston Mountain | Ark | Nov. 28, Dec. 4–6, 1862. |
| Bottom's Bridge | Va | July 2, Aug. 28, 1863. |
| Bowling Green | Ky | Feb. 1, 15, 1862. |
| Boyd's Station | Ala | March 18, 1865. |
| Boyd's Station | Nev | June 3, 1865. |
| Boydton Road | Va | Oct. 27, 28, 1864, March 31, 1865. |
| Boyken's Mills | S. C | April 18, 1864, April 18, 1865. |
| Bradford's Springs | S. C | April 18, 1865. |
| Bradyville | Tenn | March 1, May 16, 1863. |
| Branchville, or Joy Ford | Ark | Jan. 17, 19, 1864. |
| Brandenburg | Ky | July 8, 1863. |
| Brandon | Miss | July 13–20, 1863. |
| Brandon Station | Miss | July 19, 1863. |
| Brandon Station | Va | Aug. 20, 1862, June 9, Aug. 1–3, Sept. 6, Nov. 8, 1863. |
| Brashear City | La | March 18, June 23, 1863. |
| Brawley Fork | Tenn | March 25, 1865. |
| Brazil Creek | I. T | Oct. 11, 1863. |
| Brazos de Santiago | Texas | Nov. 2, 1863. |
| Brentsville | Va | Feb. 14, 1863, Feb. 14, 1864. |
| Brentville | Tenn | Dec. 9, 1862. |
| Brentwood | Tenn | March 25, 1863, Dec. 15, 16, 1864. |
| Brewer's Lane | Ark | Sept. 11, 1864. |
| Briar | Mo | March 26, 1862. |
| Brice's Crossroads | Miss | June 10, 1864. |

| | | |
|---|---|---|
| Bridgeport | Ala | April 29, 1862. |
| Bridgeport Ferry | Miss | July 1, 2, 1863. |
| Brier Creek | Ga | Dec 4, 1864. |
| Briggen Creek | S. C | Feb. 25, 1865. |
| Brimstone Creek | Tenn | Sept. 10, 1863. |
| Bristoe Station | Va | Oct. 14, 1863, April 15, 1864. |
| Bristol | Tenn | Sept. 21, 1863, Dec. 14, 1864. |
| Britton's Lane | Tenn | Sept. 1, 1862. |
| Broad River | S. C | April 8, 1863. |
| Broad Run | Va | April 1, 1863. |
| Brooklyn | Kans | Aug. 21, 1863. |
| Brook's Turnpike | Va | March 1, 1864. |
| Browne's Crossroads | Ga | Nov. 27–29, 1864. |
| Brown's Ferry | Tenn | Oct. 27, 1863. |
| Brown's Gap | Va | Sept. 26, 1864. |
| Brown's Springs | Mo | July 27, 1862. |
| Brownsville | Ark | July 25, Aug. 25, Sept. 14, 16, 1863, Aug. 25, Oct. 30, 1864. |
| Brownsville | Miss | June 18, Oct. 15–23, 1863, Sept. 28, 1864. |
| Brownsville | Tenn | July 25, 29, 1862. |
| Brunswick | Mo | Aug. 17, 1861. |
| Bryant's Plantation | Fla | Oct. 21, 1864. |
| Buchanan | Va | June 14, 1864. |
| Buckhannon | W. Va | July 6, 1861, July 26, 1862. |
| Buckhead Creek | Ga | Nov. 27, 29, 1864. |
| Buckland Mills | Va | Oct. 19, 1863. |
| Buckstone Station | Ga | May 23, 1862. |
| Buffalo | Va | Sept. 27, 1862. |
| Buffalo Creek | W. Va | Nov. 26, 1864. |
| Buffalo Gap | W. Va | June 6, 1864. |
| Buffalo Hill | Ky | Oct. 4, 1861. |
| Buffalo Mills | Mo | Oct. 22, 1861. |
| Buffalo Mountain | Va | Dec. 13, 1861. |
| Buffington Island, or Saint George's Creek | Ohio | July 19, 1863. |
| Buford's Gap | Va | June 21, 1864. |
| Buford's Station | Tenn | Dec. 23, 1864. |
| Bull Bayou | Ark | Aug. 26, 1864. |
| Bull Creek | Ark | Aug. 6, 27, 1864. |
| Bull Pasture Mountain | Va | May 8, 1862. |
| Bull Run, first | Va | July 21, 1861. |
| Bull Run, second | Va | Aug. 28–30, 1862. |
| Bull Run Bridge | Va | Aug. 27, 1862. |
| Bull's Gap | Tenn | Sept. 24, Nov. 13, 1864. |
| Bulltown | Va | Oct. 13, 1863. |
| Bunker Hill | Va | July 17, 1861. |
| Burkesville | Ky | July 2, 1863. |
| Burke's Station | Va | March 10, 1862. |
| Burned Church | Ga | May 26, 1864. |
| Burnt Hickory | Ga | May 24–June 4, July 4, 5, 1864. |
| Burnt Ordinary | Va | Jan. 19, 1863. |
| Burton's Ford | Va | March 1, 1864. |
| Bushy Creek | Ark | Dec. 9, 1861. |
| Bushy Creek | Mo | May 28, 1863. |
| Butler | Mo | Oct., Nov. 20, 1861, May 15, 26, Oct. 29, 1862. |
| Butler's Bridge | N. C | Dec. 12, 1864. |
| Butler Creek | Ala | Nov. 17, 1864. |
| Butler Creek | Tenn | Nov. 22, 1864. |
| Buzzard Roost | Ga | Feb. 25–27, 1864. |
| Buzzard Roost Block House | Ga | Oct. 13, 1864. |
| Buzzard Roost Gap | Ga | May 8, 1864. |
| Byhalia | Miss | Oct. 12, 1863. |
| Cabin Creek | I. T | July 1, 2, 5, 20, 1863, Sept. 19, Nov. 4, 1864. |

| | | |
|---|---|---|
| Cabin Point | Va | Aug. 5, 1864. |
| Cabletown | Va | March 10, 1864. |
| Cacapon Bridge | Va | Sept. 6, 1862. |
| Cache River | Ark | April 22, 1864. |
| Cache River Bridge | Ark | May 28, 1862. |
| Caddo Gap | Ark | Dec. 4, 1863, Jan. 26, Feb. 12, 16, 1864. |
| Caddo Mountains | Ark | Feb. 12, 1864. |
| Cahawba River | Ga | April 8, 1865. |
| Cainsville | Tenn | Feb. 15, 1863. |
| Cajon De Arivaypo | N. Mex. | May 7, 1863. |
| Calf Killer Creek | Tenn | Feb. 23, 1864. |
| Calf Killer River | Tenn | March 18, 1864. |
| Calhoun | Mo | Jan. 4, 1862. |
| Calhoun, or Haguewood Prairie | Tenn | Sept. 26, 1863. |
| Calhoun Station | La | May 18, 1864. |
| California | Mo | Oct. 9, 10, 1864. |
| California House | Mo | Oct. 18, 1862. |
| Cambridge | Mo | Sept. 26, 1862. |
| Camden | Ark | April 2, 15, 16, 18, 24, 1864. |
| Camden, or South Mills | N. C | April 19, 1862. |
| Camden Point | Mo | July 13, 1864. |
| Cameron | Mo | Oct. 12, 1861. |
| Cameron | Va | Jan. 27, 1864. |
| Campaign in Northern Georgia | | May 5–Sept. 8, 1864. |
| Camp Alleghany, Buffalo Mt | W. Va | Dec. 13, 1861. |
| Camp Babcock | Ark | Nov. 25, 1862. |
| Campbell's Station | Tenn | Nov. 16, 1863. |
| Campbellton | Ga | July 28, 1864. |
| Campbellville | Tenn | Sept. 5, Nov. 24, Dec. 24, 1864. |
| Camp Cole | Mo | June 18, 1861. |
| Camp Crittenden | Mo | Sept. 22, 1861. |
| Camp Jackson | Mo | May 10, 1861. |
| Camp Marengo | La | Sept. 14, 1864. |
| Camp Moore | La | May 15, 1863. |
| Campti | La | March 26, April 4, 1824. |
| Camp Verdigris | I. T | Sept. 2, 1864. |
| Canadian River | I. T | Aug. 21, 1864. |
| Cane Creek | Ala | Oct. 26, 1863, June 10, 1864. |
| Cane Hill | Ark | Nov. 28, Dec. 20, 1862, Jan. 2, 1863. |
| Cane River | La | April 24, 1864. |
| Cane River Crossing | La | April 23, 1864. |
| Cañon De Chelly | | Jan. —, 1864. |
| Canton | Ky | Aug. 22, 1864. |
| Canton | Miss | July 11–18, Sept. 28, Oct. 15, 1863, Feb. 24–March 2, 1864. |
| Cape Girardeau | Mo | April 26, 1863, Feb. 5, 1864. |
| Capture of Fort Hell | Va | Sept. 10, 1864. |
| Capture of Rebel Ram Fair Play | La | Aug. 18, 1862. |
| Capture of tug Columbia | Fla | May 23, 1864. |
| Carnifax Ferry | Va | Sept. 10, 1861. |
| Carrick's Ford | W. Va | July 14, 1861. |
| Carrion Crow Bayou | La | Nov. 3, 18, 1863. |
| Carroll County | Ark | April 4, 1863. |
| Carrollton | Ark | March —, 1863. |
| Carrollton Store | Va | March 13, 1864. |
| Carsville | Va | Oct. 15, 1862, Jan 30, May 15–18, 1863. |
| Carter's Creek | Tenn | April 27, 1863. |
| Carter's Farm | Va | July 20, 1864. |
| Carter's Station | Ark | Sept. 27, 1864. |
| Carter's Station | Tenn | Dec. 30, 1862, Sept. 22, 1863, April 25, 26, 1864. |
| Carthage | Ark | Nov. 27, 1862. |
| Carthage | La | Jan. 23, 1863. |

Carthage ........ Mo ....... July 5, 1861, March 23, 1862, Jan. 13, May 16, 24, June 27, 28, Oct. 2, 1863, Sept. 22, Oct. 26, 1864.
Cass County ........ Mo ....... Nov. 3, 1862.
Cassville ........ Ga ........ May 19–22, 1864.
Cassville ........ Mo ....... Sept. 21, 1862.
Cassville Station ........ Ga ........ May 25, 1864.
Castor River ........ Mo ....... April 29, 1863.
Catawba River ........ N. C...... April 19. 1865.
Catlett's Station ........ Va ........ Aug. 21, 22, Oct. 24, 1862, Jan. 10, 1863.
Cedar Bluffs ........ Colo ..... May 3, 1864.
Cedar Creek, or Middletown ........ Va ........ Oct. 19. 1864.
Cedar Fork ........ U. T ...... April 2, 1863.
Cedar Keys ........ Fla ...... Feb. 16, 1865.
Cedar Mountain, or Slaughter Mountain, Southwest Mountain ........ Va ........ Aug. 9, 1862.
Cedar Run ........ Va ........ Aug. 9, 1862.
Cedar Run Church ........ Va ........ Oct. 17, 1864.
Cedar Springs ........ Va ........ Nov. 12, 1864.
Celina ........ Ky ....... April 20, 1863.
Celina ........ Tenn..... Dec. 7, 1863.
Centralia ........ Mo ....... Sept. 27, 1864.
Centre Creek ........ Mo ....... Feb. 20, 1865.
Centreville ........ Ala ..... April 1, 1865.
Centreville ........ La ........ April 13, 1863.
Centreville ........ Tenn..... Nov. 3, 1863, Sept. 29, 1864.
Chackahoola Station ........ La ........ June 24, 1863.
Chalk Bluffs ........ Ark ...... May 15, 1862, March 15, 19, April 1, 30, May 1, 1863.
Chambersburg ........ Pa ........ July 30, 1864.
Champion Hill ........ Miss...... May 16, 1863, Feb. 4, 1864.
Chancellorsville ........ Va ........ May 1–5, 1863.
Chantilly, or Ox Hill ........ Va ........ Sept. 1, 1862.
Chapel Hill ........ Tenn..... March 2, 4, 1863.
Chapin's Farm ........ Va ........ Sept. 29, 30, Nov. 4, 1864.
Chaplin Hills ........ Ky ....... Oct 8, 1862.
Chapmansville ........ W. Va... Sept. 25, 1861.
Chariton Bridge ........ Mo ....... Aug. 3, 1862.
Chariton River ........ Mo ....... Aug. 9, 1862.
Charles City Crossroads ........ Va ....... June 30, 1862, Nov. 16, 1863, Oct. 1, 1864.
Charleston ........ Ills........ March 28, 1864.
Charleston ........ Mo ....... Jan. 8, 1862.
Charleston ........ S. C...... Feb. 18, 1865.
Charleston ........ Tenn..... Dec. 28, 1863.
Charleston ........ Va ........ Oct. 6, 16, Dec. 1, 1862.
Charlestown, or Bird's Point ........ Mo ....... Aug. 19, 1861.
Charlestown ........ W. Va... May 28, Sept. 12, 1862, Oct. 8, 18, 1863, June 27, 1864.
Chattahoochie River ........ Ga ........ July 3–12, 1864.
Chattanooga ........ Tenn..... Aug. 21, Nov. 23–25, 1863, Feb. —, 1865.
Cheat Mountain ........ W. Va... Sept. 12, 13, 1861.
Cheek's Crossroads ........ Tenn..... March 14, 1864.
Cheese Cake Church ........ Va ........ May 4, 1862.
Cheraw ........ S. C...... March 2, 3, 1865.
Cherokee Nation ........ I. T ...... Jan. 18, 1863.
Cherokee Station ........ Ala ....... April 17, Oct. 21, 29, 1863.
Cherry Creek ........ Miss...... July 10, 1864.
Cherry Grove ........ Mo ....... June 26, 1862.
Cherry Grove ........ Va ........ April 14, 1864.
Chesterfield ........ S. C ...... March 2, 1865.
Chester Gap ........ Va ........ Nov. 5, 1862, July 21, 22, 1863.
Chester Station ........ Va ........ Nov. 17, 1864.

| | | |
|---|---|---|
| Chewa Station | Ga | July 18, 1864. |
| Chickahominy | Va | May 24, June 27, 1862. |
| Chickamicomico | N. C. | Oct. 5, 1861. |
| Chickamauga | Ga | Sept. 19–23, 1863. |
| Chickamauga Station | Ga | Nov. 26, 1863. |
| Chickasaw Bayou | Miss | Dec. 28, 29, 1862. |
| Chickasaw Bluffs | Miss | Dec. 29, 1862. |
| Childsburg | Va | May 9, 1864. |
| Chippewa Steamer | Ark | Feb. 17, 1865. |
| Choctaw Nation | I. T | Oct. 7, Nov. 9, 1863. |
| Christmas Prairie | Cal | Dec. 26, 1863. |
| Chulahoma | Miss | Nov. 30, 1862. |
| Chunky Station | Miss | Feb. 12, 1864. |
| Church-in-the-Woods | Va | Aug. 6, 1862. |
| City Belle Steamer | La | May 3, 1864. |
| City Point | Va | May 6, June —, 1864. |
| Civiques Ferry | La | May 10, 1863. |
| Clarendon | Ark | Aug. 13, 1862, March 15, June 25–30, July 14, 1864. |
| Clarendon Road | Ark | Jan. 15, 1863. |
| Clarke's Hollow | W. Va | May 1, 1862. |
| Clarke's Neck | Ky | Aug. 27, 1863. |
| Clarkson | Mo | Oct. 28, 1862. |
| Clarksville | Ark | Oct. 28, Nov. 8, 24, 1863, May 18, Sept. 28, 1864, Jan. 18, 1865. |
| Clarksville | Tenn | Aug. 19, Sept. 7, 1862. |
| Clay County | Mo | July 4, 1864. |
| Claysville | Ala | March 14, 1864. |
| Clayton | Ala | March 14, 1864. |
| Clear Creek | Ark | Aug. 19, 1862, Feb. 11, 1865. |
| Clear Creek | Mo | Aug. 2, 1862, May 16, 1864. |
| Clear Fork | Nev | Aug. 29, 1865. |
| Clear Lake | Ark | March 11, 1865. |
| Clear Springs | Md | July 29, 1864. |
| Clendenin's Raid | Va | May 20–28, 1863. |
| Cleveland | Tenn | Nov. 27, Dec. 22, 1863, April 2, 13, Aug. 17, 1864. |
| Clinch Mountain | Tenn | Dec. 6, 1863. |
| Clinton | Ga | Nov. 22, 1864. |
| Clinton | La | Dec. 28, 1862, June 4, 1863, May 1, Aug. 25, Nov. 15, 1864, March —, 1865. |
| Clinton | Miss | July 8, 16, Oct. 17, 1863, Feb. 5, July 4, 7, 1864. |
| Clinton | Mo | July 9, 1862. |
| Clinton | N. C | May 19, 1862. |
| Cloutersville | La | April 23, 24, 1864. |
| Clover Hill | Va | April 8, 9, 1865. |
| Cloyd's Mountain | Va | May 9, 10, 1864. |
| Coahoma County | Miss | Aug. 2, 1862. |
| Cochran's Crossroads | Miss | Sept. 10, 1862. |
| Coffeeville | Miss | Dec. 5, 1862. |
| Cold Harbor | Va | June 27, 1862, May 31–June 12, 1864. |
| Cold Knob Mountain, or Frankfort and Sinking Creek | Va | Nov. 26, 1862. |
| Coldwater | Miss | May 11, July 24, Nov. 8, 9, Sept. 10, 1862, Feb. 19, April 19, July 28, Aug. 21, 1863. |
| Coldwater Creek | Miss | Sept. 8, 11, 1862. |
| Coldwater Grove | Mo | Oct. 24, 1864. |
| Coldwater | Tenn | April 19, 1863. |
| Coldwater Station | Miss | Nov. 29, 1862. |
| Coldwater Station | Tenn | March 17, 1863. |
| Cole Camp | Mo | Oct. 5, 1862, June 8, 1863. |

| | | |
|---|---|---|
| Cole County | Mo | Oct. 6, 1864. |
| Cole Creek | Miss | Oct. 4, 1864. |
| Coleman's | Miss | March 5, 1864. |
| Coleman's Plantation | Miss | July 4, 5, 1864. |
| College Hill, or Oxford Hill and Hurricane Creek | Miss | Aug. 21, 22, 1864. |
| Colliersville | Miss | June 23, 1864. |
| Colliersville | Tenn | Oct. 11, 25, Nov. 3, Dec. 27, 28, 1863. |
| Columbia | Ark | June 2, 1864. |
| Columbia | Ky | July 3, 1863. |
| Columbia | La | Feb. 4, June 6, 1864. |
| Columbia | S. C | Feb. 15–18, 1865. |
| Columbia | Tenn | Sept. 9, 1862, Nov. 24–29, Dec. 19, 1864. |
| Columbus | Ga | April 16, 1865. |
| Columbus | Mo | Jan. 9, July 23, 1862. |
| Combahee River | S. C | Jan. 25, 1865. |
| Comfort | N. C | July 6, 1863. |
| Como | Miss | Oct. 7, 1863. |
| Como | Tenn | Sept. 19, 1863. |
| Concha's Springs | N. Mex | July 22, 1863. |
| Concordia Bayou | La | Aug. 5, 1864. |
| Conee Creek | La | Aug. 25, 1864. |
| Congaree Creek | S. C | Feb. 15, 1865. |
| Construction Train | Tenn | Jan. 25, 1863. |
| Convalescent Correll | Miss | July 7, 1863. |
| Conyersville | Tenn | Sept. 5, 1863. |
| Cook's Cañon | Nev | July 24, 1863. |
| Coon Creek, or Lamar | Mo | Aug 24, 1862. |
| Coosa Creek | Ala | April 1, 1865. |
| Coosa River | Ala | July 13, 1864. |
| Coosa River | Ga | Oct. 25, 1864. |
| Coosaw River | S. C | Dec. 4, 1864. |
| Corinth | Miss | April 30–May 30, Oct. 3, 4, 1862, Aug. 16, 1863, June 10, 1864. |
| Corydon | Ind | July 9, 1863. |
| Cottage Grove | Tenn | March 21, 1863. |
| Cotton Gap | Ark | Sept. 1, 1863. |
| Cotton Hill | W. Va | Sept. 11, 1862. |
| Cotton Plant | Ark | July 7, 1862, April 21, 1864. |
| Courtland | Ala | July 25, 27, 1864. |
| Courtland | Tenn | Aug. 32, 1862. |
| Courtland Bridge | Ala | July 25, 1862. |
| Courtney's Plantation | Miss | April 11, 1863. |
| Cove Creek | Ark | Nov. 18, 1862. |
| Cove Mountain, or Grassy Lick | Va | May 9, 10, 1864. |
| Covington | Tenn | March 10, 1863. |
| Cow Creek | Kans | Nov. 14–28, 1864, June 12, 1865. |
| Cowskin Creek | Mo | Aug. 5, 7, 1864. |
| Coxe's Bridge | N. C | March 24, 1865. |
| Coyle Tavern | Va | Aug. 24, 1863. |
| Crab Orchard | Ky | Aug. 22, 1862. |
| Craig's Meeting House | Va | May 5, 1864. |
| Crampton's Ferry | Mo | Aug. 11, 1862. |
| Crampton's Gap | Md | Sept. 14, 1862. |
| Crane Creek | Mo | Oct. 29, 30, 1864. |
| Crawford County | Ark | Aug. 11, 1864. |
| Crawford County | Mo | Nov. 25, 1862. |
| Creek Agency | I. T | Oct. 15, 25, 1863. |
| Creelsborough | Ky | Dec. 7, 1863. |
| Crew's Farm | Va | July 1, 1862. |
| Cripple Creek, or Bradyville | Tenn | May 16, 1863. |
| Crooked Creek | Mo | Aug. 24, 1862. |
| Crooked River | Oreg | May 18, 1864. |

| | | |
|---|---|---|
| Crooked Run | Va | Aug. 16, 1864. |
| Cross Bayou | La | Sept. 14, 1863. |
| Cross Hollow, or Oxford Bend | Ark | Oct. 18, 28, 1862. |
| Cross Keys, or Union Church | Va | June 8, 1862. |
| Cross Lanes, or Summerville | W. Va | Aug. 26, 1861. |
| Cross Timbers | Mo | July 28, 1862, Oct. 16, 1863. |
| Croton Springs | A. T | July 14, 1865. |
| Crump's Hill, or Piney Woods | La | April 2, 1864. |
| Crump's Landing, or Adamsville | Tenn | April 4, 1862. |
| Culpeper | Va | Sept. 13, Oct. 12, 13, 1863. |
| Culp's House | Ga | June 22, 1864. |
| Cumberland, Flock's Mills | Md | Aug. 1, 1864. |
| Cumberland Gap | Tenn | June 18, 1862, Sept. 9, 1863, Jan. 29, Feb. 22, 1864. |
| Cumberland Iron-Works | Tenn | Aug. 26, 1862, Feb. 3, 1863. |
| Cumberland Mountain | Tenn | April 28, 1852. |
| Cuyler's Plantation | Ga | Dec. 9, 1864. |
| Cynthiana | Ky | July 17, 1862, June 10, 11, 1864. |
| Cypress Bridge | Ky | Nov. 17, 1861 |
| Dabney's Mills, or Rowanty Creek and Vaughn Road | Va | Feb. 5–7, 1865. |
| Dallas | Ark | Jan. 28. 1864. |
| Dallas, or Burnt Hickory, Altoona Hills, New Hope Church, Pumpkin Vine Creek | Ga | May 25–June 5, 1864. |
| Dallas | Mo | Sept. 2, 1861, Aug. 24, 1862. |
| Dallas County | Mo | Sept. 19, 1864. |
| Dallas | N. C | April 19, 1865. |
| Dalton | Ga | May 9, Aug. 14–16, Oct. 13, 1864. |
| Dam No. 4, Potomac | Va | Dec. 11, 1861. |
| Dandridge | Tenn | Jan. 16, 17, 1864. |
| Danville | Ark | March 28, 1864. |
| Danville | Ky | Aug. 26, 1862, March 24, 1863. |
| Danville | Miss | June 6, 1864. |
| Darbytown Road | Va | Oct. 7, 13, 1864. |
| Dardanelle | Ark | Sept. 9, 12, 1863, May 10, Nov. 29, 1864, Jan. 14, 1865. |
| Darksville | Va | July 19, Sept. 3, 1864. |
| Darnestown | Va | Sept. 15, 1861. |
| Davis Bend | La | June 2, 29, 1864. |
| Davis's Crossroads | Ga | Sept. 11, 1863. |
| Davis's Mills | Miss | Dec. 21, 1862, March 14, 1863. |
| Day's Gap | Ala | April 30, 1863. |
| Dayton | Ark | Dec. 23, 1861. |
| Dayton | Mo | April 27, 1864. |
| Dead Buffalo Lake | D. T | July 26, 1863. |
| Deatonsville | Va | April 6, 1865. |
| Decatur | Ala | March 7, April 17, May 26, 27, Aug. 18, Oct. 26-29, Dec. 27, 28, 1864. |
| Decatur | Ga | July 22, Aug. 5, 1864. |
| Decatur | Miss | Feb. 12, 1864. |
| Decatur | Tenn | Aug. 18, 1864. |
| Deep Bottom | Va | July 21, 27, 28, Aug. 14–19, Sept. 2, 6, Oct. 1, 31, 1864. |
| Deep Creek | N. C | Feb. 5, 1864. |
| Deep River Bridge | N. C | April 4, 1865. |
| Deep Water Creek | Mo | Oct. 15, 1863. |
| Deer Creek | Miss | Feb. 23, March 21, April 8–12, 1863. |
| Deer Creek | D. T | May 21, 1865. |
| Denver | Kan | Sept. 7, 1864. |
| Des Allemands | La | Sept. 9, 1862. |
| Des Arcs | Ark | Jan. 16, 1863, July 26–Dec. 6, 1864. |

| Place | State | Date |
|---|---|---|
| Deserted House, or Carsville and Kelly's Ford | Va | Jan. 30, 1863. |
| Destruction Rebel Ram Albemarle | | Oct. 28, 1864. |
| Devaux Neck, or Tillafinny River, Mason's Bridge, and Gregory's Farm | S. C. | Dec. 6–9, 1864. |
| Devil's Back-bone, or Fort Smith and Cotton Gap | Ark | Sept. 1, 1863. |
| Diamond Grove | Mo | April 14, 1862, June 3, Aug. 21, 1864. |
| Dickson Station | Ala | April 19–23, Oct. 20, 1863. |
| Dinwiddie Court-House | Va | March 31, 1865. |
| Ditch Bayou | La | June 6, 1864. |
| Dobbin's Ferry, or La Vergne | Tenn | Dec. 9, 1862. |
| Donaldsonville | La | June 28, July 13, 1863, Feb. 8, Aug. 5, 1864. |
| Doniphan | Mo | Sept. 17–20, 1864. |
| Doubtful Cañon | A. T | May 4, 1864. |
| Douglas Landing | Ark | Feb. 22, 1865. |
| Dover | Mo | Oct. 20, 1864. |
| Dover | Tenn | Feb. 14–16, 1862. |
| Dover Road | N. C. | April 28, 1863. |
| Downer's Bridge | Va | May 20, 1864. |
| Drainesville | Va | Nov. 26, Dec. 20, 1861, Feb. 22, 1864. |
| Draft Riots | N.Y.C. | July 13–15, 1863. |
| Dresden | Ky | May 5, 1862. |
| Dresden | Tenn | May 5, 1862. |
| Dripping Springs | Ark | Dec. 28, 29, 1862. |
| Droop Mountain | Va | Nov. 6, 1863. |
| Drury's Bluff | Va | May 10–16, 20, 1864. |
| Dry Creek | Va | Aug. 29, 1863. |
| Dry Fork Creek | Mo | July 5, 1861. |
| Dry Forks | Mo | July 5, 1861. |
| Dry Forks | W. Va | Jan. 8, 1862. |
| Dry Wood, or Fort Scott | Mo | Sept. 2, 1861, Nov. 9, 1862, Oct. 29, 1864. |
| Duck Creek | S. C | Feb. —, 1865. |
| Duck River Island | Tenn | April 26, 1863. |
| Dug Gap | Ga | Sept. 11, 1863, May 7, 1864. |
| Dug Springs | Mo | Aug. 2, 1861. |
| Dukedom | Ky | Feb. 28, 1864. |
| Dumfries | Va | Dec. 27, 1862. |
| Dunbar's Plantation | La | April 15, 1863. |
| Dunksburg | Mo | Dec. 4, 1861. |
| Dunn's Bayou | La | May 5, 1864. |
| Dunn's Lake | Fla | Feb. 5, 1865. |
| Durhamville | Tenn | Sept 17, 1862. |
| Dutch Gap | Va | Aug. 5, 1863, Aug. 24, Sept. 7, Nov. 17, 1864. |
| Dutch Mills | Ark | April 14, 1864. |
| Dutton's Hill, or Somerset | Ky | March 30, 1863. |
| Duvall's Bluff | Ark | Jan. 16, Dec. 12, 1863, Aug. 21, Sept. 6, 1864. |
| Duvall's Mills | Va | Dec. 1, 1864. |
| Dyersburg | Tenn | Jan. 30, 1863. |
| Eagleville | Tenn | March 2, 1863. |
| East Pascagoula | Miss | April 9, 1863. |
| East Point | Ga | Sept. 5, 1864. |
| East Point | Miss | Oct 10, 1864. |
| Eastport | Miss | Oct. 10, Nov. 11, 1864. |
| Ebenezer Creek | Ga | Dec. 7, 1864. |
| Ebenezer Church | Ala | April 1, 1865. |
| Eden Station | Ga | Dec. 7–9, 1864. |
| Edgefield Junction | Tenn | Aug. 20, 1862. |
| Edisto Island | S. C. | April 18, 1862. |

| Place | State | Date |
|---|---|---|
| Edward's Ferry | Md | July —, 1861. |
| Edward's Ferry | Va | June 17, Oct. 21, 1861. |
| Edward's Station | Miss | May 16, 1863. |
| Eel River | Cal | May 3, 1863. |
| Egypt Station | Miss | Dec. 28, 1864. |
| Elizabeth City | N. C | Feb 10, 1862. |
| Elizabethtown | Ark | Oct. 1, 1863. |
| Elizabethtown | Ky | Dec. 27, 1862, Dec. 16, 24, 1864. |
| Eliott's Mills, or Camp Crittenden | Mo | Sept. 22, 1861. |
| Elk Creek | Nev | Aug. 15, 1864. |
| Elk Fork | Ky | Dec. 28, 1862. |
| Elkhorn Tavern | Ark | March 8, Oct. 16, 1862. |
| Elkin's Ford | Ark | April 4–6, 1864. |
| Elk River | Tenn | July 2, 14, 1863. |
| Elk Shute | Mo | Aug. 3, 4, 1864. |
| Elkton | Ky | Dec. 12, 1864. |
| Elkton Station | Ala | May 9, 1862. |
| Elkwater | W. Va | Sept. 11, 1861. |
| Ellison's Mills | Va | June 26, 1862. |
| Ellistown | Miss | July 16, 21, 1864. |
| Eminence | Mo | June 17, 1862. |
| Enterprise | Mo | Aug 7, 1864. |
| Eudoro Church | Ark | May 9, 1864. |
| Evacuation Battery Gregg and Ft. Wagner | S. C | Sept. 7, 1863. |
| Evacuation of Corinth | Miss | May 30, 1862. |
| Evlington Heights | Va | July 3, 1862. |
| Expedition from Vicksburg to Jackson | Miss | July 3–9, 1864. |
| Expedition from Vicksburg to Meridian | Miss | Feb. 3–March 5, 1864. |
| Expedition into Western North Carolina | | Dec. 9, 1864–Jan. 14, 1865, Jan. 29–Feb. 11, 1865. |
| Expedition to Black Bayou | Miss | April 5–10, 1863. |
| Expedition to Hamilton | N. C. | Dec. 9–12, 1864. |
| Expedition to Jacksonville | Fla | March 29, 1863. |
| Expedition to Steele's Bayou | Miss | March 16–22, 1863. |
| Expedition up Yazoo River | Miss | Feb. 1–March 8, 1864. |
| Explosion of Ammunition, City Point | Va | Aug. 9, 1864. |
| Explosion of Magazine, Fort Fisher | N. C. | Jan. 16, 1865. |
| Ezra Chapel | Ga | July 28, 1864. |
| | | |
| Fairburn | Ga | Aug. 18, 1864. |
| Fairfax | Va | July 13, 1862, June 27, 1863. |
| Fairfax Court-House | Va | June 1, 1861, March 8, 1863. |
| Fairfax Station | Va | Sept. 17, 1864. |
| Fairfield | Pa | July 3, 5, 1863. |
| Fairfield | Tenn | June 29, 1863. |
| Fair Gardens, or French Broad and Kelly's Ford | Tenn | Jan. 27, 28, 1864. |
| Fairmount | W. Va | April 29, 1863. |
| Fair Oaks | Va | May 31, June 1, 1862, Oct. 27, 28, 1864. |
| Falling Waters, or Haynesville and Martinsburg | Md | July 2, 1861, July 14, 1863. |
| Fall of Petersburgh | Va | April 2, 1865. |
| Falmouth | Va | April 18, 1862. |
| Farmington | Miss | May 3, 9, 26, 28, 1862. |
| Farmville | Va | April 7, 1865. |
| Farr's Mills | Ark | July 14, 1864. |
| Fayette | Miss | Nov. 22, Dec. 22, 1863, Oct. 3, 1864. |
| Fayette | Mo | Oct. 7, 1862, July 1, Sept. 24, Nov. 18, 1864. |
| Fayetteville | Ark | July 15, Oct. 24, 27, 28, Dec. 7, 1862, April 18, 1863, May 19, June 24, Aug. 28, Oct. 28, 1864. |

Fayetteville ........ N. C..... March 13, 1865.
Fayetteville ........ Tenn .... Nov. 1, 1863.
Fayetteville ........ W. Va ... Sept. 10, Nov. 15, 1862, May 17–20, 1863.
Federal Point ........ N. C.... Feb. 11, 1865.
Ferry's Landing ........ Ark ...... Sept. 7, 1863.
Fiker's Ferry ........ Ala ..... April 8, 1865.
Fillmore ........ Va ...... Oct. 4, 1864.
Fish Bayou ........ La ........ June 5, 1864.
Fish Creek ........ Nev ...... Jan. 22, 1866.
Fisher's Hill ........ Va ...... Aug. 15, Sept. 22, Oct. 9, 1864.
Fishing Creek ........ Ky ........ Jan. 19, 20, 1862, May 25, 1863.
Fish Springs ........ Tenn .... Jan. 23, 1863.
Fitzhugh's Crossing ........ Va ....... April 29, 30, 1863.
Fitzhugh's Woods ........ Ark ...... April 1, 1864.
Five Forks ........ Va ....... April 1, 1865.
Five-Mile Creek ........ Ala ...... March 31, 1865.
Five Points ........ Va ....... Jan. 1, 1864.
Flat-Lick Fords ........ Ky ........ Feb. 14, 1862.
Flat Shoals ........ Ga ........ July 28, 1864.
Flint Creek ........ Ark ...... March 6, 1864.
Flint River ........ Ga ........ Sept. 1, 1864.
Flock's Mills ........ Md ........ August 1, 1864.
Florence ........ Ala ...... May 27, 1863, Jan. 26, Apr. 13, Oct. 6, 1864.
Florence ........ Ky ........ Sept. 17, 1862.
Florence ........ Mo ........ July 10, 1863.
Florence ........ S. C ...... March 3, 1865.
Florida ........ Mo ........ May 22, July 22, 1862.
Flowing Springs ........ Va ....... Aug. 21, 1864.
Floyd ........ La ........ July —, 1864.
Floyd's Fork ........ Ky ........ Oct. 1, 1862.
Forsyth ........ Mo ....... July 22, 1861, August 2, 1862.
Fort Abercrombie ........ D. T ..... Sept. 3, 6, 23, 25, 1862.
Fort Adams ........ La ....... Oct. 7, 1864.
Fort Anderson ........ Ky ........ March 25, 1864.
Fort Anderson ........ N. C ..... Feb. 18, 1865.
Fort Bisland ........ La ....... April 12, 1863.
Fort Blair ........ Ark ...... Oct. 6, 1863.
Fort Blakely ........ Ala ...... March 31–April 9, 1865.
Fort Blunt ........ I. T ...... March 27–June 19, 1863.
Fort Brady ........ Va ....... Jan. 24, 1865.
Fort Brown Road ........ Texas ... Dec. 14, 1862.
Fort Burnham ........ Va ....... Dec. 10, 1864, Jan. 24, 1865.
Fort Cobb ........ I. T ...... Oct. 21, 1862.
Fort Cottonwood ........ N. T ..... Aug. 28, Sept. 18, 1864.
Fort Craig ........ N. Mex.. Aug. 23, Sept. 6, 1861, Feb. 20, May 23, 1862.
Fort Darling ........ Va ....... May 12–16, 1864.
Fort Davidson, or Ironton ........ Mo ....... Sept. 26, 27, 1864.
Fort De Russy ........ La ........ March 14, 1864.
Fort Donelson ........ Tenn .... Feb. 13–16, Aug. 25, 1862, Feb. 3, 1863, Oct. 11, 1864.
Fort Esperanza ........ Texas ... Nov. 30, 1862, Nov. 27–29, 1863.
Fort Fillmore ........ N. Mex . July 27, 1861, Aug. 7, 1862.
Fort Fisher ........ N. C ..... Dec. 25, 1864, Jan. 13–15, 1865.
Fort Gaines ........ Ala ...... Aug. 2–23, 1864.
Fort Gibson ........ I. T...... Oct. 15, 1862, Feb. 28, May 20, 25, Dec. 26, 1863, Sept. 16, 18, 1864, Sept. —, 1865.
Fort Grant ........ A. T ..... Jan. 21, 1866.
Fort Halleck ........ D. T ..... Feb. 20, 1863, July 4, 1865.
Fort Hatteras ........ N. C ..... Aug. 28, 29, 1861.
Fort Hell ........ Va ....... Sept. 28, Nov. 5, 1864.
Fort Henry ........ Tenn .... Feb. 6, 1862.
Fort Hill ........ Miss ...... June 25, 28, 1863.

Fort Hindman........Ark......Jan. 11, 1863.
Fort Johnson........S. C......June 16, 1862, July 2, 1864.
Fort Jones........Ky........Feb. 18, 1865.
Fort Kelly........W. Va...Nov. 28, 1864.
Fort Larned........Kans.....May 22, 1865.
Fort Leavenworth........Kans.....Oct. 20–26, 1864.
Fort Lyons, or Sand Creek........I. T......Dec. 9, 1864.
Fort Lyons........Va.......June 9, 1863.
Fort Macon........N. C.....April 25, 1862.
Fort McAllister........Ga........Dec. 13, 1864.
Fort McCook........Ala.......Aug. 27, 1862.
Fort Morgan........Ala.......Aug. 5–23, 1864.
Fort Myers........Fla........Feb. 20, 1865.
Fort Pemberton........Miss......March 13–April 5, 1863.
Fort Pillow........Tenn....March 16, April 12, 1864.
Fort Pocahontas........Va.......Aug. —, 1864.
Fort Pulaski........Ga.......April 10, 1862.
Fort Rice........D. T.....Sept. 27,1864,July 28,30,1865.
Fort Ridgely........Minn.....Aug. 20, 22, 1862.
Fort Sanders........Tenn....Nov. 29, 1863.
Fort Scott........Kans.....Sept. 1, 3, 1861, Oct. 22, 28, 1864.
Fort Scott........Mo.......Sept. 2, 1861.
Fort Sedwick, or Fort Hell........Va.......Sept. 28, Nov. 5, 1864.
Fort Smith........Ark......May 15,Aug. 31, Sept. 1,1863, July 29, 31, Aug. 24, 27, Sept. 1, 11, Dec. 24, 1864.
Fort Steadman........Va.......March 25, 1865.
Fort Stevens........D. C.....July 12, 1864.
Fort Sumner........N. Mex..Jan. 4, 1864.
Fort Sumter........S. C......April 12, 13, 1861.
Fort Taylor........Fla.......Aug. 21, 1864.
Fort Taylor........Ga........April 16, 1865.
Fort Wagner........S. C......July 10–Sept. 6, 1863.
Forty Hills, or Hankinson's Ferry........Miss......May 3, 1863.
Foster's Bridge........N. C.....Dec. 10, 1864.
Foster's expedition to Goldsborough........N. C.....Dec. 12–18, 1862.
Fouch La Faix Mountain........Ark......Nov. 11, 1863.
Fourteen-Mile Creek........I. T......Oct. 30, 1863.
Fourteen-Mile Creek........Miss......May 12, 1863.
Fox Creek........Mo........March 7, 1862.
Frankfort........Ky....... June 10, 1864.
Frankfort........Va.......Nov. 26, 1862.
Franklin........La........May 25, 1863.
Franklin........Miss......Jan. 2, 1865.
Franklin........Mo........Oct. 13, 1862, Oct. 1, 1864.
Franklin........Tenn....Dec. 12, 1862, Feb. 1, March 9, 25, April 10, 27, June 4, 1863, Sept. 2, Nov. 30, Dec. 17, 1864.
Franklin........Va.......Oct. 31, Dec. 2, 1862.
Franklin Creek........Miss......Dec. 18, 1864.
Franklin's Crossing........Va.......June 5, 1863.
Frazier's Farm........Va.......June 30, 1862.
Frederick........Md........Sept. 12, 1862.
Fredericksburgh........Mo........July 17, 1864.
Fredericksburgh........Va.......Nov. 9, Dec. 11–16, 1862.
Fredericksburgh Road........Va.......May 16–20, 1864.
Fredericktown........Mo........Oct. 17–21, 1861.
Freeman's Ford........Va.......Aug. 24, 1862.
Frémont's Orchard........Col.......April 12, 1864.
French Broad........Tenn....Jan. 27, 1864.
French Point........Mo.......May 15, 1863.
Frog Bayou........Ark......July 1, 1864.
Front Royal........Va.......May 23,30.1862, Sept. 21,1864.
Frying Pan........Va........June 4, 1863.

| | | |
|---|---|---|
| Fulton | Ga | Oct. 13, 1864. |
| Fulton | Mo | July 17, 1861. |
| Funkstown | Md | July 12, 13, 1863. |
| Gainesville | Fla | Feb. 14, Aug. 17, 1864. |
| Gainesville | Va | Aug. 28–29, 1862. |
| Gaines' Mill | Va | June 27, 1862, June 2, 1864. |
| Gallatin | Tenn | Aug. 12, Oct. 1, 1862. |
| Galveston | Texas | Jan. 1, 1863. |
| Garrettsburgh | Ky | Nov. 6, 1862. |
| Gaucha Mountain | Cal | July 22, 1865. |
| Gauley's Bridge | W. Va | Nov. 10, 1861. |
| Geiger Lake | Ky | Sept. 3, 1862 |
| Georgia Landing | La | Oct. 27, 1862. |
| Germantown | Tenn | June 25, 1862, Jan. 27, April 1, 1863. |
| Gettysburg | Pa | July 1–3, 1863. |
| Ghent | Ky | Aug. 29, 1864. |
| Gila River | N. Mex | Nov. 5, 1863. |
| Glade Springs | Va | Dec. 15, 1864. |
| Gladesville | Va | Oct. 2, 1864. |
| Glasgow | Ky | Oct. 5, Dec. 24, 1862, Oct. 5, 1863, Oct. 15, 1864, March 25, 1865. |
| Glasgow | Mo | Oct. 15, 1864. |
| Glass Bridge | Tenn | Sept. 2, 1864. |
| Glendale | Ala | Feb. 22, 1863. |
| Glendale | Miss | May 8, 1862, April 14, 1863. |
| Glendale | Va | June 30, 1862. |
| Glorietta | N. Mex | March 26–28, 1862. |
| Gloucester | Va | Nov. 17, 1862. |
| Gloucester Point | Va | Feb. 10, 1863. |
| Golding's Farm | Va | June 27, 1862. |
| Goldsborough | N. C | Dec. 17, 1862, March 21–24, 1865 |
| Golgotha | Ga | June 16, 1864. |
| Goodrich's Landing | La | June 30, 1863, March 24, July 16, 1864. |
| Good's Landing | Miss | Dec. 16–25, 1864. |
| Goose Creek | Va | Oct. 22, 1861, Sept. 17, 1862. |
| Gov. Moore's Plantation | La | May 2, 1864. |
| Grafton | W. Va | Aug. 13, 1861. |
| Grahamsville | S. C | Nov. 30, 1864. |
| Granby | Mo | Sept. 24, 1862. |
| Grand Coteau, or Bayou Bordeau and Carrion Crow Bayou | La | Nov. 3, 1863. |
| Grand Ecore | La | April 3, 1864. |
| Grand Gulf | Miss | April 29, 1863, Jan. 16–18, July 16, 17, 1864. |
| Grand Haze | Ark | July 4, 1862. |
| Grand Lake | Ark | June 16, 1863. |
| Grand Pass | I. T | July 7, 1863. |
| Grand Prairie | Ark | July 6, 1862. |
| Grand Prairie | Mo | Oct. 24, 1862. |
| Grand River | Mo | Nov. 30, 1861, Aug. 10–13, 1862. |
| Grant's Creek | N. C | April 12, 1865. |
| Grass Lick | W. Va | April 23, 1862. |
| Grassy Lick | Va | May 9, 10, 1864. |
| Gravel Hill | Va | Aug. 14, 1864. |
| Gravelly Run | Va | March 31, 1865. |
| Graysville | Ga | Sept. 10, 1863. |
| Greasy Creek | Ky | May 11, 1863. |
| Great Bear Creek | Ala | April 17, 1863. |
| Great Bethel, or Big Bethel | Va | June 10, 1861, April 4, 1862. |
| Great Cacapon Bridge | Va | Jan. 4, 1862. |

| | | |
|---|---|---|
| Great Falls | Va | July 7, Sept. 4, 1861. |
| Greenbrier | W. Va | Oct. 3, 1861. |
| Greencastle | Pa | June 20, 1863. |
| Greenleaf Prairie | I. T | June 16, Nov. 12, 1863. |
| Greenland Gap | W. Va | April 25, 1863. |
| Greenland Gap Road | W. Va | June 6, 1864. |
| Green River Bridge, or Tebb's Bend | Ky | July 4, 1863. |
| Green's Chapel | Ky | Dec. 25, 1862. |
| Green Springs Depot | W. Va | Aug. 2, 1864. |
| Greenville | Miss | May 20, 27, 1864. |
| Greenville | Mo | July 26, 1862. |
| Greenville | N. C | Nov. 25, Dec. 30, 1863. |
| Greeneville | Tenn | Sept. 4, Oct. 12, 1864. |
| Greenville Road | Ky | Nov. 5, 1862. |
| Greenville Road | N. C | May 31, 1862. |
| Greenville Springs Road | La | Sept. 19, Oct. 5, 1863. |
| Greenwich | Va | May 30, 1863. |
| Gregory's Farm | S. C | Dec. 5, 9, 1864. |
| Grenada | Miss | Aug. 13, 1863. |
| Greysville | Ga | Nov. 27, 1863. |
| Grierson's expedition from La Grange, Tenn., to Baton Rouge | La | April 17–May 2, 1863. |
| Griswoldville | Ga | Nov. 22, 1864. |
| Grosse Tete Bayou | La | Feb. 19, March 30, 1864. |
| Ground Squirrel Church and Bridge | Va | May 10, 1864. |
| Grouse Creek | Cal | May 23, 1864. |
| Groveton | Va | Aug. 29, 1862. |
| Guerrilla warfare in Missouri | Mo | July 20–Sept. 20, 1862. |
| Gum Slough | Ark | March 16, 1863. |
| Gum Swamp | N. C. | May 22, 1863. |
| Gunboats on James River | Va | Oct 22, 1864. |
| Gunter's Bridge | S. C | Feb. 14, 1865. |
| Guntown | Miss | May 4, 1863, June 10, 1864. |
| Guyandotte | W. Va | Nov. 10, 1861. |
| Guy's Gap | Tenn | June 27, 1863. |
| | | |
| Hagar's Mountain | Md | July 7, 1864. |
| Hagerstown | Md | July 6, 11, 1863, July 5, 1864. |
| Haguewood Prairie | Tenn | Sept. 26, 1863. |
| Half-Moon Battery | N. C | Jan. 19, 1865. |
| Half Mount | Ky | April 14, 1864. |
| Hall Island | S. C | Nov. 24, 1863. |
| Hall's Ferry | Miss | May 13, 1863. |
| Halltown | Va | July 15, 1863, Aug. 24–27, 1864. |
| Hamburg | Tenn | May 30, 1863. |
| Hamburg Landing | Ala | May 29, 1863. |
| Hamilton | N. C | July 9, 1862. |
| Hamilton | Va | March 21, 1865. |
| Hammack's Mills | W. Va | July 3, 1864. |
| Hampton | Va | Aug. 7, 1861. |
| Hampton Roads | Va | March 9, 1862. |
| Hancock | Va | Jan. 4, 1862. |
| Hanging Rock | W. Va | Sept. 23, 1861. |
| Hankinson's Ferry | Miss | May 3, 1863. |
| Hanover | Pa | June 30, 1863. |
| Hanover C. H | Va | May 27, 1862, May 29–31, 1864. |
| Hanoverton | Va | May 27–31, 1864. |
| Hardy County | W. Va | Jan. 5, 1863. |
| Harney Lake Valley | Oregon | April 7, 1864, Sept. 23, 1865. |
| Harper's Farm | Va | April 6, 1865. |
| Harper's Ferry | Va | April 18, Oct. 11, 1861, May 28, Sept. 12–15, 1862, Oct. 5, 1863. |
| Harper's Ferry Bridge | Va | July 7, 1863. |
| Harpeth River | Tenn | March 2, 4, April 10, 1863. |

Harrison ........................................................Mo . .....Sept. 27, 30, 1864.
Harrisonburg ..................................................Va........June 6, 1862.
Harrison's Field .............................................Ga........Dec. 9, 1864.
Harrison's Island.............................................Va........Oct. 21, 1861.
Harrisonville .................................................Mo .......July 18, 25, 26, 1861, Nov. 3, 1862, Oct. 24, 1863.
Harrodsburg ...................................................Ky........Oct. 10, 1862, Oct. 21, 1864.
Hartsville ......................................................Mo .......Jan. 11, May 23, 1863.
Hartsville.......................................................Tenn.....Dec. 7, 1862.
Hartwood Church.............................................Va........Nov. 28, 1862, Feb. 25, 1863.
Hatcher's Run.................................................Va........Oct. 27, 28, 1864, Feb. 5-7, 1865.
Hatchie ..........................................................Miss .....Oct. 5, 1862.
Hatchie River..................................................Miss .....Aug. 10, 1864.
Hawe's Shop....................................................Va........May 28, June 2, 1864.
Hawk's Nest....................................................W. Va...Aug. 20, 1861.
Haxal's, or Evlington Heights ...........................Va........July 3, 1862.
Haymarket ......................................................Va........Oct. 18, 1862, Oct. 19, 1863.
Hayne's Bluff ..................................................Miss ......April 29–May 2, 1863, Feb. 3, April —, 1864.
Haynesville ....................................................Md........July 2, 1861.
Hazel Bottom ..................................................Mo .......Oct. 14, 1862.
Hedgesville ....................................................Va........Oct. 22, 1862, Oct. 15, 1863.
Helena...........................................................Ark ......Aug. 11–14, Sept. 20, Oct. 11, 18, Dec. 5, 1862, May 25, Jan. 15, July 4, 1863, Aug. 2, 1864.
Henderson .....................................................Ky........July 21, Sept. 25, 1864.
Henderson's Hills, or Bayou Rapids...........La ........March 21, 1864.
Henderson's Mill .............................................Tenn.....Oct. 11, 1863.
Hendrick's......................................................Miss .....Sept. 15, 1863.
Henrytown .....................................................Mo .......Oct. 13, 1861.
Hermitage ......................................................Mo .......Nov. 2, 1864.
Hernando........................................................Miss......Apr. 18, May 28, June 20, 1863.
Hiampom Valley .............................................Cal ......Oct. 10, 1863.
Hickory Grove ................................................Mo .......Aug. 23, Sept. 19, 1862.
Hickory Hills...................................................S. C......Feb. 1, 1865.
Hicksford .......................................................Va........Dec. 9, 1864.
High Bridge....................................................Va........April 6, 1865.
Hillsborough...................................................Ala ......April 17, 1863.
Hillsboro' .......................................................Ga........July 31, 1864.
Hillsboro' .......................................................Ky........Oct. 8, 1861.
Hillsborough ...................................................Miss......Feb. 10, 1864.
Hill's Plantation..............................................Ark .... July 7, 1862.
Hill's Plantation..............................................Miss......June 22, 1863.
Hodgeville ......................................................Ky........Oct. 23, 1861.
Holland House ................................................Va........May 15, 16, 1863.
Hollow Tree Gap.............................................Tenn.....Dec. 17, 1864.
Holly River .....................................................W. Va...April 17, 1862.
Holly Springs .................................................Miss......Nov. 12, 28, Dec. 20, 1862, April 17, 1863, May 24, Aug. 1, 8, 27, 28, 1864.
Holston River..................................................Tenn.....Nov. 15, 1863, Feb, 20, 1864.
Honey Hill, or Grahamsville .............................S. C......Nov. 30, 1864.
Honey Springs ................................................Kans ....July 17, Aug. 22, 1863.
Hoover's Gap .................................................Tenn.....June 24, 1863.
Hopkinsville ...................................................Ky .......Nov. 6, 1862, Dec. 12, 16, 1864.
Hornersville ...................................................Mo.......Sept 20, 1863.
Hornsboro'......................................................S C......March 3, 1865.
Horse Creek....................................................D. T .....June 14, 1865.
Horse Creek....................................................Mo........Sept. 17, 1863.
Horse-Head Creek...........................................Ark ......Feb. 17, 1864.
Horse-Shoe Bend, or Greasy Creek...............Ky .......May 11, 1863.
Horton's Mills.................................................N C.....April 27, 1862.
Hot Springs....................................................Ark ......Feb. 4, 1864.
Howard County ...............................................Mo .......Aug. 28, 1862, Aug. 28, 1864.

| Place | State | Date |
|---|---|---|
| Howell's Ferry | Ga | July 1, 1864. |
| Howe's Ford, or Weaver's Stores | Ky | April 28, 1863. |
| Hudnot's Plantation | La | May 1, 1864. |
| Hudson | Mo | Dec. 21, 1861. |
| Hudsonville, or Cold Water | Miss | Nov. 8, 1862. |
| Huff's Ferry | Tenn | Nov. 14, 1863. |
| Humansville | Mo | March 26, Aug. 12, 1862, Oct. 16, 17, 1863. |
| Humboldt | Tenn | Dec. 20, 1862. |
| Hunnewell | Mo | Jan. 3, 1862. |
| Hunter's Mills | Va | Nov. 26, 1861. |
| Huntersville | Va | Jan. 4, 1862. |
| Huntsville | Ala | April 11, 1862, Oct. 1, 1864. |
| Huntsville | Mo | Nov. 9, 1862. |
| Huntsville | Tenn | Nov. 11, 1862. |
| Hurricane Bridge | W. Va | March 28, 1863. |
| Hurricane Creek | Ark | Oct. 23, 1864. |
| Hurricane Creek | Miss | Aug. 14, 16, 22, Oct. 23, 1864. |
| Hutchinson | Minn | Sept. 3, 4, 1862. |
| Illinois Creek | Ark | Dec. 7, 1862. |
| Independence | Mo | June 17, Nov. 29, 1861, Feb. 18, March 22, Aug. 11, 1862, Feb. 3. 8, Mar. 23, April 23, 24, 1863, Feb. 19, Oct. 22, 24, 26, 1864. |
| Indian Bay | Ark | Feb. 16, April 13, 1864. |
| Indian City Village | La | Aug. 6, 1864. |
| Indiantown, or Sandy Swamp | N. C | Dec. 18, 1863. |
| Indian Village | D. T | March 27, 1863. |
| Indian Village | La | Jan. 27, 1863. |
| Ingham's Mills | Miss | Oct. 12, 1863. |
| Ingraham's Plantation | Miss | Oct. 10, 1863. |
| Irish Bend | La | April 12, 14, 1863. |
| Iron Bridge | I. T | June 19, 1864. |
| Iron County | Mo | Sept. 11, 1862. |
| Ironton | Mo | Sept. 26, 27, 1864. |
| Irvine | Ky | July 30, 1863. |
| Irwinsville | Ga | May 10, 1865. |
| Island Mound | Mo | Oct. 27, 29, 1862. |
| Island No. 76 | Miss | Jan. 20, 1864. |
| Island No. 10 | Tenn | April 8, Oct. 17, 1862, Oct. 16, 1863. |
| Isle of Wight C. H | Va | Dec. 22, 1862. |
| Issequena County | Miss | July 10, Aug. 17, 1864. |
| Iuka | Miss | Sept. 13, 20, 1862, July 7, 9, 14, 1863. |
| Ivy Ford | Ark | Jan. 19, 1864, Jan. 8, 1865. |
| Ivy Hills | Miss | Feb. 22, 1864. |
| Jacinto | Miss | Aug. 13, 1863. |
| Jackson | Ark | Aug. 3, 1862, April 26, 1863. |
| Jackson | La | Aug. 3, 1863, Oct. 5, Nov. 21, 1864. |
| Jackson | Miss | May 14, July 10–17, 29, 1863, Feb. 5, July 5–8, 1864. |
| Jackson | Mo | April 9, 1862, April 27, 1863. |
| Jackson | Tenn | Dec. 18, 1862, July 13, 1863. |
| Jacksonboro' | Tenn | March 10, 1862. |
| Jackson County | Mo | June 2, 1862, April 5, 1863. |
| Jackson Crossroads | La | June 20, 1863. |
| Jacksonport | Ark | Dec. 23, 1863, April 24 Aug. 26, 1864. |
| Jackson's Ford | Ala | July 14, 1864. |
| Jacksonville | Fla | March 29, 1863, May 1, 28, 1864, April 4, 1865. |

| Place | State | Date |
|---|---|---|
| Jack's Shop | Tenn | Sept. 22, 1863. |
| Jack's Shop | Va | Dec 23, 1864. |
| James City, or Robertson's Run | Va | Oct. 10, 1863. |
| James Island | S. C | June 10–13, 1862, July 16, 1863, May 21, July 1, 2, 5, 7, 1864, Feb. 10, 1865. |
| Jarrett's Station | Va | May 9, 1864. |
| Jasper | Tenn | June 4, 1862. |
| Jasper County | Mo | June 10, Oct. 5, 1863. |
| Jenken's Ferry | Ark | April 15, 30, May 4, 1864. |
| Jenk's Bridge | Ga | Dec. 7–9, 1864. |
| Jennie's Creek, or Paintsville | Ky | Jan. 7, 1862. |
| Jefferson | Tenn | Dec. 30, 1862. |
| Jefferson City | Mo | Oct. 7, Nov. 3, 1864. |
| Jeffersonton | Va | Oct. 12, 1863. |
| Jeffersonville, or Abb's Valley | Va | May 8, 1864. |
| Jeff. Thompson surrendered | Ark | May 11, 1865. |
| Jericho Ford | Va | May 23–27, 1864. |
| Jerusalem Plank Road | Va | June 22, 23, 1864. |
| Jettersville | Va | April 5, 1865. |
| John Day's River | Oregon | July 12, 1864, April 16, 1865. |
| John's Island | S. C | July 5–9, 1864. |
| Johnson County | Mo | July 16, 1864. |
| Johnson Depot | Tenn | Sept. 22, 1863. |
| Johnson's Mills | Tenn | Feb. 22, 1864. |
| Johnsonville | Tenn | Sept. 25, Nov. 4–5, 1864. |
| Johnston surrendered | N. C | April 26, 1865. |
| Johnstown | Mo | Nov. 24, 1861. |
| Jonesboro' | Ark | Aug. 3, 1862. |
| Jonesboro' | Ga | Aug. 19, 20, 31, Sept. 1, 7, 1864. |
| Jonesboro' | Mo | Aug. 21, 22, 1861, Oct. 12, 14, 1863. |
| Jones' Bridge | Va | June 23, 1864. |
| Jones' Crossroads | Miss | May 3, 1863. |
| Jones' Ford | Miss | July 6, 1863. |
| Jones' Ford | Tenn | July 2, 1863. |
| Jones' Hay Station | Ark | Aug. 24, 1864. |
| Jones' Plantation | Ga | Nov. 27–29, 1864. |
| Jonesville | Va | Jan. 3, 1864. |
| Jornado del Muerto | N. Mex | June 16, 1863. |
| Joy's Ford | Ark | Jan. 8, 1865. |
| Julesburg | I. T | Jan. 7, 1865. |
| Jumpertown | Miss | Nov. 5, 1862. |
| Kansas City | Mo | Nov. 22, 1864. |
| Kautz's raid in Virginia | | May 4–13, 1864. |
| Kautz's raid on R. R | Va | May 12–17, 1864. |
| Kearneysville | Va | Aug. 25, 1864. |
| Kearnstown | Va | March 23, 1862. |
| Keller's Bridge | Ky | June 10, 1864. |
| Kelly's Ford | Tenn | Jan. 27, 1864. |
| Kelly's Ford | Va | Aug. 21, 1862, March 17, Aug. 1–3, Nov. 7, 1863. |
| Kelly's Island | Va | June 26, 1861. |
| Kelly's Store | Va | Jan 30, 1863. |
| Kenesaw Mountain, or Lost Mountain, Big Shanty, Marietta, and Nose's Creek | Ga | June 10–July 2, 1864. |
| Kernstown | Va | July 23, 1864. |
| Kettle Run | Va | Aug. 27, 1862. |
| Keysville | Cal | April 19, 1863 |
| Keytesville | Mo | Feb. 17, 26, 1862. |
| Kilpatrick's raid in Virginia | | Feb. 28–March 4, 1864. |
| Kilpatrick's raid on railroad | Ga | Aug. 18–23, 1864. |
| Kincaels | Tenn | Nov. 6, 1863. |
| Kinderhook | Tenn | Aug. 11, 1862. |

| Place | State | Date |
|---|---|---|
| King George County | Va | Aug. 24, 1863. |
| King George Court-House | Va | Dec 2, 1862. |
| King's Creek | Miss | July 9, 1864. |
| Kingsport | Tenn | Dec. 13, 1864. |
| King's River | Ark | April 16, 1864. |
| King's School-House | Va | June 25, 1862. |
| Kingston | Ga | May 18, 24, Oct. 12, 1864. |
| Kingston | N. C. | Dec. 14, 1862, March 14, 1865. |
| Kingston | Tenn | Nov. 26, 1863, Aug. 26, 1864. |
| Kingsville | Mo | June 12, 1864. |
| Kirby Smith surrendered | | May 26, 1865. |
| Kirksville | Mo | Aug. 5, 6, 26, 1862. |
| Knob Gap | Tenn | Dec. 26, 1862. |
| Knob Noster | Mo | Jan. 22, 1862. |
| Knoxville. (See also Siege of) | Tenn | Sept. 10, 1863. |
| Kock's Plantation | La | July 13, 1863. |
| Kossuth | Miss | Aug 27, 1862. |
| | | |
| Labadieville, or Thibodeauxville and Georgia Landing | La | Oct. 27, 1862. |
| Lacey's Springs | Va | Dec. 20, 1864. |
| Ladija | Ala | Oct. 30, 1864. |
| La Fayette | Ga | June —, 1864. |
| La Fayette | Tenn | Dec. 25, 1863, June 9, 24, 1864. |
| La Fayette County | Mo | June 14, 1864. |
| La Fourche Crossing | La | June 20, 21, 1863. |
| La Grange | Ark | Sept 6, Oct. 11, Nov. 7, Dec. 30, 1862, Jan. 3, May 1, 1863. |
| La Grange | Tenn | Nov. 11, 1862, July 16, 1863. |
| Lake Chicot, or Ditch and Fish Bayous, Columbia and Old River Lake | La | June 6, 1864. |
| Lake Chicot | La | July 6, 7, 1864. |
| Lake City | Fla | Feb. 12, 1864. |
| Lake Providence | La | Feb. 10, May 27, June 10, 29, 1863 |
| Lake Village | Ark | Feb. 10, 1864. |
| Lamar | Miss | Nov 12, 1862. |
| Lamar | Mo | Aug. 24, Nov. 5, 1862. |
| Lamb's Ferry | Tenn | Dec. 25, 1864. |
| Lamonica Springs | N. Mex. | Sept. 4, 1865. |
| Lancaster | Ky | Oct. 14, 1862. |
| Lancaster | Mo | Nov. 24, 1861. |
| Lane's Prairie | Mo | July 26, 1861, May 26, 1864. |
| Languelle Ferry | Ark | Aug. 3, 1862. |
| Lattamore's Mills | Ga | June 20, 1864. |
| Lauderdale Springs | Miss | Feb. 16, 1864. |
| Laurel Hill, or Bealington | W. Va | July 8, 1861. |
| La Vergne | Tenn | Oct. 7, Nov. 27, Dec. 9, 1862, Jan. 1, 1863, Sept. 1, 1864. |
| Lawrence | Kan | July 27, Aug. 21, 1863. |
| Lawrenceburg | Ky | Oct. 9, 1862. |
| Lawrenceburg | Ohio | July 14, 1863 |
| Lawrenceburg | Tenn | Nov. 4, 1863, Nov. 22, 27, Dec. 22, 1864. |
| Lay's Ferry | Ga | May 15, 1864. |
| Leasburg | Mo | Sept. 29, 30, Oct. 1, 28, 1864. |
| Leatherwood | Ky | Nov. 6, 1862. |
| Lebanon | Ala | Feb. 3, 6, 1864. |
| Lebanon | Ky | July 12, 1862, July 5, 1863, July 30, 1864. |
| Lebanon | Tenn | May 5, Nov. 11, Dec. 6, 1862, Feb. 8, 1863. |
| Leesburg | Va | Oct. 21, 1861. |
| Leesburg Road | Va | Sept. 17, 1862. |
| Lee's Creek | Ark | Aug. 1, 1864. |
| Lee's Mills | Va | Apr. 16, 1862, July 12, 30, 1864. |

| Place | State | Date |
|---|---|---|
| Lee Springs | Va | Aug 23, 1862. |
| Lee surrendered | Va | April 9, 1865. |
| Leesville | Mo | March 19, 1862. |
| Leetown | Va | March 7, 1862, July 3, 1864. |
| Legare's Point | S. C | June 3, 1862. |
| Leighton | Ala | April 24, 1863. |
| Leiper's Ferry | Tenn | Oct. 28, 1863. |
| Leland's Point | Ark | May 27, 1864. |
| Lenoirs | Tenn | Nov. 15, 1863. |
| Lett's Tan-yard | Ga | Sept. 13, 1863. |
| Lewinsville | Va | Sept. 11, 1861. |
| Lewisburgh | Ark | Jan. 17, 1864. |
| Lewisburg | Va | May 23, 1862. |
| Lexington | Ky | Oct. 17, 1862, July 28, 1863, June 10, 1864. |
| Lexington | Mo | Aug. 29, Sept. 12–20, 1861, March 12, Oct. 17, 1862, Feb. 22, June 14, Oct. 19, 21, 1864. |
| Lexington | Tenn | Dec. 18, 1862, June 29, 1863. |
| Lexington | W. Va | June 10, 11, 1864. |
| Liberty | La | Nov. 21, 1864. |
| Liberty | Mo | Oct. 6, 1862. |
| Liberty | Va | June 20, 1864. |
| Liberty Creek | La | Nov. 15, 1864. |
| Liberty Gap, or Beech Grove | Tenn | June 25, 1863. |
| Liberty Landing | Mo | Oct. 6, 1862. |
| Liberty Mills | Va | Oct. 15, 1863. |
| Liberty Post-Office | Ark | April 15, 1864. |
| Lick Creek | Ark | Jan. 12, 1863. |
| Lick Creek | Tenn | April 24, 1862. |
| Licking | Mo | May 4, 1862. |
| Limestone Station | Tenn | Sept. 5, 1863. |
| Linden | Tenn | May 12, 1863. |
| Linden | Va | May 15, 1862. |
| Linn Creek | Mo | Oct. 15, 1861. |
| Linn Creek | Va | Feb. 8, 1862. |
| Liscomb's Hill | Cal | June 6, 1862. |
| Little Bear Creek | Ala | Nov. 28, Dec. 12, 1862. |
| Little Blue | D. T | Aug 12, 1864. |
| Little Blue | Mo | Nov. 11, 1861, April 12, 1862, July 6, Oct. 21, 1864. |
| Little Cacapon | Va | April 10, 1864. |
| Little Creek | N. C | Nov. 3, 1862. |
| Little Harpeth | Tenn | March 25, 1863. |
| Little Lermio | Colo | Aug. 5, 1865. |
| Little Missouri River | Ark | Jan. 25, April 4, 6, 1864. |
| Little Osage River | Kan | Oct. 25, 1864. |
| Little Pond | Tenn | Aug 30, 1862. |
| Little Red River | Ark | June 5, 25, 1862. |
| Little River | Tenn | Oct. 20, 1864. |
| Little Rock | Ark | Sept. 10, 1863, April 26, May 28, 1864. |
| Little Rock Landing | Tenn | April 26, 1863. |
| Little Rock Road | Ark | April 2, 1863. |
| Little Salkahatchie | S C | Feb. 5, 1865. |
| Little Santa Fé | Mo | Nov. 6, 20, 1861, March 23, 1862. |
| Little Washington | Va | Nov. 15, 1862. |
| Liverpool Heights | Miss | Feb 3, 1864. |
| Livingston | Miss | March 27, 1864. |
| Lockbridge's Mills, or Dresden | Ky | May 5, 1862 |
| Lock's Ford | Va | Sept. 13, 1864. |
| Locust Grove | I. T | July 3, 1862. |
| Locust Grove | Va | Nov. 26–28, 1863. |
| Logan's Crossroads | Ky | Jan. 19, 20, 1862. |
| London Lane | Ala | April 25, 1863. |
| Lone Jack | Mo | Aug. 11, 15, 16, '62, Nov. 1, '64. |

| Place | State | Date |
|---|---|---|
| Longview | Ark | March 26, 30, 1864. |
| Lookout Mountain | Tenn | Nov. 24, 1863. |
| Lookout Station | Mo | Aug. 20, 1861. |
| Lost Creek | Mo | April 15, 1862. |
| Lost Mountain | Ga | June 9–30, 1864. |
| Lotspeach Farm | Mo | July 8, 1862. |
| Lotus Steamer | Ark | Jan. 17, 1865. |
| Loudon Creek | Tenn | Nov. 15, 1863. |
| Loudon Heights | Va | Jan. 10, 1864. |
| Louisa C. H | Va | May 1, 1863. |
| Louisville | Tenn | Nov. 28, 1863. |
| Lovejoy's Station | Ga | July 29,30, Aug. 20, Sept. 2-6, Nov. 16, 1864. |
| Lovettsville | Va | Aug. 8, 1861, Oct. 21, 1862. |
| Low Creek | W. Va | June 21, 1863. |
| Lowndesborough | Ala | April 10, 1865. |
| Lowtonville | S. C | Feb. —, 1865. |
| Lucas Bend | Ky | Sept. 26, 1861. |
| Lumkin's Mills | Miss | Nov. 28, 30, 1862. |
| Luna Landing | Ark | Feb 22, 1864. |
| Lundy's Lane | Ala | April 17, 1863. |
| Luray | Va | June 30, July 12, 1862, Sept. 24, 1864. |
| Lynchburg | Va | June 17, 18, 1864. |
| Lynch's Creek | S. C | Feb 26, 1865. |
| Lynnville | Tenn | Nov. 24, Dec. 23, 1864. |
| Macon | Ga | July 30, Nov. 20, 24, 1864, April 20, 1865. |
| Macon | Mo | Feb. 12, 1865. |
| Madeline Plains | Cal | Nov. 17, 1862. |
| Madison | Ark | April 4, 1863. |
| Madison C. H | Va | Dec 20, 1864. |
| Madison Station | Ala | May 17, Nov. 26, 1864. |
| Madisonville | Ky | Aug. 26, Oct. 5, 1862. |
| Madisonville | La | Jan. 7, 1864. |
| Mad River | Cal | July 11, 1863. |
| Magnolia | Tenn | Jan. 7. 1865. |
| Malhuer River | Oreg | July 9, 1865. |
| Malvern Hill | Va | July 1, Aug. 5, 1862, July 27, 28, 1864 |
| Manassas | Va | Aug 30, 1862. |
| Manassas Gap | Va | Nov. 5, 1862, July 21, 1863. |
| Manassas Junction | Va | Oct. 24, 1862. |
| Manchester | Tenn | Aug 29, 1862, March 17, 1864. |
| Mansfield | La | April 8, 1864. |
| Mansura, or Avoyells Prairie, Marksville, Morreausville | La | May 13–17, 1864. |
| Maplesville | Ala | April 1, 1865 |
| Maria des Cygnes | Kans | Aug. 31, 1863, Oct. 25, 1864. |
| Marianna | Fla | Sept. 27, 1864. |
| Mariana | Ark | Nov 7, 1862 |
| Marie's County | Mo | May 26, 1864. |
| Marietta | Ga | July 3, 4, 1864. |
| Marietta | Miss | Aug. 31. 1862. |
| Marion | Miss | Feb 17, 1864. |
| Marion | Va | Dec. 16, 18, 1864. |
| Marion County | Fla | March 10, 1865. |
| Markham | Va | Nov 5, 1862. |
| Mark's Mills | Ark | April 5, 25, 1864. |
| Marksville | La | May 14–16. 1864. |
| Marrowbone, or Burkesville | Ky | July 2, 1863. |
| Marshall | Mo | July 28, Oct 12, 13, 1863. |
| Marshfield | Mo | Feb. 14, Oct 20, 1862. |
| Martinsburg | Md | July 2, 1861. |
| Martinsburg | Mo | July 17, 18, 1861. |

| | | |
|---|---|---|
| Martinsburg | Va | Sept., 1862, June 14, 1863, |
| Martin's Creek | Ark | Aug 19, Sept. 18, 1864, Jan. 7, 1864. |
| Maryland Heights | Va | July 4–7, 1864. |
| Marysville | Tenn | Nov. 14, 1863. |
| Mason's Bridge | S. C | Dec. 6–9, 1864. |
| Mason's Neck | Va | Feb 24, 1862. |
| Massacre at Centralia | Mo | Sept. 27, 1864. |
| Massacre on Railroad | Mo | Sept. 27, 1864. |
| Massacre on Sam Gaty | Mo | March 30, 1863. |
| Matagorda Bay | Texas | Dec. 29, 30, 1863. |
| Matapony, or Thornburg | Va | August 6, 1862. |
| Mathias Point | Va | June 27, 1861. |
| Matote | Cal | May 26, 1864. |
| Mayfield | Ky | January 12, 1864. |
| Mayre's Heights | Va | May 3, 1863. |
| Maysville | Ala | Aug 28, Oct. 13, 1863. |
| Maysville | Ark | October 22, 1862. |
| Mazzard Prairie | Ark | July 27, 1864. |
| McAfee's Crossroads | Ga | June 12, 1864. |
| McConnellsburg | Pa | June 24, 28, 1863. |
| McCook's raid in Georgia | | July 26–31, 1864. |
| McCullough's Store | Mo | July 26, Aug. 3, 1861. |
| McDonald County | Mo | August 5, 1864. |
| McDowell, or Bull Pasture Mountain | Va | May 8, 1862 |
| McGuire's Ferry | Ark | Sept. 23, 1862. |
| McKay's Point | S. C | Dec. 22, 1864. |
| McLean's Ford, or Liberty Mills | Va | October 15, 1863. |
| McMinnville | Tenn | Aug. 30, 1862, April 20, Sept. 28, Oct. 3, 1863. |
| Meadow Bluff | W. Va | Dec. 12, 1863. |
| Meadow Bridge | Va | May 12, 1864. |
| Mechanicksburg | Miss | May 29, June 4, 7, 1863. |
| Mechanicsville | Miss | May 24, 29, 1863. |
| Mechanicsville, or Ellison's Mills | Va | June 26, 1862. |
| Medalia | Minn | April 16, 1863. |
| Medley | W. Va | Jan. 20, 1864. |
| Medoc | Mo | Aug. 23, 1861. |
| Meffleton Lodge | Ark | June 29, 1864. |
| Memphis | Mo | July 18, 1862. |
| Memphis | Tenn | June 6, 1862, May 2, Aug. 21, Dec 14, 1864. |
| Mendon Station | Tenn | Aug. 31, Oct. 10, 1862. |
| Meridian | Miss | Feb 9–19, 1864. |
| Merrill's Crossing | Mo | Oct. 12, 13, 1863. |
| Merriweather's Ferry | Tenn | Aug. 15, 1862. |
| Mesilla | N. Mex | Aug. 3, 1861. |
| Messenger's Bridge | Miss | Oct 5, 1863. |
| Messenger's Ferry | Miss | July 1, 2, 1863. |
| Metamora | Miss | Oct. 5, 1862. |
| Metley's Ford | Tenn | Nov. 4, 1863. |
| Mexico | Mo | July 15, 1861. |
| Mezcal River | Cal | May 29, 1864. |
| Michel's Creek | Miss | May 5, 1863. |
| Middleburg | Miss | Dec. 24, 1862. |
| Middleburg | Tenn | Sept 21, 1862. |
| Middleburg | Va | March 28, 1862, June 19, 1863. |
| Middle Creek | Ky | Jan. 10, 1862. |
| Middle Creek Fork, or Buckhannon | Va | July 6, 1861. |
| Middleton | Md | July 7, 1864. |
| Middleton | Tenn | Jan. 5, 31, May 21, June 24, 1863, Jan. 14, 1864. |
| Middletown | Va | May 24, 1862, June 11, 1863, Oct. 19, 1864. |
| Middle Yager | Cal | June 28, 1863. |
| Milford, or Shawnee Mound, Blackwater | Mo | Dec. 18, 1861. |

| | | |
|---|---|---|
| Milford | Va | July 2, 1862. |
| Milford Station | Va | May 20, 1864. |
| Mill Creek | Ga | May 7, 1864. |
| Mill Creek | Mo | April 24, 1863. |
| Mill Creek | Tenn | Nov. 27, 1862. |
| Mill Creek Valley | W. Va | Nov. 13, 1863. |
| Millen Grove | Ga | Dec. 1, 1864. |
| Milliken's Bend, or Ashland | La | June 5–7, 1863. |
| Mill Point | W. Va | Nov. 5, 1863. |
| Mill Springs, or Beech Grove, Fishing Creek, Logan's Crossroads | Ky | Jan. 19, 20, 1862. |
| Millsville, or Wentzville | Mo | July 16, 1861. |
| Milltown Bluff | S. C | July 10, 1863. |
| Millwood | Va | Dec. 17, 1864. |
| Milton | Fla | Oct 26, 1864. |
| Milton | Tenn | Feb 18, 1863. |
| Mine Creek | Kans | Oct 25, 1864. |
| Mineral Point | Mo | Sept 27, 1864. |
| Mine Run | Va | Nov. 26, Dec. 2, 1863. |
| Mine Explosion, Petersburg | Va | July 30, 1864. |
| Mingo Swamp | Mo | Feb. 3, 1863. |
| Missionary Ridge | Tenn | Nov. 25, 1863. |
| Mississippi City | Miss | March 8, 1862. |
| Mississippi Springs | Miss | May 13, 1863. |
| Missouri River | D. T | July 30, 1863. |
| Mitchell's Creek | Fla | Dec. 17, 1864. |
| Mitchell's Station | Va | Aug. 9, 1862. |
| Mobile. (See also Siege of) | Ala | Dec. 22, 1864. |
| Mocassin Gap | Va | Dec. 24, 1864. |
| Moffatt's Station | Ark | Sept. 27, 1863. |
| Monaqua Springs | Mo | March 25, 1862. |
| Monday Hollow | Mo | Oct 13, 1861. |
| Monetis Bluff | La | April 23, 1864. |
| Monocacy | Md | July 9, 1864. |
| Monroe County | Mo | Sept. 16, Oct. 4, 1862. |
| Monroe's Crossroads | N. C | March 10, 1865. |
| Monroe Station | Mo | July 9, 10, 1861. |
| Monterey | Ky | June 11, 1862. |
| Monterey | Tenn | April 28, May 13, 1862. |
| Monterey | Va | April 12, 1862. |
| Monterey Gap | Md | July 4, 1863. |
| Montevallo | Ala | March 13, 30, 31, 1865. |
| Montevallo | Mo | April 14, Aug. 6, 1862. |
| Montgomery | Ala | April 12, 13, 1865. |
| Montgomery | Ga | July 18, 1864. |
| Monticello | Ky | May 1, June 9, 1863. |
| Monticello | Ark | Jan. 16, March 18, 1864. |
| Moorefield | W. Va | Nov. 9, 1862, Jan. 3, Sept. 5, 11, 1863, Feb. 4, Aug. 7, 1864. |
| Moore's Bluff | Miss | Sept. 29, 1864. |
| Moore's Mills | Mo | July 24, 28, 29, 1862. |
| Moreau Bottom | Mo | Oct. 7, 1864. |
| Moresburg | Tenn | Dec. 10, 1863. |
| Morgan County | Tenn | Feb. 2, 1862. |
| Morgan's Mills | Ark | Feb. 9, 1864. |
| Morgan's raid from Kentucky, into Indiana and Ohio | | July 1–26, 1863. |
| Morgansville | Ky | Sept. 2, 1862. |
| Morgantown | Ky | Oct. 29, 1861, Oct. 24, 1862. |
| Morganzia | La | Sept. 29, 1863, May 18, 30, Nov. 23, 1864. |
| Morning Sun | Tenn | July 1, 1862. |
| Moro Bottom | Ark | April 25, 1864. |
| Moro Creek | Ark | April 26, 1864. |
| Moreausville | La | May 14–16, 1864. |

Morristown.......................................Mo.......Sept. 17, 1861.
Morristown.......................................Tenn.....Dec. 1, 1861, Dec. 10, 1863. Oct. 28, 1864.
Morton.......................................Miss......Feb. 7, 8, 1864.
Morton's Ford.......................................Va........Feb. 6, 1864.
Moscow.......................................Ark......April 15, 1864.
Moscow.......................................Tenn.....Feb. 18, Nov. 4, Dec. 2, 3, 1863, June 15, 1864.
Moscow Station, or Wolf River Bridge........Miss......Dec 4, 1863.
Mossy Creek.......................................Ga........Oct. 3, 1864.
Mossy Creek.......................................Tenn.....Dec. 29, 1863, Jan. 13, 1864.
Mossy Creek Station.......................................Tenn.....Dec. 24, 1863.
Moulton.......................................Ala.......May 28, 29, 1864.
Mound Plantation.......................................La........June 29, 1863.
Mountain Fork.......................................Ark......Feb 4, 1864.
Mountain Grove.......................................Mo.......March 9, 1862.
Mountain Home.......................................Mo.......Oct. 17, 1862.
Mountain Store.......................................Mo.......July 25, 26, 1862, May 26, 1863.
Mount Carmel.......................................Tenn.....Nov. 29, 1864.
Mount Clio.......................................S. C......Feb 26, 1865.
Mount Crawford.......................................Va........June 5, 1864, Feb 29, 1865.
Mount Elba.......................................Ark......March 30, 1864.
Mount Elba Ferry.......................................Ark......April 26, 1864.
Mount Ivy, or Ivy Hills.......................................Miss......Feb. 22, 1864.
Mount Jackson.......................................Va........Nov. 17, 1863.
Mount Pleasant.......................................Ala.......April 1, 1865.
Mount Pleasant.......................................Miss......May 21, 1864.
Mount Pleasent Landing.......................................La........May 15, 1864.
Mount Sterling.......................................Ky........July 29, 1862, March 22, 1863, June 9, 1864.
Mount Tabor Church.......................................N. C.....July 26, 1863.
Mount Vernon.......................................Ark......May 11, 1863.
Mount Vernon.......................................Mo.......Sept. 30, 1864.
Mount Washington.......................................Ky........Oct 2, 1862.
Mount Zion.......................................Mo.......Dec. 28, 1861.
Mount Zion Church.......................................Va.......July 6, 1864.
Mouth of Monocacy.......................................Md........Oct. 11, 1862.
Mud Creek.......................................Ala.......Jan 5, 1865.
Muddy Run.......................................Va........Nov. 8, 1863.
Mud Springs.......................................I. T......Feb. 8, 1865.
Mulberry Gap, or Wyerman's Mills.......................................Tenn.....Feb. 22, 1864.
Muldraugh's Hill.......................................Ky........Dec. 28, 1862.
Mumford's Station.......................................Ala.......April 23, 1865.
Munfordsville.......................................Ky........Dec. 17, 1861, Sept. 14, 16, 21, 1862.
Munson's Hill.......................................Va.......August 31, Sept. 29, 1861.
Murfreesboro'.......................................Tenn.....July 13, Dec 31, 1862–Jan. 3, June 6, 1863, Sept. 3, Dec. 5, 6, 7, 15, 24, 1864.
Murfreesboro' Road.......................................Tenn.....Oct. 4, 1863.
Muscle Shoals.......................................Ala.......Oct. 30, 1864.
Mustang Island.......................................Texas...Nov. 17, 1863.
Myerstown.......................................Va.......Nov. 18, 1864.

Nashville and Northwestern Railroad........Tenn.....Sept. 4, 1864.
Namozin Church.......................................Va.......April 3, 1865.
Nansemond.......................................Va.......April 14, 1863.
Nansemond River.......................................Va.......May 3, 1863.
Narrows.......................................Ga........Oct. 11, 1864.
Nashville.......................................Tenn.....March 9. July 21. Nov. 5, 1862, May 24, Dec. 2–22, 1864.
Natchez.......................................Miss......Nov. 11. Dec. 7, 10, 1863, April 25, 1864.
Natchitoches.......................................La........Mar. 31, April 19, May 5, 1864.

Natural Bridge.......... Fla ......March 6, 1865.
Nauvoo.......... Ala ......Jan. 2, 1865.
Near Alexandria.......... La ........May 1-8, 1864.
Near Blue Springs.......... Tenn.....Oct. 5, 1863.
Near Boliver Heights.......... Va ........July 14, 1863.
Near Brownsville.......... Ark ......Oct. 30, 1864.
Near Canton.......... Miss......Feb. 27, 28, 1864.
Near Culpeper.......... Va........July 12, 1862.
Near Dalton.......... Ga........Jan. 21, 1864.
Near Decatur.......... Tenn.....July 15. 1862.
Near Lebanon.......... Mo.......March 12, 1862.
Near Memphis.......... Tenn.....Oct. 4, 1864.
Near Nashville.......... Tenn.....March 8, Oct. 20, 1862.
Near New Berne.......... N. C.....Feb. 27, 1863.
Near Pine Bluff.......... Ark ......Sept. —, 1864.
Near Point Washington.......... Fla ......Feb. 9, 1864.
Near Romney.......... Va ........Feb. 16, 1863.
Near Snicker's Gap.......... Va ........Aug. 13, 1864.
Near the Rappahannock.......... Va........April 1, 1864.
Near Tunica Bend.......... La ........April 22, 1864.
Near Walkertown.......... Va ........March 2, 1864.
Near Yazoo City.......... Miss......Feb. 28, 1864.
Nelson's Farm.......... Va ........June 30, 1862.
Neosho.......... Mo .......April 26, May 31, Sept. 1-4, Dec. 15, 1862, March 2, Oct. 4, Nov. 5, 1863, June 3, Nov. 10, 1864.
Neuse River.......... N. C.....April 10, 1865.
New Albany.......... Miss......April 19, Oct. 5, 1863, July 10, 1864.
Newark.......... Mo.......Aug. 1, 1862.
New Baltimore.......... Va ......Nov. 5, 1862.
New Berne.......... N. C ....March 14, May 22, Nov. 11, 1862, March 14, 1863, Feb. 1-4, 29, 1864.
New Bridge.......... Va........May 24, 1862.
New Cider Mills.......... Tenn.....Nov. 29, 1864.
New Creek.......... W. Va...June 17, 1861, Aug. 4, 1864.
New Creek Valley.......... W. Va...Feb. 1, 1864.
New Hope.......... Ky........July 11, 1862.
New Hope.......... Va ........Nov 28. 1863.
New Hope Church.......... Ga........May 25-June 5, 1864.
New Kent Court-House.......... Va ........May 9, 1862, March 2, 1864.
New Lisbon.......... Ohio .....July 26, 1863.
New Madrid.......... Mo.......March 3-6, 14, 1862, Aug. 7, 1863.
New Madrid Bend.......... Tenn.....Oct. 22, 1863.
New Market.......... Va ........May 15, July 27, 28, Oct. 7, '64.
New Market Bridge.......... Va........Dec 22, 1861.
New Market Crossroads.......... Va........June 30, 1862.
New Market Heights.......... Va........June 24, Sept. 28-30, 1864.
Newnan.......... Ga .......July 30, 31, 1864.
Newport Barracks.......... N. C.....Feb. 1-3, 1864.
Newport News.......... Va........July 5, 1861.
New Providence.......... Tenn....Sept. 6, 1862.
New River.......... La .......Feb. 9, 1864.
New River Bridge.......... Va........May 9, 10, 1864.
Newtonia.......... Mo .......Aug. 5, Sept. 13, 30, Oct. 4, 5, 7, 1862, Sept 27, 1863, Oct. 28-30, 1864.
Newton.......... La .......Oct. 4, 1863.
Newtown.......... Va .......May 24, 1862, Nov. 12, 1864.
Newton County.......... Mo.......Feb. 10, 1863.
New Ulm.......... Minn....Aug. 25, 26, 1862.
Nickajack Creek, or Smyrna and Vining Station.......... Ga........July 1-10, 1864.

Nickajack Trace....................Ga........April 23, 1864.
Nineveh....................Va........Nov. 12, 1864.
Niobrara....................Neb......Dec. 4, 1863
Nolansville....................Md........Sept. 9, 1862.
Nolensville....................Tenn....Dec. 26, 1862, Feb. 15, 1863.
Norfolk....................Va........May 10, 1862.
North Anna River....................Va........July 23, 1862.
North Anna River, or Taylor's Bridge and
Jericho Ford....................Va........May 23-27, 1864.
Northeast River....................N. C.....Jan. 17, 1863
North Fork....................Va........March 6, 1865.
North Mountain....................Va........July 3, 1864.
Northport....................Ala........April 3, 1865.
North Shenandoah....................Va........Oct —, 1864.
Nose's Creek....................Ga........June 17, Oct. 1-3, 1864.
Nottaway Court-House....................Va........June 23, 1864.
Nueces River....................Tex......Aug. 10, 1862.

Oak Grove, or King's School-House and The
Orchards....................Va........June 25, 1862.
Oak Hills....................Mo........Aug. 10, 1861.
Oakland....................Miss......Dec 3, 8, 1862.
Ocean Pond....................Fla........Feb. 20, 1864.
Occoquan....................Va........March 5, Dec. 19, 28, 1862.
Occoquan Bridge....................Va........Jan 29, 1862.
Occoquan Creek....................Va........Nov. 12, 1861.
Occupation of Atlanta....................Ga........Sept. 2, 1864.
Occupation of Camden....................Ark......April 15, 16, 1864.
Offett's Knob....................Mo........April 28, 1864.
Ogeeche River, or Jenk's Bridge, and Eden,
and Poole's Stations....................Ga........Dec. 7-9, 1864.
Okalona....................Ark......April 3, 1864.
Okalona....................Miss......Feb. 22, 1864.
Old Church....................Va........June 13, 1862, May 30, June
10, 11, 1864.
Old Fort Wayne, or Maysville....................Ark......Aug 22, 1862.
Old Oaks....................La........May 18, 1864.
Old Randolph....................Mo........Sept. 14, 1861.
Old River....................La........Feb. 10, 1863, May 22, 1864.
Old River Lake....................Ark......June 5, 6, 1864.
Olive Branch....................La........March 6, 1865.
Olive Hill....................Ky........Oct. 2, 1862.
Olustee, or Ocean Pond and Silver Lake...Fla........Feb. 20, 1864.
Oostenaula....................Ga........May 13-16, 1864.
Opelousas....................La........Oct. 21, 1863
Opequan....................Va........Sept. 19, 1864.
Operations at Mine Run....................Va........Nov. 26-28, 1863.
Orangeburgh....................S. C......Feb. 12, 1865.
Orange Court-House....................Va........July 25, Aug. 2, 1862.
Orange Grove....................Va........Nov. 26-28, 1863.
Orchard Knob....................Tenn....Nov. 23, 1863.
Oregon County....................Mo........Oct. 23, 1863, March 19, 1864.
Oregon Mountains....................Oreg....Jan. 28, 1864
Orleans....................Ind........June 17, 1863.
Osage, or Island Mounds....................Mo........Oct. 29, 1862
Osage Mission....................Kan......Sept. 26, 1864.
Osage River....................Mo........Oct. 6, 1864.
Osceola....................Ark......Aug. 2, 4, 1864.
Osceola....................Mo........Sept. 20, 21, 1861, May 27,
1862.
Otter Creek....................Va........June 16, 1864
Overall's Creek....................Tenn....Dec. 4, 1864
Overton's Hills....................Tenn....Dec. 15, 16, 1864.
Owensborough....................Ky........Aug. 27, 1864.
Owensburgh....................Ky........Sept. 19, 20, 1862.
Owen's Crossroads....................S. C......Feb. 2, 1865.

| Place | State | Date |
|---|---|---|
| Owen's River | Cal | April 9, 1862. |
| Owen's Valley | Cal | March 3, 19, April 10, 1863. |
| Oxford | Miss | Dec 3, 1862, Aug. 12, 19, 22, 23, 1864. |
| Oxford Bend | Ark | Oct. 28, 1862. |
| Ox Hill | Va | Sept. 1, 1862. |
| Ozark | Ark | Oct. 29, 1863, July 14, 15, 1864. |
| Ozark | Mo | Aug. 2, Dec. 2, 1862. |
| Painsville | Ky | Jan. 7, 1862 |
| Paint Rock Railroad Bridge | Ark | April 28, 1862. |
| Paintsville | Ky | April 13, 1864. |
| Palaquemine, or Indian City Village | La | Aug 6, 1864. |
| Palmer's Creek | Va | May 12–16, 1864. |
| Palmetto Ranche | Texas | May 13, 1865. |
| Palmyra | Mo | Nov 18, 1861. |
| Palmyra | Tenn | Nov 13, 1863. |
| Palo Alto | Miss | April 21, 22, 1863. |
| Panther Creek | Mo | Aug. 8, 1862. |
| Panther Gap | W. Va | June 3, 1864. |
| Panther Springs | Tenn | March 5, 1864. |
| Papinsville | Kan | Sept. 5, 1861. |
| Papinsville, or Osceola | Mo | Sept 21, 22, 1861. |
| Paris | Ky | July 30, 1862, March 11, July 29, 1863. |
| Paris | Tenn | March 11, April 10, 1862, Sept. 13, 1863. |
| Parker's Crossroads, or Red Mound | Tenn | Dec. 30, 1862. |
| Parkersville | Mo | July 17, 19, 1861, Dec. 6, 1862. |
| Pass Christian | Miss | April 4, 1862. |
| Pasquotank | N. C | Aug 18, 1863. |
| Pass Manchas | La | March 20, 1864. |
| Pattacassey Creek, or Mount Taber Church | N. C | July 26, 1863. |
| Patten | Mo | July 26, 1862. |
| Patterson | Mo | April 20, 1863. |
| Patterson Creek, or Kelly's Island | Va | June 26, 1861, Feb. 3, 1864. |
| Pattersonville | La | March 28, 1863. |
| Pawnee Forks | Kans | Nov 25, 1864. |
| Pawnee Reservation | | June 20, 1863. |
| Payne's Plantation | Miss | Aug 18, 1863. |
| Payne's Tavern | Va | Nov 26–28, 1863. |
| Peach Orchard, or Allen's Farm | Va | June 29, 1862. |
| Peach-Tree Creek | Ga | July 19, 20, 1864. |
| Pea Ridge | Ark | March 6–8, 1862. |
| Pea-Vine Creek | Ga | Nov 27, 1863. |
| Pechacho Pass | D. T | April 15, 1862. |
| Pembescott Bayou | Ark | April 8, 1864. |
| Pendleton | Mo | Oct 29, 1864. |
| Pensacola | Fla | Nov 23, 1861, April 2, 1864. |
| Peralto | N. Mex | April 15, 1862. |
| Perry County | Ky | Nov. 9, 1862. |
| Perryville | Ark | Aug. 26, 1863. |
| Perryville | Ky | Oct. 6, 7, 8, 1862. |
| Perryville | I. T | Aug. 26, 1863. |
| Petersburgh | Tenn | March 2, 4, 1863. |
| Petersburgh | Va | June 10, 1864–April 3, 1865. |
| Petersburgh | W. Va | Sept. 7, 1861, Jan. 8, 1864. |
| Petit Jean | Ark | July 12, 1864. |
| Philadelphia | Tenn | Oct. 20, 22, 26, 1863. |
| Philimont | Va | Nov. 1, 1862. |
| Philippi | W. Va | June 3, 1861. |
| Phillip's Creek | Miss | May 21, 1862. |
| Piedmont, or Mount Crawford | Va | June 5, 1864. |
| Piedmont Station | Va | May 16, 1863. |
| Pierce's Point | Fla | Oct 18, 1864. |
| Pierson's Farm | Va | June 16, 1864. |

Pigeon-Roost Creek........ Miss...... May 14, 1863.

Piketown, or Try Mountain........ Ky....... Nov. 9, 1861.

Pikeville........ Ark...... June 25–29, 1864.

Pikeville........ Ky....... April 15, 1863.

Pilot Knob........ Mo........ Sept. 26–29, Oct. 26, 1864.

Pinal Creek........ Ariz. T.. Aug 1, 5, 1864.

Pinckney Island........ S. C...... Aug. 21, 1862.

Pine-Barren Creek........ Ala....... Dec. 17–19, 1864, Mar. 25, '65.

Pine-Barren Fork........ Fla........ Dec 17, 18, 1864.

Pine Bluff........ Ark...... Oct 25, 1863, Jan. 19, May 1, 21, June 27, July 2, 1864.

Pine Bluff........ Tenn..... Aug. 19, 1864.

Pine Forest........ Nev...... Nov. 17, 1865.

Pine Knob........ Ga........ June 19, 1864

Pine Mountain........ Ga....... June 14, 1864.

Pineville........ Mo....... Nov. 19, 1862, Aug. 13, 1863.

Piney Factory........ Tenn.... Nov 3, 1863.

Piney Woods........ La........ April 2, 1864.

Pink Hill........ Mo........ June 11, 1862.

Pinos Altos........ Ariz. T.. Feb. 27, 1864.

Pinos Altos Mines........ Ariz. T.. Jan. 29, 1863.

Pittman's Ferry........ Ark...... July 20, Nov. 25, 1862.

Pittman's Ferry........ Mo........ Oct. 27, 1862.

Pittsburg Landing, or Shiloh........ Tenn..... March 2, April 6, 7, 1862.

Plain's Store........ La........ May 21, 1863, April 7, 1864.

Plantersville, or Ebenezer Church and Maplesville........ Ala...... April 1, 1865.

Platte Bridge........ Dak...... June 3, July 26, 1865.

Platte City........ Mo........ July 3, 1864.

Plattsburg........ Mo....... Oct. 27, 1861.

Plaquemine........ La........ June 18, 1863, June 28, Aug. 6, 1864.

Pleasant Glove........ La........ April 8, 1864.

Pleasant Hills........ La........ April 9, 1864.

Pleasant Hill........ Mo....... July 8, 11, 1862, May 25, 28, 1864.

Pleasant Hill Landing........ La........ April 12, 1864.

Pleasant Ridge........ Ala...... April 6, 1865.

Plenitude........ Miss...... July 10, 1864.

Plymouth........ N. C...... Sept. 2, 1862, Nov. 26, 1863, April 1, 17–20, 1864.

Pocahontas........ Ark...... Aug 22, 1863.

Pocahontas........ Mo....... Feb 10, 1864.

Pocotaligo........ S. C...... May 29, Oct 22, 1862, Jan. 14–16, 1865.

Point Lick........ Ky....... Oct. 23, 1862.

Point Lookout........ Va........ May 13, 1864.

Point of Rocks........ Kan..... Jan. 20, 1865.

Point of Rocks........ Md....... Aug. 5, 1861, June 9, July 4, 1864.

Point Pleasant........ La........ June 25, 1864.

Point Pleasant........ W. Va... March 30, 1863.

Poison Springs........ Ark...... April 18, 1864.

Polk's Plantation........ Ark...... May 25, 1863

Pollocksville........ N. C..... April 14, 1862, Jan. 17, 1863.

Ponchatoula........ La........ Sept 14, 1862, March 24, May 13, 1863.

Pond Creek........ Ky....... May 16, 1864.

Pond Spring........ Ala...... Dec 29, 1864

Pontotoc........ Miss...... July 11, 1864.

Poole's Station........ Ga....... Dec 7–9, 1864.

Poolesville........ Md....... Sept 7, 1862

Pope's Campaign in Virginia........ Va........ Aug. 23–Sept. 1, 1862.

Poplar Springs Church........ Va........ Sept. 30, Oct 1, 1864.

Port Gibson........ Miss...... May 1, Dec. 26, 1863, July 7, 15, Oct. 1, 1864.

| Place | State | Date |
|---|---|---|
| Port Hudson | La | March 14, May 22–July 9, 1863. |
| Port Republic | Va | June 9, 1862. |
| Port Royal | S. C | Nov. 7, 1861, Jan. 1, 1862. |
| Port Walthall | Va | June 16, 17, 1864. |
| Potosi | Mo | Aug. 10, 1861. |
| Pound Gap | Ky | April 19, 1864. |
| Pound Gap, or Sounding Gap | Tenn | March 14, 1862. |
| Pound Gap Expedition | Tenn | July 6, 1863. |
| Powder River | Dak | Sept. 5–11, 1865. |
| Powder's Mill | Mo | Oct. 3, 1864 |
| Powder Springs | Ga | June 20, 1864. |
| Powder Springs Creek | Ga | Oct. 1–3, 1864. |
| Powell's River Bridge | Tenn | Feb. 22, 1864. |
| Powhatan | Va | Jan. 25, 1865. |
| Prairie Chapel | Mo | Sept. 4, 1862. |
| Prairie D'Ann | Ark | April 10–13, 1864. |
| Prairie Grove, or Fayetteville and Illinois Creek | Ark | Dec. 7, 1862. |
| Prairie Station | Miss | Feb. 21, 1863, Feb. 20, 1864. |
| Preble's Farm | Va | Sept. 30, Oct. 1, 1864. |
| Prentis | Miss | Sept. 20, 1862. |
| Prestonburg | Ky | Jan. 10, 1862. |
| Price's Invasion of Missouri | | Sept. 24–Oct. 28, 1864. |
| Prince's Place | Mo | Oct. 6, 1864. |
| Princeton | Ark | Dec 6, 8, 1863, April 29, Oct. 23, 1864 |
| Princeton | Ky | June 10, 1864. |
| Princeton | W. Va | May 15–18, 1862, May 6, 1864. |
| Pritchard's Mills, or Darnestown | Md | Sept. 15, 1861. |
| Proctor's Creek | Va | May 12–16, 1864. |
| Pueblo Colorado | N. Mex | Aug. 18, 1863. |
| Pulaski | Ala | July 15, 1863. |
| Pulaski | Tenn | May 4, 1862, May 13, Sept. 26, 27, Dec. 25, 1864. |
| Pumpkin Vine Creek | Ga | May 25 June 4, 1864. |
| Putnam | Mo | Sept. 1, 1862. |
| Putnam's Ferry | Mo | April 2, 1862. |
| Pyramid Lake | Nev | May 14, 1865. |
| Quaker Bridge, or Comfort | N. C | July 6, 1863. |
| Quaker Road | Va | March 29, 1865. |
| Qualltown, or Deep Creek | N. C | Feb. 5, 1864. |
| Quicksand Creek | Ky | April 6, 1864. |
| Quincy | Mo | Nov. 1, 1864. |
| Raccoon Ford | Ala | Oct. 30, 1864. |
| Raccoon Ford | Va | Sept. 14, 19, 1863, Nov. 26, 1863. |
| Raceland | La | June 22, 1862. |
| Raid—Rocky Mount | N. C | July 18–21, 1863. |
| Raid—Tar River | N. C | July 18–21, 1863. |
| Raid to Gordonsville | Va | Dec. 8–28, 1864. |
| Raleigh | N. C | April 7, 13, 1865. |
| Randolph County | Mo | May 8, 1864. |
| Rapidan | Va | Oct. 10, 17, 1863, Mar. 1, 1864. |
| Rapidan Station | Va | May 1, 1863. |
| Rappahannock Bridge | Va | Nov. 8, 1862, Oct. 24, 1863. |
| Rappahannock Crossing | Va | Oct 22, 1863. |
| Rappahannock Station | Va | Aug. 20–23, 1862, Aug. 1, 2, 1863, Nov. 7, 1863. |
| Rawle's Mills, or Little Creek | N. C | Nov. 3, 1862. |
| Raymond | Miss | May 12, 1863, Feb. 4, 1864. |
| Raytown | Mo | June 23, 1862. |
| Readyville | Tenn | Aug. 28, 1862, Sept. 7, 1864. |
| Ream's Station | Va | June 22, 29, Aug. 25, 1864. |
| Reconnoissance, Darbytown Road | Va | Oct. 13, 1864. |

| | | |
|---|---|---|
| Reconnoissance on Charles City Crossroads | Va | Oct. 1, 1864. |
| Reconnoissance on Corinth Road | Miss | April 8, 1862. |
| Reconnoissance to Boydton Road | Va | Oct. 8, 1864. |
| Reconnoissance to Hatcher's Run | Va | Dec. 8, 9, 1864. |
| Reconnoissance to Strasburg | Va | Oct 13, 1864. |
| Rector's Farm | Ark | Dec. 19, 1864. |
| Rectortown, or Five Points | Va | Jan. 1, 1864. |
| Red Bone | Miss | April 21, 1864. |
| Red Bone Church | Mo | Sept 25, 1863. |
| Red Clay | Ga | May 3, 1864. |
| Red Hill | Ala | Jan. 14, 1865. |
| Red House | W.Va | July 12, 1861. |
| Red Mound | Tenn | Dec. 30, 1862. |
| Red Oaks | Ga | Aug. 19, 20, 28, 1864. |
| Red River expedition | La | May —, 1864. |
| Redoubt before Yorktown | Va | April 26, 1862. |
| Redwood | Cal | Aug. 4, 1863. |
| Redwood | Minn | Aug. 18, 1862. |
| Redwood Creek | Cal | July 7, 1863. |
| Reed's Mountains | Ark | Dec. 5, 1862. |
| Reedy Creek | W. Va | May 13, 1862. |
| Renick | Mo | Nov. 1, 1861. |
| Rensey's Ferry | Mo | May 31, 1862. |
| Rerock | Ariz | March 24, 1865. |
| Resaca | Ga | May 13–16, Oct. 12, 1864. |
| Reynold's Plantation | Ga | Nov. 27–29, 1864. |
| Rhea's Mills | Ark | Nov 7, 1862. |
| Rheartown | Tenn | Oct. 11, 1863. |
| Richfield | Mo | May 19, 1863. |
| Richland | Ark | May 3, 1864. |
| Richland | Tenn | Oct 23, 1862, Sept. 26, 1864. |
| Richmond | Ky | Aug. 30, 1862, July 28, 1863. |
| Richmond | La | March 30, June 15, 1863. |
| Richmond | Miss | June 14, 1863. |
| Richmond | Va | Sept 29, 30, Oct. 28, 29, 1864, March 30–April 3, 1865. |
| Richmond and Petersburgh Railroad | Va | May 6, 7, 1864. |
| Rich Mountain | W. Va | July 11, 1861. |
| Rickett's Hill | Tenn | Aug. 6, Sept. 7, 1862. |
| Riddle's Shop | Va | June 13, 1864. |
| Rienzi | Miss | Aug. 19, 26, Sept. 9, 18, 1862. |
| Rincon de Mascaras | N. Mex | Dec. 11, 1863. |
| Ringgold | Ga | Sept. 11, Nov. 27, 1863. |
| Rio De Los Animos | N. Mex | July 19, 1863. |
| Rio Hondo | N. Mex | July 18, 1863. |
| Rio Verde | Ariz | Oct. 13, 1865. |
| Ripley | Miss | July 7, Dec. 1, 1863, June 7, 11, July 7, 1864. |
| Ripley | Tenn | Jan. 8, 1863. |
| River's Bridge | S. C | Feb. 3–9, 1865. |
| Roache's Plantation | Miss | March 31, 1864. |
| Roanoke | Mo | Sept. 6, 1862. |
| Roanoke Island | N. C | Feb. 8, 1862. |
| Roan's Tan-yard | Mo | Jan. 8, 1862. |
| Robertson's Run | Va | Oct. 10, 1863. |
| Robertson's Tavern | Va | Nov. 28, 1863. |
| Robinson's Mills | Miss | Oct. 17, 1863. |
| Rocheport | Mo | June 1, 18, 1863. |
| Rock Cañon | Nev | Feb. 15, 1866. |
| Rock Creek | Dak | July 1, 1865. |
| Rockford | Tenn | Nov. 14, 1863. |
| Rock House | W. Va | Feb. 12, 1864. |
| Rockingham | N. C | March 7, 1865. |
| Rockport | Ark | March 25, 1864. |
| Rockport | Mo | Sept. 23, 1864. |
| Rockville | Md | Sept. 22, 1863. |

| | | |
|---|---|---|
| Rocky Bluff | Mo | Aug. 7, 1862. |
| Rocky Creek Church | Ga | Dec. 2, 1864. |
| Rocky Crossing | Miss | June 20, 1863. |
| Rocky Face Ridge | Ga | Feb. 23–27, March 5–9, May 8–12, 1864. |
| Rocky Gap | Ky | June 9, 1863. |
| Rocky Gap | Va | Aug. 26, 1863. |
| Rodgersville | Tenn | Aug. 22, 1864. |
| Rodney | Miss | Dec. 17, 24, 1863, March 4, Aug. 1, 1864. |
| Rogersville | Ala | May 13, 1862. |
| Rsgersville | Tenn | Nov. 6, 1863. |
| Rolla | Mo | Aug. 1, Nov. 1, 1864. |
| Rolling Fork | Miss | Nov. 22, 1864. |
| Rolling Prairie | Ark | Jan. 23, Feb. 4, 1864 |
| Rome | Ga | May 17, 18, Oct. 13, 1864. |
| Rome Crossroads | Ga | May 16, 1864. |
| Romney, or Hanging Rock | W. Va | June 11, Sept. 23, Oct. 26, 1861. |
| Rood's Hill | Va | May 14, Nov. 22, 1864. |
| Rosecrans's campaign in Tennessee | | June 23–30, 1863. |
| Roseville | Ark | Nov. 12, 1863, March 29, April 4, 5, 15, 1864. |
| Roseville Creek | Ark | March 20, 1864. |
| Ross Landing | Ark | Feb. 14, 1864. |
| Round Away Bayou | La | March 30, 1863. |
| Round Hill | Ark | July 7, 1862. |
| Round Hill | Tenn | Aug. 28, 1862. |
| Rousseau's campaign in Tennessee | | June 23–30, 1863. |
| Rousseau's pursuit of Wheeler in Tennessee | | Sept. 1–8, 1864. |
| Rousseau's raid in Alabama and Georgia | | July 11–22, 1864. |
| Rover | Tenn | Jan. 31, June 23, 1863. |
| Rowanty Creek | Va | Feb. 5, 7, 1865. |
| Rowlett's Station, or Munfordsville and Woodsonville | Ky | Dec. 17, 1861. |
| Ruckersville | Miss | Oct. 6, 1862. |
| Rural Hills | Tenn | Nov. 18, 1862. |
| Rush Creek | I. T | Feb. 9, 1865. |
| Russell's House | Miss | May 17, 1862. |
| Russellville | Ky | July 29, Sept. 30, 1862. |
| Russellville | Mo | Oct. 9, 1864. |
| Russellville | Tenn | July 1, 1862. |
| Rutherford's Creek | Tenn | March 10, 1863, Dec. 19, 1864. |
| | | |
| Sabine Crossroads, or Mansfield and Pleasant Grove | La | April 8, 1864. |
| Sabine Pass | La | Sept. 8, 1863. |
| Sacramento | Ky | Dec. 28, 1861. |
| Sacramento Mountains | N. Mex | Aug. 25, 1864, July 1, 1865. |
| Sage Creek | D. T | April 21, 1865. |
| Sailor's Creek, or Harper's Farm and Deatonsville | Va | April 6, 1865. |
| Salem, or Spring River | Ark | March 18, 1862. |
| Salem | Miss | Oct. 8, 1863, June 11, 1864. |
| Salem | Mo | Dec. 3, '61, July 6, Aug. 9, '62. |
| Salem | N. C | April 3, 1865. |
| Salem | Va | Nov. 5, 1862, June 21, 1864. |
| Salem Cemetery | Tenn | Dec. 18, 1862. |
| Salem Church | Va | June 2, 1864. |
| Salem Pike | Tenn | March 21, 1863. |
| Salem Heights | Va | May 3, 4, 1863. |
| Salin | I. T | Dec. 2, 1862. |
| Saline County | Mo | July 30, 1863. |
| Saline River | Ark | May 4, 1864, May —, 1865. |
| Salisbury | Tenn | Aug. 11, 1862, April 16, Dec. 3, 1873. |

Salkehatchie ......S. C......Feb. 9, 1865.
Salkehatchie River......S. C......Feb. 6, 1865.
Salt Lick......Va......Oct. 14, 1863.
Salt Springs......Ga......Oct. 1, 1864.
Saltville......Va......Oct. 2, Dec. 20, 1864.
Salyersville......Ky......Nov. 30, 1863.
Samaria Church......Va......June 15, 24, 1864.
Sam Jones surrendered......Fla......May 10, 1865.
San Andres Mountain......N. Mex..July 1, 1865.
San Carlos River......Cal......May 27, 1864.
Sand Creek......I. T......Dec. 9, 1864.
Sandersville, or Buffalo Creek......Ga......Nov. 26, 1864.
Sand Mountain......Ala......April 30, 1863, Jan. 27, 1865.
Sandy Swamp......N. C......Dec. 18, 1863.
Sangster's Station......Va......Dec. 15, 1863.
Santa Fe......Mo......July 24, 25, 1862.
Santa Rosa......Fla......Oct. 9, 1861.
Saratoga......Ky......Oct. 26, 1861.
Sartoria......Miss......June 4, 1863.
Sauk Centre......Minn......Sept. 10, 1862.
Saulsbury......Miss......July 2, 1864.
Saunders......Fla......May 19, 1864.
Savage's Station......Va......June 29, 1862.
Savannah......Ga......Dec. 10–21, 1864.
Savannah......Tenn......April 16, 1862.
Scarytown......W. Va....July 17, 1861.
Scatterville......Ark......July 10, Aug. 3, 1862.
Scottsborough......Ala......Jan. 8, 1865.
Scott's Farm......Ark......Feb. 12, 1864.
Scott's Ford......Mo......Oct. 14, 1863.
Scott's Mills Road......Tenn......Jan 27, 1864.
Scottsville......Ala......April 2, 3, 1865.
Scrougesville......Tenn......Nov. 27, 1862.
Scullyville......I. T......April 16, 1864.
Seabrook's Point......S. C......June 1, 1862.
Searcy......Ark......June 3, July 4, Sept. 6, 13, 1864.
Searcy Landing......Ark......May 19, 1862.
Secessionville......S. C......June 16, 1862, July 16, 1863.
Second assault on Fort Wagner......S. C......July 18, 1863.
Second assault on Port Hudson......La......June 14, 1863.
Second assault on Vicksburg......Miss......May 20, 1863.
Section 37, Nashville and N. W. R. R......Tenn......Nov. 24, 1864.
Sedalia......Mo......April 9, 1863, Oct. 15, 1864.
Selma......Ala......April 2, 1865.
Senatobia......Miss......May 25, 1863.
Seneca......Md......June 11, 1863.
Seneca Station......I. T......Sept. 14, 1863.
Seven days, includes Chickahominy, Peach Orchard, and Savage Station......Va......June 26–July 1, 1862.
Seven Pines......Va......May 31, June 1, 1862.
Shady Springs......W. Va...Aug. 28, 1862, July 14, 1863.
Shanghai......Mo......Sept. 27, Oct. 13, 1861.
Shannon Hill......Va......May 4, 1863.
Sharon......Miss......Feb. 27, 1864.
Sharpsburgh......Md......Sept. 17, 1862.
Shawnee Mound......Mo......Dec. 18, 1861.
Shawneetown......Kans......June 6, 1863.
Shelbina......Mo......Sept. 4, 1861.
Shelburne......Mo......Sept. 15, 1862.
Shelby Depot......Tenn......Oct. 23, 1862.
Shelbyville......Tenn......June 27, 1863.
Shelbyville Pike......Tenn......June 4, Oct. 7, 1863.
Shell's Mills......Ark......Oct. 16, 1862.
Shepherdstown......W. Va...Oct. 1, 1862, July 16, 1863, Aug. 25, 1864.

| | | |
|---|---|---|
| Shepherdsville | Ky | Sept. 21, 1862. |
| Sheridan's raid in Virginia | | May 9–13, 1864, Feb. 27–Mar. 25, 1865. |
| Sherwood | Mo | May 18, 1863. |
| Shiloh | Tenn | April 6, 7, 1862. |
| Ship's Gap | Ga | Oct. 16, 1864. |
| Shirley's Ford | Mo | Sept. 20, 1862. |
| Shoal Creek | Ala | Nov. 9, 1864. |
| Sibley's Landing | Mo | Oct. 6, 1862. |
| Siege of Atlanta | Ga | July 28–Sept. 2, 1864. |
| Siege of Knoxville | Tenn | Nov. 17–Dec. 4, 1863. |
| Siege of Mobile | Ala. | March 26–April 9, 1865. |
| Siege of Petersburg | Va | June 15, 1864–April 2, 1865. |
| Siege of Port Hudson | La | May 27–July 9, 1863. |
| Siege of Savannah | Ga | Dec. 10–21, 1864. |
| Siege of Suffolk | Va | April 12–May 4, 1863. |
| Siege of Vicksburg | Miss | May 18–July 4, 1863. |
| Siege of Yorktown | Va | April 5–May 3, 1862. |
| Silver Creek | Ala | Nov. 9, 1864. |
| Silver Creek | Ga | Oct. 13, 1864. |
| Silver Creek, or Roan's Tan-yard and Sugar Creek | Mo | Jan. 8, 1862. |
| Silver Lake | Fla | Feb. 20, 1864. |
| Silver Run | N. C | March 13, 1865. |
| Simmsport | La | May 18, Oct. 6, 1864. |
| Simpsonville | Ky | Jan. 25, 1865, |
| Sinking Creek | Va | Nov. 26, 1862. |
| Sinkpole Woods | Mo | March 23, 1862. |
| Sipsey Swamp | Ala | April 6, 1865. |
| Six-Mile Creek | Ala | March 31, 1865. |
| Six-Mile House | Va | Aug. 18–21, 1864. |
| Skeet, or Swan's Quarter | N. C | March 4, 1863. |
| Skull Valley. | A. T | May 26, 1865. |
| Slatersville, or New Kent C. H. | Va | May 9. 1862. |
| Slaughterville | Ky | Sept. 3, 1862. |
| Slaughter Mountain | Va | Aug. 9, 1862. |
| Smithfield | Ky | Jan. 5, 1865. |
| Smithfield | Va | Feb. 13, Sept. 15, 1863, Feb. 1, April 14, Aug. 25, 29, 30, 1864. |
| Smithsburg. | Md | July 4, 1863. |
| Smith's expedition from Tennessee to Miss | | July 5–18, 1864. |
| Smith's Farm | N. C | March 16, 1865. |
| Smith's raids from Tennessee to Mississippi | | Feb. 10–25, 1864. |
| Smith's Station | I. T | May 12, 1864. |
| Smithville | Ark | June 18, 1862. |
| Smoky Hill | Col | May 16, 1864. |
| Smoky Hill Crossing | Kans | Aug. 16, 1864. |
| Smyrna | Ga | July 2–5, 1864. |
| Snaggy Point | La | May 3, 1864. |
| Snake Creek Gap | Ga | May 8–10, Oct. 15, 1864. |
| Snia Hills | Mo | April 29, May 21, 1864. |
| Snicker's Gap | Va | Nov. 2, 1862, July 17, 1864. |
| Snicker's Gap Pike | Va | Aug. 19, 1864. |
| Snicker's Ferry | Va | July 18, 1864. |
| Snow Hill | Tenn | April 2, 3, 1863. |
| Snyder's Bluff | Miss | April 30, 1863. |
| Soldier's Grove | Cal | Sept. 26, 1864. |
| Solomon's Gap | Md | July 7, 1864. |
| Somerset | Ky | March 30, 1863. |
| Somerville | Tenn | Jan. 3, Mar. 29, 1863. |
| Somerville Heights. | Va | May 7, 1862. |
| Sounding Gap | Tenn | March 14, 1862. |
| South Anna | Va | June 26, 1863, March 15, 1865. |
| South Branch Edisto River | S. C | Feb. 9, 1865. |
| South Branch Watonwan | Minn | April 16, 1863. |

| Place | State | Date |
|---|---|---|
| South Fork | Fla | Feb. 9, 10, 1864. |
| South Mills | N. C | April 19, 1862. |
| South Mountain | Md | Sept. 14, 1862. |
| South Quay | Va | April 17, 1863. |
| South Quay Bridge | Va | May 1, 1863. |
| South Tunnel | Tenn | Oct. 10, 1864. |
| South Union | Ky | May 13, 1863. |
| Southwest Creek | N. C | Dec. 13, 1862. |
| Southwest Mountain | Va | Aug. 9, 1862. |
| Spanish Fork Cañon | Utah | April 15, 1863. |
| Spanish Fork | Ala | March 26–April 8, 1865. |
| Sparta | Tenn | Aug. 4, 1862, Aug. 9, Nov. 26, 1863. |
| Sperryville | Va | July 5, 1862. |
| Spoonville | Ark | April 2, 1864. |
| Sporting Hill | Pa | June 30, 1863. |
| Spottsylvania | Va | May 8–21, 1864. |
| Spottsylvania Court-House | Va | April 30, 1863. |
| Spring Creek | I. T | June 6, 1863. |
| Spring Creek | Mo | Aug. 23, 1862. |
| Springfield | Mo | Aug. 10, Oct. 5, 25, 1861, Feb. 13, 1862, Jan. 7, 8, Dec. 16, 1863. |
| Springfield | W. Va | Feb. 3, 1864. |
| Springfield Landing | La | July 2, 1863. |
| Spring Hill | Mo | Oct. 27, 1861. |
| Spring Hill | Tenn | March 4, 5, 1863, Nov. 29, 1864. |
| Spring River | Ark | March 18, 1862, Feb. 9, 1864. |
| Spring River | Mo | Sept. 1, 1862, Feb. 19, 1863. |
| Stahel's reconnoissance in Virginia | | Nov. 30, 1862. |
| Standardsville | Va | March 1, 1864. |
| Stanford, or Lancaster | Ky | Oct. 14, 1862. |
| State Creek | Ky | June 11, 1863. |
| Statesboro | Ga | Dec. 4, 1864. |
| St. Augustine | Fla | Dec. 30, 1863. |
| Staunton Bridge | Va | June 24, 1864. |
| Staunton Road | Va | June 1, 2, 1862. |
| St Catherine's Creek | Miss | July 28, 1863. |
| St. Charles | Ark | June 17, 1862, June 25, 29, '64. |
| Steamer Clara Bell | Miss | July 24, 1864. |
| Sterling's Farm | La | Sept. 12, 29, 1863. |
| Stevensburgh | Va | Nov. 7, 1863. |
| Steven's Gap | Ga. | Sept. 11, 1863. |
| Stevenson | Ala | Aug. 31, 1862. |
| Stevenson's Depot | Va | July 20, 1864. |
| Stewart's Creek | Tenn | Dec. 29, 1862, Jan. 1, 1863. |
| St. Francis County | Mo | April 8, 1863. |
| St. Francis River | Mo | April 30, May 1, 1863. |
| St. George's Creek | Ohio | July 19, 1863. |
| St. John's River | S. C | May 23, 1864. |
| St. Louis, streets of | Mo | May 10, 1861. |
| St. Mary's River | Fla | Feb. 9, 10, 1864. |
| St. Mary's Trestle | Fla | July 26, 1864. |
| Stockade at Stone River | Tenn | Oct 5, 1863. |
| Stockton | Mo | Aug. 9, 1862. |
| Stoneman's raid in Virginia | | April 27, May 8, 1863. |
| Stoneman's raid to Macon | Ga | July 26–31, 1864. |
| Stoneman's raid from Tennessee to Virginia | | Dec. 12–21, 1864. |
| Stoneman's raid in Va. and N. C | | March 20, April 6, 1865. |
| Stone River, or Murfreesborough | Tenn | Dec. 31, 1862, to Jan. 3, 1863. |
| Stone's Farm | Ark | April 5, 1864. |
| Stone's Ferry | Ala | July 5, 1864. |
| Stony Creek | Va | June 28, 1864. |
| Stony Creek Station | Va. | May 7, Oct. 11, Dec. 1, 1864. |
| Stony Lake | Dak | July 28, 1863. |
| Stony Point | Ark | May 20, 1864. |

Strasburgh .......... Va....... Mar. 27, June 1, 2, 1862, Oct. 9, 1864.
Strasburgh Road .......... Va ....... Feb. 26, April 23, 1863.
Strawberry Plains .......... Tenn..... Jan. 10, 1864.
Strawberry Plains .......... Va ........ Aug. 14–18, 1864.
Streight's raid from Alabama to Georgia .......... April 27, May 3, 1863.
St. Stephen's .......... S. C...... March 1, 1865.
Stuumptown .......... Mo ....... Aug. 2, 1863.
Sturgeon .......... Mo ....... Sept. 22, 1862.
St. Vrain's Old Fort .......... N. Mex. Nov. 25, 1864.
Suffolk. (See also siege of) .......... Va ....... Dec. 28, 1862, April, 4, May 15, 16, 1863, March 9, 1864.
Sugar Creek .......... Ark ...... Oct. 17, 1862.
Sugar Creek .......... Mo ....... Jan. 8, Feb. 17, 18, 1862.
Sugar Creek .......... Tenn.... Oct. 9, 1863, Dec. 25, 26, 1864.
Sugar-Loaf Battery .......... N. C..... Feb. 11, 1865.
Sugar-Loaf Hill .......... N. C..... Jan. 9, 1865.
Sugar-Loaf Mountain .......... Md ....... Sept. 10, 1862.
Sugar Valley .......... Ga ....... May 13–16, 1864.
Sulphur Branch Trestle .......... Ala ..... Sept. 25, 1864.
Sulphur Springs .......... Ala ...... Jan. 25, 1864.
Sulphur Springs .......... Va ....... Aug. 25, 1862.
Sulphur Springs Bridge .......... Va ....... Aug. 11, 1864.
Summerville .......... Miss ..... Nov. 26, 1862.
Summerville .......... Tenn .... Dec. 24, 25, 1863.
Summerville .......... Va ....... Feb. 9, 1863.
Summerville .......... W. Va... Aug. 26, 1861.
Summit Point .......... Va ....... Aug. 21, 1864.
Sumterville .......... S. C...... March 23, April 9, 1865.
Sunnyside Landing .......... Ark ...... June 7, 1864.
Supply Train .......... Tenn..... Oct. 23, 1863.
Sutton .......... Va ....... Sept 22, 1863.
Suwano Gap .......... N. C..... April 23, 1865.
Swallow's Bluff .......... Tenn .... Sept. 30, 1863.
Swan Lake .......... Ark ...... April 23, 1864.
Swan's Quarter .......... N. C ..... March 4, 1863.
Sweetwater .......... Ga ....... Oct. 1–3, 1864.
Sweetwater .......... Tenn..... Oct. 24, 1863.
Swift Creek .......... S. C...... April 19, 1865.
Swift Creek, or Arrowfield Church .......... Va ....... May 8–10, 1864.
Swift Creek Bridge .......... N. C...... June 27, 1862.
Switzer's Mill .......... Mo ....... Aug. 10, 1862.
Sycamore Church .......... Va ....... Aug. 3, 1862, Sept. 16, 1864.
Sykestown .......... Mo ....... March 1, 1862.
Sylamore .......... Ark ...... May 28, 29, 1862.
Sylvan Grove .......... Ga ....... Nov. 26, 1864.
Syracuse .......... Mo ....... Oct. 14, 1863.

Taberville .......... Ark ...... Aug. 11, 1862.
Taberville .......... Mo ....... Aug. 2, 1862.
Table Mountain .......... Nev ...... May 20, 1865.
Tabourville .......... Ark ...... July 20, 1862.
Tah-kah-o-kuty .......... Dak...... July 28, 1864.
Tahlequah .......... I. T...... March 30, 1863.
Talbot's Ferry .......... Ark ...... April 19, 1862.
Talbot's Station .......... Tenn .... Dec. 29, 1863.
Tallahatchie .......... Fla....... June 18, 1862.
Tallahatchie River .......... Miss ..... Aug. 7–9, 1864.
Talladega .......... Ala....... April 22, 1865.
Tanner's Bridge .......... Ga ....... May 15, 1864.
Taylor's Bridge .......... Va ....... May 25–27, 1864.
Taylor's Ford .......... Tenn .... Nov. 10, 1861.
Taylor's Hole Creek .......... March 15, 1865.
Taylor's Ridge .......... Ga ....... Nov. 27, 1863.
Taylor surrendered .......... May 4, 1865.
Taylorsville .......... Ky ....... April 18, 1865.

| | | |
|---|---|---|
| Taylorsville | Va | Feb. 29, 1864. |
| Tazewell | Tenn | Aug. 6, 1862, Jan 24, 1864. |
| Tebb's Bend | Ky | July 4, 1863. |
| Ten Islands, or Jackson's Ford | Ala | July 14, 1864 |
| Ten miles from Columbus | Ky | Jan. 18, 1865. |
| Terre Noir Creek | Ark | April 2, 1864. |
| Terrisville | Tenn | Jan. 14, 1864. |
| Texas County | Mo | Sept. 12, 1863. |
| The Cedars | Tenn | Dec. 5–8, 1864. |
| The Island | Mo | March 30, 1863. |
| The Orchards | Va | June 25, 1862. |
| Thibodeauxville | La | Oct 27, 1862. |
| Thomas Place | Cal | June 28, 1864. |
| Thomas Ranche | Cal | Nov. 12, 1863. |
| Thomas Station | Ga | Nov. 27–29, Dec. 3, 1864. |
| Thompson Cove | Tenn | Oct 3, 1863. |
| Thompson's Station, or Spring Hill and Unionville | Tenn | March 4, 5, 1863. |
| Thornburg | Va | Aug. 6, 1862. |
| Thorn Hill | Ala | Jan. 3, 1865. |
| Thoroughfare Gap | Va | April 2, Oct. 17, Nov. 5, 1862. |
| Tickfaw River | Miss | May 1, 1863. |
| Tillafinny River | S. C | Dec. 6–9, 1864. |
| Tilton | Ga | Oct. 13, 1864. |
| Tilton | Tenn | May 13, 1864. |
| Timber Hill | I. T | Nov. 19, 1864. |
| Tobbert's Ferry | Ark | March 20, 1865. |
| Tobosofkee | Ga | April 20, 1865. |
| Todd's Tavern | Va | May 8, 1864. |
| Tolopotomy | Va | May 28–31, 1864. |
| Tompkinsville | Ky | July 9, 1862, April 23, 1863. |
| Tom's Brook, or Fisher's Hill, Strasburgh, and Woodstock | Va | Oct. 9, 1864. |
| Tongue River | Dak | Aug. 29, 1865. |
| Toon's Station | Tenn | Aug. 31, 1862. |
| Torpedo explosion | N C | May 26, 1864. |
| Town Creek | Ala | April 27, 28, 1863. |
| Town Creek | N C | Feb 20, 1865. |
| Township | Fla | Jan. 26, 1863. |
| Tracy City | Tenn | Jan. 20, 1864. |
| Training Post | Ark | Oct 24, 1864. |
| Tranter's Creek | N. C | June 5, 1862. |
| Treadwell's Plantation | Miss | Oct. 20, 1863 |
| Trenches, front of Petersburg | Va | June 20–Dec. 31, 1864. |
| Trenton | Ark | Oct. 14, 1862. |
| Trenton | N. C | Dec. 12, 1862. |
| Trenton | Tenn | Aug. 7, Dec. 20, 1862. |
| Trenton Bridge | N. C | May 14, 1862. |
| Trevillian Station | Va | June 11, 12, 1864. |
| Trinity | Ala | July 24, 1862. |
| Trinity River | Cal | Nov. 13, 1863. |
| Trion | Ala | April 1, 1865. |
| Triplet's Bridge | Ky | June 16, 1863. |
| Triune | Tenn | June 9, 1863. |
| Try Mountain | Ky | Nov. 9, 1861. |
| Tule Rosa Valley | Cal | Feb. 26, 1863. |
| Tulip | Ark | Oct 10, 1863. |
| Tullahoma | Tenn | July 1, 1863. |
| Tunnel Hill | Ga | Jan. 28, Feb. 25–27, May 7, 1864. |
| Tunnel Hill | Miss | Feb. 13, 1864. |
| Tunnel Mountain | Miss | Feb. 7, 1864. |
| Tunstall Station | Va | June 14, 1862, May 4, 1863, March 3, 1864. |
| Tupelo | Miss | May 6, 1863, July 13–15, 25, 1864. |

| | | |
|---|---|---|
| Turkey Bend | Va | June 30, 1862. |
| Turkey Island Bridge | Va | July 20, 1862. |
| Turman's Ferry | Ky | Jan. 9, 1864. |
| Turnback Creek | Mo | April 26, 1862. |
| Turner's Gap | Md | Sept. 14, 1862. |
| Tuscahoma | Miss | May 15, 1863. |
| Tuscaloosa | Ala | April 4, 1865. |
| Tuscumbia | Ala | Feb. 22, April 24, Oct. 24–27, 1863. |
| Tuscumbia | Miss | May 30, 1862. |
| Tuscumbia Creek | Miss | May 30, Oct. 5, 1862. |
| Tuscumbia River | Ala | Oct. 5, 1862. |
| Twelve miles from Yazoo City | Miss | Dec. 1, 1864. |
| Two Hills | Dak | Aug. 8, 1864. |
| Tyree Springs | Tenn | Nov. 7, 8, 1862. |
| | | |
| Union | Miss | Feb. 21, 22, 1864. |
| Union | Va | Nov. 3, 1862. |
| Union Church | Miss | April 28, 1863. |
| Union Church | Va | June 8, 1862. |
| Union City | Ky | March 24, 1864. |
| Union City | Tenn | March 30, 1862, July 10, Nov. 19, 1863. |
| Union Mills | Mo | Aug. 20, 1862. |
| Union Station | Tenn | Nov. 1–4, 1864. |
| Unionville | Tenn | March 4, 5, 1863. |
| University Place | Tenn | July 4, 1863. |
| Upper Missouri River | Ark | Oct. 10, 1862. |
| Upperville | Va | Nov. 3, 1862, June 21, Sept. 25, 1863. |
| Upton Hill | Va | Oct. 12, 1861. |
| Utoy Creek | Ga | Aug. 5, 6, 1864. |
| | | |
| Vache Grass | Ark | Sept. 26, 1864. |
| Valley Station | Colo | Jan. 15, 1865. |
| Valverde, or Fort Craig | N. Mex. | Feb. 21, 1862. |
| Van Buren | Ark | Dec 21, 28, 1862, Aug. 12, 1864 |
| Van Buren County | Ark | March 25, 1864. |
| Vance's Store | Ark | Oct. 2, 1863. |
| Van Wert | Ga | Oct. 10, 1864. |
| Varnell's Station | Ga | May 7, 9, 1864. |
| Vaughan Road | Va | Feb. 5–7, 1865. |
| Vaughan | Miss | May 12, 1864. |
| Vaught's Hill | Tenn | March 20, 1863. |
| Vera Cruz | Ark | Nov. 3, 1864. |
| Vermilion Bayou | La | April 17, Oct. 10, Nov. 30, 1863. |
| Verona | Ind | July 12, 1863. |
| Verona | Miss | Dec. 25, 1864. |
| Vicksburg | Miss | May 18–July 4, Aug. 27, 1863, Feb. 13, July 4, 1864. |
| Vidalia | La | Sept. 14, 1863, Feb. 7, July 22, 1864. |
| Vienna | Va | June 17, Dec. 3, 1861, Sept. 2, 1862. |
| Village Creek | Ark | June 27, 1862. |
| Vincent's Crossroads, or Bay Springs | Miss | Oct. 26, 1863. |
| Vinegar Hill | S. C | Aug. 26, 1863. |
| Vining Station | Ga | July 2–5, 1864. |
| | | |
| Wachita Indian Agency | Tex | Feb. 10, 1863. |
| Waddell's Farm | Ark | June 12, 27, 1862. |
| Waldesburg | Mo | Dec. 24, 1861. |
| Waldron | Ark | Sept, 11, Oct. 6, Dec. 30, 1863, Feb. 1, 1864. |

| Place | State | Date |
|---|---|---|
| Walker's Ford | W. Va | Dec. 2, 1863. |
| Walkersvillle | Mo | April 2, 14, 1862. |
| Wallace's Ferry | Ark | July 26, 1864. |
| Wall Bridge | Va | May 5, 1864. |
| Wall Hill | Miss | Feb. 12, 1864. |
| Walnut Creek | Mo | Aug. 8, 1862. |
| Walnut Grove Church | Ga | June 24, 1863. |
| Walthal | Va | June 16, 1864. |
| Wapping Heights | Va | July 23, 1863. |
| Wardensville | Va | May 28, 1862. |
| Warm Springs | N. Mex. | June 20, 1863. |
| Warm Springs | N. C | Nov. 26, 1863. |
| Warm Springs | Tenn | Aug. 19, 1863. |
| Warrensburg | Mo | Oct. 18, 1861, March 26, 28, April 8, June 17, 1862, May 28, 1864. |
| Warrenton Junction | Va | Sept. 26. 1862, May 3, 14, 1863. |
| Warrenton Springs | Va | Oct. 12, 13, 1863. |
| Warsaw | Mo | Oct. 16, 1861, April 8, 17, 28, 1862, Oct. 8, 1863. |
| Warsaw | N. C. | April 6, 1865. |
| Wartrace | Tenn | Oct. 5, 1863. |
| Washington | N. C. | Sept. 6, 1862, March 30–April 4, Nov. 1, 1863. |
| Waterford | Miss | Nov. 29, 30, 1862, Aug. 16, 17, 1864. |
| Waterford | Va | Aug. 7, 1863. |
| Waterloo | La | Oct. 20, 1864. |
| Waterloo Bridge | Va | Aug. 23, 1862. |
| Water Proof | La | Nov. 21, 1863, Feb. 14, 15, April 20, 1864. |
| Water Valley | Miss | Dec. 4, 1862. |
| Waugh's Farm | Ark | Feb. 19, 1864. |
| Wauhatchie | Tenn | Oct. 27, 1863. |
| Wautauga Bridge | Tenn | December 30, 1862, April 25, 26, 1864. |
| Waverly | Tenn | Oct. 23. 1862, April 10, 1863. |
| Wayne County | Mo | April 26, 1864. |
| Wayne Court-House | W. Va | April 26, 27, 1861. |
| Waynesboro' | Ga | Nov. 27–29, Dec. 4,-1864. |
| Waynesboro' | Va | Sept. 28, Oct. 2, 1864, March 2, 1865. |
| Waynesville | Mo | Aug. 25, 1863. |
| Weaver's Store | Ky | April 28, 1863. |
| Webber's Falls | I. T | April 11, 26, Sept. 9, Oct. 12, 1863. |
| Welaka | Fla | May 19, 1864. |
| Weldon Railroad | Va | June 22, 23, Aug. 18, 22, 1864. |
| Weldon Railroad Expedition | Va | Dec. 7–11, 1864. |
| Wellington | Mo | July 8, 1864. |
| Wentzville | Mo | July 15, 17, 1861. |
| West Branch | Va | April 14, 1863. |
| West Liberty | Ky | Oct. 23, 1861 |
| Westminster | Md | June 29, 1863. |
| Weston | W. Va | Aug. 31, 1862. |
| West Plains | Mo | Feb. 18, 1862. |
| West Point | Ark | Aug. 14, 1863, June 16, July 28, Aug. 5, 1864. |
| West Point | Ga | April 16, 1865. |
| West Point | Miss | Feb. 21, 1864. |
| West Point | Mo | Oct. —, 1861, Aug. 14, 1863, Oct. 26, 1864. |
| West Point | Va | May 7, 8, 1862. |
| West Point Railroad | Ga | July 18, 1864. |
| Westport | Mo | June 17, 1863, Oct. 23, 1864. |
| Westprairie | Mo | July 23, 1862. |

Wet Glaze, or Henrytown, Monday's Hollow, and Shanghai..........Mo.......Oct. 13, 1861.
Weyer's Cave..........Va.......Sept. 27, 1864.
Whiphy..........S. C......Feb. —, 1865.
Whistler's Station..........Ala......April 13, 1865.
White County..........Ark......Feb. 9, 1864.
White County..........Tenn.....Jan. 16, 1864.
Whitehall..........N. C......Dec. 16, 1862.
White House..........Va.......June 20, 1864.
White House Landing..........Va.......June 21, 1864.
Whitemarsh, or Wilmington Island..........Ga.......April 16, 1862.
White Mountains..........Dak......Nov. 25, 1862.
White-Oak Creek..........Ark......April 14, Aug. 11, 1864.
White-Oak Ridge..........Ky.......Aug. 19, 1862.
White-Oak Road..........Va.......March 31, 1865.
White-Oak Swamp, or Glendale, Charles City Crossroads, Nelson's Farm, Frazier's Farm, Turkey Bend, and New Market Crossroads..........Va.......June 30, 1862.
White-Oak Swamp Bridge..........Va.......Aug. 4, 1862, June 13, 1864.
White Post..........Va.......June 13, Aug. 11, Dec. 6, 1864.
White River..........Ark......May 6, 1862, April 26, 1863, June 22, 24, Oct. 22, 1864.
White River..........Mo......Aug. 4, 1862, April 17, 1863.
White River..........Dak......June 17, 1865.
White Sulphur Springs..........Va.......Nov. 15, 1862, Oct. 12, 13, 1863.
White's Bridge..........Va.......May 9, 1864
White's Ford..........Va.......Sept. 21, 1863.
Whiteside..........Fla.......July 27, 1864.
White Stone Hill..........Dak......Sept. 3–5, 1863.
White Water..........Mo.......April 24, 1863.
Whitlen's Mill..........Ark......Oct. 8, 1864.
Whittaker's Mills..........Va.......April 11, 1863.
Wier Bottom Church..........Va.......May 12–16, June 16, 1864.
Wild Cat..........Ky.......Oct. 21, 1861.
Wilderness..........Va.......May 5–7, 1864.
Wilcox's Bridge..........N. C......March 8–10, 1865.
Wiliston..........S. C......Feb 8, 1865.
William's Bridge..........La.......June 27, 1862.
Williamsburg..........Ky.......Oct. 28, 1862.
Williamsburg..........Va.......May 5, July 11, Sept. 9, 1862, Feb. 7, Mar. 29, 1863, Mar. 4, 1864.
Williamsburg Road..........Va.......June 18, 1862.
Williamsport..........Md.......Sept 20, 1862, July 6, 1863.
Williamsport..........Tenn.....Aug. 11, 1862.
Willicomack..........Va.......April 3, 1865.
Willis' Church..........Va.......June 29, 1862.
Willmarsh Island..........S. C......Feb 22, 1864.
Willow Creek..........Cal.......Nov. 17, 1863.
Wilmington..........N. C......Feb. 22, 1865
Wilmington Island..........Ga.......April 16, 1862.
Wilson's Creek..........Ky.......June 13, 1863.
Wilson's Creek, or Springfield and Oak Hills..Mo.......Aug. 10, 1861.
Wilson's Farm..........La.......April 7, 1864.
Wilson,s Landing..........Va.......June 11, 1864.
Wilson's raid on Weldon Railroad..........Va.......June 22–30, 1864.
Wilson's raid, Alabama to..........Ga.......March 22–April 24, 1865.
Wilson's Wharf Landing..........Va.......May 24. 1864.
Winchester..........Va.......March 23, May 25, 1862, May 19, June 13, 15, 1863, July 20, 24, Aug. 17, Sept. 19, 1864.
Wireman's Shoals..........Ky.......Dec. 4, 1862.
Wirt Court-House..........W. Va...Nov. 19, 1861.
Wittsburgh..........Ark......June 6, 1864.
Wolf Creek Bridge..........Miss.....Sept. 23, 1862.

| | | |
|---|---|---|
| Wolf River | Tenn | April 8, 1864. |
| Wolf River Bridge | Miss | Dec. 4, 1863. |
| Woodbury | Ky | Oct. 29, 1861. |
| Woodbury | Tenn | Jan. 24, April 2, 3, 1863. |
| Wood Creek | Mo | Jan 11, 1863. |
| Wood Lake | Minn | Sept. 23, 1862. |
| Woodsonville | Ky | Dec. 17, 1861. |
| Woodstock | Va | Sept 23, Oct. 9, 1864. |
| Woodville | Miss | Oct. 6, 1864. |
| Woodville | Tenn | Oct. 21, 1862. |
| Wormley's Gap | Va | Aug. 29, 1864. |
| Worthington | W. Va | Sept. 2, 1861. |
| Wright County | Mo | July 22, 1864. |
| Wyatts | Miss | Oct. 13, 1863, Feb. 5, 1864. |
| Wyerman's Mills | Tenn | Feb. 22, 1864 |
| Wyoming Court-House | W. Va | Aug. —, 1862. |
| Wytheville | Va | July 18, 1863, Dec. 16, 1864, April 3, 1865. |
| | | |
| Yate's Ford | Ky | Aug. 31, 1862. |
| Yazoo City | Miss | July 13, Sept. 27, Oct. 31, 1863, March 5, May 13, Dec. 1, 1864, March 15, 1865. |
| Yazoo City expedition | Miss | May 4–13, 1864. |
| Yazoo expedition | Miss | Feb. 28, 1864. |
| Yazoo Pass | Miss | Feb 16–20, 1863 |
| Yellow Bayou | La | May 10, 18, 19, 1864. |
| Yellow Medicine, or Wood Lake | Minn | Sept. 23, 1862. |
| Yellow Tavern | Va | May 11, Oct. 1–5, 1864. |
| Yellville | Ark | June 25, 1862, March —, 1863. |
| Yemasse | S. C | Oct. 22, 1862. |
| Yorktown | Va | April 5-May 4, 1862. |
| Young's Crossroads | N. C | July 26, 1862. |
| | | |
| Zollicoffer | Tenn | Sept. 24, 1863. |
| Zuni | Va | Dec. 12, 1862. |

## BATTLES PARTICIPATED IN BY THE NAVY.

| | | |
|---|---|---|
| Apalachicola River | Fla | Oct. 15, 1862. |
| Aquia Creek Batteries | Va | March 16, 1862. |
| Attempt to destroy rebel ram Arkansas | | July 15, 1862. |
| Bayou Teche | La | Nov. 3, 1862, Jan. 14, 1863. |
| Bombardment of Fort Sumter | S. C | April 7, 1863. |
| Burning of Royal Yacht | Texas | Nov. 7, 1861. |
| Bute La Rose | La | April 20, 1863. |
| Cape Fear River | N. C | Oct 11, 1862. |
| Capture of Atlanta | Ga | June 17, 1863. |
| Chuckatuck | Va | April 23, 1863. |
| Cobb's Point | N. C | Feb. 10, 1862. |
| Coggin's Point | Va | July 31, 1862. |
| Cypress Bend | Miss | June 22, 1863. |
| Destruction of two blockade-runners in Tampa Bay | | Oct. 17, 1863. |
| Dunn's Bayou | La | May 5, 1864. |
| Duvall's Bluff | Ark | Jan. 16, 1863. |
| Empress, United States Steamer | Miss | Aug. 10, 1864. |
| Expedition up Yazoo River | Miss | Feb 1–March 8, 1864. |
| Fort Anderson | N. C | Feb. 18, 1865. |
| Fort Darling | Va | May 15, 1862. |
| Fort De Russy | La | March 14, 1864. |
| Fort Fisher | N. C | Dec. 25, 1864, Jan. 13–15, 1865. |
| Fort Gaines | Ala | Aug. 2-23, 1864. |

Fort Heiman........................................Tenn.....Oct. 28, 1864.
Fort Macon........................................N. C.....April 25, 1862.
Fort McAlister........................................Ga........Feb. 1, March 3, 1863.
Fort Morgan........................................Ala......Aug 5–23, 1864.
Fort Pemberton........................................Miss......March 13–April 5, 1863.
Fort Pillow........................................Tenn.....April 14, May 10, June 4, 1862.
Fort Wright........................................Tenn.....June 4, 1862.
Forts Jackson and Saint Philip, and capture
of New Orleans........................................La........April 18–28, 1862.
Galveston........................................Texas...Jan. 1, 1863.
Gordon's Landing, Red River........................La........Feb. 14, 1863.
Hampton Roads........................................Va........March 9, 1862.
Harrisonburg........................................La........March 2, 1864.
Hatteras, and Alabama off........................Texas...Jan. 11, 1863.
Island No. 10........................................Tenn.....April 8, 1862.
James River........................................Va........May 6, June 21, 1864.
Judah, rebel ram, destroyed........................Fla.......Sept 14, 1861.
Kearsarge and Alabama, off Cherbourg......France..June 19, 1864.
Legarsville........................................S. C......Dec 25, 1863.
Little Rock Landing........................................Tenn.....April 24, 1863.
Loss of Housatonic, Charleston....................S. C......Feb. 17, 1864.
Matagorda Bay........................................Texas...Dec. 29, 30, 1863.
Mississippi River, below Vicksburg............Miss......Feb. 24, 1863.
Mosquito Inlet........................................Fla......March 21, 1862.
Night attack on Fort Sumter........................S. C......Sept. 8, 1863.
Off Charleston Bar........................................S. C......Jan. 31, 1863.
Pattersonville........................................La........March 28, 1863.
Pittsburg Landing........................................Tenn.....March 2, 1862.
Plymouth........................................N. C.....Oct. 31, 1864.
Port Hudson........................................La........March 14, 1863.
Ram Albemarle........................................N. C.....May 5, 1864.
Reconnoisance to Franklin, on Blackwater.Va........Oct 3, 1862.
Red River........................................La........April 26, 1864.
Running the Vicksburg batteries....................Miss......April 16, 1863.
Sabine Pass........................................La........Sept. 8, 1863.
Sabine Pass........................................Texas...April 18, 1863.
Siege of Port Hudson........................................La........May 27–July 9, 1863.
Siege of Vicksburg........................................Miss......May 18–July 4, 1863.
Vicksburg........................................Miss......June 26–29, 1862.
Yazoo City........................................Miss......July 13, 1863.

# LIST OF IMPORTANT BATTLES.

The following is a list of the important battles, taken from the *Official Chronological Summary of Engagements and Battles*, as compiled by the SURGEON-GENERAL, U. S. A., giving the number of killed, wounded, and missing, in both armies, Union troops engaged, with the names of the Generals killed and wounded:

ATLANTA, GEORGIA, (*Hood's 1st Sortie.*) July 22, 1864.
Union losses—Killed, 500; wounded, 2,141; missing, 1,000.
Confederate losses—Killed, 2,482; wounded, 4,000; missing, 2,017.
Union Troops engaged—15th, 16th, and 17th Corps, Army of the Tenn.; Maj.-Gen. McPherson, of the Military Div. of the Miss.
Maj.-Gen. J. B. McPherson, and Brig.-Gen. L. Greathouse, U. S. A., killed.

ANTIETAM, MD. September 16 and 17, 1862.
Union losses—Killed, 2,010; wounded, 9,416; missing, 1,043.
Confed. losses—Killed, 3,500; wounded, 16,399; missing, 6,000.
U. T. engaged—1st, 2d, 5th, 6th, 9th, and 12th Corps, Couch's Div. 4th Corps, and Pleasanton's Div. of Cav., Army of the Potomac.
Brig.-Gen. J. K. F. Mansfield, killed; Maj.-Gens. Richardson and Hooker, and Brigadier-Generals Rodman, Weber, Sedgwick, Hartsuff, Dana, and Meagher, U. S. A., wounded.
Brigadier-Generals L. O'B. Branch, G. B. Anderson, and W. E. Starke, killed; Maj.-Gen. R. H. Anderson, Brigadier-Generals Toombs, Lawton, Ripley, Rodes, Gregg, Armistead, and Ransom, C. S. A., wounded.

BENTONVILLE, N. C. March 19 to 21, 1865.
Union losses—Killed, 191; wounded, 1,168; missing, 287.
Confed. losses—Killed, 267; wounded, 1,200; missing, 1,625.
U. T. engaged—14th, 15th, 17th, and 20th Corps, and Kilpatrick's Cav. Div.

BRICE'S CROSSROADS, MISS. June 10, 1864.
Union losses—Killed, 223; wounded, 394; missing, 1,623.
Confed. losses—Killed, 131; wounded, 475; missing, ——.
U. T. engaged—4th Mo.; 2d N. J.; 19th Penn.; 7th and 9th Ill.; 7th Ind.; 3d and 4th Iowa, and 10th Kans. Cav; 9th Minn.; 81st, 95th, 108th, 113th, 114th, and 120th Ill.; 72d and 95th Ohio, and 93d Ind. Vols.; 1st Ill.; 6th Ind., and Co. E, 2d Ill. batteries; 59th and 55th U. S. C. T., and battery F, 2d U. S. C. Art.

BOYDTON AND WHITE-OAK ROADS, VA. March 31, 1865.
Union losses—Killed, 177; wounded, 1,134; missing, 556.
Confed. losses—Killed, —; wounded, 1,000; missing, 235.
U. T. engaged—2d and 5th Corps, Army of the Potomac.

BULL RUN, (1st,) VA. July 21, 1861.
Union losses—Killed, 481; wounded, 1,011; missing, 1,460.
Confed. losses—Killed, 269; wounded, 1,483; missing, —.
U. T. engaged—2d Me.; 2d N. H.; 2d Vt.; 1st, 4th, and 5th Mass.; 1st and 2d R. I.; 1st, 2d, and 3d Conn.; 8th, 11th, 12th, 13th, 16th, 18th, 27th, 29th, 31st, 32d, 35th, 38th, and 39th N. Y. Vols.; 2d, 8th, 14th, 69th, 71st, and 79th N. Y. Militia; 27th Pa. Vols; 1st, 2d, and 3d Mich.; 1st Minn.; 1st and 2d Ohio; 2d Wis. Vols; detachments of the 2d, 3d, and 8th U. S. I., and a battalion of Marines; of artillery—batteries D, E, G, and M, 2d Art; E, 3d Art.; D, 5th Art; and the 2d R. I. battery; of cavalry—detachments from the 1st and 2d Dragoons.
Among the killed were Brig.-Gens. B. E. Bee and Barton, C. S. A.

BULL RUN, (2d.) VA. August 28–30, 1862.
Union losses—Killed, 800; wounded, 4,000; missing, 3,000.
Confed. losses—Killed, 700; wounded 3,000; missing, —.

U. T. engaged—1st and 3d Corps, Army of Va.; Hooker's and Kearney's Divs. 3d and 5th Corps, and Reynolds' Div. 1st Corps, Army of the Potomac, and the 9th Corps.

Brig.-Gens. Tower and Schenck, U. S. V., wounded, and Field, Trimble, and Mahone, C. S. A., wounded.

CAMPAIGN IN NORTHERN GEORGIA, (*From Chattanooga to Atlanta.*) May 5 to September 8, 1864.

Union losses—Killed, 5,284; wounded, 26,129; missing, 5,786.
Confed. losses—Not known.
U. T. engaged—Armies of the Cumberland, Tennessee, and Ohio.

CEDAR CREEK, VA. October 19, 1864.

Union losses—Killed, 588; wounded, 3,516; missing, 1.891.
Confed. losses—Killed and wounded, 3 000; missing, 1,200.
U. T. engaged—6th and 8th Corps; 1st and 2d Divs. 19th Corps; 1st Div. Merritt's and 3d Div. Cust r's Cav. and Cav. of the Armies of the Potomac, West Virginia, and the Middle Military Division.

Brig-Gens. Bidwell and Thorburn, killed; Maj.-Gens Wright, Ricketts and Grover, and acting Brig-Gens. Kitchen. McKenzie, Penrose, Hamlin, Devens, Duval, and Lowell, U. S. A., wounded.

Maj-Gen. Ramseur, killed; and Maj-Gens. Battle and Connor, C. S. A., wounded.

CEDAR MOUNTAIN, VA. August 9, 1862.

Union losses—Killed, 450; wounded, 660; missing 290.
Confed. losses—Killed, 229; wounded, 1 047; missing, 31.
U. T. engaged—2d and 3d Corps, Army of the Potomac.
Brig.-Gens. Auger Carroll. and Geary, U. S. A., wounded.
Brig-Gen. C. S Winder, C. S. A., killed.

CHATTANOOGA, TENN. November 23 to 25, 1863.

Union losses—Killed, 757; wounded, 4,529; missing, 330.
Confed losses—Killed, 361; wounded. 2,181; missing. 6,142.
U. T engaged—4th and 14th Corps, Army of the Cumberland; 11th and one Division 12th Corps, and 15th Corps. Army of the Tennessee.
Brig.-Gens. J. M. Corse. G. A. Smith and Mathias, U. S A., wounded.

CHAMPION HILLS, MISS. May 16, 1863.

Union losses—Killed 426; wounded, 1.842; missing, 189.
Confed. losses—Killed and wounded. 2,500; missing, 1,800.
U. T. engaged—17th Corps and one Division 13th Corps.

CHANCELLORVILLE, VA. May 1 to 5, 1863.

Union losses—Killed, 1,512; wounded, 9,518; missing. 5.000.
Confed. losses—Killed. 1,581; wounded, 8,700; missing, 2,000.
U. T. engaged—1st, 2d, 3d, 5th. 6th, 11th, and 12th Corps, Army of the Potomac.

Maj.-Gen Hiram G Berry and Brig.-Gen. A. W. Whipple, killed; Brig.-Gens. Devan and Kirby U S. A, wounded

Brig.-Gen E. F. Paxton, killed; Lieut. Gen J. S. Jackson. Maj.-Gen. A. P. Hill, and Brig.-Gens. Hoke, Nichols, Ramseur, McGowan, Heth, and Pender, C. S. A., wounded.

CHICKAMAUGA, GA. September 19 to 23, 1863.

Union losses—Killed. 1,644; wounded, 9,262; missing. 4,945
Confed. losses—Killed, 2,389; wounded, 13,412; missing, 2,003.
U. T engaged—14th, 20th, 21st Corps, and Reserve Corps, Army of the Cumberland.

Brig.-Gen. W. H Lytle, killed; Brig.-Gens. Starkweather, Whittaker, and King. U. S A., wounded.

Brig.-Gens. Preston Smith Deshler, and B. H Helm killed; Maj.-Gen. J. B. Hood, and Brig.-Gens. Adams, Brown, Gregg. McNair. Bunn, Preston, Cleburne, Benning, and Clayton, C. S A., wounded.

COLD HARBOR, VA. June 1 to 12, 1864.

Union losses—Killed, 1,905; wounded, 10,570; missing. 2,456.
Confed. losses—Killed ——; wounded. 1,200; missing, 500.
U. T. engaged—2d, 5th, 6th, and 9th Corps, and Sheridan's Cavalry, Army of the Potomac, and 18th Corps, Army of the James.

Brig.-Gens. Brookes and Byrnes, killed; and Tyler, Stannard, and Johnson, U. S A., wounded.
Brig -Gens. G E. Doles and Keitt, killed; and Kirkland, Finnegan, Saw, and Lane, C. S. A., wounded.

CORINTH, MISS. October 3 and 4, 1862.
Union losses—Killed, 315; wounded, 1,812; missing, 232.
Confed. losses—Killed, 2,017; wounded 7,854; missing, 4,350.
U. T. engaged—McKean's, Davies's, Hamilton's, and Stanley's Divisions, Army of the Mississippi.
Brig.-Gen. P A Hackleman, killed; Brig.-Gen. Oglesby, wounded.

DADNEY'S MILLS, HATCHER'S RUN, VA. February 5 to 7, 1865.
Union losses—Killed, 232; wounded, 1,062; missing, 186.
Confed. losses—Killed, wounded and missing, 1,200.
U. T. engaged—2d and 5th and 1st Division 6th Corps, and 2d Division Cavalry, Army of the Potomac.
Brig.-Gens. Morrow, Davis, Smythe, Gregg, Ayres, Sickel, and Gwynn, U. S. A., wounded.
Gen. Pegram, killed; and Brig.-Gen. Sorrell, C. S. A., wounded.

FALL OF PETERSBURG, VA. April 2, 1865.
Union losses—Killed, 296; wounded, 2,565; missing, 500.
Confed losses—Killed, —; wounded, —; missing, 3,000.
U. T. engaged—2d, 6th, and 9th Corps, Army of the Potomac; 24th Corps, Army of the James.
Maj -Gens. Grant and Potter, Brig.-Gens. Chamberlain, Dennison, Sickels, Madill, and McDougall, U. S A, wounded.
Lieut.-Gen D. H Hill, C. S. A., killed.

FIVE FORKS, VA. April 1, 1865.
Union losses—Killed, 124; wounded, 706; missing, 54.
Confed losses—Killed and wounded, 3,000; missing, 5 500.
U. T. engaged—5th Corps, Division of Cavalry, Army of the James, and Merritt's Cavalry Corps.
Brig.-Gen. Winthrop, U. S. A., killed.

FORT DARLING, DRURY'S BLUFF, VA. May 12 to 16, 1864.
Union losses—Killed, 422; wounded, 2,380; missing, 210.
Confed. losses—Killed. 400; wounded, 2,000; missing, 100.
U. T. engaged—10th and 18th Corps, Army of Va. and N C.

FORT DONELSON, TENN. Feb. 14 to 16, 1862.
Union losses—Killed, 446; wounded, 1,735; missing, 150
Confed. losses—Killed, 231; wounded, 1,007; missing, 13,829.
U. T engaged—17th and 25th Ky; 11th, 25th, 31st, and 44th Ind.; 2d, 7th, 12th. and 14th Iowa; 1st Neb.; 58th and 76th Ohio; 8th and 13th Mo.; 8th Wis.; 8th, 9th, 11th, 12th, 17th, 18th, 20th, 28th, 29th, 30th, 31st, 41st. 45th, 46th. 48th, 49th, 57th, and 58th Ill. Vols.; Batteries B and D. 1st, and D and E, 2d Ill. Art.; four companies Ill. Cav.; Birges' Sharpshooters, and six gunboats.

FORT STEVENS, (BRIGHTWOOD,) WASHINGTON, D. C. July 12, 1864.
Union losses—Killed, 54; wounded, 319; missing, —.
Confed. losses—Killed, wounded and missing, 500.
U. T. engaged—1st and 2d Divs. 6th Corps, 22d Corps, convalescents, marines, home guards, and citizens, commanded by Gen. Augur.

FRONT OF PETERSBURG, VA. July 1 to 31, 1864.
Union losses—Killed, 419; wounded, 2,076; missing, 1,200.
Confed. losses—Not given.
U. T. engaged—2d, 5th, and 9th Corps, Army of the Potomac; 10th and 18th Corps, Army of the James.

FRANKLIN, TENN. November 30, 1864.
Union losses—Killed, 189; wounded, 1,033; missing, 1,104.
Confed. losses—Killed, 1,750; wounded, 3,800; missing, 702.
U. T. engaged—4th Corps, Army of the Cumberland; 23d Corps, Army of the Ohio.
Maj.-Gens. Stanley and Bradley, U. S. A., wounded.

Maj.-Gen. Cleborne, Brig.-Gens. Adams, John Williams, Strahl, Geist, and Granberry, killed; Maj.-Gen. J. Bowen, Brig.-Gens. S. Carter, Manigault, Quarles, Cockerelle, and Scott, C. S. A., wounded.

FREDERICKSBURG, VA. December 13, 1862.
Union losses—Killed, 1,180; wounded, 9,028; missing, 2,145.
Confed. losses—Killed, 579; wounded, 3,870; missing, 127.
U. T. engaged—1st, 2d, 3d, 5th, 6th, and 9th Corps, Army of the Potomac.
Brig.-Gens. C. F. Jackson and G. D. Bayard, killed, and Gibson and Vinton, U. S A., wounded; Brig.-Gen. T. R. R. Cobb, killed, and Maxcy Gregg, C. S. A., wounded.

GETTYSBURG, PA. July 1 to 3, 1863.
Union losses—Killed, 2,834; wounded, 13,709; missing, 6,643.
Confed. losses—Killed, 3 500; wounded, 14.500; missing, 13 621.
U. T. engaged—1st, 2d 3d, 5th, 6th, 11th, and 12th Corps, and Cav. Corps, Army of the Potomac.
Maj-Gen. John F. Reynolds, Brig.-Gens. S H. Weed, Kosciusko, Zook, and Elon J Farnsworth, killed; Maj.-Gens D. E. Sickels and W S Hancock, and Brig.-Gens Paul, T. A. Rowley, J. Gibbons, and F. C. Barlow, U. S. A., wounded.
Maj-Gen Pender, Brig-Gens R. B. Gurnett, W. Barksdale, and Semmes, killed; Maj-Gens Hood, Trimble, and Heth, Brig.-Gens Kemper, Scales, G. T. Anderson, Hampton, J. M. Jones, Jenkins, Pettigrew, and Posey, C. S. A., wounded.

GROVETON AND GAINESVILLE, VA. August 28 and 29, 1862.
Union losses—Killed, wounded, and missing, 7,000.
Confed. losses—Killed, wounded, and missing, 7,000.
U. T. engaged—1st and 3d Corps, Army of Virginia; 9th Corps, Hooker's and Kearney's Divs of 3d, and Reynold's Div 1st Corps, Army of Potomac.
Maj.-Gen. Ewell and Brig-Gen. Taliaferro, C. S. A., wounded.

HARPER'S FERRY, VA. September 12 to 15, 1862.
Union losses—Killed, 80; wounded, 120; missing, 11,583.
Confed. losses—Killed and wounded, 500.

HATCHER'S RUN, SOUTH SIDE RAILROAD, VA. October 27, 1864.
Union losses—Killed, 156; wounded, 1,047; missing, 699.
Confed Losses—Killed, 200; wounded, 600; missing, 200.
U. T. engaged—5th and 9th Corps; 2d and 3d Div., 2d Corps, and 2d Cav. Div., Army of the Potomac.

JACKSON, MISS July 9 to 16, 1863.
Union losses—Killed, 100; wounded, 800; missing, 100.
Confed. losses—Killed, 71; wounded, 504; missing, 764.

KENESAW MOUNTAIN, GA. June 9 to 30, 1864.
Union losses—Killed, 1,370; wounded, 6,500; missing, 800.
Confed. losses—Killed and wounded, 1 100; missing, 3,500.
U. T. engaged—4th, 14th, and 20th Corps, Army of the Cumberland; 15th, 16th, and 17th Corps, Army of the Tenn.; 23d Corps, Army of the Ohio; Army of the Mil. Div. of the Miss
Brig.-Gen C. G. Harker, killed; and Brig.-Gen Daniel McCook, U. S A. dangerously wounded
Lieut-Gen. Polk, C S A, killed.

MINE EXPLOSION AT PETERSBURG, VA. July 30, 1864.
Union losses—Killed, 419; wounded, 1,679; missing, 1,910.
Confed. losses—Killed, 400; wounded, 600; missing, 200.
U. T engaged—9th Corps, supported by the 18th Corps, with the 2d and 5th Corps in reserve.

NEW MARKET, VA May 15, 1864.
Union losses—Killed, 120; wounded 560; missing, 240
Confed losses—Killed, 85; wounded, 320; missing. —

NEW MARKET HEIGHTS VA. September 28 to 30, 1864.
Union losses—Killed, 400; wounded, 2 029; missing —.
Confed. losses—Killed, wounded and missing, 2,000.
U T. engaged—10th and 18th Corps. and Kautz Cav. Brig., Army of James.
Gen. Burnham, killed, and Maj.-Gens Ord and Stannard, wounded.

NORTH ANN RIVER, VA. May 23 to 27, 1864.
Union losses—Killed, 223; wounded, 1,460; missing, 290.
Confed. losses.—Killed, —; wounded, 2,000; missing, —.
U. T. engaged—2d, 5th, and 9th Corps, Army of the Potomac.

OLUSTEE, FLA. February 20, 1864.
Union losses—Killed, 193; wounded, 1,175; missing, 460.
Confed. losses—Killed, 100; wounded, 400; missing, —.
U. T. engaged—47th, 48th, and 115th N. Y.; 7th Conn., 7th N. H., and 40th Mass. Vols.; 1st Mass. Cav.; 54th Mass., 1st N. C. and 8th U. S. Colored Troops; 1st and 3d U. S. and 3d R. I. Art.

PEACH TREE CREEK, GA. July 20, 1864.
Union losses—Killed, 300; wounded, 1,410; missing, —.
Confed. losses—Killed, 1,113; wounded, 2,500; missing, 1,183.
U. T. engaged—4th, 14th, and 20th Corps, Army of the Cumb.; Gen. G. H. Thomas, of the Army of the Mil. Div. of Miss, commanding
Brig.-Gens. W. S. Featherstone, A. L. Long, J. J. Pettis, and G. M. Stevens, C. S. A., killed.

PEA RIDGE, ARK. March 6 to 8, 1862.
Union losses—Killed, 203; wounded, 972; missing, 174.
Confed. losses—Killed, 1,100; wounded, 2,500; missing, 1,600.

PERRYVILLE, KY. October 8, 1862.
Union losses—Killed, 916; wounded, 2,943; missing, 489.
Confed. losses—Killed, 1,300; wounded, 3,000; missing, 200.
U. T. engaged—1st and 3d Corps, Army of the Ohio.
Brig.-Gens. J. S. Jackson and Wm R. Terrill, U. S. A., killed.
Brig.-Gens. Wood, Cleburne, and Brown, C. S. A., wounded.

PETERSBURG, VA. June 15 to 19, 1864.
Union losses—Killed, 1,298; wounded, 7,474; missing, 1,814
Confed. losses—Not known.
U. T. engaged—10th and 18th Corps, Army of the James; 2d, 5th, 6th, and 9th Corps, Army of the Potomac.

PETERSBURG, (Fall of) VA. April 2, 1865.
Union losses—Killed, 296; wounded, 2,565; missing, 500.
Confed. losses—Killed, —; wounded, —; missing, 3,000
U. T. engaged—2d, 6th, and 9th Corps, Army of the Potomac; 24th Corps, Army of the James.
Maj.-Gens. L. A. Grant and Potter, and Brig.-Gens. Sickels, Chamberlain, Dennison, Madill, and McDougall, U. S. A., wounded.
Lieut.-Gen. D. H. Hill, C. S. A., killed.

PLEASANT HILLS, LA. April 9, 1864.
Union losses—Killed, 100; wounded, 700; missing, 300.
Confed. losses.—Killed, 300; wounded, 1,200; missing, 500.
U. T. engaged—1st and 3d Div. 16th Corps; 1st Div. 19th Corps, and A. L. Lee's Cav. Div.

RESACA, GA. May 13 to 16, 1864.
Union losses—Killed, 600; wounded, 2,147; missing, —.
Confed. losses—Killed, 300; wounded, 1,500; missing, 1,000.
U. T. engaged—4th, 14th, 20th Corps, and Cav., Army of the Cumb.; 15th and 16th Corps, Army of the Tenn; 23d Corps, Army of the Ohio.
Maj.-Gen. Kilpatrick, commanding the 3d Cav. Div., U. S. A., wounded, and Brig.-Gen. B. G. Wadkins, C. S. A., killed.

RICHMOND, KY. Aug. 30, 1862.
Union losses—Killed, 200; wounded, 700; missing, 4,000.
Confed. losses—Killed, 250; wounded, 500; missing, —.
U. T. engaged—6th and 7th Ky. Cav., 95th Ohio, 18th Ky., 12th, 16th, 55th, 66th, 69th, and 71st Ind. Vols; and batteries D and G, Mich. Art.

SABINE CROSSROADS, LA. April 8, 1864.
Union losses—Killed, 200; wounded, 900; missing, 1,800.
Confed. losses—Killed, 300; wounded, 1,200; missing, —.
U. T. engaged—3d and 4th Div. 13th Corps; 1st Div. 19th Corps, and A. L. Lee's Cav. Div.; Army of the Gulf.
Maj.-Gen. Franklin, and Brig.-Gen. Ransom, U. S. A., wounded; Maj.-Gen. A. Mouton, and Brig.-Gen. M. M. Parsons, C. S. A., killed.

SAILOR'S CREEK, VA. April 6, 1865.

Union losses—Killed, 166; wounded, 1,014; missing, —.

Confed. losses—Killed and wounded, 1,000; missing, 6,000.

U. T. engaged—Cav. Corps, 2d and 6th Corps, Army of the Potomac.

SEVEN DAYS' RETREAT. June 26 to July 1, 1862.

Union losses—Killed 1,582; wounded, 7,709; missing, 5,958.

Confed. losses—Killed, 2,820; wounded, 14,011; missing, 752.

U. T. engaged—1st, 2d, 3d, 4th, 5th, 6th Corps, Stoneman's Cav. Corps, and Engineers, Army of the Potomac.

SEVEN PINES AND FAIR OAKS, VA. May 31 and June 1, 1862.

Union losses—Killed, 890; wounded, 3,627; missing, 1,222.

Confed. losses—Killed, 2,800; wounded, 3,897; missing, 1,300.

U. T. engaged—2d, 3d, and 4th Corps, Army of Potomac.

Brig.-Gens. Wessells, Nagle, and O. O. Howard, U. S. A., wounded, Gen. J. E. Johnson, (commanding,) and Brig.-Gen. R. E. Rhodes, wounded; Brig.-Gen. Robert Hatton, killed, and J. J. Pettigrew, C. S. A., captured.

SHILOH, TENN. April 6 and 7, 1862.

Union losses—Killed, 1,735; wounded, 7,882; missing, 3,956.

Confed. losses—Killed, 1,728; wounded. 8,012; missing, 959.

U. T. engaged—1st, 2d, 3d, 4th, 5th, and 6th Divs., Army of the Dist. of West Tenn.; 2d, 4th, and 5th Divs., and 21st Brig. of the 6th Div., Army of the Ohio; and gun-boats Tyler and Lexington.

Gens W. T. Sherman and W. H. L. Wallace, wounded; Gen. B. M. Prentiss, U. S. A., captured.

Maj.-Gen. A. S. Johnson, (Commander-in-chief,) and Brig.-Gen. A. H. Gladden, killed; Maj.-Gen. W. S. Cheatham, Brig.-Gens. C. Clark, B. R. Johnson, and J. S. Bowen, C. S. A., wounded.

SIEGE OF VICKSBURG, MISS. May 18 to July 4, 1863.

Union losses—Killed, 545; wounded, 3,688; missing, 303.

Confed losses—Killed, —; wounded, —; missing, 31,277.

U. T. engaged—13th, 15th, and 17th Corps, assisted by the navy on the Mississippi river; after the assault of the 16th Cops, the 2d Div. of the 9th Corps and a div. from the Dep't of the Mo. were added to the forces; on July, 4, 1863, the Confederates surrendered.

Brig.-Gen. Green, killed, and Brig.-Gen. Baldwin, C. S. A., wounded.

SIEGE OF PORT HUDSON, LA. May 27 to July 9, 1863.

Union lossses—Killed, 500; wounded, 2,500; missing, —.

Confed. losses—Killed, 100; wounded, 700; missing, 6,408.

U. T. engaged—Maj.-Gens. Weitzel's, Grover's, Paine's, Augur's and Dwight's Divs. of the 19th Corps; Maj.-Gen. Banks' Army of the Gulf, assisted by the navy. Confederates surrendered July 9, 1863.

Brig.-Gens. W. T. Sherman and H. E. Paine, U. S. A., wounded.

SIX-MILE HOUSE, WELDON RAILROAD, VA. August 18, 19, and 21, 1864.

Union losses—Killed, 212; wounded, 1,155; missing, 3,176.

Confed. losses—Killed, not known; wounded, 2,000; missing, 2,000.

U. T. engaged—Kautz's Cav. and the 2d Cav. Div., 5th and 9th Corps, Army of the Potomac.

Brig.-Gens. Saunders and Lamar killed; Gens. Claigman, Barton, Finnegan, and Anderson, C. S. A., wounded.

SPOTTSYLVANIA C. H., VA. May 8 to 21, 1864.

Union losses—Killed, 2,146; wounded, 7,956; missing, 2,577.

Confed. losses—Killed 1,000; wounded, 5,000; missing 3,000.

U. T. engaged—2d, 5th, 6th, and 9th Corps, and Cav. Corps, Army of the Potomac.

Maj.-Gen. J. Sedgwick, Brig.-Gens. J. C. Rice, J. J. Owens, and T. G. Stevenson, killed; Brig.-Gens. Robertson, Bartlett, Morris, and Baxter, U. S. A., wounded

Gens Daniels and Perrin, killed; Gens. Hayes and Walker, wounded; Brig.-Gen. G. H. Stewart and Maj -Gen. Ed. Johnson, C. S. A., captured.

STONE RIVER, TENN. December, 31, 1862, to January 3, 1863.

Union losses—Killed, 1,533; wounded, 7 245, missing, 2,800.

Confed. losses—Killed and wounded, 9,000; missing, 2,000.

U. T. engaged—McCook's Corps, right wing, Thomas' Corps, center, and Crittenden's Corps, left wing, Army of the Cumberland.

Brig.-Gen Sill, killed; Brig.-Gen. Kirk, U. S. A., wounded.
Brig.-Gens. Raines and Hanson, killed; Brig -Gens. Chalmers and Davis, C. S. A., wounded.

**Strawberry Plains** (Deep Bottom Run,) Va. August 14 to 18, 1864.
Union losses—Killed, 400; wounded, 1,755; missing, 1,400.
Confed. losses—Killed, not known; wounded, 1,000; missing, 100.
U. T. engaged—2d Cav. Div, 2d Corps, Army of the Potomac, and 10th Corps, Army of the James.
Gen. Chaplin, U. S. V., and Gen. Girard, C. S. A., killed.

**Turner's and Crampton's Gap, South Mountain, Md.** Sept. 14, 1862.
Union losses—Killed 443; wounded, 1,806; missing, 76.
Confed. losses—Killed, 500; wounded, 2,343; missing, 1,500.
U. T. engaged—1st, 6th, and 9th Corps, Army of the Potomac.
Maj -Gen. J. L. Reno. U. S. A., killed; Brig.-Gen. R. E. Garland, C. S. A., killed.

**Wauhatchie, Tenn.** October 27, 1863.
Union losses—Killed, 76; wounded, 339; missing, 22.
Confed. losses—Killed, 300; wounded, 1,200; missing, 100.
U. T. engaged—11th Corps and 2d Div. 12th Corps, Gen. Hooker commanding.

**Weldon Railroad, Va.**, (*Also known as Jerusalem Plank-Road.*) June 22 and 23, 1864.
Union losses—Killed, 604; wounded, 2,494; missing, 2,217.
Confed. losses—Killed, not known; wounded, 300; missing, 200.
U. T. engaged—2d and 6th Corps, and 1st Div. of the 5th Corps, Army of the Potomac.

**Wilderness, Va** May 5 to 7, 1864.
Union losses—Killed, 3,288; wounded, 9,278; missing, 6,784.
Confed. losses—Killed, 2,000; wounded, 6,000; missing, 3,400.
U. T. engaged—2d, 5th, 6th, and 9th Corps, and Cav. Corps, Army of the Potomac.
Brig.-Gens. James S. Wadsworth, Alex. Hays, and A. S. Webb, killed; and Brig.-Gens Getty and Carroll, U S. A., wounded.
Gens. J. M. Jones and Pickett, killed, and Gens. Longstreet, Pegram, Stafford, Hunter, and Jennings, C. S. A., wounded.

**Wilson's Creek, Mo.** August 10, 1861.
Union losses—Killed, 223; wounded, 721; missing, 291.
Confed. losses—Killed, 265; wounded, 800; missing, 30.
U. T. engaged—6th and 10th Mo Cav., and 2d Kans. Mounted Vols.; one Co. 1st U. S. Inf.; detachments 1st and 2d U. S. Inf'ty; 1st Iowa; 1st Kans.; 1st, 2d, 3d, and 5th Missouri Home Guards; 1st Mo., and Battery F, 2d U. S. Art.
Brig.-Gen. Nathaniel Lyon, U. S. A., killed.

# CHRONOLOGICAL RECORD OF THE REBELLION.

---

**1860.**

Nov. 9. An attempt to seize the arms in Fort Moultrie.

11. Senator Hammond, of S. C., resigned.

18. Georgia Legislature appropriated $1,000,000 to arm the State; Major Anderson sent to Fort Moultrie to relieve Col. Gardner.

Dec. 1. Great secession meeting in Memphis.

3. Congress met; President Buchanan denied the right of a State to secede.

10. Howell Cobb, Sec'y of the Treasury, resigned; Senator Clay, of Ala., resigned.

13. An extra session of the Cabinet was held to consider the question of re-inforcing Fort Moultrie; President Buchanan opposed it, and reinforcements were not sent.

14. Gen. Cass, Sec'y of State, resigned.

18. The Crittenden compromise introduced in the U. S. Senate.

20. South Carolina Convention adopted a secession ordinance by a unanimous vote.

24. South Carolina members of Congress resigned.

26. Maj. Anderson left Fort Moultrie and took possession of Fort Sumter.

27. The State troops of S. C. seized the Gov't property in Charleston and took possession of Castle Pinckney and Fort Moultrie.

29. John B. Floyd, Sec'y of War, resigned.

30. U. S. Arsenal at Charleston seized by State troops.

**1861.**

Jan. 2. Gov. Ellis, of N. C., took possession of Fort Macon.

3. Georgia State troops seized Fort Pulaski.

4. U. S. Arsenal at Mt Vernon, Ala., seized by State troops.

5. Forts Morgan and Gaines, Ala., seized by State troops.

6. U. S. Arsenal at Apalachicola, Fla., seized by State troops.

7. Fort Marion, Fla., seized by State troops.

8. Jacob Thompson, Sec'y of the Interior, resigned.

9. Steamer Star of the West, with supplies for Fort Sumter, fired on by Confederate batteries in Charleston harbor, and driven back; Fort Johnston, N. C., seized by the citizens of Smithville; Mississippi adopted the ordinance of secession.

10. Florida adopted the ordinance of secession; U. S. troops transferred from Fort Barrancas to Fort Pickens, Fla.; Fort Caswell, N. C., seized by the citizens of Smithville and Wilmington.

11. P. B. Thomas, Sec'y of the Treasury, resigned, and was succeeded by John A. Dix, of N. Y.; Governor of Louisiana seized Forts Philip, Jackson, Pike, and Macomb and the U. S. Arsenal at Baton Rouge; Governor of South Carolina demanded the surrender of Fort Sumter, which Major Anderson refused; Alabama adopted the ordinance of secession.

12. Florida State troops took possession of Pensacola Navy Yard and Forts Barrancas and McRee; surrender of Fort Pickens demanded.

13. Lieut. Slemmer, in command of Fort Pickens, refused to obey Commodore Armstrong's order to surrender the fort to the Florida troops.

16. Col. Hayne, of S. C., demanded of President Buchanan the surrender of Fort Sumter, which was refused.

18. Virginia appropriated $1,000,000 for the defense of the State.

20. Forts on Ship Island, Miss., seized by State troops.

21. Jefferson Davis resigned his seat in the U. S. Senate—Members of Congress from Ala. resigned.

23. Members of Congress from Ga. resigned.

24. The Confederates seized the U. S. arsenal at Augusta, Ga.

26. Oglethorpe barracks at Savannah, Ga., and Fort Jackson seized by State troops.

29. Kansas admitted into the Union.

**1861.**

Jan. 30. The N. C. legislature submitted the convention question to the people; this was the first instance of the will of the people being consulted in regard to the question of secession.

Feb. 1. Texas passed an ordinance of secession, to be submitted to the will of the people; La. seized the U. S. Mint and custom house at New Orleans.

4. Delegates from the seceded States met at Montgomery, Ala., to organize a Confederate Government; the Peace Congress met at Washington, D. C.; Ex-President Tyler being chosen president.

7. The Choctaw Nation declared its adherence to the Southern Confederacy.

8. U. S. arsenal at Little Rock, Ark., seized.

9. Jefferson Davis and A. H Stephens were elected Provisional President and Vice-President of the Confederate States.

16. U. S. arsenal and barracks at San Antonio, Tex., seized by Confederates.

18. Gen. Twiggs surrendered U. S Government property in Texas, valued at $1,200,000, to the Confederacy.

19. Gen. Twiggs superseded by Col. Waite, U. S. A; Fort Kearney, Kans., seized.

March 1. Gen. Twiggs expelled from U. S. Army; the Peace Congress adjourned; the Confederate Government assumed control of military affairs at Charleston, S. C.

3. Gen. Beauregard, C. S. A., took command of the troops at Charleston, S. C.

4. The ordinance of secession was passed by the Texas convention after having been submitted to the people.

11. Gen. Bragg assumed command of the Confederate forces in Florida.

22. Col. Wm. W. Loring, U. S. A., assumed command of the Department of New Mexico.

28. Vote of Louisiana on secession made public; 20,448 for, 17,926 against.

30. Miss. convention ratified Confederate constitution by a vote of 78 to 70.

April 3. South Carolina convention ratified the Confederate constitution by a vote of 114 to 16.

4. Virginia convention, by a vote of 89 to 45 refused to submit an ordinance of secession to the people.

7. All intercourse between Fort Sumter and Charleston, S. C. stopped by order of Gen. Beauregard, C. S. A.

8. The U. S. Government notified the South Carolina authorities that provisions would be sent to Maj. Anderson, at Fort Sumter, by force if necessary; the State Department refused to recognize the commissioners from the Confederate States.

11. United States troops were stationed at Washington, D. C.; the Confederate commissioners left Washington, D. C; Gen. Beauregard demanded the surrender of Fort Sumter, Maj. Anderson refused.

12. Bombardment of Fort Sumter—Fort Moultrie opened fire at 4 o'clock a. m., Fort Sumter did not reply until 7 o'clock; Maj. Anderson had under his command 111 men, including officers, musicians, and laborers.

13. The bombardment continued; by noon most of the wood work was on fire; Gen. Wigfall came with a flag of truce, and arrangements were made for evacuating the fort; the terms were that the garrison should take all its individual and company property; that they should march out with their side arms in their own way, at their own time, and that they should salute their flag, and take it with them; Daniel Hough, private Bat. E, 1st U. S. Art., was killed by the premature explosion of a cannon while saluting the Union flag on Fort Sumter at the evacuation; he was buried on the 15th, with all the honors of war, by order of Gen. Beauregard, C. S A.; he was the first soldier killed in the war; Col. Harvey Brown, 2d U. S. Art., assumed command of the Department of Florida.

14. Maj. Anderson and his men sailed for New York.

15. President Lincoln issued a proclamation commanding all persons in arms against the Government to disperse within twenty days, and also called for 75,000 troops; President Lincoln called an extra session of congress to meet July 4th; the governor of North Carolina refused to furnish the quota of militia to the United States; Fort Macon, N. C., seized by State troops.

**1861.**

Apr. 16. The Confederate Government called for 32.000 men; the Governors of Ky., Va., Tenn. and Mo. refused to furnish troops under President Lincoln's proclamation.

17. Virginia convention adopted the ordinance of secession to be submitted to the people; Jefferson Davis issued a proclamation offering letters of marque and reprisal to all who wished to engage in privateering.

18. U. S arsenal at Harper's Ferry, Va., destroyed by Lieut. Jones to prevent it falling into the hands of the Confederates; Col. Cake with 400 men of the 25th Pa. Vols. arrived in Washington, D. C.—the first volunteer troops to enter the city for its defense.

19. The 6th Mass. Vols. was attacked by a mob while passing through Baltimore, Md, and three soldiers were killed; the soldiers fired on the mob, killing 11 and wounding many; Maj-Gen. Robert Patterson, Pa. militia, was assigned to command of the States of Del., Md., Pa., and D C.; Philadelphia appropriated $1,000,000 to equip volunteers and support their families.

20. Several bridges on the Northern Pennsylvania R R. destroyed by Maryland Confederates to prevent the passage of troops to Washington; the 4th Mass. arrived at Fortress Monroe, Va; the Gosport navy yard destroyed, and several war vessels scuttled by Gen. McCauley to prevent them falling into the hands of the Confederates; the Cumberland was towed out; Gen. Butler's command arrived at Annapolis, Md; U. S. arsenal at Liberty, Mo, seized by Confederates.

21. The Government took possession of the Philadelphia and Baltimore R. R.; Senator Andrew Johnson, of Tenn., mobbed at Lynchburg, Va.; Col. Van Dorn, C. S. A., assumed command in Texas

22. U. S. arsenal at Fayetteville, N. C., seized by State troops; Governor of Ark. refused to furnish quota of militia to U. S.

23. Fort Smith, Ark., seized by Confederates; Maj.-Gen. R. E. Lee assigned to command of the State military and naval forces in Va.; U. S. officers at San Antonio, Tex., seized by Confederates as prisoners of war.

25. Maj. Sibley surrendered 420 U. S. troops to Col. Van Dorn, C. S. A, at Saluria, Texas; Gov. Letcher proclaimed Virginia a member of the Southern Confederacy.

26. Maj.-Gen. Jos. E. Johnston assigned to command of Virginia State forces in and about Richmond.

27. All officers of the U. S. Army were required to take the oath of allegiance to the U. S; Brig.-Gen. B. F. Butler, Mass. militia, assigned to command of department of Annapolis; Col. K. F. Mansfield, U. S A., assigned to command of department of Washington.

29. Maryland House of Delegates rejected the ordinance of secession by a vote of 63 to 13.

May 1–3. Gov. Letcher, of Va, called for volunteers for the Confederate Army.

3. President Lincoln called for 42,000 three-years' vols., 22,000 for the regular army, and 18,000 seamen; fourteen companies of Ky. Vols. offered their services to the U S. Secretary of War, notwithstanding the Governor's refusal; Connecticut Legislature appropriated $2.000.000 for military purposes.

4. U. S. ordnance stores seized at Kansas City, Mo.

5. Gen. Butler took possession of the Relay House, Md.; Alexandria, Va., abandoned by Confederates.

6. Confederate capital removed to Richmond, Va; ordinance of secession adopted by Arkansas and Tennessee.

7. Route between Philadelphia, Harrisburgh, and Washington, via Baltimore, re-established.

10. A Confederate force of 800 men surrendered to Capt. (afterward Gen.) Lyon at St. Louis.

11. Riot at St. Louis, Mo; blockade of Charleston, S. C, established by Steamer Niagara.

13. Gen. Geo. B. McClellan, U. S. A, assumed command of department of the Ohio; Baltimore, Md., occupied by U. S. troops.

14. A vessel loaded with arms for the Confederate States and a large number of guns seized at Baltimore by Gen. B. F. Butler.

16. A bridge on the Baltimore and Ohio R R. destroyed; Gen. Scott ordered that Arlington Heights, Va., be fortified.

**1861.**

May 17. Confederate spies arrested in Washington; Adams Express Company prohibited from carrying letters or packages south of Washington.

20. Gov. Magoffin declared the neutrality of Kentucky; ordinance of secession adopted by North Carolina.

22. Gen. B. F. Butler assigned to command of Fortress Monroe, Va.

24. 13,000 U. S. troops crossed the Potomac into Virginia; Alexandria and Arlington Heights occupied; Col E. E Ellsworth, of the 11th N. Y. Inf , (First Fire Zouaves,) killed by Jackson, a hotel-keeper, who was instantly shot by Francis E Brownell.

25. Union troops destroyed seven bridges and five miles of railroad between Alexandria and Leesburg, Va.

26. West Virginia gave a large majority in favor of the Union; New Orleans blockaded by U. S Sloop of War Brooklyn; all postal service in the seceded States suspended.

28. Brig Gen. Irwin McDowell, U. S. A , assumed command of Department of Northeastern Virginia.

31. The steamers Freeborn and Anacosta engaged the Confederate batteries at Aquia Creek, Va.

June 2. Gen. Beauregard assumed command of the Confederate forces at Manassas Junction, Va

3. Hon. Stephen A Douglas died at Chicago; the voluntary contributions in the Northern States to carry on the war amounted to over thirty-two million dollars

6. A company of Confederate cavalry captured at Alexandria, Va , took the oath of allegiance.

8. Virginia State troops transferred to Confederate States.

11. Col. Canby, U. S. A., reported that Col Loring had abandoned the command of the Department of New Mexico

15. Confederates evacuated Harper's Ferry, armory machinery taken to Richmond; the brig Perry arrived at New York with the privateer Savannah, captured June 4.

17. Wheeling convention unanimously declared Western Virginia independent of the Confederate portion of the State; a train of cars with 275 Ohio volunteers was fired into near Vienna, Va , and 8 men killed and 12 wounded.

20. Union convention elected Frank D. Pierpont governor of Virginia; Gen. McClellan assumed command in person of the army in Western Virginia.

23. Forty-eight locomotives, valued at $400.000 and belonging to the Baltimore & Ohio Railroad, were destroyed by the Confederates.

26. President Lincoln acknowledged the Wheeling government of Virginia.

27. George P. Kane, marshal of Baltimore police, arrested by Gen. Banks and sent to Fort McHenry.

29. Confederates made a dash at Harper's Ferry, destroying several boats and the railroad bridge.

July 1. Arrest of Baltimore police commissioners; orders issued for raising United States troops in Kentucky and Tennessee.

4. Congress met in extra session; Confederates seized the Louisville & Nashville Railroad.

8. Brig.-Gen. Henry H. Sibley, C. S A , ordered to Texas to expel Union forces from New Mexico.

11. The following members were expelled from the United States Senate: J. M. Mason and R. M Hunter, of Va.; T. L. Clingman and Thos. Bragg, of N. C.; L. T. Wigfall and J. U. Hemphill, of Tex ; C. B. Mitchell and W. K. Sebastian, of Ark ; and A. O. F. Nicholson, of Tenn.

15. Military forces, stores, etc., of Ark , transferred to Confederate States.

16. President Lincoln authorized to call the militia and accept the services of 500.000 men.

20. Confederate congress met at Richmond.

21. Gen. Banks superseded Gen. Patterson in the command of the Department of the Shenandoah, headquarters in the field.

22. The three months' volunteers began to return home.

23. Department of Maryland created, and Gen. John A. Dix placed in command, headquarters at Baltimore; Brig -Gen. W. S. Rosecrans

**1861.**

assumed command of the Department of Ohio, embracing a portion of Western Virginia.

July 25. Gen. Fremont appointed to command of Western Department, headquarters at St. Louis; Gen. John A. Dix assumed command of Department of Pennsylvania.

26. Fort Fillmore, N. Mex., treacherously surrendered to the Confederates by Maj. Lynde, U. S. A.

27. Gen. McClellan took command of the Division of the Potomac.

Aug. 1. Gen. R. E. Lee, C. S. A., commanding in Western Virginia.

3. Congress passed the confiscation bill and a bill to raise $20,000,000 by direct taxation.

5. The Alvarado burned off Fernandina, Fla., by the United States vessel Vincennes.

6. Extra session of Congress closed.

7. Village of Hampton, Va., burned by Confederates.

8. Brig.-Gen. U. S. Grant assumed command of the district of Ironton, Mo.

10. Gen. Lyon killed at the battle of Wilson Creek, Mo.

14. Gen. Fremont declared martial law in St. Louis.

15. Jefferson Davis ordered all Northern men to leave the South in forty days.

17. Gen. Wool took command at Fortress Monroe.

20. Maj.-Gen. McClellan assumed command of the Army of the Potomac.

30. "Emancipation Proclamation" issued by Gen. Fremont.

Sept. 1. Gen. Grant assumed command in Southern Missouri.

2. Destruction of United States dry dock at Pensacola, Fla.

6. Paducah, Ky., occupied by Union troops.

11. President Lincoln modified Gen. Fremont's "Emancipation Proclamation."

12. Col. J. A. Washington, proprietor of Mt. Vernon, killed at battle of Cheat Mountain, W. Va.

12–17. Arrest of members of Maryland legislature and other citizens of that State.

14. Descent upon Pensacola navy yard by United States gunboats.

18. Col. Frank Blair arrested by order of Gen. Fremont; Maryland legislature closed by provost marshal—secession members sent to Fort McHenry; Bowling Green, Ky., occupied by Confederates.

19. Gov. Morehead, Reuben Merritt and M. A. Barr arrested in Louisville, Ky., for treason.

21. John C. Breckenridge fled from Frankfort, Ky., to join the Confederates; Gen. A. S. Johnston, C. S. A., called upon Tennessee to furnish 30,000 men.

22. Arkansas and Mississippi called upon to furnish 10,000 men each for the Confederate army.

Oct. 1. Department of New England constituted—Gen. Butler, U. S. A., in command.

7. The Confederate ironclad steamer Merrimac made its first appearance in sight of Fortress Monroe.

8. Brig.-Gen W. T. Sherman superseded Gen. Anderson in command of Department of the Cumberland.

9. Col. Geary with 400 Pennsylvania troops crossed the Potomac at Harper's Ferry and seized 21,000 bushels of wheat.

11. The Confederate steamer Theodore escaped from Charleston, S. C., with Mason and Slidell on board, the Confederate commissioners to Europe; Brig.-Gen. W. S. Rosecrans assumed command of the Department of Western Virginia.

21. Col. Baker killed at battle of Ball's Bluff, Va.

29. The second naval expedition, consisting of 80 vessels and 15,000 men, sailed from Fortress Monroe, commanded by Com. Dupont and Gen. Sherman.

Nov. 1. Gen. Scott resigned as commander-in-chief of the armies of the United States; Gen. McClellan appointed in his place.

2. Gen. Hunter superseded Gen. Fremont in command of the Western Department.

5. Gen. R. E. Lee. C. S. A., assigned to command of the Department of South Carolina, Georgia and Eastern Florida.

8–18. Revolt of Unionists in East Tennessee.

**1861.**

Nov. 15. United States frigate San Jacinto arrived at Fortress Monroe with Mason and Slidell.

18. Confederate congress met.

19. Gen. A S. Johnston, C. S A., called upon Tennessee to furnish all the troops that could be armed.

27. Gen. McClellan directed the observance of the Sabbath in all the camps of the United States Army.

Dec. 3. Congress met.

4. John C. Breckenridge expelled from the U. S. Senate.

9. Confederate Congress passed a bill admitting Kentucky into the Southern Confederacy.

18. Gen. Pope captured 1,300 Confederates, a number of horses and wagons, and 1,000 stand of arms, at Millford, Mo.

20. Stone fleet sunk in Charleston Harbor by Union forces; another one sunk Jan. 20, 1862.

21. Brig.-Gen. Henry A. Wise assigned to command of Confederate forces in North Carolinia.

27. Mason and Slidell surrendered to the British Minister.

**1862.**

Jan. 1. Mason and Slidell left Fort Warren for England, in the British steamer Rinaldo.

11. Simon Cameron resigned as Secretary of War, and E. M. Stanton appointed.

19. Battle of Mill Spring Kentucky, Gen. Zollicoffer, C. S. A., killed.

Feb. 5. Jesse D. Bright of Indiana expelled from the U. S. Senate.

8. Battle of Roanoke Island, Gen. Burnside captured six forts, taking about 3,000 small arms and destroying all the Confederate fleet, except two vessels, 2,500 prisoners and a large quantity of ammunition were captured.

9. Gen. C. P. Stone arrested and sent to Fort Lafayette.

13. Gen Curtis took possession of Springfield, Mo.

22. Jefferson Davis inaugurated President and A. H. Stephens, Vice-President of the Southern Confederacy.

25. Nashville, Tenn., occupied by Union troops.

March 3. Gen. R E Lee's army called to Richmond, Va.

4. Andrew Johnson appointed military governer of Tennessee.

8. Confederate steamers Merrimac, Jamestown and Yorktown attacked the Union fleet in Hampton Roads, destroying the Cumberland and Congress, and damaging several other vessels

9. Duel of the Monitor and Merrimac in Hampton Roads, after three hours' fighting the Merrimac was towed under the protection of the battery at Sewell's Point, but did not renew the contest. The Monitor was uninjured.

11. Gen. McClellan relieved of the command of the armies of the United States, but retained command of the Army of the Potomac.

11–12. Winchester, Va., abandoned by Confederates and occupied by Union forces.

13. Army Corps organized in Department of Potomac, Gens. McDowell, Sumner, Heintzelman, Keyes and Banks assigned as commanders. Gen. R. E. Lee charged with the military operations of the armies of the Confederacy.

14. Brig.-Gen. Rosecrans, U. S. A., assumed command of the Mountain Department.

20. Gen. Benjamin F. Butler assumed command of the Department of the Gulf.

April 7. Maj.-Gen. A. S. Johnston, C. S. A., killed at the battle of Shiloh, Tenn.

9. Jacksonville, Fla., evacuated by Union forces.

10–11. Fort Pulaski commanding the approach to Savannah, surrendered after a bombardment of thirty hours. The Merrimac made her second appearance in Hampton Roads and destroyed three small vessels. Congress abolished slavery in the District of Columbia.

18–28. Bombardment and capture of Forts Jackson and St. Philip on the Mississippi.

24. The Union fleet having removed the obstructions in the Mississippi, passed Forts Jackson and St. Philip on the way to New Orleans.

**1862.**

April 25. Commodore Farragut arrived at New Orleans and took possession of the city. Gen C. F. Smith died at Savannah, Tenn.

May 9–12. Confederates evacuated Pensacola, Fla., and destroyed the Navy Yard.

10. The Union forces took possession of Norfolk, Va. The result of this movement was the destruction of the iron-clad Merrimac and the capture of a number of guns and a large amount of ammunition. Gosport Navy Yard destroyed by Confederates.

30. Union troops took possession of Corinth, Miss.

June 6. Gun-boat engagement on the Mississippi, near Memphis. Seven Confederate boats were destroyed or captured. After the naval battle Memphis surrendered to the Union troops; Gen. Ashby, C. S. A., killed.

18. Union troops occupied Cumberland Gap, Tenn.

26. Gen. Pope assigned to the command of the Army of Virginia; commencement of the seven days' fight before Richmond.

27. Bombardment of Vicksburg commenced; Gen. Fremont relieved of his command.

July 1. Battle of Malvern Hill, and last of the Richmond battles; President Lincoln called for 300,000 additional volunteers.

11. Gen. Halleck appointed commander of all the land forces of the United States; the Confederate General Morgan entered Glasgow, Ky., and called upon the Kentuckians to rise.

18. A band of Confederates entered Newburgh, Ind., destroyed hospital stores, and captured 250 stand of arms; Gen. Twiggs died.

21. John S. Phelps appointed Military Governor of Arkansas.

22. Siege of Vicksburg abandoned

Aug. 3. The Confederate General Jeff Thompson defeated near Memphis, Tenn.; Gen Halleck ordered Gen. McClellan to evacuate the peninsula of Virginia.

4. The Secretary of War ordered a draft of 300,000 men; the Confederate ram Arkansas destroyed by her crew.

5. Gen. Robert McCook killed by Confederates while wounded and riding in an ambulance

16. Gen. McClellan evacuated Harrison's Landing, Va.

19. Gen. Wright placed in command of the Department of the Ohio; Col. Rodney Mason surrendered Clarksville, Tenn, to an inferior force without firing a gun.

27. Federal gunboats destroyed the Confederate works at City Point, Va.

Sept. 1. The Union troops evacuated Lexington. Ky.

2. Gen McClellan appointed to the command of the troops for the defense of Washington.

5. Confederates began crossing the Potomac into Maryland.

6. Col. Lowe recaptured Clarksville, Tenn.

7. Gen. Banks assigned to the command of the fortifications in and around Washington; Gen. McClellan took the field at the head of the Army of the Potomac.

14. Battle of South Mountain, Md.; Gen. Reno killed.

15. Harper's Ferry surrendered, after two days' fighting, to the enemy, with all the garrison, consisting of 8,000 men.

16. Mumfordsville, Ky., captured by the Confederates; about 4,000 prisoners taken.

18. Confederates recrossed the Potomac into Virginia, having been in Maryland two weeks; the Confederates evacuated Harper's Ferry.

19. Gen. McCook recaptured Mumfordsville, Ky.

22. President Lincoln's Emancipation Proclamation issued.

29. Gen. Nelson was shot by Gen. Jeff. C. Davis at Louisville, Ky.

Oct. 10. Confederate cavalry, under Gen. Stuart, entered Chambersburg, Pa., and captured a quantity of small arms and clothing.

18. Gen. Morgan, C. S. A., occupied Lexington, Ky.

22. Confederate salt works in Florida destroyed.

30. Gen. Rosecrans assumed command of the Army of the Cumberland; Gen. Mitchell died at Port Royal, S. C.

Nov. 5. Gen. McClellan relieved of the command of the Army of the Potomac, and Gen. Burnside put in his place.

11. Under the cartel the following United States officers were exchanged:

**1862.**

Brigadier-generals, 3; colonels, 18; lieutenant-colonels, 19; captains, 431; lieutenants, 545. Confederate officers: Colonels, 27; lieutenant-colonels, 17; captains, 467; lieutenants, 1,085. About 24,000 privates were also exchanged, leaving a balance due the United States of 6,000 privates.

Nov. 16. President Lincoln enjoined on the United States forces the orderly observance of the Sabbath.

22. All political State prisoners released.

Dec. 6. Gen. Banks' expedition sailed for New Orleans.

7. Confederate General Morgan captured the 104th Illinois, the 106th and 108th Ohio, and a number of the 2d Indiana cavalry at Hartsville, Tenn.

11. The City of Fredericksburg bombarded by Union troops, under cover of which they crossed the Rappahannock.

13. An expedition under Commodore Parker destroyed the Confederate salt works; also, five schooners and two sloops in Mob Jack Bay.

31. West Virginia admitted into the Union as a State, taking effect June 20, 1863; the steamer Monitor foundered on the coast of South Carolina.

**1863.**

Jan. 1. The steamer Harriet Lane was captured by the Confederates at the attack on Galveston, Texas; and the Westfall, which had got aground, was destroyed to prevent her falling into their hands; Commodore Renshaw perishing with his vessel by reason of premature explosion.

12. Three Federal transports on the Cumberland River were captured by the enemy; the gunboat Slidel, which was in company, surrendered without firing a gun.

28. Gen. Burnside relieved of the command of the Army of the Potomac and Gen. Hooker appointed in his place; Gen. Sumner and Gen. Franklin were relieved from duty in the Army of the Potomac.

Feb. 2. The Federal ram Queen of the West ran the blockade at Vicksburg, Miss., but was captured a few days after by the Confederates.

13. The ironclad Indianola ran the blockade at Vicksburg, and was captured.

18. Gunboats commenced the bombardment of Vicksburg.

26. A train of twenty-eight cars on the L. & N. R. R. captured by the rebels at Woodburn, Ky., and destroyed.

27. The Confederate steamer Nashville, while attempting to run the blockade, got aground near Fort McAllister, Ga., and was destroyed by the blockading fleet.

March 9. A band of Confederate cavalry passed through the Union lines, entered Fairfax, Va., and captured Gen. Stoughton and a few privates.

13. Commodore Farragut's fleet attempted to pass the Confederate batteries at Port Hudson, La., but only a part of the vessels succeeded; the Mississippi got aground and was destroyed.

17. Two hundred cavalry, under command of Gen. Averill, crossed the Rappahannock near Kelly's Ford, where but a single horssman could cross at once, and, in the face of a terrible fire from rifle pits and sharpshooters, charged the Confederates in their intrenchmeants killing or capturing nearly the whole force. They then encountered Stuart's cavalry and, after a desperate hand-to-hand fight of five hours, routed them, with great loss, capturing 80 prisoners.

20. Maj.-Gen. Burnside appointed to command of the Department of the Ohio; the negro brigade took Jacksonville, Fla.

April 6. Gen. Mitchell, with 300 cavalry, dashed into a Confederate camp near Nashville on a saber charge, capturing 5, killing 15, and capturing all their tents, arms, horses, and equipments.

7. Attack on Charleston—The Federal fleet was composed of 9 ironclad vessels, under the command of Commodore Dupont; the fight began on the afternoon of the 7th and lasted about two hours. The Keokuk was so badly damaged that she sank in a few hours. Several other vessels were temporarily disabled. The fleet was then withdrawn.

17. Gen. Banks' command left Baton Rouge, fought three battles, two on land and one on Grand Lake, capturing 2,000 prisoners; six vessels of Porter's fleet ran by the Confederate batteries at Vicksburg, Miss.

18. Fayetteville, Ark., attacked by 3,900 Confederates with four pieces of artillery; Union forces numbered but 2,000. The Confederates were repulsed.

**1863.**

Apr. 22. The Federal ram Queen of the West, was captured in Grand Lake, with Capt. Fuller and all her officers and crew, numbering 90. Gen. McClellan's staff disbanded. The Baltimore & Ohio Railroad destroyed between Cumberland and Grafton. The advance guard of Marmaduke's army, under command of Col. Newton, was surprised, the entire regiment being either killed or captured by the Union forces under Vandever.

May 2. Grierson's Raid—On the morning of the 17th of April, 1863, the 6th & 7th Ill. Cav., 900 strong, under Col. Grierson of the 6th (together with 6 pieces of artillery,) set out from Lagrange, Tenn. and pursuing in the main a southerly course, marched through the center of Miss., destroying as they went railroads, bridges, cars, locomotives and stores of all kinds, belonging to the Confederates. They traveled on an average of forty miles per day; they reached Baton Rouge, La., on the evening of May 2; they traveled nearly 800 miles in sixteen days, and traversed seventeen counties. They brought into Baton Rouge over 1,000 horses and a large number of cattle; 500 negroes followed them.

3. Fredericksburg, Va.—The second attempt to capture Fredericksburg was made by the Army of the Potomac under Gen. Hooker and failed.

5. Vallandigham arrested by order of Gen. Burnside at his residence in Dayton, Ohio. Office of the Dayton Journal destroyed by the mob. Suffolk, Va., abandoned by the Confederate troops and the fortifications destroyed. One hundred prominent secessionists of St. Louis sent South.

8. Col. Streight's command of 1,700 men captured by Forrest's cavalry, two miles from Cedar Bluff, Ga., after severe fighting. Confederate Gen. Van Dorn killed by Dr. Peters, in Maury County, Tenn.

10. Confederate Gen. Stonewall Jackson died at Richmond, Va., of wounds and pneumonia.

11. Buell court of inquiry adjourned after a session of 165 days.

13. Grant defeated Joseph E. Johnson and captured Jackson, Miss., with 7 cannon, and large quantities of military stores, besides 400 prisoners; the State Capitol was destroyed by fire.

24. Austin, Miss., burned by Col. Ellet's marine brigade.

25. Vallandigham delivered to the rebels at Murfreesboro, Tenn.; Confederate Navy Yard at Yazoo City, destroyed.

28. The gun-boat Cincinnati sunk by the Confederate batteries near Vicksburg; she went down with her flag flying; 25 men were killed and wounded, and 15 drowned.

29. An immense train consisting of 600 wagons, 3,000 horses and mules, 1,500 head of cattle, and 6,000 negroes from the Teche country, La., arrived within Gen. Banks' lines.

June 1. Gen. Hunter removed from the command of the Dept. of the South; Gen. Gilmore succeeded him.

3. Col. Montgomery, of the 2d S. C. (colored) regt., made a brilliant raid at the head of 200 men, up the Coosaw River, and about 25 miles into the interior, bringing back 725 negroes, a fine lot of blooded horses, and other property valued at $600,000.

11. The famous blockade runner, Herald, was sunk at midnight by a broadside from our blockading fleet off Charleston.

17. The Confederate ram, Atlanta, was decoyed into Wilmington waters, off the coast of S. C., and captured. after a brief fight, by the Weehauken, commanded by Capt. John Rodgers.

21. Gen. McClernand removed by Grant and Gen. Ord put in his place.

26. Rear Admiral Foote died in New York city.

28. Gen. Hooker was relieved of his command of the Army of the Potomac at his own request and Gen. Meade succeeded him.

July 1. Gettysburg, Pa.—In the latter part of June the Confederate Army, under Gen. Lee, invaded Pennsylvania; on the 1st July they were attacked by Gen. Meade, near Gettysburg, and after a three days' battle were driven from the field, leaving 5,000 killed and wounded; Meade took 20,000 prisoners; Missouri passed the ordinance of emancipation; Rosecrans drove Bragg from Tullahoma, Tenn.

4. Vicksburg—The siege of Vicksburg by the Union Army, under Grant, commenced May 18, and was pressed forward with almost unprece-

**1863.**

dented vigor until July 4, when Pemberton surrendered to Gen. Grant 27,000 prisoners, 132 cannon, and 50,000 stand of arms

July 5. John Morgan captured Lebanon, Ky., with 400 prisoners.

8. Morgan's raid—Morgan, with 5,000 cav. and 4 pieces of artillery, crossed the Ohio river into Harrison Co., Ind., and marched rapidly through the southern part of the State into Ohio, committing numerous depredations; on the 18th he was overtaken by the troops under Cols. Hobson and Judah, near Pomeroy, who captured all his artillery and 1,300 prisoners; with a mere fragment of his command, he retreated to Columbiana Co., Ohio, where, on the 20th, he surrendered to Gen. Shackleford.

17. Gen. Sherman attacked Jackson, Miss., routed Johnson and occupied the city; large stores were captured, also 40 locomotives, and all the rolling stock of 3 railroads; Gen. Ransom occupied Natchez, Miss.

20. A cavalry force, sent out by the Union Gen. Foster, struck the Wilmington & Weldon Railroad in North Carolina; burned the bridge over Tar River, and seized a large quantity of cotton.

23. Kentucky again invaded by the Confederates; Kit Carson with a part of the 1st N. M. Reg., defeated the Navajoe Indians near Fort Canby.

Aug. 17. An immense quantity of Confederate stores at Grenada, Miss., were destroyed by Lieut. Col. Phillips, of the 9th Ill. mounted Inf.; he burned the depot and machine shops, tore up the railroad track, and destroyed 57 locomotives, and more than 400 cars.

20. The town of Lawrence, Kan., was surprised in the middle of the night by 300 guerillas, who had collected in Cass Co., Mo., under the leadership of Quantrill; the town was set on fire and 182 buildings burned to the ground, and $2,000,000 worth of property destroyed: 191 persons were killed, many of whom were helpless women and children; 581 were wounded; after the departure of the guerillas, the citizens organized under Gen. James H. Lane, and pursued them to their headquarters at Grand River, Mo., where they scattered in various directions; about 80 of the murderers were killed.

22 Col. Woodson's cavalry made a successful onslaught upon numerous guerilla bands in Arkansas, capturing Jeff. Thompson, with his entire staff.

Sept. 1. Little Rock, Ark., abandoned by the Confederates.

4. Gen. Burnside occupied Knoxville, Tenn., and was hailed with delight by the inhabitants.

9. Gen. Crittenden's Div. of Rosecran's army entered Chattanooga, Tenn.

10. Gen. Burnside captured Cumberland Gap, with 2,000 prisoners and 14 pieces of artillery, under the command of Maj.-Gen. Frazer; Gen. Steele took possession of Little Rock, Ark.

Oct. 20. The Departments of the Cumberland and Mississippi were consolidated, and placed under the command of Gen. Grant; Gen. Rosecrans was removed and Gen. Thomas appointed in his place.

Nov. 17. Gen. Longstreet commenced the siege of Knoxville, Tenn., which lasted until December 4.

**1864.**

Feb. 9. A large number of prisoners, including Col. Streight, escaped from Libby prison.

15. Gen. W. T. Sherman, with his command, arrived at Meridian, Miss., on his great raid into the heart of the South; after destroying railroads and stores, he returned to Vicksburg, Miss., with immense booty.

March 8. Gen. Grant was formally presented by President Lincoln with his commission as Lieut. Gen., and on the 12th was assigned to the command of the armies of the United States.

14. The Union forces under Gen. A. J. Smith captured Fort DeRussey, La., on Red River, with 325 prisoners, 12 pieces of artillery, 2,000 barrels of powder, etc

25. About 5,000 Confederates under Forrester captured Paducah, Ky., and fired the place.

28. The 54th Ill. Reg. attacked by Coles Co. copperheads, at Charleston, Ill.

April 12. Fort Pillow—Gen. Forrest overpowered the Union forces at Fort Pillow; compelled them to surrender, and immediately after commenced an indiscriminate massacre of wounded, both colored and white, not excepting women and children who had taken refuge in the fort.

**1864.**

April 17, 18. At Plymouth, N. C., the Confederate ram and a battery sunk three Union gunboats.

23. The governors of Ohio, Illinois, Iowa, Wisconsin and Indiana offered to raise for the General Government 85,000 men for 100 days.

26. The Government accepted the services of the 100 days' men and appropriated $20,000,000 for their payment.

May 5. Draft ordered in Massachusetts, New Jersey, Ohio, Minnesota, Kentucky and Maryland.

6. Gen. Grant crossed the Rapidan and Lee fell back toward Richmond.

7. After three days' hard fighting Lee's forces retreated, leaving 3,000 killed and 10 000 wounded on the field.

13. Gen. Sheridan with cavalry reached the rear of the enemy near Hanover Junction, Va., breaking two railroads, capturing several locomotives and destroying Lee's depot of supplies at Beaver Dam, Va., containing over 1,000,000 rations.

15. Sherman after two days' fighting forced Johnson to evacuate Resaca, Ga.

23. The Confederate Gen. John Morgan entered Kentucky with 4,000 men.

June 5. Sherman flanked Johnson and captured Ackworth, Ga.

7. Union convention at Baltimore.

8. Abraham Lincoln and Gov. Andrew Johnson were nominated for President and Vice-President.

11. Morgan demanded of Gov. Bramlette the surrender of Frankfort, Ky., which the governor refused.

12. Gen. Hancock drove the Confederates from Bottoms Bridge, Va., at the point of the bayonet.

15. Gen. Smith attacked by a force of 15.000 men.

23. Confederates attacked Wright and Hancock; captured three full regiments, after which they were repulsed.

27. Gen. Sherman made an unsuccessful attack on the enemy, losing from 2,000 to 3 000 men.

30. Secretary Chase resigned and Hon. Wm. P. Fessenden was appointed to fill the vacancy.

July 10. Confederates invade Maryland.

13, 15. The Confederates under Gen. Forrest defeated in five different battles near Pontotoc, Miss.

17. The Confederate army was driven within the fortifications at Atlanta.

22. A great battle was fought before Atlanta, resulting in the complete defeat of the Confederates.

25. Gen. Crook overtook the Confederates retreating from the Maryland raid and recaptured a large amount of stores; after a severe fight on the 23d and 24th Gen. Averill was compelled to fall back to Harper's Ferry.

30. A mine containing six tons of powder, under the Confederate forts at Petersburg was exploded destroying the fort and garrison.

Aug. 5. The Confederate ram Tennessee was captured and several other vessels destroyed. Shortly after Fort Gaines, Ala., surrendered and Fort Powell was evacuated.

18. The Weldon Railroad seized by Gen. Grant.

23. Fort Morgan, Ala., surrendered.

Sept. 2. The Federals took possession of Atlanta.

5. The Confederate Gen. John Morgan was killed near Greenville, Tenn.

28. Gen Grant advanced his lines on the north side of the James River to within seven miles of Richmond. The Confederates under Gen. Price invaded Mo.

Oct. 7. The pirate vessel Florida was captured by the U. S. steamer Wachusett.

19. Gen. Sheridan gained his fourth victory over the Confederates under Early at Cedar Creek, Va.

30. Gen Hood made three attacks on Decatur, Ala., but repulsed each time.

Nov. 3. The Confederate ram Albemarle destroyed by Lt. Cushing.

8. The Presidential election took place; Lincoln and Johnson received 212, McClellan and Pendleton 21 electoral votes.

Nov. 16 Gen. Sherman left Atlanta and began his march to the sea.

Dec. 13. Fort McAllister, Ga., captured by Gen. Sherman.

20. Confederates under Gen. Breckenridge defeated in Southwestern Virginia, and the salt works were destroyed.

**1864.**

Dec. 21. Gen. Sherman entered the city of Savannah, capturing 150 cannon, 30,000 bales of cotton and other stores.

29. Hood's army recrossed the Tennessee River, thus ending the Tennessee campaign.

**1865.**

Jan. 3. Mass. ratified the constitutional amendment.

8. Gen. Butler was removed from the command of the army of the James and was succeeded by Gen. Ord.

16. Fort Fisher, near Wilmington N C ,was captured with all its equipments.

20. Confederates evacuated Corinth, Miss.

21. Peace rumors.

27 Confederate incendiaries set fire to the city of Savannah, Ga.

31. Gen. R. E. Lee appointed Commander-in-chief of the Confederate forces by Jefferson Davis.

Feb. 1. Illinois ratified the constitutional amendment.

2. Maryland, Michigan, New York and Rhode Island ratified the amendment.

4. Illinois Black Law was repealed.

7. Maine ratified the amendment.

12. Gen. Sherman occupied Branchville, South Carolina.

13. Indiana ratified the amendment.

17. Louisiana ratified amendment; Gen. Sherman's forces entered Columbia, South Carolina, and burned the city.

18. Charleston, S. C., evacuated by the Confederates and taken possession of by Gen. Gilmore; a great amount of valuable property was destroyed, together with six thousand bales of cotton. Ammunition stored in the railroad depot exploded, and many lives were lost; Gen. Gilmore hoisted the Union flag over Fort Sumter.

19. Fort Anderson, N. C , taken.

21. Fort Armstrong, N C., taken; Wisconsin ratified the amendment.

22. Wilmington, N. C., captured

March 2. Gen. Sheridan captured Confederate General Early, with 1,800 men, between Staunton and Charlottesville, Va.

10. Gen. Sherman occupied Fayetteville, N. C.

12 Mobile attacked.

13. Gen. Schofield occupied Kingston, N. C.

April 3. Evacuation of Richmond.

4. President Lincoln held a levee in Jefferson Davis' house.

9. Gen Lee surrendered; 26,000 Confederates missing; Mobile, Ala , taken.

12. Salisbury, N. C , taken; Columbus, Ga., taken.

13. Raleigh, N. C., taken; Gov Vance taken prisoner.

14. President Lincoln was shot at Ford's Theater, Washington, D. C , by John Wilkes Booth, the actor; the building was afterward purchased by the Government, and is now the Medical Museum; Secretary Seward was also assaulted at his residence and severely stabbed, but recovered from his wounds; Arkansas ratified the constitutional amendment.

15. President Lincoln died at the house of Mr. Peterson, No. 516 10th street, N. W., Washington, D. C., at 7:22 a. m.

16. Andrew Johnson took the oath of office, and was declared President of the United States.

17. Gen. Mosby surrendered at Berryville, Va , 700 Confederates missing.

26. Gen. J E. Johnson surrendered with 27,500 men

27. J. Wilkes Booth, the murderer of President Lincoln, was shot and captured.

May 4. Gen. Taylor surrendered—10.000 Confederates missing.

9. President Johnson issued a peace proclamation declaring the war at an end.

10. Sam Jones surrendered at Tallahassee, Fla., 8,000 Confederates missing; Jefferson Davis captured at Irwinville, Ga., by the 1st Wis. and 4th Mich. Cav.; also his wife and mother, Postmaster-General Regan, Col. Harrison, (private secretary) Col. Johnson and other military characters.

May 11. Jeff Thompson surrendered at Chalk Bluff, Ark., 7,454 Confederates missing.

**1865.**

May 24. Grand review of the Army at Washington, D. C.; Jefferson Davis indicted for treason.

26. Kirby Smith surrendered, 20,000 Confederates missing. This was the last armed Confederate organization to surrender.

31. Gen. Hood and staff surrendered.

# STATEMENT OF

IN THE VOLUNTEER AND REGULAR ARMIES OF THE UNITED STATES, AND THE COLORED MENT OF THE REBELLION

| STATES, &c. | Officers killed. | Enlisted men killed. | Officers died of wounds. | Enlisted men died of wounds. | Officers died of disease. | Enlisted men died of disease. | Officers deserted. |
|---|---|---|---|---|---|---|---|
| Maine | 116 | 1,620 | 66 | 1,069 | 65 | 5,479 | 1 |
| New Hampshire | 91 | 1,006 | 33 | 531 | 49 | 2,481 | 1 |
| Vermont | 68 | 1,133 | 39 | 662 | 34 | 2,964 | 1 |
| Massachusetts | 274 | 3,624 | 104 | 2,027 | 80 | 7,824 | 3 |
| Rhode Island | 30 | 446 | ........ | .......... | 21 | 1,052 | ...... |
| Connecticut | 97 | 1,094 | 48 | 663 | 63 | 3,246 | 2 |
| New York | 427 | 8,695 | 302 | 5,021 | 222 | 17,185 | 50 |
| New Jersey | 106 | 1,231 | 40 | 317 | 33 | 2,933 | 6 |
| Pennsylvania | 376 | 6,096 | 137 | 3,675 | 117 | 10,973 | 15 |
| Delaware | 9 | 178 | 10 | 113 | 7 | 207 | ...... |
| Maryland | 16 | 359 | 17 | 326 | 39 | 824 | ...... |
| West Virginia | 58 | 741 | 23 | 391 | 20 | 1,792 | 2 |
| District of Columbia | 3 | 43 | 1 | 8 | ........ | 244 | ...... |
| Ohio | 280 | 6,283 | 140 | 4,534 | 159 | 13,195 | 6 |
| Indiana | 294 | 3,140 | 139 | 2,244 | 220 | 13,172 | 5 |
| Illinois | 394 | 5,463 | 126 | 2,925 | 364 | 19,570 | 12 |
| Michigan | 154 | 2,554 | 68 | 1,151 | 78 | 8,421 | 6 |
| Wisconsin | 121 | 2,237 | 67 | 1,393 | 101 | 6,885 | 3 |
| Minnesota | 29 | 381 | 7 | 191 | 26 | 1,650 | ...... |
| Iowa | 146 | 1,926 | 69 | 1,303 | 127 | 8,515 | 4 |
| Missouri | 89 | 1,461 | 48 | 767 | 130 | 7,216 | 15 |
| Kentucky | 82 | 1,103 | 30 | 669 | 124 | 5.121 | 24 |
| Kansas | 34 | 762 | 12 | 192 | 26 | 2,080 | 2 |
| California | 1 | 34 | ........ | 57 | 1 | 298 | 1 |
| Tennessee | 27 | 1,264 | 11 | 920 | 11 | 2,182 | 5 |
| Mississippi | ........ | .......... | ........ | .......... | ........ | 69 | ...... |
| Alabama | 2 | 32 | ........ | 31 | 2 | 228 | ...... |
| Florida | ........ | 27 | ........ | 142 | ........ | 102 | ...... |
| Texas | ........ | 22 | ........ | 11 | ........ | 278 | ...... |
| North Carolina | ........ | 34 | 1 | 19 | 1 | 248 | 1 |
| Louisiana | 2 | 117 | 2 | 101 | 1 | 768 | ...... |
| Arkansas | 8 | 210 | 3 | 163 | 1 | 544 | 7 |
| Nevada | ........ | 8 | ........ | 2 | ........ | 225 | 1 |
| Oregon | ........ | 58 | 2 | 7 | 2 | 665 | 5 |
| Colorado | 2 | 61 | 1 | 44 | 2 | 205 | 1 |
| Indian Territory | 2 | 231 | ........ | 141 | ........ | 416 | ...... |
| Washington Territory | ........ | 14 | 4 | 11 | ........ | 107 | ...... |
| Dakota Territory | ........ | .......... | ........ | .......... | ........ | 10 | ...... |
| Nebraska Territory | 1 | 5 | ........ | 8 | 1 | 122 | 1 |
| New Mexico Territory | ........ | 7 | 1 | 15 | 1 | 159 | ...... |
| U. S. Vols. "Penitent Rebels" | ........ | 9 | ........ | 5 | ........ | 352 | ...... |
| Hancock's Corps | ........ | 7 | ........ | 2 | ........ | 406 | 1 |
| Mississippi Marine Brigade | 3 | 136 | 2 | 107 | 4 | 181 | 1 |
| Veteran Reserve Corps | 1 | 43 | ........ | 70 | 11 | 1,269 | 4 |
| Total Volunteers | 3,345 | 54,056 | 1,549 | 32,095 | 2,141 | 152,013 | 187 |
| Regular Army | 157 | 1,890 | ........ | .......... | 83 | 2,749 | 5 |
| Colored Troops | 124 | 1,790 | 46 | 1,037 | 90 | 26,211 | 24 |
| Grand Total | 3,626 | 57,736 | 1,595 | 33,132 | 2,314 | 180,973 | 216 |

# CASUALTIES

TROOPS, DIVIDED BY STATES AND INDEPENDENT ORGANIZATIONS, FROM THE COMMENCE-
TO AUGUST 1, 1865.

| Enlisted men deserted. | Officers honorably discharged. | Enlisted men honorably discharged. | Officers discharged for disability. | Enlisted men discharged for disability. | Officers dishon'y disch'd. | Enlisted men dishonorably discharged. | Officers dismissed. | Officers cashiered. | Officers resigned. | Officers miss'g in action. | Enlisted men missing in action. | Aggregate casualties. | Number of men enlisted during the war in which these casualties occurred; term of service from three months to three years. |
|---|---|---|---|---|---|---|---|---|---|---|---|---|---|
| 2,840 | 378 | 9,293 | 192 | 6,450 | ..... | 47 | 22 | 2 | 457 | ..... | ....... | 28,097 | 64,708 |
| 3,705 | 183 | 2,409 | 8 | 2,407 | ..... | ....... | 28 | 7 | 262 | ..... | ....... | 13,201 | 33,025 |
| 1,689 | 312 | 4,417 | 93 | 4,312 | ..... | ....... | 24 | 6 | 317 | ..... | ....... | 16,071 | 32,653 |
| 8,415 | 1,149 | 11,975 | 316 | 12,500 | ..... | 11 | 103 | 8 | 797 | ..... | ....... | 49,210 | 126,236 |
| 1,674 | 47 | 342 | 28 | 2,125 | ..... | 42 | 17 | 8 | 253 | ..... | ....... | 6,085 | 21,301 |
| 6,281 | 385 | 5,451 | 51 | 4,361 | ..... | 105 | 58 | 9 | 481 | 21 | 389 | 22,805 | 53,594 |
| 35,999 | 2,530 | 32,509 | 741 | 24,167 | 176 | 455 | 292 | 67 | 2,046 | 7 | 1,407 | 132,298 | 404,748 |
| 7,183 | 191 | 2,609 | 1 | 6,908 | ..... | 47 | 89 | 1 | 599 | ..... | ....... | 22,294 | 67,186 |
| 19,032 | 1,500 | 24,970 | 562 | 16,706 | ..... | 128 | 237 | 39 | 1,121 | 30 | 1,522 | 87,236 | 323,846 |
| 958 | 35 | 842 | 13 | 456 | ..... | ....... | 5 | ..... | 35 | ..... | ....... | 2,868 | 12,171 |
| 2,981 | 83 | 1,684 | 46 | 826 | 10 | 60 | 57 | 6 | 102 | ..... | 112 | 7,548 | 42,128 |
| 1,269 | 292 | 4,404 | 34 | 2,218 | ..... | 52 | 87 | 2 | 303 | ..... | ....... | 11,798 | 32,003 |
| 701 | 3 | 350 | ...... | 218 | ..... | 6 | 1 | ..... | 12 | ..... | ....... | 1,590 | 15,181 |
| 13,603 | 624 | 15,407 | 335 | 21,545 | ..... | 105 | 157 | 16 | 1,824 | ..... | ....... | 78,213 | 307,380 |
| 7,232 | 443 | 1,552 | 70 | 17,115 | ..... | 17 | 235 | 26 | 2,664 | ..... | ....... | 48,568 | 193,285 |
| 13,034 | 771 | 1,672 | 67 | 23,864 | ..... | 223 | 257 | 13 | 3,334 | ..... | ....... | 72,291 | 255,938 |
| 6,136 | 595 | 12,564 | 210 | 9,614 | ..... | 104 | 88 | 5 | 1,015 | ..... | ....... | 42,763 | 87,613 |
| 3,230 | 424 | 10,912 | 94 | 9,219 | ..... | 7 | 57 | 3 | 1,093 | ..... | ....... | 35,846 | 90,888 |
| 493 | 146 | 1,598 | 15 | 2.859 | ..... | ....... | 26 | ..... | 229 | ..... | ...... | 7,650 | 23,999 |
| 1,474 | 65 | 21 | 11 | 9,931 | ..... | 55 | 22 | 7 | 1,304 | ..... | ....... | 24,980 | 75,780 |
| 6,983 | 340 | 7,092 | 22 | 7,827 | ..... | 182 | 127 | 12 | 1,230 | 13 | 588 | 34,142 | 108,756 |
| 6,541 | 91 | 2,047 | 38 | 4,097 | ..... | ....... | 61 | 4 | 903 | ..... | ....... | 20,935 | 74,961 |
| 1,988 | 88 | 999 | 8 | 1,849 | 1 | 94 | 43 | 4 | 281 | ..... | 35 | 8,498 | 20,097 |
| 758 | 16 | 628 | 6 | 912 | ..... | 4 | 2 | 1 | 43 | ..... | ....... | 2,762 | 7,451 |
| 2,658 | 31 | 700 | 25 | 4,015 | ..... | 5 | 8 | 3 | 112 | ..... | ....... | 11,970 | ............ |
| 124 | ........ | 5 | 1 | 21 | ..... | ....... | ....... | ..... | ........ | ..... | ....... | 220 | ............ |
| 209 | 2 | 20 | 2 | 226 | ..... | ...... | ....... | ..... | 5 | ..... | ...... | 819 | ............ |
| 173 | 4 | 30 | 3 | 69 | ..... | 1 | ....... | ..... | 10 | ..... | ....... | 561 | ............ |
| 546 | 7 | 34 | ....... | 96 | ..... | 2 | 4 | 1 | 3 | ..... | ....... | 1,004 | ............ |
| 299 | ........ | 14 | ....... | 27 | ..... | 7 | ....... | 1 | 15 | ..... | ....... | 667 | ............ |
| 1,240 | 14 | 304 | 7 | 481 | ..... | ...... | ....... | ..... | 21 | ..... | ....... | 3,058 | ............ |
| 549 | 7 | 197 | 10 | 596 | ..... | 2 | 1 | ..... | 16 | ..... | ....... | 2,314 | ............ |
| 701 | 1 | 24 | 1 | 69 | ..... | 1 | ....... | ..... | 5 | ..... | ....... | 1,038 | ............ |
| 856 | 5 | 337 | 2 | 414 | ..... | 7 | 1 | ..... | 9 | ..... | ....... | 2,370 | ............ |
| 237 | 8 | 126 | 2 | 280 | ..... | ....... | ....... | ..... | 7 | ..... | ....... | 976 | 1,762 |
| 247 | ........ | 20 | 6 | 263 | ..... | ....... | ....... | ..... | 8 | ..... | ....... | 1,334 | ............ |
| 397 | 4 | 73 | ....... | 170 | ..... | ....... | 1 | ..... | 4 | ..... | ....... | 785 | ............ |
| 12 | 1 | 6 | ...... | 205 | ..... | 1 | 1 | ..... | 2 | ..... | ....... | 238 | ............ |
| 173 | 2 | 10 | 4 | 240 | ..... | ....... | ....... | ..... | 3 | ..... | ....... | 570 | 3,157 |
| 332 | 3 | 51 | 2 | 271 | ..... | ...... | 1 | ..... | 9 | ..... | ....... | 852 | 2,395 |
| 605 | 5 | 46 | 2 | 378 | ..... | 1 | 1 | ..... | 15 | ..... | ....... | 1,419 | ............ |
| 2,348 | 1 | 209 | ....... | 182 | ..... | 8 | ....... | ..... | 19 | ..... | ....... | 3,183 | ............ |
| 219 | 4 | 123 | 5 | 233 | ..... | ...... | ....... | ..... | 13 | ..... | ......, | 1,031 | ............ |
| 3,534 | 15 | 1,688 | 5 | 8,218 | ..... | 285 | 28 | 4 | 129 | ..... | ....... | 15,304 | 60,508 |
| 170,029 | 10,805 | 159,764 | 3,058 | 209,102 | 186 | 2,023 | 2,143 | 252 | 21,090 | 72 | 4,085 | 828,307 | ............ |
| 16,360 | 2 | 1,201 | 2 | 5,089 | ..... | 275 | 122 | 6 | 390 | 33 | 1,266 | 29,637 | 67,000 |
| 12,440 | 427 | 2,378 | 166 | 6,889 | 18 | 191 | 158 | 16 | 801 | 18 | 1,275 | 54,099 | 180,017 |
| 198,829 | 11,234 | 163,343 | 3,226 | 221,080 | 204 | 2,489 | 2,423 | 274 | 22,281 | 123 | 6,626 | 912,043 | ............ |

# LIST OF PRESIDENTS AND VICE-PRESIDENTS

## From 1789 to 1885.

---

1789 to 1793.—George Washington, of Va.; inaugurated April 30, 1789; born February 22, 1732; died December 14, 1796. John Adams, of Mass., Vice-President; born October 19, 1735; died July 4, 1826.

1793 to 1797.—George Washington, inaugurated March 4, 1793. John Adams, Vice-President.

1797 to 1801.—John Adams, President; inaugurated March 4, 1797. Thomas Jefferson, of Va., Vice-President; born April 13, 1743; died July 4, 1826.

1801 to 1805.—Thomas Jefferson, President; inaugurated March 4, 1801. Aaron Burr, of N. Y., Vice-President; born February 6, 1756; died September 14, 1836.

1805 to 1809.—Thomas Jefferson, President; inaugurated March 4, 1805. George Clinton, of N. Y., Vice-President; born in 1737.

1809 to 1813.—James Madison, of Va, President; inaugurated March 4, 1809; born March 16, 1751; died June 28, 1836. George Clinton, Vice-President; died April 20, 1812.

1813 to 1817.—James Madison, of Va, President; inaugurated March 4, 1813. Elbridge Gerry, of Mass., Vice-President until his death, November 23, 1814; he was born July 17, 1744.

1817 to 1821.—James Monroe, of Va., President; inaugurated March 4, 1817; born in 1759; died July 4, 1831. Daniel D. Tompkins, of N. Y., Vice-President; born June 21, 1774; died June 11, 1825.

1821 to 1825.—James Monroe, President; inaugurated March 4, 1821. Daniel D. Tompkins, Vice-President.

1825 to 1829.—John Quincy Adams, of Mass., President; inaugurated March 4, 1825; born July 11, 1767; died February 23, 1848. John Caldwell Calhoun, of South Carolina, Vice-President; born March 18, 1782; died March 31, 1850.

1829 to 1833.—Andrew Jackson, of Tenn., President; inaugurated March 4, 1829; born March 15, 1767; died June 8, 1845. John C. Calhoun, Vice-President until his resignation, December 28, 1832.

1833 to 1837.—Andrew Jackson, President; inaugurated March 4, 1833. Martin Van Buren, of N. Y., Vice-President; born December 5, 1782

1837 to 1841.—Martin Van Buren, President; inaugurated March 4, 1837; died December 27, 1862. Richard M. Johnson, of Ky., Vice-President; born in 1780; died November 19, 1850.

1841 to 1845.—Wm. Henry Harrison, of Ohio, President until his death, April 4, 1841; inaugurated March 4, 1841; he was born February 9, 1773. John Tyler, of Va., Vice-President; born April, 1790; he became President by the death of W. H. Harrison; he took the oath of office April 6, 1841; died January 17, 1862.

1845 to 1849.—James Knox Polk, of Tenn., President; inaugurated March 4, 1845; born November 2, 1795; died June 15, 1849. Geo. Mifflin Dallas, of Pa., Vice-President, born July 10, 1792.

1849 to 1853.—Zachary Taylor, La., President; inaugurated March 4, 1849; born in 1784; died July 9, 1850. Millard Fillmore, of N. Y., Vice-President; born January 7, 1800; he became President after the death of Zachary Taylor, and took the oath of office July 10, 1850; died March 8, 1874.

1853 to 1857.—Franklin Pierce, of N. H., President; inaugurated March 5, 1853; born November 23, 1804; died October 8, 1869. William R. King, of Ala., Vice-President; born April 7, 1786, and died April 18, 1853.

1857 to 1861.—James Buchanan, of Pa., born April 22, 1791; died June 1, 1868. John C. Breckenridge, of Ky., Vice-President; born January 21, 1820.

1861 to 1865.—Abraham Lincoln, of Ill., President; inaugurated March 4, 1861; born February, 1809. Hannibal Hamlin, of Me., Vice-President; born August 27, 1809.

1865 to 1869—Abraham Lincoln, President; inaugurated March 4, 1865; died April 15, 1865. Andrew Johnson, of Tenn., Vice-President; died July 31, 1875. Upon the assassination of President Lincoln April 14, 1865, Andrew Johnson assumed the Presidency, and Lafayette S. Foster, of Conn., became Vice-President.

1869 to 1873.—Ulysses S. Grant, of Ill., President; inaugurated March, 1869; born at Mount Pleasant. Ohio, April 27, 1822. Schuyler Colfax, of Ind., Vice-President; born March 23, 1823.

1873 to 1877.—Ulysses S. Grant, President; inaugurated March 4, 1873. Henry Wilson, of Mass., Vice-President; born at Farmington, N. H., February 16, 1812; died November 22, 1875.

1877 to 1881.—Rutherford B. Hayes, of Ohio, President; born at Delaware, Ohio, October 4, 1822; inaugurated March 5, 1877. William A. Wheeler, of New York, Vice-President; born in Malone, Franklin county, New York, June 30, 1819.

1881 to 1885.—James Abram Garfield, of Ohio, inaugurated March 4, 1881, and died by the pistol of the assassin, Chas. J. Guiteau, September 19, 1881; he was born March 19, 1831. Chester A. Arthur, Vice-President; born October 5, 1830; inaugurated Vice-President March 4, 1881, and upon the death of President Garfield sworn into office September 20, 1881.

## PRESIDENTS WHO HAVE DIED IN OFFICE.

William Henry Harrison, died at 12:30 a. m., April 4, 1841, of a disease of the lungs and liver.

Zachary Taylor, died at 10:30 p. m., Sunday, July 9, 1850, at the White House, of cholera morbus.

Abraham Lincoln, was assassinated by J. Wilkes Booth, at 10:30 p. m., April 14, 1865, while at Ford's Theater, on 10th street, witnessing the performance of "Our American Cousin." He was carried to the home of Mr. Peterson, No. 516 10th street, where he died at 7:22 a. m., April 15, 1865.

James A. Garfield was assassinated by Charles J. Guiteau, at 9:30 a. m., July 2, 1881, while passing through the Baltimore and Potomac depot at Washington, D. C., to take the train for Long Branch. He lived for eighty days, suffering intensely most of the time, and died at Elberon, N. J., Monday, September 19, 1881, at 10:35 p. m.

# ROSTER OF REGIMENTAL SURGEONS.

## ALABAMA.

### 1st Cavalry—Mustered out October 20, 1865.

| Name | Rank | Residence | Service |
|---|---|---|---|
| Swaving, John G. C. | Surgeon | Pottsville, Pa. | From January, 1864. |
| Davis, Joseph H. | Ass't S. | | From August, 1864. |
| Stewart, John W. | " | | From August, 1864. |
| Stewart, Absalom B. | Surgeon | | To Jan., 1864; also 10th Mo. Inf. |
| McDavitt, Virgil | Ass't S. | | To August, 1864. |
| Smith, Stephen C. | " | | To June, 1864. |

## ARKANSAS.

### 1st Cavalry—Mustered out August 23, 1865.

| Name | Rank | Residence | Service |
|---|---|---|---|
| Caffee, Amos H. | Ass't S. | Carthage, Mo. | To Surgeon 13th Kan. Inf. Feb. 1865; Ex. S. |
| Maynard, Henry J. | Surgeon | Cheyenne, Wyoming Ty. | From June, 1863; also 59th Ill. Inf. |
| Tefft, Jonathan E. | Ass't S. | Springfield, Mo. | To January, 1865; Ex. S. |
| Hunter, Wm. | " | | To January, 1863. |

### 2d Cavalry—Mustered out August 20, 1865.

| Name | Rank | Residence | Service |
|---|---|---|---|
| Maynard, H. M. | Surgeon | Los Angeles, or Santa Ana, Cal. | From March, 1864; also 18th Iowa Inf. |
| Twiner, A. B. | Ass't S. | Searcy, Ark. | From September, 1864. |
| Hocker, John D. | " | | From November, 1863. |

### 3d Cavalry—Mustered out June 30, 1865.

| Name | Rank | Residence | Service |
|---|---|---|---|
| Madison, J. W. | Ass't S. | Lewisburg, Ark. | From January, 1864. |
| Thomas, Abner D. | Surgeon | Morrillton, Ark. | From Dec., 1863; also 2d Mo. Cav. |
| Piero, F. L. | Ass't S. | | From March, 1864. |

### 4th Cavalry—Mustered out June 30, 1865.

| Name | Rank | Residence | Service |
|---|---|---|---|
| Warferd, F. W. | Surgeon | Cicero, Ind. | A. W. M.; also 3d Iowa Cav. |
| Fryrear, A. F. | Ass't S. | | To July, 1864. |

### 1st Infantry—Mustered out August 10, 1865.

| Name | Rank | Residence | Service |
|---|---|---|---|
| Bolinger, Harvey H. | Ass't S. | St. Paul, Ark. | To April, 1864. |
| Waterman, W. B. | Surgeon | | A. W. M. |
| Campfield, Robert B. | Ass't S. | Buffalo, Kan. | From June, 1864. |
| Drake, Thomas B. | " | | To May, 1863. |

### 2d Infantry—Mustered out August 8, 1865.

| Name | Rank | Residence | Service |
|---|---|---|---|
| Hocker, Nicolas B. | Surgeon | Mount Vernon, Mo. | From February, 1864. |
| Ayers, A. R. | Ass't S. | Hannibal, Mo. | From July, 1864. |
| Bowers, William P. | " | | Dismissed Sept., 1864. |

## ARKANSAS—Continued.

### 4TH INFANTRY—Consolidated with the 2d Infantry October 28, 1864.

| Name | Rank | Address | Service |
|---|---|---|---|
| Blanchard, Basil | Ass't S. | | To October, 1864. |

## CALIFORNIA.

### 1ST CAVALRY—Mustered out from March 6 to October 19, 1866.

| Name | Rank | Address | Service |
|---|---|---|---|
| Kunkler, John E. | Surgeon | | From May, 1865. |
| Strong, Wm. E. | Ass't S. | | To January, 1865. |
| Prentiss, John H. | Surgeon | | To September, 1864. |

### 1ST BATTALION—Mustered out from March 15 to April 2, 1866. (Also called Native Cavalry Battalion.)

| Name | Rank | Address | Service |
|---|---|---|---|
| Tolman, Geo. B. | Ass't S. | Ocean View, Cal. | From May, '65; also 6th Inf. |
| Gelcich, Vincent | " | Los Angeles, Cal. | To Surg. 4th Inf. May, '65. |

### 2D CAVALRY—Mustered out from February 1 to July 12, 1866.

| Name | Rank | Address | Service |
|---|---|---|---|
| Horne, Geo. H. | Ass't S. | 874 N. 4th st., Phila., Pa. | To Surg. 2d Inf. Aug., 1865; also 1st Inf. |
| Handy, John C. | " | Tucson, Ariz. | From September, 1865. |
| Reid, Robert K. | Surgeon | | From Oct., 1864; also 3d Inf. |
| Holbrook, Chas. E. | Ass't S. | | To May, 1864. |
| Cooper, Jas. G. | " | | To October, 1865. |
| Furley, Chas. C. | " | | To January, 1863. |
| Williamson, J. M. | Surgeon | | To October, 1864. |

### 1ST INFANTRY—Mustered out from September 15 to October 21, 1866. (The 5th Infantry was consolidated with this regiment.)

| Name | Rank | Address | Service |
|---|---|---|---|
| McNulty, Jas. M. | Surgeon | San Francisco, Cal. | To Feb., 1863; Bd. Ex. S. |
| Randall, Peter W. | Ass't S. | San Quentin, Cal. | To April, 1863. |
| Horne, Geo. H. | Surgeon | 874 N. 4th st., Phila., Pa. | To Sept., 1864; also 2d Cav. and 2d Inf. |
| Cox, V. H. | Ass't S. | | To Feb., 1866; also 5th Inf. |

### 1ST BATTALION MOUNTAINEERS—Mustered out from April 25 to June 14, 1865.

| Name | Rank | Address | Service |
|---|---|---|---|
| Clark, Jonathan | Surgeon | | From June, 1863. |

### 2D BATTALION MOUNTAINEERS—Mustered out from April 16 to July 2, 1866.

| Name | Rank | Address | Service |
|---|---|---|---|
| Horne, Geo. H. | Surgeon | 874 N. 4th st., Phila., Pa. | From Sept. 1865; also 2d Cav. and 1st Inf. |
| Parry, Isaac | " | | To August, 1865. |
| Todd, S. S. | Ass't S. | | To April, 1862; also 4th Inf. |
| Flock, John | " | | To May, 1863. |
| Forsman, James | " | Healdsburg, Cal. | To Sept., 1863. |
| Cassell, F. M. | " | | From March, 1865. |

### 3D BATTALION MOUNTAINEERS—Mustered out July 27, 1866.

| Name | Rank | Address | Service |
|---|---|---|---|
| Brown, Isaac W. | Ass't S. | | To May, 1864. |
| Reid, Robert K. | Surgeon | | To Oct., 1864; also 2d Cav. |
| Kirkpatrick, C. A. | Ass't S. | | To Nov., 1864; also 8th Inf. |

## CALIFORNIA—Continued.

4TH BATTALION MOUNTAINEERS—Mustered out November 30, 1865, and from December 19, 1865, to April 18, 1866.

Elliott, Stephen F...Surgeon.....................................To March, 1862.
Tompkins, Edw'd A..Ass't S.......................................To September, 1863.
Todd, S. S.................Surgeon.....................................To April, 1865; also 2d Inf.
Gelcich, Vincent ... " Los Angeles, Cal..........To Nov., 1865; also 1st Batt. Cav.
Hoffman, David B... Ass't S.......................................To November, 1865.

5TH BATTALION MOUNTAINEERS—Mustered out from November 27 to December 14, 1864. (Veterans and recruits transferred to 1st Infantry.)

Wooster, David........Surgeon...San Francisco, Cal ........To March, 1863.
McKee, Wm. H........ " ...............................................From March, 1863.
Cox, V. H...............Ass't S.........................................From Oct., '62; also 1st Inf.
Hayes, Lewis W...... " ...............................................From March, 1863.

6TH BATTALION MOUNTAINEERS—Mustered out from Oct. 25 to Dec. 20, 1865.

Lippincott, Henry...Ass't S.....Care A. G., U. S. A........To Oct., 1865; in U. S. A.
Tolman, Geo. B........ " San Jose, Cal.................To May, 1865; also 1st Batt. Cav.
Hayes, Wm. W........Surgeon.......................................To October, 1865.
Phelps, Edward........Ass't S.........................................To Surg. 7th Inf. Jan. '65.
Deans, Wm. C......... " ...............................................To May, 1864.

7TH BATTALION MOUNTAINEERS—Mustered out from March 1 to June 28, 1866.

Phelps, Edward ......Surgeon.......................................From Jan., 1865; also 6th Inf.
Davies, Jos. W..........Ass't S.........................................To March, 1865.

8TH BATTALION MOUNTAINEERS—Mustered out October 24, 1865.

Kirkpatrick, C. A.....Surgeon.......................................From April, 1865; also 3d Inf.
Wood, Eugene H.....Ass't S.........................................From March, 1865.

## COLORADO.

1ST CAVALRY—Mustered out at different dates from Oct. 26 to Nov. 18, 1865.

Tolles, Larkin C......Ass't S.....Central City, Col............To January, 1865
Hamilton, J. F.........Surgeon...Salt Lake, Utah............From August, 1861.
Smith, Azor A.........Ass't S.........................................From June, 1863.

2D CAVALRY—Mustered out September 23, 1865.

Akin, Geo. S.............Ass't S.....Harrisonville, Mo...........To July, 1865.
Pollok, Irving J......Surgeon...Georgetown, Col............To July, 1865.
Saville, J. I.............. " ...............................................To November, 1863.

3D CAVALRY—Mustered out from December 28 to December 31, 1864.

Morrision, S. B........Surgeon.......................................To December, 1864.
Burdsall, C. S.........Ass't S.........................................To December, 1864.
Yates, C. P.............. " ...............................................To December, 1864.

## CONNECTICUT.

### 1st Cavalry—Mustered out August 2, 1865.

Hurlburt, Geo. A.. ..Surgeon...Dead ....... ....................From February, 1864.
Buck, Thos. E.........Ass't S.....2710 Jefferson avenue, St. Louis, Mo......... .........From March, 1863.
Bishop, Herbert M... " Norwich, Conn..............A. W. M.
Jarvis, Geo. C......... " Hartford, Conn..............(Not in A. G. R.;) also 7th Inf.; U. S. Ex. S.

### 1st Heavy Artillery—Mustered out September 25, 1865.

Stevens, J. H. P......Ass't S.....Norfolk, Conn................To September, 1862.
Soule, Wm............... " Jewett City, Conn.........To Sept., '62; also 21st Inf.
Bunce H. Clinton..... " Glastonbury, Conn.........To October, 1863.
Hoyt, Henry A........ " Grand Ledge, Mich.........To Dec., 1863; also 6th Inf.
Delevan, J. S........... " Albany, N. Y.................From April 16, 1864, to March, 1865.
Skinner, Samuel W..Surgeon...Toledo, Ohio. ................From June, 1861.
Matson, Nathaniel...Ass't S.....285 Franklin ave., Brooklyn, N. Y....................From April, 1864.
Thomson, Wm. H..... " Fair Haven, Conn...........From June, 1865.
Bentley, Edwin........ " Care A. G., U. S. A.........To Surg. U. S. V. Oct. 1, 1861.
Frost, Frank............ Private Co. D...Norwich or Dayville, Ct..Acted as Hospital Stew'd.
Young, Francis J..... Co. B...Bridgeport, Conn............Acted as Hospital Stew'd.
Hendricks, E. F......Ass't S.....Dead..............................To 15th Inf. Jan., '63.

### 2d Heavy Artillery, (19th Infantry)—Mustered out August 18, 1865.

Phelps, Jerem'h W...Ass't S.....Towington. Conn...........To September, 1862.
Plumb, Henry ........Surgeon...Durango, Col...................A W M.
Andrews, Judson B..Ass't S.....Utica, N. Y,.......................From July, 1863.
Hassard, Robert G... " Harwinton, Conn...........A. W. M.
Buell, Orson.............H. Stew...Norfolk, Conn.
Lawton, John W......Ass't S.....Dead..............................To Ass't S. U. S. A., April, 1863.

### Three Independent Batteries—Mustered out June 11, 1865.

Parkington, Geo. A..H. Stew...New Haven, Conn.........Alleged dead.

### 1st, 2d and 3d Infantry were 3 months organizations.

### 4th Infantry—See 1st Heavy Artillery.

### 5th Infantry—Mustered out July 19th, 1865.

Bennett, Wm. C......Surgeon...Danbury, Conn..............To June, 1863.
Bissell, Evelyn L..... " New Haven, Conn.........From March, 1864. U. S. Ex. S.
Gilson, Andrew J.....Ass't S.....Boston, Mass.....................From January, 1863.
Lewis, John B.........Surgeon...Hartford, Conn...............To Surg. U. S. V., April, 1862.
McClellan, Samuel...Ass't S.....161 W. 10th street, New York city.........................To Jan. 31, 1862; also 13th Inf.

## CONNECTICUT—Continued.

### 6TH INFANTRY—Mustered out August 21, 1865.

Robinson, Myron W..Surgeon...Colchester, Conn...........From May, 1864; has list of sick.
Dibble, Fred. L....... " New Haven, Conn.........To September, 1864.
Hoyt, Henry A........Ass't S.....Grand Ledge, Mich........From April, 1865; also 1st H. A.
Ensign, Robert E.......................Windsor, Vt..................Not in A. G. Report; states that he was Ass't Surg. for 6 months.
Bulkley, Edward......Ass't S.....Dead.

### 7TH INFANTRY—Mustered out July 20, 1865.

Jarvis, Geo. C.........Surgeon...Hartford, Conn...............From Oct., 1862; also 1st Cav. U. S. Ex. S.
Hine, Elmore C.......Ass't S.....1834 Green St., Phila, Pa..To September, 1864.
Bacon, Francis.........Surgeon...New Haven, Conn.........To Surg. U. S. V. Aug., 1862.
Porter, Horace P..... " Claremont, Minn............To 10th Inf. March, 1864.
Woodruff, Jas. H......H. Stew.........................................In 1864.
Shepard, Samuel B...Ass't S.........................................From May 22, 1864.

### 8TH INFANTRY—In service August 31, 1865.

Hamilton, Theo. E...Ass't S.....Springfield, Mass..........From June, 1864.
Stocking, Sabin....... " East Glastonbury, Conn..To April, 1864; also 17th Inf.
Storrs, Melancthon...Surgeon...Hartford, Conn.............To October, 1864.
Holcomb, H. V. C...Ass't S.....Dead...............................To Surg. 15th Inf. Aug., 1862.
Bigelow, Jas. A.......Surgeon...Ottawa, Ill....................From August, 1862.

### 9TH INFANTRY—Mustered out August 3, 1865.

McNeil, Rollin.........Surgeon...New Haven, Conn.........From January, 1865.
Lines, J. F...............Ass't S.....New Haven, Conn.........Not in A. G. R.
Avery, Geo. W......... " Hartford, Conn.............To 1st N. O. Vols. Dec., 1863.
Winsor, Ira C.......... " ...........................................To September, 1863.
Gallagher, Chas A... " Dead...............................Had records.

### 10TH INFANTRY—Mustered out August 25, 1865.

Douglass, A. T.........Surgeon...Kingston. N. Y..............To August, 1862.
Newton, Matthew T.. " Suffield, Conn...................To February, 1864.
Hart, Chas R......... " Bethel, Conn....................From November, 1864.
Pease, Loren H........Ass't S.....Thompsonville, Conn......Dismissed October, 1863.
Page, Henry A........ " ...........................................From February, 1865.
Wright, Nathan H... " Dead...............................From Jan 1865; also 26th Inf.
Porter, Horace P.....Surgeon...Claremont, Minn............To November, 1864.

### 11TH INFANTRY—In service August 31, 1865.

Rogers, Chas H........Ass't S.....Central Village, Conn.....To May, 1863.
Reynolds, Gideon P.. " Guilford Conn..................To September, 1864.
Satterlee, Dwight..... " Dunlap, Iowa..................From March, 1863.
*Mayer, Nathan....... " Hartford, Conn..............Missing March, 1862; also 16th Inf.
Whitcomb, Jas. B.....Surgeon...Dead.

---

* A. G. reports say "Maher."

## CONNECTICUT—Continued.

### 12TH INFANTRY—Mustered out August 12, 1865.

| | | | |
|---|---|---|---|
| Cumming, Jas. R | Surgeon | Bridgeport, Conn | From March, 1865. |
| Lines, Jairus F | Ass't S | New Haven, Conn | From April, 1863. |
| Fletcher, Henry J | Act. Surg | Dead | Was Lieut. Co. D. |
| Hough, E. A | H. Stew | Collinsville, Conn | To December, 1862, (P M.) |
| Carrier, Edmund | A. H. S | Canton, Conn. | |
| Brownell, Wm. R | Surgeon | Dead. | |

### 13TH INFANTRY—In service August 31, 1865.

| | | | |
|---|---|---|---|
| Clary, Geo | Surgeon | New Britain, Conn | From July, 1863. |
| Comings, Benj. N | " | New Britain, Conn | To January, 1863. |
| Clark, Lucius W | Ass't S | Rushville, Ill | From August, 1863. |
| McClellan, Sam'l | " | 161 W. 10th street, New York city. | To Jan. 1865; also 5th Inf. |

### 14TH INFANTRY—Transferred to 2d Heavy Artillery May 30, 1865.

| | | | |
|---|---|---|---|
| Jewett, Levi | Ass't S | 357 W. 14th street, New York city | To January, 1865. |
| Dudley, Fred'k A | Surgeon | Kings Ferry, N. Y | From April, 1863. |
| Tomlinson, Charles | Ass't S | Insane Asylum, Hartford Conn | From Sept., 1863. U. M. |
| Rockwell, Philo. G | " | Aiken, S. C | To March, 1863. |

### 15TH INFANTRY—Mustered out June 27, 1865. (Recruits transferred to the 7th Infantry.)

| | | | |
|---|---|---|---|
| Cowles, Edward O | Ass't S | 10 E. 4th street, New York city | From August, 1862. |
| Smith, Laban A | H. Stew | 180 Chapel street, New Haven, Conn. | |
| Holcomb, H. V. C | Surgeon | Alleged dead. | |
| Hendricks, Eli F | Ass't S | Dead | Also 1st H. A. |

### 16TH INFANTRY—Mustered out June 24, 1865.

| | | | |
|---|---|---|---|
| Mayer, Nathan | Surgeon | Hartford, Conn | From Jan, 1863; also 11th Inf. |
| Warner, Abner S | " | Wethersfield, Conn | To January, 1863. |
| Nickerson, N | Ass't S | Meriden, Conn | To 21st Inf. Jan., 1865. |
| Pease, E. M | " | Honolulu, Sandwich Islands. | To 9th U. S. C. T. Dec., 1863. |

### 17TH INFANTRY—Mustered out July 19, 1865.

| | | | |
|---|---|---|---|
| Stocking, Sabin | Surgeon | East Glastonbury, Conn | From May, 1864; also 8th Inf. |
| Turrill, Henry S | Ass't S | Care A. G. U. S. A | From February, 1864. |
| Hubbard, Robert | Surgeon | Bridgeport, Conn | To December, 1863. |
| McEwen, Robert C | Ass't S | Saratoga Springs, N. Y | To September, 1863. |
| Gregory, Elijah | " | Dead. | |

### 18TH INFANTRY—Mustered out June 27, 1865.

| | | | |
|---|---|---|---|
| Holbrook, Lowell | Surgeon | Thompson, Conn | From May, 1863. |
| Hough, H. W | Ass't S | Putnam, Conn | To March, 1863. |
| Carleton, Chas. M | Surgeon | Norwich, Conn | To April, 1863. |
| North, Wm. B | Ass't S | Dead | To May, 1864. |
| Rowe, Chas. H | " | Dead | From Sept. 1864. |

### 19TH INFANTRY—See 2d Heavy Artillery.

## CONNECTICUT—Continued.

20TH INFANTRY—Original members mustered out June 13, 1865. The rest transferred to the 5th Infantry.

Terry, J. Wadsworth..Surgeon...Englewood, N. J............From August, 1863.
Jewett, Dan Lee......Ass't S.....Watseka, Ill....................From Aug., 1862. U. S. Ex. S.
Brown, Peleg..........H. Stew...Sandwich, Mass.
Casey, Wm. B.........Surgeon...Dead.

21ST INFANTRY—Original members mustered out June 16, 1865. The rest transferred to the 10th Infantry.

Nickerson, N...........Surgeon...Meriden, Conn..................From Jan, 1865; also 16th Inf.
Tennant, Chas. J.....Ass't S.....186 Freemason street, Norfolk, Va..............From July, 1863
Soule, Wm..............Surgeon...Jewett City, Conn...........To Feb., 1863; also 1st H. A.
Lee, J. Hamilton...... " Dead..................................To October, 1864.
Parker, Julian N......H. Stew...S. Manchester, Conn.....Now M. D.
Dixon, Lewis E.......Ass't S.............................................To January 24, 1863.

22D INFANTRY, (9 months)—Mustered out July 7, 1863.

Pratt, Ambrose........Surgeon...Chester, Conn................From Dec., 1862. H. R.
Griswold, Wait R.....Ass't S.....161 Capital avenue, Hartford, Conn.......................From April, 1863.
Curtis, Jonathan S...Surgeon...Hartford, Conn..............To December, 1862.
Pease, Calvin, jr......Ass't S.....Dead.

23D INFANTRY, (9 months)—Mustered out August 31, 1863.

Trowbridge, Wm. H..Surgeon...Stamford, Conn..............From Nov., 1862. H. R.
Benedict, Geo..........Ass't S.....Bethel, Conn...................From March, 1863.
Lyon, Ransom P...... " Dead.........................................To 28th Inf., Nov. 1862.
Dalton, Geo. O........ " ..................................................From Nov. 14, 1862.

24TH INFANTRY, (9 months)—Mustered out September 30, 1863.

Dyer, Benj. W.........H. Stew...Cor. 4th ave. and 30th st., New York city.............Druggist.
Warren, Levi...........Surgeon.. Dead.
Warren, Hiram........Ass't S.....Ellenville, N. Y.

25TH INFANTRY, (9 months)—Mustered out August 26, 1863.

Woods, Wm. B........Surgeon...Somers, Conn.................A. W. M.—H. R.
Gould, Joseph R......H. Stew...Belchertown, Mass.

26TH INFANTRY (9 months)—Mustered out August 17, 1863. (No. H. R, and none with A. G. of Conn.)

Woodward, Ashbel...Surgeon...Franklin, Conn..............From November, 1862.
Phinney, Elisha......Ass't S.....Norwich or Yantic, Conn..From November, 1862.
Wright, Nathan H... " Dead......................................From March, 1863; also 10th Inf.

27TH INFANTRY (9 months)—Mustered out July 27, 1863.

McDonald, Wm. O...Surgeon...117 W. 44th st., N.Y. city..To Surg. U. S. V., May, 1863; also 65th N. Y. Inf.; U. S. Ex. S.
Hills, Thos. M.........Ass't S.....Willimantic, Conn.........Dismissed Feb. 2, 1863.
Treadway, Fred'k S.. " Dead.

## CONNECTICUT—Continued.

### 28th Infantry (9 months)—Mustered out August 28, 1863.

| | | | |
|---|---|---|---|
| Rockwell, Henry | Ass't S. | Port Chester, N. Y. | A. W. M. |
| Lyon, R. P | " | Dead. | Also 23d Inf. |
| Pease, Levi S | " | Dead. | |

### 29th Infantry (Colored)—Mustered out October 24, 1865.

| | | | |
|---|---|---|---|
| Rand, John M | Ass't S. | Detroit, Mich | From February, 1864. |
| Hyde, Joel W | " | 215 Schemerhorn street, Brooklyn, N. Y. | From September, 1864. |
| Stevenson, J. F | Surgeon | Dead. | |
| Crandall, Wm. B | Ass't S. | | To Surg. 23d U. S. C. T., June, 1864. |

## DAKOTA.

### 1st Cavalry—Mustered out May 9, 1865.

| | | | |
|---|---|---|---|
| Wilson, Franklin | Ass't S. | Yankton, Dakota | Not in A. G. R. |

## DELAWARE.

### 1st Battalion Cavalry—Mustered out June 30, 1865.

| | | | |
|---|---|---|---|
| Stewart, Wm | | Princess Anne, Md | Not in A. G. R. |
| McKee, Robert B | Ass't S. | Northumberland, Pa | To June, 1865. |
| Shields, Isaac C | Surgeon | 413 Walnut st., Phila., Pa. | To June, 1864. |
| Hamilton, Wm. N | " | | To Feb., 1863; also 5th Inf. |
| *Kemp, J. McK | Ass't S. | Delaware City, Del | In June, 1863. |

### 1st Infantry—Mustered out July 12, 1865.

| | | | |
|---|---|---|---|
| Maull, D. W | Surgeon | Wilmington, Del | To April, 1865; U. S. Ex. S |
| McCullough, J. W | " | Died March, 1881. | |
| Owens, Fred J | Ass't S. | Vernon, Del | To August, 1864. |
| Groves, Benj B | " | New Castle, Del | From June, 1865. |
| Beun, John E | " | | To April, 1863. |
| Marshall, Samuel | " | | To January, 1863. |

### 2d Infantry—Companies A to G mustered out; rest transferred to 1st Infantry July 1, 1864.

| | | | |
|---|---|---|---|
| Houston, David H | Surgeon | Lewes, Del | From October, 1861. |
| Plunkett, Philip M | Ass't S. | Wilmington, Del | A. W. M. |
| Claypoole, John C | " | | To March, 1865. |
| Babb, Wm. T | " | | To April, 1862. |

### 3d Infantry—Mustered out June 3, 1865.

| | | | |
|---|---|---|---|
| Dawson, Thos. E | Ass't S. | Frederica, Del | To September, 1862. |
| Marshall, Wm | Surgeon | Milford, Del | To September, 1862; also 6th Inf. |
| Wolf, David E | Ass't S. | Georgetown, Del | From October, 1862. |
| Houston, Jos. M | " | | From October, 1862. |

### 4th Infantry—Mustered out June 3, 1865.

| | | | |
|---|---|---|---|
| Smith, Linton | Surgeon | Wilmington, Del | From October, 1864. |
| Lyons, Jas. B | Ass't S. | | To December, 1862. |

* Belonged to the 1st Maryland Infantry (E. S.)

## DELAWARE—Continued.

5TH INFANTRY—Mustered out at different dates from August 6 to 12, 1863.

Hamilton, Wm. N....Surgeon..........................................From June, 1863; also 1st Cav.
Chandler, Jos. H......Ass't S.....Centreville, Del.................From June, 1863.
Naudain, C. B......... " Jennerville, Pa..............From July, 1863.

6TH INFANTRY—Mustered out at different dates from August 22 to September 5, 1863.

Marshall, Wm .........Surgeon...Milford, Del ..... ............From June, 1863; also 3d Inf.
Collens, Wm. T.......Ass't S.....Smyrna, Del.................From June, 1863.
Melvin, Walter ........ " Kennedyville, Md...........From June, 1863.

## DISTRICT OF COLUMBIA.

1ST CAVALRY—Mustered out October 26, 1865.

Northrup, Geo. J.....Ass't S.....Marquette, Mich ............To 1st Me. Cav., August 27, 1864.

1ST INFANTRY—Consolidated with 2d Infantry, February 28, 1865.

Hines, C. M..............Surgeon...Dead.................................To January, 1864.
Meade, Francis W.... " U. S. Marine Hospital, San Francisco, Cal. From Feb., 1864, to Feb. 28, 1865; also 2d Inf.

2D INFANTRY—Mustered out September 12, 1865.

Craigen, Wm. J........Ass't S.....Cumberland, Md.............From October, 1863.
Woodbury, Geo E... " Methuen, Mass ..............From November, 1862.
Marsh, A. R ...........H. Stew...Newark, N. J.
Meade, Francis W....Surgeon...Marine Hosp., San Francisco, Cal. From Feb., 1864; also 1st Inf.
Lane, Edward G......Ass't S............................................To October, 1862.
Hootee, L. C........... " .............................................To May, 1862.
Baldwin, W. O.........Surgeon.........................................To October, 1864.
Keasbey, John B...... " .............................................To February, 1863.

## FLORIDA.

1ST CAVALRY—Mustered out November 17, 1865.

Rossvally, Max........Surgeon..........................................Dismissed Dec., 1864.

2D CAVALRY—Mustered out November 25, 1865.

Gould, T. F ............Surgeon...Jacksonville, Fla............Not in A. G. R.

## ILLINOIS.

1ST CAVALRY—Mustered out July 14, 1862, and December 22, 1862.

Bluthardt, Theo. J...Ass't S.....43 S Peoria st., Chicago, Ill. To Surg. 23d Mo. Inf., April, 1862.
Parker, Henry...... ..Surgeon...Alleged dead. A. W. M.
Kirk, Wm ...............A. A. S ...Atlanta, Ill.

## ILLINOIS—Continued.

### 2D CAVALRY—Mustered out November 22, 1865.

Jones, D. C..............Surgeon...Topeka, Kans..................From October, 1864.
Williams, Joel G......Ass't S..... ..................................From February, 1865.
Cutts, Joseph B.... ..Surgeon...Polo, Ill.............................To September, 1864.
Crane, Andrew J.....Ass't S.....Alleged dead ..................To September. 1862.
Kendall, Reese P.....A. A. S ...Atlanta, Ill.......................Also 11th U. S. C. T.

### 3D CAVALRY—Mustered out September 5, 1864, and October 10, 1865.

Bigelow, A..............Surgeon...Toledo, Ohio...................To October, 1862.
Hunt, J. S............... " 139 E. Madison st., Chicago, Ill...........................From November, 1862.
Orvis, Chas..............Ass't S.....Alleged dead .................From May, 1863
Irwin, Chas. N ........ " Mt. Sterling, Ill ............To September, 1864.
Lanphear, A. H.......Surgeon...Atchison, Kansas, or Springfield, Ill............To December, 1861.

### 4TH CAVALRY—Consolidated with the 12th Cavalry June 14, 1865.

Beadle, Wm. T.........Ass't S.... Bushnell, Ill...................To Surg. 3d U. S. Cav., Nov., 1863
Luce, Hiram C.........Surgeon ..Bloomington, Ill............To November, 1864.
Goodrich, Chas. G ...Ass't S..............................................To May, 1865.
Dow, Darius A.........Surgeon..............................................To April, 1862.
Parsons, Ralph D.....H. Stew...Lake Village, Ind.

### 5TH CAVALRY—Mustered out October 27, 1865.

Ensey, J. B..............Surgeon...Alleged dead .................To December, 1864.
Higgins, C. W ......... " Toledo, Ohio.....................To February, 1863.
Watts, Wm.............. " Alleged dead.....................From March, 1865.
Kendall, Chas. B......Ass't S..............................................A. W. M.

### 6TH CAVALRY—Mustered out November 5, 1865.

Agnew, A. B...........Surgeon...Lamoth, or New Columbia. Ill ......................From March, 1865.
Corbus, J. R............ Ass't S.....La Salle, or Amboy, Ill...From April 1865.
Niglas, J. N.............Surgeon...Peoria, Ill ..........................To January, 1865.
Ray, T. D ................H. Stew...Frankfort, Ill.
Whitmore, Jas. S .....Ass't S..............................................To May, 1862.
Nixon, Madison G.... " ..............................................From April, 1865.
Robinson, H. C........H. Stew...De Soto, Ill.

### 7TH CAVALRY—Mustered out November 4, 1865.

Rigg, Thos. J...........Surgeon...Mt. Carmel, Ill ..............From January, 1865.
Gilbert, A. J............Ass't S..............................................Dismissed Sept., 1864.
Norred, Chas. H...... " Middletown, Ill ..............From April, 1865.
Nesmith, Milton W .. " Waukon, Ia., or Capron, Ill.............................From April, 1865.
Rankin, Clark D .....Surgeon...Alleged dead .................To June. 1862.
Stahl, Daniel........... " ..............................................To Surg., U. S. V., Sept., 1864; also 10th Inf.
Mahr, J. M .............H. Stew...Montana, Kan..................

### 8TH CAVALRY—Mustered out July 17, 1865.

Crawford, S. K........Ass't S.....Warsaw, Mo.....................To June, 1863; also 17th Cav
Hard, Abner.............Surgeon...Aurora, Ill........................From Sept., 1861. H. R.
Nelson, E. L...........Ass't S.....Nevada, Mo.......................From June, 1864.
Stull, Theo. W......... " Dead......................................From February, 1864.

## ILLINOIS—Continued.

### 9TH CAVALRY—Mustered out October 31, 1865.

Bracket, J. W.........Surgeon...Rochester, Ind................To June, 1863.
Christy, Geo. B........ " Alleged dead.................From March, 1863; also 32d Inf.
Hemenway, Stacy.... " Fort Klamath, Oregon....Now A. A. Surg., U. S. A.; also 41st U. S. C. T.
Knox, Wm. A......... " ..................................To January, 1862.
Holliday, Frank A...Ass't S..........................................From February, 1865.
Quast, John M.........H. Stew...931 Autum St., St. Louis, Mo.

### 10TH CAVALRY—The 15th Cavalry was consolidated with this regiment January 26, 1865. Mustered out November 22, 1865.

Wilson, W. E...........Surgeon...Denver, Colo................To October, 1864.
Skilling, J. H...........Ass't S.....Manchester, Ill...............To Aug. 1865; also 15th Cav.
Lathrop, E. L.......... " ................................. From December, 1864.
Shutt, Augustus A...Surgeon......................................To June, 1865.
Adams, Henry F......Ass't S.........................................To December, 1864.
Duncan, Wm. S.. .... " ..................................Dismissed Oct., 1864.
Hofferkamp, H.........H. Stew...Springfield, Ill.

### 11TH CAVALRY—Mustered out September 30, 1865.

Stratton, R. F.........Surgeon...St. Joseph, Mich.............From October, 1862.
Wilcox, J. L............Ass't S.....Loami, Ill.........................From May, 1863.
McMasters, Jas.........Surgeon.........................................To May, 1862.

### 12TH CAVALRY—The 4th Cavalry consolidated with this regiment June 14, 1865. Mustered out May 29, 1886.

McCarthy, Jno.........Ass't S.....Halstead and Randolph Sts., Chicago, Ill.........To February, 1865. D.
Morgan, Asa............Surgeon...Alleged dead.....................From June, 1865; also 1st Iowa Cav.
Foster, Robert J...... " ..................................To June, 1865.
Wentworth, C. E.....Ass't S.........................................To August, 1864.
Higgins, John..........Surgeon...Crown Point, Ind...........To February, 1865.
Morgan, Albert W....Ass't S.........................................To Surg. 37th Inf. March, 1866.
Bedford, Franklin....H. Stew...Compton, Ill.

### 13TH CAVALRY—Mustered out August 31, 1865.

Burks, Jas. F.......... Ass't S.....Cairo, Ill., or Eldorado...To September, 1864.
Storck, Chas.............Surgeon...251 Erie S ., Chicago, Ill..To June, 1863; also 24th Inf.
Willard, E. R..........Ass't S.....65 Watter St., Wilmington, Ill.....................From August, 1863.
Foster, Frank J........ " Carmi. Ill.......................From Apr., 1864 Ex. S.
Lake, Leonard L...... " Belvidere, Ill...................To February, 1862; also 15th Inf.
Bockee, Jacob......... " ..................................To Surg. U. S. V., May, 1862.
Austin, H................ " ..................................To May, 1863.
Carman, J. H...........A. Ass't S. Avoca, Iowa.

### 14TH CAVALRY—Mustered out July 31, 1865.

Bailhache, P. H........Surgeon...U. S. Marine Hospital Ser. From March, 1863; also 19th Inf.
Wilkins, Jno. I.........Ass't S.....Tiskilwa, Ill......................From April, 1863.
Wilson, Geo. A......... " Peoria, Ill.........................To April, 1865.

ILLINOIS—Continued.

15TH CAVALRY—Consolidated with 10th Cavalry January 10, 1865.

Moore, David N........Surgeon...Carlisle, Md....................To January, 1865.
Skilling, Josiah H.....Ass't S.....Manchester, Ill...............From June, 1863; also 10th Cav.
Durham, Jas. A...... H. Stew...Benton, Ill.
Neal, Aaron............ " "
Green, Rob't H.......A. Ass't S.Alma, Ark.

16TH CAVALRY—Mustered out August 19, 1865.

Webber, N. W.........Surgeon...Detroit, Mich................From August, 1864.
Strangland, E. C......Ass't S.......................................From April, 1865.
Parker, Henry........ Surgeon.......................................To June, 1864.

17TH CAVALRY—Mustered out from November 23 to December 22, 1865.

Crawford, S. K........Surgeon...Warsaw, Mo......................To November, 1865; also 8th Cav.
Dow, Samuel A.......Ass't S.....Peoria, Ill........................To November, 1865.

1ST LIGHT ARTILLERY.

Buckner, R. M.........H. Stew...Bolivar, or Buffalo, Mo.
Turner, Wm. D.......Ass't S.....Huntley, Ill......................To Surg. 97th Inf., April 1863; also Col. 11th U. S. C. T.
Woodworth, J. M.....Surgeon.......................................From April, 1863.
Andrews, Edmund... " 6 16th St., Chicago, Ill ...To January, 1863.
Kirk, Wm. F...........Ass't S.....Atlanta, Ill......................Missing since Feb. 28, 1863.

2D LIGHT ARTILLERY.

Ransom, Giles P......Ass't S.....Roscoe, Ill.......................To January, 1863.
Williams, Hezekiah...Surgeon.......................................To February, 1863.

7TH INFANTRY—Mustered out July 9, 1865.

Leonard, Wm. L......Surgeon...Winterset, Iowa.............From Dec., 1863; also 39th Iowa Inf. G.
McFarland, G. B......Ass't S.......................................Dismissed Oct., 1863.
Hamilton, James...... " .......................................To Surg. 120th Inf., Dec., 1863.
Burton, Elijah P...... " .......................................To Surg. 12th Inf., Mar., 1865.
Metcalf, Richard L...Surgeon...712 Locust St., St. Louis, Mo..........................To September, 1863.

8TH INFANTRY—Mustered out May 4, 1866.

Phipps, John M.......Ass't S.....1316 Walnut St., Evansville, Ind..........................To February, 1863.
Trowbridge, S. T......Surgeon...Vera Cruz, Mex.............To July, 1864. U. S. Consul.
Denison, Chas. N..... " Newburgh or Argenta, Ill...........................From October, 1864.
Buck, Wilber P........Ass't S.....Moweaqua, Ill..............From January, 1864; also 17th Inf.
Spalding, C. M........ " .......................................From March, 1865.
Chamberlain, M. A...H. Stew...Winthrop, Iowa.

## ILLINOIS—Continued.

### 9TH INFANTRY—Mustered out August 20, 1864, and July 9, 1865.

| Name | Rank | Residence | Remarks |
|---|---|---|---|
| Allen, Wm. A | Ass't S | Greenville, Ill | To August, 1864. |
| Bundy, S. H | | Metropotis or Carbondale, Ill. | Not in A. G. R. |
| Craig, W. D | Ass't S | Aledo, Ill | To August, 1864. |
| Guelich, Emil | Surgeon | Alton, Ill | To August, 1864. |
| Hamilton, S. M | " | Monmouth, Ill | To April, 1862. U. S. Ex. S. |
| Bigger, David P | " | | From May, 1865; also 102d Inf. |

### 10TH INFANTRY—Mustered out July 4, 1865.

| Name | Rank | Residence | Remarks |
|---|---|---|---|
| Craig, John W | Ass't S | Quincy, Ill | From May, 1862. |
| Ritchey, A. L | Surgeon | 488 S. Market St., Nashville, Tenn | From April, 1865; also 16th Inf. |
| Reeder, I. H | Ass't S | Lacon, Ill | To September, 1864. |
| Stahl, Daniel | " | Alleged dead | To Aug., 1862; also 7th Cav. |
| Everett, Sam'l W | Surgeon | " | To October, 1861. |
| Nichols, Wm P | Ass't S | | From December, 1864. |
| Payne, Henry R | Surgeon | Kansas City, Mo | To November, 1864. |

### 11TH INFANTRY—Mustered out July 14, 1865, and recruits transferred to 8th and 46th Infantry.

| Name | Rank | Residence | Remarks |
|---|---|---|---|
| Hopkins, Myron | Ass't S | Yorkville, Ill | From October, 1864. |
| Long, Owen M | Surgeon | 933 K St , N.W., Washington, D. C | To May, 1864. |
| Hunt, Oliver G | " | State Centre, Iowa | From June, 1864. |
| Briggs, Wm D | Ass't S | | From February, 1865. |
| Dewey, Geo. H | " | Marine, Ill | To May, 1864; also 109th Inf. |

### 12TH INFANTRY—Mustered out July 10, 1865, and recruits transferred to 8th and 46th Infantry.

| Name | Rank | Residence | Remarks |
|---|---|---|---|
| Cady, Wm. F | Surgeon | La Fayette, Ind | To October, 1864. |
| Newell, Wm M | Ass't S | Charles City, Iowa | From July, 1863. |
| Wardner, Horace | Surgeon | Anna. Ill | To April, 1862. |
| Burton, Elijah P | " | New York, Iowa | From March, 1865; also 7th Inf. |
| Swan, Sam'l M | Ass't S | | To Surg. 111th Inf. July, 1864. |

### 13TH INFANTRY—Mustered out June 18, 1864, and recruits transferred to 56th Infantry.

| Name | Rank | Residence | Remarks |
|---|---|---|---|
| Plummer, S. C | Surgeon | Rock Island, Ill | From May, 1861. |
| Thompson, C. A | Ass't S | Jefferson City, Mo | From December, 1862. |
| Hunt, I. Spofford | " | | To July, 1861. |
| Salter, Henry F | " | Poweshiek Co., Iowa | To July, 1863. |
| Law, David H | " | Dixon, Iowa | To November, 1862. |

### 14TH INFANTRY—Mustered out September 16, 1865.

| Name | Rank | Residence | Remarks |
|---|---|---|---|
| Chafee, N. F | Ass't S | Clayton, Mich | To November, 1864. |
| Allen, Geo. T | Surgeon | Alleged dead | To Brig. Surg. Apr ,1862. |
| Kersting, F. W | Ass't S | | To June, 1862. |
| Boyd, Henry W | Surgeon | Alleged dead | From March, 1865; also 144th Inf. |
| Drake, M. C | Ass't S | | To Dec., 1863; also 15th Inf. |
| Davidson, Sam'l A | " | Bradford, Ill | From March, 1865. |
| Stevenson, B. F | Surgeon | Alleged dead | To June, 1864. |

## ILLINOIS—Continued.

### 15TH INFANTRY—Mustered out September 16, 1865.

| Name | Rank | Address | Service |
|---|---|---|---|
| Lake, L. L. | Ass't S. | Belvidere, Ill | To July, 1863; also 13th Cav. |
| Wright, O. P. B. | " | Bradford, Wis | From July, 1865. |
| Buck, Harmon A. | " | | To March, 1862. |
| McKim, Wm. J. | Surgeon | Alleged dead | To March, 1865. |
| Drake, Moses C. | Ass't S. | | To Oct., 1864; also 14th Inf. |

### 16TH INFANTRY—Mustered out July 8, 1865.

| Name | Rank | Address | Service |
|---|---|---|---|
| Githens, Wm. H. | Ass't S. | Hamilton, Ill | To June, 1862; also 78th Inf. |
| Ritchey, A. L. | " | 488 S. Market st., Nashville, Tenn. | To Surg. 10th Inf. April, 1865. |
| Trush, Jacob | " | 144 Broadway, Cincinnati, Ohio, or Dallas, Ill. | To September, 1864. |
| Watson, Louis | Surgeon | Ellis, Kans., or Quincy, Ill | To December, 1864. |
| Dodds, F. S. | Ass't S. | Anna, Ill. | To November, 1864. |

### 17TH INFANTRY—Mustered out June 4, 1864, and veterans and recruits transferred to 8th Infantry.

| Name | Rank | Address | Service |
|---|---|---|---|
| Buck, Wilber P. | Ass't S. | Moweaqua, Ill | From Jan. 1864; also 8th Inf. |
| McDowell, J. R. | H. Stew. | Lewiston, Ill. | |
| Tompkins, C. B. | Surgeon | Lewiston, Ill | To June, 1864. |
| Kellogg, Lucius D. | " | | To June, 1863. |
| Penniman, H. H. | Ass't S. | | To Surg. 5th U. S. C. H. Artillery Nov., 1863. |

### 18TH INFANTRY—Mustered out July 8 and December 16, 1865.

| Name | Rank | Address | Service |
|---|---|---|---|
| Hipolite, Wm. W. | Ass't S. | Devall's Bluff, Ark | To July 1863; also 29th Wis. Inf. and 11th U. S. C. T. |
| Ormsby, O. B. | " | Murphysborough, Ill | To June, 1863. |
| Burr, C. S. | Surgeon | | From November, 1865. |
| Watson, F. W. | Ass't S. | Eureka, Kans. | To September, 1865; also 141st Inf. |
| Davis, Henry W. | Surgeon | Alleged dead | To June, 1864. |
| Layman, S. J. | A. Ass't S. | Tamaroa, Ill. | |

### 19TH INFANTRY—Mustered out July 8 and 9, 1864.

| Name | Rank | Address | Service |
|---|---|---|---|
| Bogue, R. G. | Surgeon | 9 Wash. Place, Chicago, Ill | From August, 1861. |
| Bailhache, P. H. | Ass't S. | U. S. Marine Hos. Service. | To Feb., 1863; also 14th Cav |
| Little, Chas. F. | " | | From February, 1863. |
| Southwick, G. W. | " | | To October, 1863. |

### 20TH INFANTRY—Mustered out July 20, 1865.

| Name | Rank | Address | Service |
|---|---|---|---|
| Goodbrake, Chris. | Surgeon | Clinton, Ill | To September, 1864. |
| Richards, Rolla T. | " | | From November, 1864. |
| Bailey, F. K. | Ass't S. | | To September, 1862. |

### *21ST INFANTRY—Mustered out December 16, 1865.

| Name | Rank | Address | Service |
|---|---|---|---|
| Reat, James L. | Surgeon | Tuscola, Ill. | From August, 1864. |
| Seeley, E. M. | " | Pittsfield, Ill | To May 1864. |
| Ten Broeck, S. B. | Ass't S. | Paris, Ill | To January, 1863. |
| Link, John E. | " | Terre Haute, Ind. | To June, 1864. |

*General Grant's old regiment.

ILLINOIS—Continued.

22D INFANTRY—Mustered out July 7, 1864; veterans and recruits transferred to 42d Infantry.

Brown, Isaac W.......Ass't S.....Winchester, Kans, or Sparta, Ill................From February, 1863.
Woodward, Benj......Surgeon...Olathe, Kans................From October, 1862.
Fitzer, John...........Ass't S.....................................To November, 1861.
Collins, Russell J..... " ................................From August, 1862.
Coatsworth, Geo......Surgeon.....................................To May, 1862.

23D INFANTRY—Mustered out July 24, 1865.

Taylor, John S........Surgeon...Chicago, Ill.................. From January, 1865.
Wyner, Wm. D........ " ..................................To December, 1862.
Gregg, Patrick......... " Rock Island, Ill.............To September, 1864.
Stinson, Chas. W......Ass't S.....................................To September, 1864.
Jared, L. D............. " ..................................From March, 1865.

24TH INFANTRY—Mustered out August 6, 8, and 15, 1864, and July 31, 1865.

Stork has.............Ass't S.....494 W. Lake Street, Chicago, Ill......................To March, 1862; also 13th Cav.
Wild, Theo ............ " 327 Milwaukee avenue, Chicago, Ill ..............To August, 1864.
*Fuller, S. L............Surgeon...88 Griswold Street, Detroit, Mich................To August, 1864.
Wagner, Wm.......... " Chicago, Ill......................To November, 1863.
Thomas, Jerome B...Ass't S.....Nat'l Mil. Home, Dayton, Ohio ......................To August, 1864.

25TH INFANTRY—Mustered out September 5, 1864, and September 21, 1865.

Brown, Myron S......Ass't S.....Urbana, Ill.......................To September, 1864.
Brown, R. H........... " Kirksville, Mo ..............To January, 1863.
Blount, Jos.............Surgeon...Byron, Ill.........................To December, 1863.
Clark, Dexter S........ " Rockford, Ill.. ...............To September, 1864.
Winans, Henry C..... " ..................................To December, 1861.
McHugh, John.........Ass't S.....................................To October, 1861.

26TH INFANTRY—Mustered out July 20, 1865.

Taylor, M. K..........Surgeon...Care A. G., U. S. A........To Surg. U. S. V. Aug., 1862.
Whitehill, Jas. C...... " ..................................To Surg. U. S. V. Nov., 1862.
Sheldon, Samuel A...Ass't S.....Irving, Wis ....................To January, 1865.
Woodward, Chas. E.. " ..................................To July, 1863.
Reilly, Frank W......Surgeon.....................................To May, 1865.
Mann, Harvey A......Ass't S.....................................From May, 1865.
Steel, Ezra A........... " ..................................To October, 1862.

27TH INFANTRY—Mustered out September 20, 1864; veterans and recruits transferred to 9th Infantry.

Bowman, E. H.........Surgeon...Pawnee Agency, I. T., or Andalusia, Ill.............From September, 1861.
Dickerhoff, A. J.......Ass't S.....Victoria, Mo.....................From February, 1863.
Barrell, Henry C...... " ..................................To Surg. 38th Inf. Dec., 1863.

---

*In charge of Pioneer Corps, Army of the Cumberland.

ILLINOIS—Continued.

28TH INFANTRY—Mustered out March 15, 1866.

| Name | Rank | Residence | Remarks |
|---|---|---|---|
| Kemper, John | Surgeon | Industry, or Galesburg, Ill | From November, 1864. |
| Kelly, A. W | " | Leadville, Colo., or Chicago, Ill | To August, 1864. |
| Sloan, Robert J | Ass't S | | From January, 1866. |
| Bringhurst, James | Surgeon | | From May, 1862. |
| West, Wm. F | " | Alleged dead | To April, 1863. |

29TH INFANTRY—Mustered out August 31 and September 1, 1864, and November 6, 1865.

| Name | Rank | Residence | Remarks |
|---|---|---|---|
| Bumstead, S. J | Ass't S | Decatur, Ill | From July, 1863; also 131st Inf. |
| Cheaney, S. L | Surgeon | Harrisburgh, Ill | To October, 1865. |
| Johnson, F. F | Ass't S | Stonefort, or Eldorado, Ill | To March, 1862. |
| Cheaney, Philip B | " | Alleged dead | From May, 1863. |
| Tuttle, J. W | Surgeon | | To October, 1862. |
| Mills, Lucius | Ass't S | | To August, 1863. |
| Downey, Jacob | H. Stew | Braddock, Pa. | |
| Neil, Andrew J | " | Harrisburg, Ill. | |

30TH INFANTRY—Mustered out July 17, 1865

| Name | Rank | Residence | Remarks |
|---|---|---|---|
| Gordon, Wm. A | Surgeon | Chester, Ill | To August, 1864. |
| Feland, Wm | Ass't S | Hopkinsville, Ky | To December, 1863. |
| Moore, David N | Surgeon | | To March, 1863. |

31ST INFANTRY—Mustered out July 19, 1865.

| Name | Rank | Residence | Remarks |
|---|---|---|---|
| Million, J. L | Surgeon | Springfield, Ill | To January, 1863. |
| Van Dyke, E | Ass't S | Shelbyville, Ill | To August, 1864. |
| Whitnell, David T | Surgeon | | To June, 1864. |
| Suhfras, Gustave | " | | From January, 1865. |
| Dunn, David M | H. Stew | Minneapolis, Kans | From June, 1862, to May, 1865. |

32D INFANTRY—Mustered out September 16, 1865.

| Name | Rank | Residence | Remarks |
|---|---|---|---|
| Gilmer, John G | Ass't S | Lincoln, or Concordia, Kans | To April, 1865. D. |
| King, W. H. H | " | Jacksonville, Ill | From April, 1865. |
| Christy, Geo. B | " | Dunlap, Iowa | To Nov., 1862; also 9th Cav. |
| Edgar, Wm. S | Surgeon | Alleged dead | To August, 1865. |

33D INFANTRY—Mustered out November 24, 1865.

| Name | Rank | Residence | Remarks |
|---|---|---|---|
| Antis, H. T | Ass't S | Geneseo, Ill | To 47th Inf. June, 1865. |
| Rex, Geo. P | Surgeon | Reaville, N. J | From August, 1861. |
| Rex, Oliver P | Ass't S | | From September, 1865. |
| May, Edwin | " | | To 98th Inf. Aug., 1864. |
| Wallace, Hugh L | " | | To October, 1865. |
| Abbott, Nathan H | " | | To November, 1862. |

34TH INFANTRY—Mustered out July 12, 1865.

| Name | Rank | Residence | Remarks |
|---|---|---|---|
| Hewett, Geo. W | Ass't S | Said to be dead. | |
| Barker, Franklin | " | | From May, 1865. |
| Herrick, Orson Q | Surgeon | | To January, 1865. |
| Hostetter, John L | " | Alleged dead | From May, 1865. |
| Hudson, A. S | " | | To March, 1862. |
| McNeil, Francis A | " | | To October, 1861. |
| Johns, C. A | H. Stew | Penrose, Ill. | |

ILLINOIS—Continued.

35TH INFANTRY—Mustered out September 27, 1864, and January 2, 1865.

Chenowith, W. J......Surgeon...Decatur, Ill..................To December, 1862.
Hawley, S. B.......... " ..................................From Dec., 1862; 36th Inf.
Tidball, David L......Ass't S..................................From September, 1861.
Wylie, J. D.............. " ..................................From December, 1862.
Dewatney, J. F........H. Stew...Boody, Ill......................Now M. D.
Allen, J. N..............A. Ass't S.Mt. Sterling, Ill.

36TH INFANTRY—Mustered out October 8, 1865.

Hatch, J. A.............Surgeon...Kentland, Ind..............From May, 1865.
Pierce, Wm. P.........Ass't S.....Hoopeston, or Lamont, Ill..............................To 88th Inf. Feb., 1863.
Lytle, Francis W......Surgeon...Lebanon, Ill..................To April, 1865; H. R.; also 51st Inf.
Hawley, Sidney B.....Ass't S..................................To Sept., 1862; also 35th Inf.
Young, Delos W......Surgeon..................................To February, 1863.
Charles, Edward W..Ass't S..................................From Aug., 1865; also 60th Inf.

37TH INFANTRY—Mustered out May 15, 1866.

Murphey, John........Ass't S..................................To 92d U. S. C. T. Oct., 1863.
Clark, E. A............. " ..................................To 8th Mo. Cav. March, 1863.
Humeston, L. F.......Surgeon...Alleged dead...................To September, 1864.
Morgan, Albert W.... " ..................................From March, 1866; also 12th Cav.

38TH INFANTRY—Mustered out March 20, 1866.

DeBall, J. M............Ass't S....Gerley, or Fontana, Kan..To January, 1866.
Stewart, D. W.......... " Ottumwa, Iowa..............Jo January, 1863.
Tichenor, E. J.......... " Lebanon, Ohio.................To July, 1863.
Barrell, Henry C......Surgeon...Alleged dead...................From Jan., 1864; also 27th Inf.
Teed, John L........... " Kansas City, Mo..............To June, 1863.

39TH INFANTRY—Mustered out December 6, 1865.

Clark, Chas. M.........Surgeon...Marengo, or Selma, Ill., Kans..............................From June, 1865. H. R.
Woodward, Wm......Ass't S..................................To 58th Inf. April, 1865.
Blake, Samuel C......Surgeon..................................To June, 1862.
Crozier, James.........Ass't S..................................From December, 1862.

40TH INFANTRY—Mustered out July 24, 1865.

Edwards, J. W........Ass't S.....Mendota, Ill....................To September, 1864.
Elliott, Wm. M.......Surgeon...Alleged dead....................To February, 1864.
Thompson, Sam W... " ..................................To June, 1862.
Graham, Wm........... " Dead.................................From April, 1864.
Turner, Will E........Ass't S.....Ft. Benton, Montana......From May, 1865.

41ST INFANTRY—Mustered out August 20, 1864; veterans and recruits consolidated with 53d Infantry December 31, 1864.

Coleman, J. W.........Ass't S.....Monticello. Ill..................To November. 1864.
Gray Wm. M...........Surgeon...Lebanon, Ohio, or Petersburg. Ill.................To March, 1862; also 60th and 63d Inf.
Carle, Chas.............. " Alleged dead....................To Aug., 1864; also 46th Inf.
Warmoth, Geo. M....Ass't S.....Perkins, Ky.....................From Dec., 1862; also 53d Inf.

## ILLINOIS—Continued.

### 42D INFANTRY—Mustered out December 16, 1865.

Goddard, J. H.........Surgeon...Sedgwick, Kans..............From May, 1865. H. R.
Hanson, Zenas P...... " 44 S. Curtis street, Chicago, Ill.............................From May, 1863.
Roller, E. O. F.........Ass't S.....129 22d st., Chicago, Ill...To 55th Inf. Nov., 1861.
Mills, Andrew J...... " Halstead, Kans.............To April, 1865.
Fitch, T. D...............Surgeon......................................To April, 1863.
Powell, E............... " ..........................................To January, 1862.

### 43D INFANTRY—Mustered out from August 26, 1864, to May 8, 1865, and November 30, 1865.

Starklaff, H. M.........Surgeon...Main and Shermer streets, Station B, St. Louis, Mo. To December, 1864.
Hartmann, A. K......Ass't S.....St. Louis, Mo. (79).........To December, 1864.
Funk, Julius............ " ..........................................To March, 1864.

### 44TH INFANTRY—Mustered out September 25, 1865.

Radmore, Chas. C....Surgeon...Lincoln, Nebr..............To Dec., 1861; also 107th Inf.
*Carter, Wm. D.......Ass't S.....Nashville, Ill...............From October, 1862.
Weitze, Ferdinand...Surgeon...Alleged dead...............To April, 1863.
Merrifield, Emery A. " Macon City, Mo.............From May, 1863; also 58th Inf.

### 45TH INFANTRY—Mustered out July 12, 1865.

Gaskill, J. R. M.......Surgeon...Maine Mills, Minn..........From July, 1865.
Ormsby, O. B.......... " Murphysboro, Ill.............To October, 1864.
Conant, John..........Ass't S.....................................To December, 1863.
Lyman, Wm............ " ..........................................To July, 1863.
Riley, Frank W........ " ..........................................To February, 1863.
Kittoe, Edward D ...Surgeon...Alleged dead..................To April, 1863.

### 46TH INFANTRY—Mustered out January 20, 1866.

Bradshaw, B. H.......Surgeon...Orangeville, Ill..............From Dec., 1864. H. R.
De Witt, Julius N....Ass't S.....................................From December, 1864.
Carle, Charles......... " ..........................................To 41st Inf., April, 1862.
De Puy, Elias C ......Surgeon...Alleged dead..................To November, 1864.

### 47TH INFANTRY—Mustered out January 21, 1866.

Antis, Henry T........Surgeon...Geneseo, Ill...................From June, 1865; also 33d Inf.
Andrews, L. M........Ass't S.....Alleged dead..................To October, 1864.
Lucas, Geo. L ... .....Surgeon...Albion, Idaho.................To October, 1864.
Babb, Timothy.........Ass't S.....................................To August, 1863.

### 48TH INFANTRY—Mustered out August 15, 1865.

Goslin, Asher..........Surgeon...Oregon, Mo.....................To October, 1864.
Hill, Wm................ " Bloomington, Ill.............To April, 1862.
Shearer, M. M......... " Santa Rosa, Cal..............From Feb., 1865. H. R.
Young, S. J ............Ass't S.....Terre Haute, Ind............To 79th Inf. Feb., 1863.
Rogers, Lemuel H ... " Mackinaw, Ill..................To April, 1865.
Williams, Thomas.... " ..........................................To March, 1863.
Corwin, Eden M....... " ..........................................To September, 1864.

### 49TH INFANTRY—Mustered out September 9, 1865.

Beattie, A. B..........Ass't S.....Red Bud, Ill.....................To April, 1862.
Medcalf, Wm. H......Surgeon...Chicago, Ill......................To January, 1865.
Marlow, And.......................Coultersville, Ill...............Not in A. G. R.
Mercer, S. F. F........Surgeon ..Antone, Kans..................A. W. M
Black, James A........Ass't S.....................................From March, 1863.

* Charges fee.

ILLINOIS—Continued.

50TH INFANTRY—Mustered out July 13, 1865.

Kendall, H. W.........Surgeon...514 Main st., Quincy, Ill..To October, 1864.
Williams, Jas. A...... " ............................ .....From December, 1864.
Bane, Gardner H.....Ass't S.......................................To November, 1862.
Pickett, Albert G..... " Shelbyville, Ind., (old)....To October, 1864.

51ST INFANTRY—Mustered out September 25, 1865.

Hunt, Wm. C. ........Surgeon...293 Chicago avenue, Chicago, Ill.......................To April, 1862.
Magee, Thos. L........ " Prairie City, Ill..............From May, 1863. "G."
Scott, John H.........Ass't S.....Alleged dead..................From July, 1865.
Lytle, Francis W..... " Lebanon, Ill........................To 36th Inf. May, 1863.
Elliott, Wm. W........ " Damiansville or Jamestown, Ill.....................To June, 1865.
Weeks, J. F ............Surgeon...........................................To April, 1863.
Pashley, John S ......Ass't S............................................To November, 1862.

52D INFANTRY—Mustered out July 6, 1865.

Humphrey, Wesley...Ass't S.....Moberly, Mo.....................To 55th U. S. C. T. May, 1863. Ex. S.
Rohr, Geo. W..........Surgeon...Rockford, Ill......................From June, 1864.
Guild, P. K..............Ass't S ....Alleged dead .................To March, 1862.
Arndt, Peter F....... " ...............................................From August, 1864.
Winchester, Edgar...Surgeon...Alleged dead..................To April, 1864.
Angell, Leland H..... " Alleged dead .................To March, 1862.
Hitchcock, Geo. J.....H. Stew...Rockford, Ill.. ...............From Oct. 1861, to Dec., 1864.

53D INFANTRY—Mustered out July 22, 1865.

Welch, Wm. W........Surgeon.. Galesburg,or Wataga, Ill. To January, 1865.
Harris, J. O ............Ass't S ....Ottawa, Ill .........................To November, 1862.
Warmoth, Geo. M.....Surgeon...Perkins, Ky .......................From Feb., 1865; also 41st Inf.
Zeising, Henry.........Ass't S.............................................From March, 1865.
Smith, Geo. O ......... " ...............................................To November, 1864.

54TH INFANTRY—Mustered out October 15, 1865.

Chapman, N. W ......Ass't S.....Tuscola. Ill.........................To October, 1862.
Lee, E. A ................Surgeon...Alleged dead ....................To May, 1865.
Dodge, Josiah H......Ass't S ....Pana, Ill ...............................Missing Dec., 1862. "D."
Johnson, Charles T.. " Vermillion, Ill.................From August, 1865.
Wilkins, Thos.......... " ...............................................To May, 1862.
Lycan, Leander.......Surgeon...Atlantic, Iowa..................From June, 1865.
Field, L. J...............H. Stew...Elliottstown, Ill.

55TH INFANTRY—Mustered out August 14, 1865.

Winne, Chas............Ass't S.....Kansas City, Mo............To 77th Inf. Dec., 1862.
Newell, Orlando W.. " Henry, Ill.........................To August, 1863.
Roler, E. O. F.........Surgeon...129 22d st., Chicago, Ill...To Oct., 1864; also 42d Inf. U. S. Ex. S.
Tompkins, John B ...Ass't S.....Elmwood, Ill.....................From May, 1865.
Smith, John T......... " Linn, Iowa. .......................To January, 1865.
Tompkins, Chas B...Surgeon.......................................... From December, 1864.

56TH INFANTRY (Mechanic Fusileers)—Mustered out January 28, February 1 and 5, 1862.

Higgins, John..........Surgeon...........................................From November, 1861.
Norton, John C.......Ass't S............................................From December, 1861.

ILLINOIS—Continued.

56TH INFANTRY—On the expiration of service the original members, (except veterans,) en route to the State to be mustered out, were lost at sea on board the steamer General Lyon, off Cape Hatteras, N. C., March 31, 1865. Veterans and recruits were mustered out August 12, 1865.

Poindexter, R.........Ass't S.....Thompsonville, Ill.........To October, 1862.
Thompson, F. B......Surgeon...Albion, Ill..........................To November, 1862.
Whitmire, Jas L...... " Metamora, Ill.....................To July, 1863.
Morris, Geo..............Ass't S..................................................To November, 1864.

57TH INFANTRY—Mustered out July 7, 1865.

Zearing, James R.....Surgeon...Dead..................................From September, 1861.
Crossly, Geo W........Ass't S.....Alleged dead....................To March, 1865.
Bishop, Isaac N........ " ..................................................From June, 1863.

58TH INFANTRY—Mustered out February 7, 1865, and April 1, 1866.

Crawford, H. M........Surgeon...St. Charles, Ill..................To February, 1865. G.
Heidemann, G. F.....Ass't S.....Elmhurst, Ill.....................To February, 1865. G.
Harvey, Jos. E........ " Cherokee Co., Kans........From May, 1865.
Woodward, Wm......Surgeon...Dead..................................From April, 1865.
Merrifield, Emery A..Ass't S...................................................To 44th Inf. May, 1863.
Leslie, A. G............ " ..................................................From May, 1865.
Manning, Leonard...H. Stew...Garfield, Kans..............From Jan., 1864, to Nov., 1865.

59TH INFANTRY—Mustered out December 8, 1865.

Bunce, Chas.............Surgeon...Woodhull, Ill.....................From September, 1863.
Kerr, Chas...............Ass't S.....Pawnee, Ill.........................From April, 1865.
McChesney, C..........................68 W. 11th st., Cincinnati, O..........................Not in A. G. R.
Maynard, Henry J...Ass't S....Cheyenne, W. T............To 1st Ark. Sept., 1862.
Kelley, Alonzo W.....Surgeon..................................................To August, 1863.

60TH INFANTRY—Mustered out July 31, 1865.

Doods, F. S.............Ass't S....Anna, Ill..........................To November, 1864.
Gray, W. M.............Surgeon...Lebanon, O., or Petersburg, Ill A. W. M.; also 41st and 63d Inf.
Miller, J. T............... " Urbana, Ill.......................To November, 1862.
Shirriff, John A.......Ass't S..................................................To May, 1863.
Charles, Edward W.. " ..................................................From April, 1865; also 36th Inf.

61ST INFANTRY—Mustered out September 8, 1865.

Anthony, Julius P...Surgeon...Sterling, Ill.......................From Nov., 1863; also 127th Inf. Alleged dead.
Knapp, Geo. H.........Ass't S....5th and Olive streets, St. Louis, Mo. To February, 1864.
Clemmens, L. D......Surgeon...Alleged dead.................To August, 1862.

62D INFANTRY—Mustered out May 2, 1865, and March 6, 1866.

Bridges, V. R..........Ass't S....Mattoon, Ill......................To 126th Inf., Dec., 1863.
McKinney, J. W......Surgeon...Camargo, Ill......................To August, 1862; also 63d Infantry
Rhodes, O. H..........................Baldwin, Ill......................Not in A. G. R.
Hatch, Seth C.........Surgeon...Barry, Ill..........................From Jan., 1866. Dead.
Wundt, C. L............ " ..................................................To February, 1863.

## ILLINOIS—Continued.

### 63D INFANTRY—Mustered out July 13, 1865.

McKinney, J. W......Surgeon...Camargo, Ill......................To April, 1865; also 62d Inf.
Robinson, H. C........H. Stew...De Soto, Ill.
Hall, Lyman............Ass't S....Savoy, Ill.......................Dismissed Dec , 1862.
Gray, Wm. M..........Surgeon...Lebanon, Ohio...............To Sept., 1862; also 41st and 60th Inf.
Lodge, Alex. A........ " ..................................From June, 1865.
Barton, Edward E...H. Stew...Urbana, Kans.

### 64TH INFANTRY—Mustered out July 11, 1865.

Roesch, Otto E........Ass't S....Jerseyville, Ill...............From August, 1864.
Mix, H. A................Surgeon...Oregon, Ill......................From May, 1865.
Stewart, J. T.......... " 705 Main st., Peoria, Ill...To December, 1864.
Holton, Noble.........Ass't S....Peoria, Ill.......................To April, 1863.

### 65TH INFANTRY—Mustered out July 13, 1865.

Brown, Ira...............Surgeon...Milford, Ill, (old)............To May, 1865.
Parks, Geo. H......... " ..................................To July, 1864.
Mesler, Henry T......Ass't S.............................................To April, 1863.
Bostock, F. H.........H. Stew...Chatsworth, Ill.

### 66TH INFANTRY—Mustered out April 26, and July 7, 1865.

Pogue, Jos.................Surgeon...Edwardsville, Ill...........From August, 1862.
Whitmore, J. S......................Metamora, Ill.................Not in A. G. R.
Stephenson, R. H.....Ass't S....Petersburgh, Ill.............A. W. M.
Young, John W.......Surgeon.............................................Dismissed August, 1862.
Vogel, Edward........Ass't S....Addison, Ill.....................To June, 1863.

67TH to the 71ST INFANTRY were Three Months' organizations.

### 72D INFANTRY—Part mustered out August, 7, 1865, the rest transferred to 33d Infantry.

Bucher, Chas. A......Ass't S....439 Madison street, Chicago, or Batavia, Ill. From August, 1864.
Powell, Edwin.........Surgeon...Chicago, Ill.......................From August, 1862.
Durham, Benj., Jr...Ass't S.............................................To Ass't S. U. S. V. June, 1864.
Beers, Edwin A...... " .............................................To April, 1864.

### 73D INFANTRY—Mustered out June 12, 1865.

Pond, George O......Surgeon...Camp Point, Ill...............From August, 1862.
Stephenson, R. E....Ass't S.............................................To November, 1863.
Rich, Kendall E...... " .............................................To September, 1863.
McPherson, H. C..... " .............................................From May, 1864.

### 74TH INFANTRY—Part mustered out June 10, 1865, the rest transferred to 36th Infantry.

Strong, Henry.........Ass't S....Iola, Kans.........................To March, 1863; H. R.; also 90th Inf.
Cotes, Albert L........ " .............................................From January, 1865.
Ellinwood, Chas N...Surgeon.............................................From September, 1862.
Fisher, Chesseldon...Ass't S.............................................To 75th Inf. July, 1863.

### 75TH INFANTRY—Mustered out June 12, 1865.

Corbus, J. C............Ass't S....Mendota, Ill.....................To January, 1863.
Phillips, G. W.........Surgeon...West Las Animas, Colo...To May, 1863
Ravenot, O. P. F..... " 83 13th and Place sts., Chicago, Ill. From February, 1865.
Uutley, Henry.........Ass't S....Sterling, Ill.......................To December, 1862.
Fisher Chesseldon....Surgeon.............................................To Nov., 1864; also 74th Inf.

## ILLINOIS—Continued.

76TH INFANTRY—Part mustered out July 22, 1865, the rest transferred to 37th Infantry.

| Name | Rank | Address | Remarks |
|---|---|---|---|
| Ridgway, E | Ass't S | Morris, Ill | From August, 1862. Alleged dead. |
| Blades, Franklin | Surgeon | Iroquois, Co., Ill | To March, 1864. |
| Babcock, Wm. A | " | Alleged dead | From May, 1864 |

77TH INFANTRY—Mustered out July 10, 1865.

| Name | Rank | Address | Remarks |
|---|---|---|---|
| Allen, Joel | H. Stew | Nebraska, Ill | Also 84th Inf. |
| Stoner, John | Ass't S | Tyronza, Ark., or Minonk, Ill. | A. W. M. |
| Winne, Chas | Surgeon | Sandwich, Ill., or Kansas City, Mo. | From Dec; 1862; also 55th Inf. |
| Sigler, Wm. T | Ass't S | | To 130th Inf., June, 1865. |
| Cowan, J. M | " | | To January, 1865. |

78TH INFANTRY—Part mustered out June 7, 1865; the rest transferred to 34th Infantry.

| Name | Rank | Address | Remarks |
|---|---|---|---|
| Githens, Wm. H | Ass't S | Hamilton, Ill | From May, 1863; also 11th Inf. |
| Moss, Sam'l C | Surgeon | Burlington, Iowa | From August, 1863. |
| McIntire, E. S | Ass't S | | To March, 1863. |
| Jordan, Thos. M | Surgeon | 156 Washington street, Chicago, Ill. | To April, 1863. |
| Creel, D. M | H. Stew | Industry, Ill. | |

79TH INFANTRY—Part mustered out June 12, 1865; the rest transferred to 42d Infantry.

| Name | Rank | Address | Remarks |
|---|---|---|---|
| Young, S. J | Surgeon | Terre Haute, Ind | To Feb., 1865; also 48th Inf. |
| Wheeler, Thos. J | " | Sandborn, Ill | From March, 1865 |
| McAllister, Henry C | Ass't S | Muscatine, Iowa | To 98th Inf., June, 1863. |
| Ringland, Geo A | " | Kansas, Ill. | |
| Hester, Benj. R | H. Stew | Ridge Farm, Ill. | |

80TH INFANTRY—Part mustered out June 10, 1865; the rest transferred to 38th Infantry.

| Name | Rank | Address | Remarks |
|---|---|---|---|
| Clendenin, Moses W | Ass't S | Rockwood, Ill | To May, 1865. |
| McDill, David | Surgeon | Burlington, Iowa | From July, 1864; also 84th Inf. |
| Abbott, Nathan W | " | 145 S. Clark street, Chicago, Ill. | To April, 1864. Dead. |
| Barrey, E. M H | Ass't S | | To July, 1864. |
| Rogers, E | " | | To February, 1863. |

81ST INFANTRY—Part mustered out August 5, 1865; the rest transferred to 58th Infantry.

| Name | Rank | Address | Remarks |
|---|---|---|---|
| Dyer, Lewis | Surgeon | Duquoin, Ill | From August, 1862. |
| Hamilton, Samuel | Ass't S | Thompsonville, Ill | To December, 1862. |
| Groesbeck, John W | " | Harvard, Ill | From December, 1864. |
| Neely, Isaac M | " | | To June, 1863. |

82D INFANTRY—Mustered out June 9, 1865.

| Name | Rank | Address | Remarks |
|---|---|---|---|
| Brendel, Emil | Ass't S | Cedar Rapids, Iowa, or Peoria, Ill. | To May, 1863. |
| Boerner, Chas. E | Surgeon | Venedy, or Johanesburgh, Ill. | From March, 1864. |
| *Schloetzer, Geo | " | Chicago, Ill., or Good Heart, Mich. | To January, 1864. |
| Deitzel, Herman | Ass't S | | From April, 1865. |
| Brown, John R | " | | Dismissed July, 1863. |
| Bergh, Oscar J | " | | To January, 1863. |

* Charges fee $25.

## ILLINOIS—Continued.

83D INFANTRY—Mustered out June 26, 1865; recruits transferred to 61st Infantry.

Cooper, E. H ........... Ass't S..... Henderson, Ill................ From May, 1865.
Cooper, E. S............ Surgeon... Henderson, Ill.......... .... From November, 1862.
Cuthbert, W. L........ Ass't S..... Monmouth, Ill.................. From January, 1863.
Morris, Richard ........ " Lawrence, Kans ............ To Surgeon 103d Inf., Nov., 1862.
McClanahan, J. P..... " Alexis, Ill........................ To April, 1864.

84TH INFANTRY—Part mustered out June 8, 1865; the rest transferred to 21st, Infantry.

McDill, David.......... Ass't S..... Des Moines, or Burlington, Iowa. To Surgeon 80th Inf. June, 1864.
Marshall, S. W......... " Keithsburg, or Sparta, Ill.. From January, 1865.
Marshall, E. L......... " Keithsburg, Ill............... To February, 1863.
Hunter, Frank W..... " .................................... To September, 1864.
Kyle, Jas. P ............ Surgeon... Alleged dead ........ ........ From September, 1862
Blackburn, Alex ...... H. Stew... Lafayette, Ind
Allen, Joel .............. " Nebraska, Ill ................ Also 77th Inf.
Robinson, Jos. W..... " Sheldon, Ill.

85TH INFANTRY—Mustered out June 5, 1865.

Dieffenbacher, P. L.. Surgeon... Havana, Ill ..................... From July, 1864.
Patterson, Jas. C ..... Ass't S.......................................... To April, 1864.
Southwick, G. W...... " .................................... To May, 1865.

86TH INFANTRY—Part mustered out June 6, 1865; the rest transferred to 34th Infantry.

Gregory, John......... Ass't S..... Farmington, Ill............. To Dec., 1863; also 15th U. S. C. T. Dead.
Hooton, M. M.......... Surgeon... Centralia, Ill ................. From August, 1862.
Guth, Israel J.......... Ass't S.......................................... From August, 1862.

87TH INFANTRY—Mustered out June 16, 1865.

Berry, Daniel........... Ass't S..... Carmi, Ill ....................... From May, 1864. H. R.
Stewart, E. L.. ....... Surgeon... Carmi, Ill ....................... From Oct., 1862. H. R.
Poindexter, John ..... Ass't S .......................................... To 77th U. S. C. T., January, 1864.
Handley, J. L.......... H. Stew... Fairfield, Ill.

88TH INFANTRY—Mustered out June 9, 1865.

Pierce, Wm. P ........ Surgeon... Hoopeston, or Lamont, Ill. From Feb., 1863; also 36th Inf.
Rankin, A C ........... Ass't S..... Pullman, or Oakalla, Ill.. To March, 1863.
Forshee, Thos. W..... " Madison, Ind ................. To January, 1865.
Burdick. Frank N..... " .................................... To November, 1862.
Kopp, Fred'k E........ " .................................... From February, 1865.

89TH INFANTRY—Part mustered out June 10, 1865; the rest transferred to 59th Infantry.

Hance, Samuel F...... Surgeon... Minneapolis, Minn......... To March, 1863.
Tuttle, H. B............ " Denver, Colo ................. From May, 1863.
Thombs, P. R ......... Ass't S..... Pueblo, Colo.................. From June, 1863.

90TH INFANTRY—Part mustered out June 6, 1865, the rest transferred to 48th Infantry.

Hinkley, Darwin...... Ass't S.... Leland, Ill ...................... To February, 1864.
Thompson, C. A...... Surgeon... Jefferson City, Mo......... From September, 1864.
Strong, Henry......... " Iola, Kans....................... To July, 1864; also 74th Inf.
Davison, Jas. B.... .. Ass't S.......................................... To March, 1863.
Scott, John H. ........ " .................................... From August, 1864.

## ILLINOIS—Continued.

91ST INFANTRY—Part mustered out July 12, 1865, the rest transferred to 28th Infantry.

| | | | |
|---|---|---|---|
| LeRoy, David | Surgeon | La Salle, or Streator, Ill. | From Sept., 1862. D. |
| Day, Wm. T | Ass't S. | Alleged dead | To April, 1864. |
| Miller James N | " | | From December, 1864. |
| Philips, Edgar L | " | | To September, 1863. |

92D INFANTRY—Part mustered out June 21, 1865, the rest transferred to 65th Infantry.

| | | | |
|---|---|---|---|
| Helm, Clinton | Surgeon | Rockford, Ill | From September, 1862. |
| Winston, Thomas | Ass't S. | Forreston, Ill | To July, 1864. |
| Stephenson, Nathan | " | Alleged dead | From October, 1862. |

93D INFANTRY—Mustered out June 2 and 12, 1865.

| | | | |
|---|---|---|---|
| Hopkins, Samuel A | Surgeon | Peoria, Ill | To December, 1864. |
| Huyett, Jos | " | Milan, Ill | To July, 1863. D. |
| Griswold, Chas A | " | Fulton, Ill | From March, 1865. |

94TH INFANTRY—Part mustered out July 17, 1865, the rest transferred to 33d Infantry.

| | | | |
|---|---|---|---|
| Payne, Selden M | Ass't S. | Chenoa, or Lexington, Ill. | To December, 1862. |
| Ross, J. C | Surgeon | Lincoln, Ill | From November, 1862. |
| Skaggs, L. H | Ass't S. | Ellsworth, Ill | From May, 1863. |
| *Stewart, A. E | " | Bloomington, or Randolph, Ill. | From August, 1862. G. |

95TH INFANTRY—Part mustered out August 17, 1865, the rest transferred to 47th Infantry.

| | | | |
|---|---|---|---|
| Giddings, Josiah | Ass't S. | Logan, Iowa | From May, 1863. |
| Green, John W | Surgeon | Marengo, Ill | From May, 1863. H. R. |
| Suiter, Walter F | Ass't S. | Davenport, Iowa | A W. M. |
| Woodward, Geo. N | Surgeon | Alleged dead | To March, 1863. |
| Merritt, Ansel D | Ass't S. | Alleged dead | To March, 1863. |

96TH INFANTRY—Part mustered out June 10, 1865, the rest transferred to 21st Infantry.

| | | | |
|---|---|---|---|
| Evans, Moses | Ass't S. | Waukegan, Ill | From September, 1862. |
| Martin, Chas | Surgeon | St. Joseph, Mo | To February. 1863. |
| Pierce, B. G | " | Warren, Ill | From April, 1863. |
| Sheffield. D. A | Ass't S. | Apple River, Ill | To February, 1863. |
| Wares, M | | Waukegan, Ill | Not in A. G R. |
| Byers, Fred'k W | Ass't S. | | From May, 1863. |

97TH INFANTRY—Part mustered out July 29, 1865, the rest transferred to 37th Infantry.

| | | | |
|---|---|---|---|
| Davis, Chas | Surgeon | Godfrey, or Alton, Ill | From July, 1864; says he will not testify. |
| Smith, C. M | Ass't S. | Tecumseh, Neb., or Alton, Ill. | From September, 1864. |
| Turner, Wm. D | Surgeon | Huntley, Ill | To April, 1864; also 1st Light Artillery. |
| Willard, Samuel | " | | To February, 1863. |

*Examined recruits, now Deputy Clerk of Court.

ILLINOIS—Continued.

98TH INFANTRY—Mustered out June 27, 1885.

Barnes, A. T..........Surgeon...Bloomington, Ill.............From August 1864; also 1st Lieut. 15th Inf.
Groves, John N.......Ass't S....Effingham, Ill................From September. 1864.
McAllister, Henry C..Surgeon....................................To June, 1864, also 79th Inf.
Lackey, Robt. M...... " ....................................To May. 1863.
Vertrees, Samuel W..Ass't S....................................Dismissed May, 1863.

99TH INFANTRY—Mustered out July 31, 1865.

Ledlie, J. H.............Surgeon...Pittsfield, Ill.................To Ass't S.. U. S. V., June, 1864.
McNeall, A. E.........Ass't S....Bowensburg, Ill.............To July 1863.
Spencer, A. F.......... " Pittsfield, Ill.....................To August. 1863.
May, Edwin.............Surgeon....................................From August, 1864; also 33d Inf
Curtis, John T.........Ass't S....................................From July, 1864.

100TH INFANTRY—Part mustered out June 12, 1865, the rest transferred to 51st Infantry.

Harvey, Geo. E........Ass't S....Camden, Ill....................From November, 1864.
Hiese, A. W............Surgeon...Joliet, Ill.........................To April 1864.
Woodruff, H T........Ass't S....Howard, Ill......................From June. 1864
Harwood, Elvis........ " Alleged dead....................To January, 1863.

101ST INFANTRY—Mustered out June 7, 1865.

Kimber, A. L...........Surgeon...Waverly, Ill......................To November. 1864.
Roberts, Clark......... " Winchester, Ill.................To April, 1864; U. S. Ex S
Smith, Geo E. ....... " Bloomington, Ill............To December, 1862
Robbins, Henry C.... " Creston, Ill. ....................From December. 1864.
Miner, Jas...............Ass't S ...Winchester, Ill.................To January, 1863.
Henderson, Eliel F... " ....................................From April, 1865.

102D INFANTRY—Part mustered out June 5, 1865, the rest transferred to 16th Infantry.

Rice. D B...............Surgeon...Roseburgh, Oregon.........To July, 1863.
Bigger. David P.......Ass't S....................................To Surg. 9th Inf. May,'65.
Stanway, Thos. S..... " Alleged dead....................To August 1864
Hamilton, Wm ........Surgeon...Alleged dead....................From October, 1863.

103D INFANTRY—Mustered out June 21, 1865.

Morris, Richard........Surgeon..Lawrence, Kan.................From November. 1862; H R; also 83d Inf.
Fleming, T. H.......................Canton, Ill........................Not in A. G R
Buck. Sidney S........Ass't S.....Maquon, Ill........................From October, 1862.
Van Brunt, Jas. W... " Pinckneyville, Ill.. ........From October, 1862.

104TH INFANTRY—Mustered out June 6, 1865.

Dyer, Reuben F .....Surgeon...Ottawa, Ill........................From November, 1862.
Freeman, Julius A...Ass't S....................................To July, 1863.

105TH INFANTRY—Mustered out June 7. 1865.

Beggs, Geo. W.........Ass't S....Sioux City, Ill.............From April, 1863
Waterman, Alfred...Surgeon...West Side, Iowa..............From July, 1864
Belfrage, Jno. B......H. Stew...Sargent's Bluff, Iowa.

ILLINOIS—Continued.

106TH INFANTRY—Mustered out June 12, 1865.

| | | | |
|---|---|---|---|
| Ellsworth, P. H | Surgeon | Hot Springs, Ark | From July, 1864. U. S. Ex. S. |
| Lamphear, Albert H. | " | Atchison, Kan | To April, 1863. |
| Bettelhum, B. J. | " | | To June, 1864. |

107TH INFANTRY—Mustered out June —, 1865.

| | | | |
|---|---|---|---|
| Coffin, Nelson G | Ass't S. | Monticello, Ill | From September, 1862. |
| Wright, John | Surgeon | Clinton, Ill | From November, 1862. |
| Radmore, Chas. C | Ass't S. | Lincoln, Neb | To 114th U. S. C. T. July, 1864; also 44th Inf. |

108TH INFANTRY—Part mustered out August 5, 1865; the rest transferred to 47th Infantry.

| | | | |
|---|---|---|---|
| Conover, R. A | Surgeon | Peculiar, Mo | From December, 1863. |
| Goodwin, A. E | " | Rockford, Ill | To August, 1863. |
| Kinnear, A. H | Ass't S. | Metamora, Ill | From February, 1864. |
| Hoover, Isaac L | " | | To February, 1863. |
| Cary, John | Surgeon | | To January, 1863. |
| Fursman, Henry C | H. Stew | Colorado Springs, Col. | |

109TH INFANTRY—Mustered out April 10, 1863, on account of desertion of men and incompetency of officers, except company K, transferred to 11th Infantry. (237 desertions in seven months.)

| | | | |
|---|---|---|---|
| Dewey, John S | Surgeon | Troy, Ill | To December, 1863. Alleged dead. |
| Dewey, Geo. H | Ass't S. | Marine, Ill | To 11th Infantry. |
| Henley, John H | " | | To May, 1864. |

110TH INFANTRY—Mustered out June 8, 1865.

| | | | |
|---|---|---|---|
| Hickman, Z | Ass't S. | Benton, Ill | To February, 1863. |
| Plummer, H. S | " | Mt. Vernon, Ill | To May, 1863. |
| Pace, W. C | Surgeon | Ashley, Ill | From September, 1862. |
| Munsell, John G | Ass't S. | Troy, Ill | From April, 1864. |
| Wall, David | " | Marine, Ill | To March, 1864. |
| Stevenson, Wm. M | H. Stew | Ashley, Ill. | |

111TH INFANTRY—Part mustered out June 6 and 7, 1865, the rest transferred to 48th Infantry.

| | | | |
|---|---|---|---|
| Hawley, Thos. S | Ass't S. | 3071 Easton avenue, St. Louis, Mo. | To 11th Mo. Inf. June, 1863 |
| Rainey, J. K | " | St. Augustine, Fla., or Salem, Ill. | From July, 1862. |
| Swan, Samuel M | Surgeon | | From July, 1864; also 12th Inf. |
| Phillips, Jas | " | | To March, 1864. |
| Middleton, E. W | H. Stew | Iuka, Ill. | |

112TH INFANTRY—Part mustered out June 20, 1865; the rest transferred to 65th Infantry.

| | | | |
|---|---|---|---|
| Miliken, L. S | Surgeon | Franklinton, N. C | A. W. M. |
| Phillips, Wesley | Ass't S. | Burnt Prairie or Liberty, Ill | From January, 1863. |
| Graw, Christian H | " | Little Rock, Ark | Missing since Oct., 1862. |
| Jones, Chas. D. H | " | | From May, 1863. |
| Spalding, John W | Surgeon | | To March, 1863. |
| Johnson, Jos. C | H. Stew | Mason City, Ill | From August, 1862, to June, 1865. |

## ILLINOIS—Continued.

### 113TH INFANTRY—Mustered out June 20, 1865.

Brown, L. B............Surgeon...Sheldon, Ill....................Said to be dead.
Bailey, Wm. N........Ass't S.....Plymouth, Ind................To 52d U. S. C. T. Dec., 1863.
Mack, Joel M............Surgeon.........................................To April, 1864.
Sulcer, Abraham A..Ass't S.........................................From November, 1864.

### 114TH INFANTRY—Part mustered out August 3, 1865, the rest transferred to 58th Infantry.

Higgins, James N.....Surgeon...Griggsville, Ill...............To August, 1863.
Van Meter, H.......... " Williamsville, Ill............From December, 1863. Dead.
Wilson, J. F............Ass't S.....Tollula, Ill .....................To July, 1863.
Copestake, J. C........ " .........................................From November, 1864.
Brownson, Aug. I....H. Stew...Williamsville, Ill.

### 115TH INFANTRY—Part mustered out June 11, 1865, the rest transferred to 21st Infantry.

Blalock, N. G..........Ass't S.....Walla Walla, Washington Territory. To July, 1863.
Loomis, C. E........... " Lee Center, Ill................From August, 1864.
Moore, E. W.............Surgeon...Decatur, Ill..................... To April, 1863.
Bane, Garner H....... " Alleged dead ................From July, 1863.

### 116TH INFANTRY—Part mustered out June 7, 1865; the rest transferred to 55th Infantry.

Barnes, I. N.............Surgeon...Decatur, Ill....................From March, 1863.
Heckelman, John A..Ass't S.....1103 St. Ange street, St. Louis, Mo. From September, 1862.
Hostetler, J. A. W... " .........................................A. W. M.

### 117TH INFANTRY—Part mustered out August 5, 1865; the rest transferred to 33d Infantry.

Jennings, Thos. C....Surgeon...East St. Louis, Ill..........A. W. M.
Wiley, D. M............. " Colorado Springs, Col.....From October, 1862.
Hood, H. H..............Ass't S.....Litchfield, Ill.................To 3d U. S. C. H. A. Sept., 1863.

### 118TH INFANTRY—Mustered out October 1, 1865.

Boude, J. K..............Ass't S.....U. S. Pension Office........A. W. M.
Reece, Madison........Surgeon...Abingdon, Ill................From December, 1862.
Nichols, Elmer.........Ass't S.........................................Dismissed July, 1864.
Corey, V. B.......... .H. Stew...West Point, Ill.

### 119TH INFANTRY—Mustered out August 26, 1865.

Byrnes, Geo. A........Ass't S.....Cooperstown, Ill............From November, 1862.
Bradbury, J. F.........H. Stew...Cooperstown, Ill.
Monroe, Thos...........Surgeon...Rushville, Ill.................To June, 1864.
Woods, Reuben........ " 25 N. Fifth st., Quincy, Ill. From July, 1864.

### 120TH INFANTRY—Mustered out September 10, 1865.

Guild, Phineas K......Surgeon...Santa Barbara, Cal.........To June, 1863.
Hamilton, James...... " .........................................From Jan., 1864; also 7th Inf.
Woodmansee, C. S...Ass't S.........................................From Sept 1864.
Wardner, P. J......... " Alleged dead..................To Aug., 1863.

### 121ST INFANTRY—Failed to complete.

ILLINOIS—Continued.

122D INFANTRY—Mustered out July 15, 1865.

| | | | |
|---|---|---|---|
| Norris, A. S | Ass't S | Farmer City, Ill | From March, 1864. |
| Seaman, M. W | Surgeon | Shipman, Ill | From Sept., 1863. |
| Knox, Wm. A | " | | To June, 1863. |
| Mathews, J. P | Ass't S | | To August, 1863. |

123D INFANTRY—Mustered out June 28, 1865.

| | | | |
|---|---|---|---|
| Ballou, Alvin | Surgeon | Grand Forks, Dak. Ter., or Princeton, Ill. | From January, 1865. |
| Kelso, H. A | Ass't S | Paxton, Ill | To February. 1864. |
| Phipps, John M | Surgeon | Brightwood, Ind | To March, 1864. |
| Allen, Horace R | " | | To May, 1863. |

124TH INFANTRY—Mustered out August 15, 1865.

| | | | |
|---|---|---|---|
| Kay, Jas. R | Surgeon | Bushnell, Ill | From July, 1864. |
| Angell, Leland H | " | | To June, 1864. |
| Jassey, John | Ass't S | | Dismissed Nov., 1864. |

125TH INFANTRY—Part mustered out June 9, 1865; the rest transferred to 60th Infantry.

| | | | |
|---|---|---|---|
| McElroy, J. J | Surgeon | Rossville, Ill | To April, 1864. H. R. |
| Mills, C. H | " | Champaign, Ill | From June, 1864. |
| Wright, Owen | Ass't S | | To April, 1865. |
| Erving, Joel T | " | | To February, 1864. |
| Sulcer, A. A | H. Stew | Ridge Farm, Ill. | |

126TH INFANTRY—Mustered out July 26, 1865.

| | | | |
|---|---|---|---|
| *Bridges, V. R | Surgeon | Mattoon, Ill | From Dec, 1863; also 62d Inf. |
| Washburne, T. D | Ass't S | Hillsboro', Ill | From Sept. 1862. H. R. |
| Mills, Erastus W | " | Kinsley, Kan | To August, 1864. |

127TH INFANTRY—Part mustered out May 31 and June 5, 1865; the rest transferred to 55th Infantry.

| | | | |
|---|---|---|---|
| Gore, J. R | Surgeon | 2606 Prairie ave., Chicago, Ill. | From Sept, 1862. |
| Anthony, J. P | Ass't S | Sterling, Ill | To 61st Inf. Oct., 1863. |
| Clark, Anson L | " | Elgin, Ill | From Sept., 1862. H. R. |
| Weld, Salem E | H. Stew | Elgin, Ill. | |

128TH INFANTRY—Consolidated with the 9th Infantry September, 1863, (700 desertions in 5 months.)

| | | | |
|---|---|---|---|
| †Bundy, S. H | | Marion, or Carbondale, Ill. | Not in A. G. R. |
| French, Geo. W | Ass't S | Logansport, Ind | To April, 1863. |

129TH INFANTRY—Mustered out June 8, 1865.

| | | | |
|---|---|---|---|
| Johns, H. C | Surgeon | Decatur, Ill | To January, 1864. |
| Walters, Wm. H | Ass't S | Decatur, Ill | To February, 1863. |
| Johnson, Darius | Surgeon | Alleged dead | To April, 1865. |
| Wood, Orlando S | " | Alleged dead | From May, 1865. |

* Attended 57 U. S. C. T. at Duvall's Bluff, Ark., from December, 1863, to February, 1864.
† Acted as Surgeon at Cairo, Ill., December, 1862, and at Mound City, Ill., January, 1863.

ILLINOIS—Continued.

130TH INFANTRY—Mustered out August 15, 1865.

Barry, E. L. H.........Ass't S.....Jerseyville, Ill..... .........To December, 1862.
Wilcox, L. K.......... " Warsaw, Ill. ........ .........To January, 1865.
Wilkins, D............... " Greenville, Ill...... .........To December, 1863.
Sigler, Wm. F......... " ..................................From May, 1863; also 77th Inf.

131ST INFANTRY—Consolidated with the 29th Infantry November, 1863.

Brown, Joseph.........Surgeon...Metropolis, Ill.................To February, 1863.
Bumstead, S. J ........Ass't S....Decatur, Ill......................From July, 1863; also 29th Inf.
McDonough, A. A.... " ..................................To September, 1863.
Lagore, Enoch.........Surgeon....................................To September, 1863.
Walker, John W......H. Stew...Metropolis, Ill.

From the 132d to the 143d INFANTRY were 100 days' organizations.

144TH INFANTRY—Mustered out July 14, 1865.

Bluthardt, Theo. J...Surgeon...43 S Peoria st., Chicago, Ill. From Sep., 1864. H. R.
Boyd, Henry W.......Ass't S....Chicago, Ill.................To 14th Inf. March, 1865.
Meacham, Jos. W..... " ..................................From February, 1865.
Brenckeman, F........ " ..................................From April, 1865.
Condon, S. B...........H. Stew...Upper Alton, Ill............

145th INFANTRY was 100 days' organization.

146TH INFANTRY—Mustered out July 8, 1865.

Brooks, John B........Ass't S....Hot Springs, Ark., or Geneseo, Ill. From October, 1864.
McMahon, R. H.......Surgeon...Quincy, Ill ....................From September, 1864.
Goosbeck, John B....Ass't S..................................From December, 1864.

147TH INFANTRY—Mustered out January 20, 1866.

*Conley, Wm. J......Ass't S....Elk Point, Dakota .........From March, 1865.
Adair, Wm R......... " ..................................To 153d Inf. March, 1865.
Van Buren, Evert....Surgeon..................................From January, 1866.
Emmons, Frank A... " ..................................To September, 1865.

148TH INFANTRY—Mustered out September 8, 1865.

Linn, David C ........Ass't S ...Fredericksville, Ill.........From March, 1865.
Smith, Frank N.......Surgeon..................................From March, 1865.
Drake, Thos. B........Ass't S..................................From April, 1865.
Edson, G. W............H. Stew...Quincy, Ill

149TH INFANTRY—Mustered out January 27, 1866.

Winston, Thos.........Surgeon...Forreston, Ill.................From March, 1865.
Mercer, Sam'l D......Ass't S ..................................From February, 1865.
Green, Adolphus...... " 715 Lafayette ave., St. Louis, Mo. From March, 1865.

150TH INFANTRY—Mustered out January 16, 1866.

Jenkins, Jos. M........Ass't S....Westfield, Iowa..............To June, 1865.
Buck, Harmon A......Surgeon..................................A. W. M.
Cox, James G..........Ass't S....Alleged dead.................From February, 1865.

---

* Charges fee $10.

ILLINOIS—Continued.

151ST INFANTRY—Mustered out January 24, 1866.

Cole, Fred'k............Ass't S....El Paso, Ill.....................From March, 1865.
Stillman, Walter D...Surgeon...Council Bluffs, Iowa......From March, 1865.
Cass, Frank D.........Ass't S.......................................To June, 1865.
Langford, Wiley C...H. Stew...Osage City, Kans............From February, 1865, to January, 1866.

152D INFANTRY—Mustered out September 11, 1865.

Catlin, E. P............Ass't S....Rockford, Ill....................From March, 1865.
Plummer, Hiram......Surgeon...Mt. Vernon, Ill...............From February, 1865.

153D INFANTRY—Mustered out September 21, 1865.

Scott, Amos.............Ass't S....Pecatonica, or Seward, Ill. From June, 1865.
Adair, Wm. R.........Surgeon.......................................From March, 1865; also 147th Infantry.
Chesbrough, H. F.....Ass't S........................................From February, 1865.

154TH INFANTRY—Mustered out September 18, 1865.

Keuchen, G. A.........Surgeon.......................................From August, 1865.
Shurtleff, Flavel......Ass't S........................................From April, 1865.

155TH INFANTRY—Mustered out September 4, 1865.

Hendee, Chas. K......Ass't S....La Clede, Ill.....................From February, 1865.
Collins, Russell J......Surgeon.......................................From February, 1865.

156TH INFANTRY—Mustered out September 20, 1865.

Godfrey, H. I..........Ass't S....La Fayette, Wis........... From March, 1865.
Hess, Wm. H...........Surgeon...41 S. Clark st, Chicago, Ill. From March, 1865.
Penfield, Wm. P......Ass't S....Alice, Iowa....................From March, 1865.

INDIANA.

1ST CAVALRY, (28th Volunteers)—Mustered out at different dates from July 22, 1862, to May 31, 1865.

Bruce, Geo W ........Ass't S....Winchester, Ind............To September, 1864; also 8th and 142d Inf'y.
Robson, John R ......2d Lt.......New Harmony, Ind.......To Ass't S. 91st Infantry December, 1862.
Cravens, Jas. W......Ass't S ...Osgood. Ind.....................To August, 1864.
Casselberry. Isaac ...Surgeon...Evansville. Ind..............Dead.
Paterson, John J......Ass't S....Rockport, Ind.................To Surgeon 46th U. S. C. T. April, 1863. Dead.
Brackett, Chas......... " ........................................To November, 1861.
Rhodes, Andrew. I...H. Stew...Pikeville. Ind.
Brecourt, I. D...........A. H. S...Indianapolis, Ind.

2D CAVALRY (41st Volunteers)—Part to 8th Cavalry April 8, 1865; the rest mustered out April 15 and August 7, 1865.

Jones, Thomas N.....Ass't S.....Anderson, Ind...............To December, 1862; also 130th Inf. Alleged dead.
Fritts, Thomas I...... " Cold Springs, Ill............To 8th Cav. June, 1865; also 3d Cav & 14th Inf.
Rutledge, Wm......... " 919 Olive st, St. Louis, Mo. To October, 1864.
Smith, Andrew J...... " Wabash, Ind...................To October, 1864.
Vaile, Joel ..............Surgeon.........................................To October, 1864.
Coggshall, Job S......A. A. S ...Winchester, Ind.

INDIANA—Continued.

3D CAVALRY (45th Volunteers)—Part to 8th Cavalry April 1, 1865; the rest mustered out April 15 and August 7, 1865.

| Name | Rank | Residence | Remarks |
|---|---|---|---|
| Beck, Elias W. H. | Surgeon | Delphi, Ind | To August, 1864; U. S. Ex. S. |
| Fritts, Thos. I | Ass't S. | Cold Springs, Ill | To 8th Cav. June, 1865; also 2d & 14th Inf. |
| Knight, James H. | " | Paragon, Ind | To August, 1864. |
| Brusie, Luther | " | Ione City, Cal. | To November, 1862. |

4TH CAVALRY (77th Volunteers)—Mustered out June 29, 1865.

| Name | Rank | Residence | Remarks |
|---|---|---|---|
| Boor, Wm. F | Surgeon | New Castle, Ind | To November, 1863; U. S. Ex. S. |
| Dodson, Jonas H | Ass't S. | Dongola, Ill | To November, 1862. |
| Garrison, Herod D. | " | 461 Clark st., Chicago, Ill. | From Apr., '64, to Je., '65. |
| Taggart, John F | Surgeon | Solon or Charlestown, Ind. | From Apr., '64, to Je., '65. |
| Thomas, Elias B | Ass't S. | La Gro, Ind | To January, 1863. |
| Bryant, James E | H. Stew. | Bedford, Ind. | |
| Moore, John G | " | Madison, Ind. | |

5TH CAVALRY (90th Volunteers)—Part mustered out June 15, 1865; the rest transferred to 6th Cavalry June 27, 1865.

| Name | Rank | Residence | Remarks |
|---|---|---|---|
| Fosdick, Albert C. | Surgeon | Liberty, Ind | Missing since February, 1864; U. S. Ex. S. |
| Hiatt, Christopher C. | Ass't S. | Ridgeville, Ind | A. W. M.; also 6th Cav. |
| Osgood, Howard G. | " | Gosport, Ind | To May, 1864. |
| Wishard, Jos. M | Surgeon | Greenwood, Ind. | A. W. M. |
| Russell, Geo. H | Ass't S. | | From November, 1864. |
| Bruner, Louis J | H. Stew. | Versailles, Ind. | |

6TH CAVALRY (71st Volunteers)—Mustered out June 17 and September 15, 1865.

| Name | Rank | Residence | Remarks |
|---|---|---|---|
| Hiatt, Christopher C. | Surgeon | Ridgeville, Ind | From July, 1865; also 5th Cav. |
| Olds, Joseph H | Ass't S. | Tucson, Ariz. Ter., or Indianapolis, Ind. | To June, 1865. |
| Spottswood, E. T. | Surgeon | Perrysville, Ind | To March, 1864. |
| Schmidt, Gustavus | Ass't S. | Ingraham, Ill | From July, 1864. Alleged dead. |
| Schell, Fred'k A | " | Spencer, Ind | To January, 1865. |
| Weir, Andrew N | Surgeon | Sullivan or Terre Haute, Ind. | To July, 1865. |
| Collett, Edward T | Ass't S. | | To February, 1863. |
| Gowdy, John K | H. Stew. | Rushville, Ind. | |

7TH CAVALRY (119th Volunteers)—Mustered out February 18, 1866.

| Name | Rank | Residence | Remarks |
|---|---|---|---|
| Benson, Julius L | Ass't S. | Jerome, Ind | Missing since July, 1864. |
| Chitwood, Joshua | Surgeon | Connersville, Ind | To February, 1866. |
| Grove, Jasper M | Ass't S. | Tipton, Ind | To June, 1864. |
| Jay, James C | " | Bryant, Ind | To Sept., 1865. Dead. |
| Freeman, Wm | Surgeon | Camden or Pennville, Ind. | Dismissed May, 1864. |
| Roether, Daniel B. | Ass't S. | New Era or Garrett City, Ind. | To August, 1865. |

8TH CAVALRY (39th Volunteers)—Mustered out July 20, 1865.

| Name | Rank | Residence | Remarks |
|---|---|---|---|
| Connett, Mahlon C | Ass't S. | Bedford, Iowa | From June, 1863. |
| Gray, John M. | Surgeon | Noblesville, Ind | From October, 1864; U. S. Ex. S. |
| Fritts, Thos I | Ass't S. | Cold Springs, Ill | Also 3d Cavalry. |
| Waterman, L. D | Surgeon | Indianapolis, Ind | To October, 1864. |
| Garver, James A. | Ass't S. | | To March, 1863; also 136th Inf. (100 days.) |
| Scott, Wm. G. | " | | To May, 1863. |

## INDIANA—Continued.

9TH CAVALRY (121st Volunteers)—Mustered out August 28, 1865.

Wellman, R. M........Surgeon...Jasper, Ind....................From May, 1864. H. R.
McChristie, John......Ass't S.....College Corner, Ohio......From May, 1864, to August, 1865.
Magann, Edwin W... " ......................................From June, 1864, to August, 1865.
Adams, T. J............H .Stew...North Salem, Ind.

10TH CAVALRY—(125th Volunteers)—Mustered out August 31, 1865.

*Culbertson, Jos. R..Ass't S.....Trenton, N. J.
Davis, Solomon........Surgeon...Columbus or Lexington, Ind. To March, 1865.
Lewis, Samuel B...... " Canaan, Ind................From August, 1864.
Houser, Jacob H......Ass't S......................................From June, 1865.

11TH CAVALRY (126th Volunteers)—Mustered out September 19, 1865.

Bushnell, Samuel B..Ass't S.....Monticello, Ind..............To January, 1865.
Crowder, Robert H...Surgeon...Sullivan, Ind.................From June, 1865. H. R.
Read, Ezra............. " Terre Haute, Ind...........To April, 1865; also 1st H. Art. Dead.
Swafford, Benj. F..... " Terre Haute, Ind...........To May, 1865.
Robinson, John A....Ass't S......................................To August, 1865.

12TH CAVALRY (127th Volunteers)—Mustered out November 10, 1865.

Browne, John T......Ass't S.....Logansport, Ind............From July, 1864. Alleged dead.
Pratt, Samuel R......Surgeon...Hebron, Ind.................From May, 1864. H. R. Charges fee.
Wood, James A.......Ass't S.....Lowell, Ind..................To October, 1864. H. R.
Clowes, D. A.......... " ......................................From July to November, 1865.

13TH CAVALRY (131st Volunteers—Mustered out November 18, 1865.

Buck, Robert H.......Surgeon...814 Wash. avenue, St. Louis, Mo. To Feb., 1865. H. R. Also 75th and 118th Inf.
Jones, John H... .....Ass't S.....Roann, Ind.......................From July, 1864, to Nov., 1865.
Kilgore, Tecumseh...Surgeon...Chesterfield, Ind.............Dead.
Morrow, Doctor F ...Ass't S.....Longton, Kans...............From August, 1864.
Walton, Allen M......Surgeon......................................To July, 1864; also 86th Inf.
Chitwork, John E....A. A. S ...Connersville, Ind..........From Jan. to June, 1865.

[For 1ST HEAVY ARTILLERY see 21st Infantry.]

*The first five regiments of Infantry were credited to the Mexican War.*

6TH INFANTRY—Mustered out September 22, 1864; veterans and recruits transferred to 68th Infantry.

Collins, Wm. A........Ass't S.....Madison, Ind..................From Sept., 1862, to Sept., 1864.
Charleton, S. H........ " Seymour, Ind................To March, 1862.
Sparks, Nathan B.... " Lovely Dale, or Monroe, Ind. To December, 1861.
†Davis, John W........ " Vincennes, Ind.............Also 1st Lieut. 20th and Ass't S. 24th Inf.
Schussler, Chas........Surgeon...Madison, Ind.................From Sept., 1861. Alleged dead.
Lattimore, Finley C..Ass't S......................................To May, 1864.

* In charge of Post Hospital at Union City, Tenn., July, August, and September, 1862.
† Belonged to the 3-months' 6th Infantry.

## INDIANA—Continued.

### 7TH INFANTRY—Mustered out September 20, 1864.

| Name | Rank | Residence | Remarks |
|---|---|---|---|
| Duffield, Jas. T. | Ass't S. | Indianapolis, Ind. | A. W. M.; also 76th Inf. Dead. |
| Gillespie, Wm. | " | Rising Sun, Ind. | To 83d Inf. Aug., 1863. |
| Linigar, Daniel B. | " | Springfield, or Whitcomb, Ind. | A. W. M. |
| New, Geo. W. | Surgeon | Indianapolis, Ind. | A. W. M.; also 7th 3-mos. G. |

### 8TH INFANTRY—Mustered out August 28, 1865.

| Name | Rank | Residence | Remarks |
|---|---|---|---|
| Bigelow, Jas. K. | Surgeon | Indianapolis, Ind. | From July, 1863. H. R. U. S. Ex. S. |
| Bruce, Geo. W. | Ass't S. | Winchester, Ind. | To January, 1863; also 1st Cav. and 142d Inf. |
| Ford, James | Surgeon | Wabash, Ind. | To January, 1863; also (3-months) 8th Inf. |
| Brown, S. Clay | Ass't S. | Topeka, Kans. | To 18th Inf. July, 1864. |

### 9TH INFANTRY—Mustered out September 28, 1865.

| Name | Rank | Residence | Remarks |
|---|---|---|---|
| Meeker, Daniel | Surgeon | La Porte, Ind. | To November, 1861; also (3-months) 9th Inf. Alleged dead. |
| Sherman, Mason G. | " | Michigan City, Ind. | From Nov., 1861; also (3-months) 9th Inf. |
| Blackstone, John K. | Ass't S. | | To March, 1862. |
| Hoffman, M. F. A. | " | | To 128th Inf. July, 1864. |
| Trigg, Jas. | A. H. S. | Michigan City, Ind. | |

### 10TH INFANTRY—Mustered out September 19, 1864.

| Name | Rank | Residence | Remarks |
|---|---|---|---|
| Avery, Increase J. | Surgeon | Richmond, Ind. | To January, 1863. |
| Killen, Jas. | Ass't S. | Montgomery, Ind. | From Feb., 1863. Dead. |
| Martin, Wm. H. | Surgeon | Rensselaer, Ind. | To May, 1863. |
| Williamson, R. A. | " | Lebanon, Ind. | From June, 1863. G. |
| *McCrea, Thos. P. | " | Logansport, Ind. | |
| *Myers, Wm. H. | Ass't S. | Ft. Wayne, Ind. | |
| Cresap, Wm. S. | Chaplain | Lebanon, Ind. | To Ass't S. 135th Inf. Nov., 1863; also 154th Inf. |
| Allen, Jos. S. | Surgeon | Dead | To October, 1862. |
| Perkins, Conrad S. | Ass't S. | | To February, 1862. |

### 11TH INFANTRY—Mustered out July 26, 1865.

| Name | Rank | Residence | Remarks |
|---|---|---|---|
| Avery, John P. | Ass't S. | Indianapolis, Ind. | From April to July, 1865. |
| Comington, J. A. | Surgeon | Indianapolis, Ind. | To September, 1864. |
| Fry, Thos. W., Sr. | " | La Fayette, Ind. | To September, 1861; also (3-months) 11th Inf. Alleged dead. |
| Rooker, Jas. J. | Ass't S. | Castleton, Ind. | To February, 1863. |
| Rockwell, Wm. | " | Elmore, Neb. | To June, 1863. |
| Thompson, John C. | Surgeon | Terre Haute, Ind. | To October, 1862. |
| Todd, Wm. A. | Ass't S. | Garden Grove, Iowa | From May to July, 1865. |
| Wilson, Jas. | " | | To February, 1865. |
| Scearce, John T. | " | Dead | From March, 1865. |
| Stahl, E. F. | H. Stew. | Mackinaw, Ill. | |
| Carther, Jas. | " | Rossville, Ind. | From Aug., 1861 to July, 1865. |

### 12TH INFANTRY—(1 year.) Mustered out May 16, 1862.

| Name | Rank | Residence | Remarks |
|---|---|---|---|
| Howard, Noble P. | Ass't S. | Greenfield, Ind. | A. W. M. |
| Lomax, Wm. | Surgeon | Marion, Ind. | A. W. M. H. R. |
| Cook, Robert M. | Ass't S. | | To October, 1861. |

* Belonged to the 3-months' 10th Infantry.

## INDIANA—Continued.

### 12TH INFANTRY—Mustered out June 8, 1865.

Lomax, Wm............Surgeon...Marion, Ind ................From May, 1862. H. R.
Campfield, John A...Ass't S.....Pike's Peak, Ind............A. W. M. Alleged dead.
Blackwell, John A...1st Lt......Foristell, Mo....................To Surg. 115th Inf. Sept., 1863.
Taylor, A. B............Ass't S.....Kansas City, Mo............Dead.

### 13TH INFANTRY—Mustered out September 5, 1865.

Chamberlin, N. A....Surgeon...La Porte, Ind....................From August, 1865.
Craig, Isaac N......... " Castleton, Ind..................To July, 1864. G.
Kennedy, H. D........Ass't S.....St. Louis, Mo.................To July, 1864.
Foster, Wm. C......... " ..........................................Dismissed October, 1862.
Gall, Alois D..........Surgeon...Dead......................................To July, 1863.
Mason, Ferdinand.... " ..........................................To February, 1862.

### 14TH INFANTRY—Mustered out June 16, 1864; veterans and recruits transferred to 20th Infantry.

Hurd, Anson ..........Surgeon...Findlay, Ohio..................To Dec., 1862; also 20th and 33d Inf. G.
McCune, Geo. W...... " Montezuma, Ind............From January, 1863. G.
McPheeters, Jos. G... " Bloomington, Ind..........To Aug., 1861; also 33d Inf.; U. S. Ex. S.
Squire, Wm. B.........Ass't S.....Worthington, Ind ..........From December, 1863.
Clippinger, Geo. W...Surgeon...Dead....................................To April, 1862.
Lambey, Louis........Ass't S...........................................To December, 1862.
Sabin, Elias H......... " ..........................................To October, 1863.
Fritts, Thos. J.........H. Stew...Cold Springs, Ill...........From June, 1861, to Jan., 1863; also 2d and 3d Cav.
Britton, Stephen.......H. Stew...Loogootee, Ind.

### 15TH INFANTRY—Mustered out June 25, 1864; veterans and recruits transferred to 17th Infantry.

Adams, Jas. R. ......Surgeon...Petersburgh, Ind...........From Aug., 1863; H. R.; also 58th Inf.
Bond, Richard C...... " Aurora, Ind ....................To August, 1862.
Youart, John M.......Ass't S.....15 Miller's Block, Indianapolis, Ind .............To May, 1863.
Anderson, Jos. V..... " ..........................................To February, 1864.
Wonsetler, Gideon ... " ..........................................A. W. M.

### 16TH INFANTRY—Part mustered out June 30, 1865; the rest transferred to 13th Cavalry.

Chittenden, Geo. F..Surgeon...Anderson, Ind...............To Feb., 1864; also one year 16th Inf.
Cullen, John C........ " Anderson, Ind...............From May, 1864.
Gatch, James D.......Ass't S.....Lawrenceburgh, Ind..... To July 1863.
Fisher, Elias..........Surgeon...Richmond, Ind ..............A. W. M.; 1 year 16th Inf. only. Alleged dead.
Spurrier, John H .....Ass't S.....Rushville, Ind ..............To Jan., 1863; also 123d Inf.
Sadler, Joseph J...... " ..........................................From, May, 1864.

### 17TH INFANTRY—Mustered out August 8, 1865.

Collins, Geo. M........Ass't S.....Tipton or Noah, Ind......From December, 1864.
Dome, David C........ " Rono, Ind ......................From March, 1865.
Hitt, John Y...........Surgeon...Greensburgh, Ind..........To January. 1862.
Kemper, G. W. H....Ass't S.....Muncie, Ind .....................To July, 1864.
Larkin, John B........Surgeon...Mitchell, Ind ...................From March, 1865. H. R.
Munford, Samuel E.. " Princeton, Ind..............To January, 1865. Ex. S.
Henry, David H.......Ass't S...........................................To August, 1861.
Winans, Richard...... " ..........................................To April, 1863.

## INDIANA—Continued.

### 18TH INFANTRY—Mustered out August 18, 1865.

| Name | Rank | Address | Service |
|---|---|---|---|
| Bigney, Peter M | Ass't S. | 66 Franklin, Cincinnati, Ohio. | From December, 1862. |
| Daughters, A. P | Surgeon | Lawrenceburg, Ind., or Moore's Hill, Ind. | To June, 1863. G. |
| Gordon, Geo W | " | Equality, Ill | To March, 1864. G. |
| Peck, Samuel W | " | Washington, Ind | To October, 1861. |
| Brown, S. Clay | " | | From July, 1864; also 8th Inf. |
| Hitchcock, John W | " | | To Dec, 1862; also 133d Inf, 100 days. |

### 19TH INFANTRY—Part mustered out July 28, 1864; the rest transferred to 20th Infantry October 19, 1864.

| Name | Rank | Address | Service |
|---|---|---|---|
| Ebersole, Jacob | Surgeon | Cincinnati, Ohio | From April, 1862, to October, 1864. |
| Greene, John N | Ass't S. | Indianapolis, Ind | To December, 1862. |
| Garver, Henry F | " | Nat'l Mil. Home, Montgomery Co., Ohio, or Billingsville, Ind. | To September, 1863. |
| Haines, Abraham B. | " | Aurora, Ind | To 20th Inf.; also 146th Inf. |
| Kendrick, Wm. H. | " | 73 N. E. st, Indianapolis, Ind. | To September, 1861. |
| Woods, Cabin J | Surgeon | Wayne Co., Ind | To March, 1862. |

### 20TH INFANTRY—Mustered out July 12, 1865.

| Name | Rank | Address | Service |
|---|---|---|---|
| Evarts, Orpheus | Surgeon | College Hill, Ohio | From July, 1861. |
| Grover, Henry C | Ass't S. | Rushford, Minn | To October, 1864. |
| Hurd, Anson | " | Findlay, Ohio | To Jan., 1862; also 14th and 33d Inf. G. |
| Prunk, Daniel H | " | Indianapolis, Ind | Dismissed Nov. 15, 1862. |
| Haines, Abraham B. | " | Aurora, Ind | To 146th Inf. April, 1865; also 19th Inf. |
| Guffin, John | " | Vermillion Co., Ill | To Surg. 156th Inf. May, 1865. |

### 21ST INFANTRY (1st Heavy Artillery)—Mustered out January 10, 1866.

| Name | Rank | Address | Service |
|---|---|---|---|
| Conn, Isaac T | Ass't S. | Evansville, Ind | From June, 1865. |
| Campbell, J. C. L | " | Loogootee, Ind | To June, 1864. |
| Davis, John B | " | New Britton, Ind | To Oct., 1864. Alleged dead. |
| Dunn, Williamson D. | " | Frankfort, Ind | To September, 1863. |
| Goldsberry, John A. | " | Annapolis or Greencastle, Ind. | To July, 1865. |
| *Hawn, Emanuel R. | " | Indianapolis, Ind | To 49th and 144th Inf. April, 1864. |
| Read, Ezra | Surgeon | Terre Haute, Ind | To Dec., 1862; also 11th Cav. Dead. |
| Sherrod, Wm. F | " | Jeffersonville, Ind | From January, 1863. |
| Woods, Daniel L | Ass't S. | | From Oct., 1865; also 153d and 138th Inf., 100 days. |

### 22D INFANTRY—Mustered out July 24, 1865.

| Name | Rank | Address | Service |
|---|---|---|---|
| Beachly, N. J. | Ass't S. | Lincoln, Neb., or Bridgeport, Ind. | To June, 1864; also Capt. 26th Inf. |
| Newland, Benj. J | Surgeon | Bedford, Ind | To November, 1862. |
| Stillwell, Joseph A | " | Brownstown, Ind | From Feb., 1863. U. S. Ex. S |
| Liddall, James P | Ass't S. | Indianapolis, Ind | To January, 1865. Dead. |
| Ireland, Wm. H | " | | From July, 1865. |

*Secretary State of Indiana.

INDIANA—Continued.

23D INFANTRY—Mustered out July 23, 1865.

Austin, Thos. R.......Surgeon...Vincennes or Terra Haute, Ind. To September, 1862.
Byrn, Spencer.........Ass't S.....Palmyra or Milton, Ind...To August, 1863.
Brucker, Magnus......Surgeon...Tell City, Ind.................Died October, 1874.
Calderwood, J. C.....Ass't S.....Salem, Ind.........................From April, 1865.
Kay, Robert............ " Greenville or Salem, Ind..To March, 1862; also 144th Inf.
McPheeters, J. S......Surgeon...Hardinsburgh or Livonia, Ind. From April, 1865.

24TH INFANTRY—Mustered out July 19 and November 15, 1865. The 67th Infantry was consolidated with this Regiment December 21, 1864.

Burton, Wm. A........Ass't S.....Mitchell, Ind..................To July, 1865; also 67th Inf.
Boynton, C. S.........Surgeon...Indianapolis, Ind............To July, 1865; also 67th Inf.
Davis, John W.........Ass't S.....Vincennes, Ind.............To May, 1862; also 1st Lt. 20th, and Ass't S. 6th Inf., 3 months.
Gray, Arthur W......Surgeon...Bridgewater, Ind...........Dead.
Jessup, Robert B...... " Vincennes, Ind............ To September, 1863.
Montgomery, G. B... " Winslow, Ind.....................From Aug, 1865, Ex. S.
Freeman, Wm. H.....H. Stew...Louisville, Ky.

25TH INFANTRY—Mustered out July 17, 1865.

Houghland, Wm. T..Ass't S.....Rockport, Ind ................Dead.
Slaughter, R. C........ " Evansville or Newburgh, Ind. To 53d Inf. May, 1862.
Thomas, Chas. L......Surgeon...Crawfordsville, Ind........From January, 1863.
White, Arthur.........Ass't S.....Rockport, Ind..............To April, 1862.
Johnson, Thos. J...... " ..........................................To August, 1863.
Walker, John T........Surgeon...Dead.........................................Also Major.

26TH INFANTRY—Mustered out January 15, 1866.

Florer, Thos. W.......Surgeon...Waxahatchie, Texas.......From November, 1862.
Short, Wesley..........Ass't S.....Gilmer, Texas...............To 1st Tex. Cav., March, 1864.
Todd, Robert N.......Surgeon...164 Park ave., Indianapolis, Ind. To June, 1862.
Torbet, Geo. A.........Ass't S.....Kansas City, Mo. .......... Dead.
Storey, Thos. H.......H. Stew...Paris, Ind.

27TH INFANTRY—Mustered out November 4, 1864; veterans and recruits transferred to 70th Infantry.

Alexander, J. H.......Ass't S.....Clifty, Ind..............................A. W. M.
Johnson, J. J...........Surgeon...Martinsville, Ind............To August, 1862.
Woolen, Green V.....Ass't S.....Indianapolis, Ind ...........From September, 1861.
Twiford, Willis H.....Surgeon.............................................To July, 1864.

28TH INFANTRY—(See 1st Cavalry.)

29TH INFANTRY—Mustered out December 2, 1865.

Brown, Jacob R.......Ass't S.....South Bend, Ind.............To November, 1862.
Confer, James M......Surgeon...Plymouth, Ind.................To December, 1863.
Humphreys, Lewis... " South Bend, Ind.............Dead.
Keen, Lorenzo S...... " La Porte, Ind...................To Jan., 1863. H. R.
McCarthy, John F.... " Valparaiso, Ind................From March, 1864.
Griffith, John C........Ass't S.....Belleville, Kans............ To August, 1864.
Heaton, Johnson F .. " ..........................................From July, 1865.

## INDIANA—Continued.

### 30TH INFANTRY—Mustered out November 25, 1865.

Meyers, Wm. H........Surgeon...Fort Wayne, Ind...........Dismissed Oct., 1862.
Miller, James..........Ass't S.....La Grange, Ind................To February, 1863.
Pearman, F. M.........Surgeon...Rose Hill or Palestine, Ind. From March, 1865.
Hutchinson, David... " Winterset, Iowa ..........To August, 1863.
Bodman, Elam.........Ass't S.....Champaign, Ill...............To January, 1864.
Freeman, Sam'l A... " ..............................To December, 1861.
Hayes, Sam'l M........ " ..............................To September, 1864.
Parks, Edward R.....Surgeon..........................To February, 1862.

### 31ST INFANTRY—Mustered out December 8, 1865.

Armstrong, Jas. B...Surgeon...Terre Haute, Ind...........To March, 1863. Dead.
Hendricks, Wm. C... " Greenwood or Franklin, Ind. To May, 1864; H. R; also 149th Inf.
McKinney, Asa W.... " Hutchinson, Kans..........From September, 1864.
Merit, Nathaniel P...Ass't S.....Wabash, Ill.. ................From October, 1864.
Morgan, James W.... " ..............................To December, 1863.

### 32D INFANTRY—(1st German Regiment)—Mustered out December 4, 1865.

Aichele, Emil...........Ass't S.....Jonesville, Ind...............To April, 1863.
Forstmeyer, Emil..... " Evansville, Ind..............Dead.
Jeancon, John A......Surgeon...Newport, Ky..................To July, 1862.
Josse, John M.... ..... " Fort Wayne, Ind.............To Sept., 1864; also 74th Inf. Alleged dead.
Kunkler, Gustave A.. " Madison, Ind ..................To September, 1863.
Blaser, Felix F.........Ass't S.....Worthington, Ind...........To March, 1863.
Krauth, Ferdinand...Surgeon...Dead.

### 33D INFANTRY—Mustered out July 21, 1865.

Bence, Robert F......Surgeon...Indianapolis, Ind .. .......From September, 1864.
Hurd, Anson ..............................Findlay, Ohio.................Not in A. G. R. for 33d; also 14th and 20th Inf.
Moffitt, John ...........Ass't S.....194 4th st., Indianapolis, Ind. From May, 1865.
McPheeters, Jos. G..Surgeon...Bloomington, Ind...........To Aug., 1864; also 14th Inf.; U. S Ex. S.
Vincent, J. K...........Ass't S.....Waverly, Ind.................To October, 1864.
Hunt, Andrew M... " ..............................To June, 1863.

### 34TH INFANTRY—Mustered out February 3, 1866.

Babbitt, Edward D..Ass't S.....Paragon, Ind.................To Jan., 1866. Alleged dead.
Bohrer, G ..............A. A. S....Sterling, Kan.................Not in A. G. R.
Grinnell, John L......Ass't S.....Peabody, Kan ................From March, 1863.
White, Jacob S........Surgeon...Michigan City, Ind.........To Dec., 1862. Dead.
Harriman, S. B........Ass't S.... Richmond, Ind..............To December, 1862.
Taylor, Daniel W.....Surgeon..........................To July, 1865.
Lenfestey, Robt. F...H. Stew...Marion, Ind.

### 35TH INFANTRY—Mustered out September 30, 1865.

Averdick, Henry G...Surgeon...Oldenburg, Ind..............From March, 1864. H. R.
Mullen, Alexander J.. " 3018 Thomas street, St. Louis, Mo. To February, 1864.
Parsons, Geo. W......Ass't S.... Rei, Ind.........................From May, 1865.
Bell, Nathaniel G..... " ..............................To November, 1864.
McCoy, Geo. H.. ..... " ..............................To April, 1862.
Moriarty, Wm. C.....H. Stew...Indianapolis, Ind.

## INDIANA—Continued.

36TH INFANTRY—Part mustered out September 21, 1864; veterans and recruits transferred to the 30th Infantry July 12, 1865.

Bosworth, Richard... Ass't S..... Winchester, Ind............ To September, 1864. U. S. Ex. S.
Kersey, Silas H........ Surgeon... Centreville, Ind............ To September, 1864.
Orr, James P.......... Ass't S..... Andersonville, Ind......... To March, 1863.
Whilsell, Joseph M... " Knightstown, Ind.......... To August, 1862.
Abbott, Chas. H...... " ................................ To September, 1864.
Bayse, Thos. S......... Surgeon... Alleged dead................ To March, 1863.
Hall, Daniel D......... Ass't S................................ To March, 1862.

37TH INFANTRY—Mustered out July 24 and 25, 1865.

Anderson, Wm......... Surgeon... Versailles, Ind.................. To October, 1864. H. R.
Goodwin, John R..... Ass't S.... Franklin Co., Ind........... To October, 1864. Alleged dead.
McClure, Samuel M.. " ................................ To February, 1864.
Redlon, Daniel M..... H. Stew... Pierceville, Ind.

38TH INFANTRY—Mustered out July 15, 1865.

Beckwith, Lod W..... Surgeon... Jeffersonville, Ind.......... To June, 1863.
Clapp, Wm. A......... " New Albany, Ind........... To June, 1862. Ex. S.
Currey, John........... " Mauckport, Ind.............. To October, 1864. G.
Mitchell, Robert...... Ass't S..... Marengo or Mitchell, Ind.. To October, 1864.
Nichols, John A...... " ................................ From January, 1865.
Whitaker, Eli D...... Surgeon................................ From April, 1865.

39TH INFANTRY—(See 8th Cavalry)

40TH INFANTRY—Mustered out December 21, 1865.

Aborn, Orin............ Ass't S..... Marshfield, Ind.............. To February, 1862.
Dunn, Williamson P.. " Frankfort, Ind................. To September, 1863. U. S. Ex. S.
Glick, Elias B......... Surgeon... La Fayette, Ind............... Died September, 1879
O'Ferrell, Robert M.. " La Fayette, Ind............... To March, 1862.
Potts, John.............. Ass't S..... Harmony, Ind.................. Cashiered Nov., 1862.
Riffle, John S.......... " Newtown, Ind.................. From December, 1862. G.

41ST INFANTRY—(See 2d Cavalry)

42D INFANTRY—Mustered out July 21, 1865.

Hornbrook, Wm. P.. Ass't S..... Union, Ind...................... To April, 1865.
Mageniss, John....... " Evansville, Ind............... Died March, 1876.
Tyner, Samuel L....... Ass't S..... Lynnville, Ind................. From June, 1865. G. H. R.
Shapley, Wm. W..... Surgeon................................ From June, 1865.
Taylor, Wm. D........ " Alleged dead.................. To November, 1864.

43D INFANTRY—Mustered out June 14, 1865.

Ellis, Hamilton E..... Surgeon... Greencastle, Ind............ To June, 1863 Dead.
Helmer, Orlando H.. Ass't S..... Tipton, Ind. (?)................ From June, 1863.
Smydth, Wm. C....... Surgeon... Worthington, Ind........... Dismissed May, 1862.
Smythe, Gonzaloa C.. " Greencastle, Ind............ From June, 1863.
Sweeney, Thos. J..... Ass't S..... Waveland, Ind................ From December, 1864.
Bogle, Christopher F.. " ................................ To November, 1864.
Culbertson, David P.. " ................................ To April, 1864.

## INDIANA—Continued.

### 44TH INFANTRY—Mustered out September 14, 1865.

| Name | Rank | Address | Remarks |
|---|---|---|---|
| Carr, Geo. W | Ass't S | Ligonier, Ind | To Surg. 129th Inf. March, 1864; also Lt.-Col. 93d Inf. |
| Plummer, Isaac N | " | Shoals, Ind | From April, 1865. |
| *Rerick, John H | Surgeon | Lagrange, Ind | From October, 1863. |
| Pardee, Chas. A | H. Stew | Wolcottsville, Ind | |
| Martin, W. W | Surgeon | Alleged dead | To August, 1863. |

### 45TH INFANTRY—(See 3d Cavalry.)

### 46TH INFANTRY—Mustered out September 4, 1865.

| Name | Rank | Address | Remarks |
|---|---|---|---|
| Haymond, Wm. A | Ass't S | Indianapolis, Ind | To December, 1862. |
| Spencer, Wm | " | Monticello, Ind | To December, 1862. |
| Underhill, J. W | Surgeon | 434 John st, Cincinati, Ohio. | From February, 1865. |
| Washburn, Israel B | " | Rensselaer. Ind | To December, 1864. |
| Coleman, Horace | Surgeon | Troy, Ohio | To July, 1863. |
| Doane, Geo. M | Ass't S | Burlington, Ind | From June, 1865. |

### 47TH INFANTRY—Mustered out October 23, 1865.

| Name | Rank | Address | Remarks |
|---|---|---|---|
| Crosby, Thos. H | Ass't S | Bluffton, Ind | To December, 1864. |
| Dicken, James L | Surgeon | Wabash or La Fontaine, Ind. | From December, 1861. |
| Stewart, Wm. J | Ass't S | | To December, 1862. |

### 48TH INFANTRY—Mustered out July 15, 1865.

| Name | Rank | Address | Remarks |
|---|---|---|---|
| Ham, L. J | Surgeon | South Bend, Ind | To April, 1864; H. R. |
| Lansing, Sylvester | Ass't S | Kingman, Kans | To 49th U. S. C. T. June, 1863. H. R |
| Kimball, Abner D | Ass't S | Xenia, Ind | From July, 1865. |
| Bryson, Frank T | Surgeon | Alleged dead | To March, 1865. |
| Loomis, Chauncey | A. H. S | La Porte, Ind. | |

### 49TH INFANTRY—Mustered out September 13, 1865.

| Name | Rank | Address | Remarks |
|---|---|---|---|
| †Hawn, Emanuel R | Surgeon | Indianapolis, Ind | To November, 1864; also 144th Inf. & 1st H. Art. |
| McCoy, James A. C | Ass't S | Snohomish, Wash. Ter | To October, 1862. |
| Monroe, Jasper R | Surgeon | Seymour, Ind | To August, 1862. |
| Pearson, Chas. D | " | 160 N. Delaware st., Indianapolis or La Fayette, Ind. | To February, 1862; also 82d Inf. |
| Ritter, John A | " | Orangeville, Ind | To September, 1863. |
| Smith, Wm. Z | Ass't S | Shoals, Ind | To June, 1864. Dead. |
| Widimer, John F. B | " | Bretzville, Ind | To July, 1863. Dead. |
| Buzett, Edward F | Surgeon | Burlington, Iowa | From April, 1865. |
| Pickthall, Arthur | Ass't S | | From July, 1865. |
| Thomas, John H | " | | To June, 1863. |

### 50TH INFANTRY—Consolidated with 52d Infantry May 26, 1865.

| Name | Rank | Address | Remarks |
|---|---|---|---|
| Durand, Amos M | Ass't S | Mt. Hope, Kans | Also Ass't S. 52d Inf. |
| ‡Hervey, Jas. W | " | Indianapolis, Ind | To February, 1863. |
| Hervey, Thos. P | " | McCordsville, Ind | To May, 1863. |
| Wells, James C | " | Mooney, Ind | To May, 1864 |
| Stewart, John L | H. Stew | New Albany, Ind | Was at Hospital No. 1, Bardstown, Ky. |
| Flack, Wm. C | Surgeon | | To January, 1865. |
| Rodman, Wm. M | A. A. S | Houston, Ind. | |

* Has a complete list of killed and wounded at Shiloh, made at the time. Examined recruits.
† Secretary of State of Indiana.
‡ In charge of Burnside Barracks, near Indianapolis, Ind., for two years.

## INDIANA—Continued.

### 51st Infantry—Mustered out December 13, 1865.

| | | | |
|---|---|---|---|
| Adams, David | Ass't S. | Edinburgh, Ind. | To November, 1862. |
| Collins, E. B. | Surgeon | 998 W. Madison st., Chicago, Ill., or Decatur, Ala. | A. W. M. |
| King, Henry R. | Ass't S. | 2603 Gravois Road, St. Louis, Mo. | From December, 1862. D. |
| Pearce, John W. | " | 998 W. Madison st., Chicago, Ill., or Decatur, Ind. | To April, 1863. |
| Easterling, Amos | " | | From June, 1865. |
| Smith, John P. | H. Stew. | Jamestown, Ind. | |

### 52d Infantry—Mustered out September 10, 1865.

| | | | |
|---|---|---|---|
| Freeman, Wm. | Ass't S. | Camden or Pennville, Ind. | To August, 1863. |
| Garrison, J. L. F. | Surgeon | Lebanon, Ind. | From May, 1865; H. R. D. |
| Martin, James W. | " | Red Oak, Iowa | To January, 1865. |
| Sexton, Marshall | " | Rushville, Ind. | To April, 1862 |
| Casterline, Amos B. | Ass't S. | Rush Co., Ind. | To December, 1862. |
| Durand, Amos M. | " | Mount Hope, Kans. | Also 50th Infantry. |
| Gard, James F. | A. H. S. | Ligonier, Ind. | |
| Martin, J. A. J. | H. Stew. | Deadwood, Dak. | |

### 53d Infantry—Mustered out July 21, 1865.

| | | | |
|---|---|---|---|
| Dukate, John S. | Ass't S. | Wheatland, Ind. | From May, 1865. |
| Davis, Solomon | Surgeon | Columbus or Cortland, Ind. | To May, 1862. Alleged dead. |
| Horner, Jacob S. | " | Corydon or Lanesville, Ind. | From May, 1865. |
| Hoagland, John S. | Ass't S. | Gentryville, Ind. | To May, 1862. Alleged dead. |
| Rose, Madison H. | Surgeon | Thornton, Ind. | To April, 1865. |
| Slaughter, Robt. C. | " | Newburgh or Evansville, Ind. | To March, 1863; also 25th Infantry. |

### 54th Infantry—(1 year.) Mustered out December 8, 1863

| | | | |
|---|---|---|---|
| Cyrus, Wm. H. | Ass't S. | Noblesville, Ind. | From April, 1863; also 54th Inf., (3 months.) |
| Davison, Henry C. | " | Hartford City, Ind. | To March, 1863. |
| Banks, Ephraim N. | Surgeon | | To March, 1863. |
| Pope, Henry E. | Ass't S. | | A. W. M. |
| Ryan, Townsend | Surgeon | | From April, 1863. |

### 55th Infantry—(3 months.)

| | | | |
|---|---|---|---|
| Preston, Albert G. | Surgeon | Greencastle, Ind. | |

### 56th Infantry—Failed to complete organization.

### 57th Infantry—Mustered out December 14, 1865.

| | | | |
|---|---|---|---|
| Brown, Jesse R. | Ass't S. | Green Fork or South Bend, Ind. | To April, 1862. |
| Crouse, Henry M. | Surgeon | Knightstown, Ind. | To September, 1863. |
| Mendenhall, Wm T. | Ass't S. | Richmond, Ind. | To Nov., 1863. Dead. |
| Mitchell, Robert S. | " | Richmond, Ind. | To September, 1863. |
| Prichet, John | Surgeon | Centreville, Ind. | To June, 1862. |
| Tillson, Hosea | " | Centreville, Ind. | To June, 1865. |
| Hochstetler, J. P. | " | | To October, 1863. |
| Jones, Harry | Ass't S. | | From September, 1865. |

## INDIANA—Continued.

### 58TH INFANTRY—Mustered out July 25, 1865.

| | | | |
|---|---|---|---|
| Adams, James R | Ass't S | Petersburgh, Ind | To Surg. 15th Inf Aug., 1863. H. R. G. |
| Blair, Wm. W | Surgeon | Princeton, Ind | To March, 1864. |
| Patten, James C | Ass't S | Princeton, Ind | From April, 1864. |
| Holstman, Sam'l E | Surgeon | Pontiac, Ind | From April, 1864. |

### 59TH INFANTRY—Mustered out July 17, 1865.

| | | | |
|---|---|---|---|
| Brown, Wilkins B. | Ass't S | Martz, Ind | To April, 1865. |
| Dixson, Wm H. | " | Knightsville, Ind | To April 1863. |
| Richards, Sam'l D | Surgeon | Patricksburgh, Ind | From July, 1865. |
| *Rogers, Dudley | " | Greencastle, Ind | To September, 1864. |
| Stueky, John M | Ass't S | Gosport, Ind | To January, 1863. |
| Fawcett, A. J. | H. Stew | Bloomfield, Ind. | |
| Taylor, James A | A. H. S | Bloomington, Ill. | |

### 60TH INFANTRY—Mustered out March 21, 1865.

| | | | |
|---|---|---|---|
| Bray, Madison J | Surgeon | Evansville, Ind | To December, 1862. |
| Hunter, James B | " | Evansville, Ind., or 2 E. 33d st., N. Y. City. | From January, 1864. |
| Slaughter, Wm. W | " | Newburgh, Ind | To June, 1864. |
| Whitehall, Alex. L | Ass't S | Attica, Ind | To August, 1863. |
| Tilman, Jonathan R | | Newburgh Ind | Not in A. G. R. |
| Welborne, T. W | A. H. S | Stewartsville, Ind. | |

### 61ST and 62D INFANTRY—Failed to organize.

### 63D INFANTRY—Mustered out May 3, and June 21, 1865.

| | | | |
|---|---|---|---|
| Garrett, Anthony | Surgeon | Delphi, Ind | To Jan., 1863. Alleged dead. |
| Jones, Caleb V | " | Covington, Ind | Dismissed Dec., 1864. |
| Jones, Geo. W | Ass't S | Danville, Ill | A. W. M. |
| Walker, Augustus C. | " | West Lebanon, Ind | A. W. M. H. R. |

### 64TH INFANTRY—Organized only as an Independent Battery of Light Artillery.

### 65TH INFANTRY—Mustered out June 22, 1865.

| | | | |
|---|---|---|---|
| Byers, Alexander R. | Surgeon | Petersburgh, Ind | To March, 1865; also 1st Lieut., 42d Inf. |
| Johnson, Samuel F | " | Dale, Ind | From May 1865. |
| Lewis, Eli | " | Princeton, Ind | Died March, 1879. |
| Scudder, John A | Ass't S | Washington, Ind | To Feb., 1864; U. S. Ex. S. |

### 66TH INFANTRY—Mustered out June 3, 1865.

| | | | |
|---|---|---|---|
| Bare, John R | Surgeon | Salem Ind | To January, 1865. |
| Field, Nathaniel | " | Jeffersonville, Ind. | Dead. |
| Simonson, James C | " | Little York, Ind | Dead. |
| Voyles, David W | " | Byrneville, Ind | To February, 1864. |
| Martin, Samuel F | Ass't S | | From May, 1865. |

### 67TH INFANTRY—Consolidated with 24th Infantry December 21, 1864.

| | | | |
|---|---|---|---|
| Boynton, Chas. S | Surgeon | Indianapolis, Ind | From April, 1864; also 24th Inf. |
| Burton, Wm. A | Ass't S | Mitchell, Ind | From May, 1863; also 24th Inf |
| Bryan, Geo. W | " | Bloomington, Ind | To May, 1863. |
| Dodd, James | " | Clear Creek, Ind | To April, 1863. |
| Gerrish, Jas. W. F | Surgeon | Seymour, Ind | To August, 1863. |

* Examined recruits.

## INDIANA—Continued.

### 68TH INFANTRY—Mustered out June 20, 1865.

Wooden, John L......Surgeon...Greensburgh, Ind.. ........From August, 1862. H. R. Ex. S.
Hodgkins, Lewis W..Ass't S....Ellsworth Me..............From August, 1863.
Meredith, Marion..... " Vinton, Iowa................From December, 1862.

### 69TH INFANTRY—Mustered out July 5, 1865.

Evans, David S..... ..Surgeon...Alleged dead..................To March, 1864.
Monteith, Jacob, S...Ass't S....Alleged dead.................A. W. M.

### 70TH INFANTRY—Mustered out June 8, 1865, and recruits transferred to 33d Infantry.

Kennedy, Leroy H...Ass't S....Danville. Ind..................To September, 1863.
Regan, Amos W......Surgeon...Mooresville, Ind ........... From August, 1862.
Smith, Wm. R.........Ass't S....Franklin, Ind.................To November, 1862.
Webb, Wm. A ......... " Franklin, Ind.. ..............To March, 1863.
Fitzgerald, J. A....... " Dead.
Watzer, Herman J...H. Stew...Vincennes, Ind.

### 71ST INFANTRY—(See 6th Cavalry.)

### 72D INFANTRY—Mustered out June 26, 1865; recruits transferred to the 44th Infantry.

Cole, Wm. C.............Surgeon...Attica, Ind.......................From Jan., 1864. H. R.
Kirkpatrick, G. W...Ass't S.....Culver's Station, Ind......From April, 1864.
Morrow, Jas. L........Surgeon...Pittsburgh, or Delphi, Ind To December, 1863.
Stearns, Elias P.......Ass't S.....Newton, Kans ..............From January, 1864.
Johnson, John B...... " Alma, Ill.........................To May, 1863.

### 73D INFANTRY—Mustered out July 1, 1865.

Brenton, Wm. H......Ass't S.....Peru, Ind.........................To March, 1863.
Myers, Seth F.........Surgeon...1536 Master st., Phila., Pa To May, 1865.
Spencer, William .....Ass't S.....Annapolis, Ind..............To 10th Tenn. Cav. Apr., 1864 Ex. S.
Applegate, Chas. H.. " Kankakee, Ill...................From November, 1864.
Pottenger. Wilson... " ..................................To December, 1863.
Spencer, Robert ......Surgeon.........................................To January, 1863.

### 74TH INFANTRY—Mustered out June 9, 1865; recruits transferred to the 22d Infantry.

Higbee, Edward S...Surgeon...Milford, Ind ....................From May, 1865. Alleged dead.
Josse, John M .........Ass't S.....Fort Wayne, Ind............To 32d Inf. Nov., 1863. Alleged dead.
Leidy, John K.........Surgeon...Warsaw, Ind.. ................Dead
Sheldon, Geo. W...... " Coopersville, Mich .........To February, 1863. D.
Bassett, John Q. A...Ass't S..........................................To March, 1863
Dodge, Henry C..... " Elkhart, Ind..................... From May, 1865.

### 75TH INFANTRY—Mustered out June 8, 1865.

Arthur, C. S.............Surgeon...Portland, Ind...................To September, 1864.
Buck, Robert H.......Ass't S.....418 Wash. avenue, St. Louis, Mo. To April 1863; also 13th Cav. and 118th Infantry (6 months.)
Shaffer, Abner H.....Surgeon...Huntington, Ind............From November, 1864.
White, James B.......Ass't S....Normandy, Ind..............A. W. M. Alleged dead.

## INDIANA—Continued.

### 76th Infantry—30 days' organization.

| Name | Rank | Address | Remarks |
|---|---|---|---|
| Davidson, Wm | Ass't S | Madison, Ind | A. W. M.; also 1st Lt. 42d Inf. |
| Duffield, Jas. T | Surgeon | Indianapolis, Ind | A. W. M.; also 7th Inf. |
| Simms, John N | Ass't S | Alleged dead | A. W. M. |

### 77th Infantry—(See 4th Cavalry.)

### 78th Infantry—60 days' organization.

| Name | Rank | Address | Remarks |
|---|---|---|---|
| Daly, Geo. P | Ass't S | Rockville, Ind | A. W. M. |

### 79th Infantry—Mustered out June 7, 1865.

| Name | Rank | Address | Remarks |
|---|---|---|---|
| McFadden, Wm. G | Surgeon | Shelbyville, Ind | From March, 1864. Ex. S. |
| Manker, Lewis | " | Bridgeport, Ind | To June, 1863. |
| Tilford, John H | Ass't S | Windom, Minn | From August, 1862. |
| Charleton, Robert | Surgeon | | To December, 1862. |

### 80th Infantry—Mustered out June 22, 1865; recruits transferred to the 129th Infantry.

| Name | Rank | Address | Remarks |
|---|---|---|---|
| Culbertson, R. H | Ass't S | Terre Haute, Ind | To January, 1864. |
| Jaquess, Geo. D | Surgeon | Helena, Ark | To Sept., 1864. Alleged dead. |
| Spain, Archibald W | Ass't S | Vigo, or Terre Haute, Ind. | From Dec., 1864, also 136th Inf. |
| Welborn, Wm. P | Surgeon | Princeton, Ind | From December, 1864. |
| Campbell, J. C. L | A. A. S | Loogootee, Ind | D. |

### 81st Infantry—Mustered out June 13, 1865; recruits transferred to the 31st Infantry.

| Name | Rank | Address | Remarks |
|---|---|---|---|
| Fouts, Wm. D | Surgeon | Jeffersonville, Ind | From Oct., 1863. H. R. |
| Ralston, Wm. G | " | Evansville, Ind | To May, 1863. |
| Wolf, Harvey S | " | Corydon, Ind | To February, 1863. |
| Kelso, Wm. H | Ass't S | | From February, 1863. |
| Kay, David G | Surgeon | | To December, 1862. |

### 82d Infantry—Mustered out June 9, 1865; recruits transferred to the 22d Infantry.

| Name | Rank | Address | Remarks |
|---|---|---|---|
| Brooks, Mordecai | Ass't S | Madison, Ind | To Oct., 1863. Died, 1881. |
| Harris, Wm. B | " | Vincennes, Ind | From January, 1865. |
| Lemon, Wm. H | Surgeon | Winchester, Kans | From June, 1863. |
| Pearson, Chas. D | " | 160 N. Delaware street, Indianapolis, Ind. | To May, 1863; also 49th Inf. |

### 83d Infantry—Mustered out June 1, 2, and 3, 1865, except Co. D, 9-months' service.

| Name | Rank | Address | Remarks |
|---|---|---|---|
| Davis, Samuel | Surgeon | 296 Lexington ave., Indianapolis, Ind. | To August, 1863. |
| Gillespie, Wm | " | Rising Sun, Ind | To March, 1864; also 7th Inf |
| Vincent, Henry C | Ass't S | Guilford, Ind | To July, 1863. |
| Weaver, Samuel M | " | Dillsborough Ind | From January, 1865. |

### 84th Infantry—Mustered out June 14, 1865; recruits transferred to the 57th Infantry.

| Name | Rank | Address | Remarks |
|---|---|---|---|
| Boyd, Samuel S | Surgeon | Dublin, Ind | To March, 1865. |
| Davis, Robert P | Ass't S | Portland, Ind | To May, 1865. |
| Kirby, Henry | Surgeon | Osage City, Kans | From April, 1865. |
| Casterline, Ziba | Ass't S | | To July, 1863. |

## INDIANA—Continued.

85TH INFANTRY—Mustered out June 12, 1865; recruits transferred to the 33d Infantry.

Hobbs, William P....Ass't S.....Knightstown, Ind..........To October, 1864. H. R.
Hobbs, Wilson.........Surgeon...Knightstown, Ind..........From September, 1862.
Johnson, Wm. W.....Ass't S.....Eureka Springs, Ark......To April, 1863; also 9th Ohio Independent Battery.
Wiles, Wm. V......... " Spencer, Ind.................From September, 1862. H. R.

86TH INFANTRY—Mustered out June 6, 1865.

Jones, Joseph.........Surgeon...San Antonio, Texas.......From December, 1862.
Van Vorhis, F. J......Ass't S.....Indianapolis, Ind...........From December, 1862.
Elliott, James S......Surgeon..................................To November, 1862.
Walton, Allen M......Ass't S.....................................To May, 1864; also 13th Cav.
Woodward, Jas. H...H. Stew...Indianapolis, Ind.

87TH INFANTRY—Mustered out June 10, 1865.

Gould, Vernon.........Ass't S.....Rochester, Ind...............From March, 1863.
Moss, Gordon D....... " Rensselaer, Ind.............To February, 1863.
Pratt, Samuel R......Surgeon...Hebron, Ind.................To February, 1863.
Triplett, Chas. E...... " Morocco, Ind................From August, 1863.
Lynch, Webster.......H. Stew...Union Mills, Ind.

88TH INFANTRY—Mustered out July 7, 1865.

Gregg, James S........Surgeon...Fort Wayne, Ind.............From January, 1863.
Teal, Norman.........Ass't S.....Kendallville, Ind............A. W. M.
Willard, Henry W...H. Stew...Dallas, Mich...................Allowed to prescribe, &c.
Eno, Newton G.......Ass't S.......................................To November, 1864.
Myers, Wm. D.........Surgeon.......................................To December, 1862.

89TH INFANTRY—Mustered out June 19, 1865; recruits transferred to the 32d Infantry.

Meeks, John A.........Ass't S.....Jonesborough, Ind.........To August, 1864.
Scott Wm.................Surgeon...Kokomo, Ind...............From February, 1865.
*Cox, Jesse T.........Ass't S.....Dallas, Texas.................From February, 1865.
Henderson, John F...Surgeon...Kokomo, Ind.................Dismissed August, 1864.

90TH INFANTRY—(See 5th Cavalry.)

91ST INFANTRY—Cos. A to G, inclusive, mustered out June 26, 1865; the rest transferred to the 124th and 128th Infantry.

Robson, Robert........Surgeon...New Harmony, Ind.......To June, 1864. Alleged dead.
Robson, John R......Ass't S.....New Harmony, Ind.......To April, 1865. Dead.

92D INFANTRY—Failed to complete its organization.

93D INFANTRY—Cos A to H mustered out August 10, 1865, the rest November 10, 1865.

Ford, John H...........Surgeon...Columbus, Ind...............To August, 1865. Alleged dead
Ruter, Rinaldo R..... " Patriot, Ind.....................To April, 1863. I.
Irwin, Geo. E.........Ass't S.....Alleged dead.................To August, 1865.

---

* Also Hospital Steward from September, 1862, to February, 1865. Private in Co. G.

INDIANA—Continued.

94TH, 95TH, and 96TH INFANTRY—Failed to complete their organization.

97TH INFANTRY—Mustered out June 9, 1865.

Hilburn, Jabez C.. ...Surgeon...Spencer, Ind..................Dead; widow has records; remarried Reed.
Murphy, Alex. D.....Ass't S.....Sullivan, Ind..................From April, 1865.
Murphy, Alex. M.....Surgeon...Sullivan, Ind..................To May, 1864. U. S. Ex. S.
McNutt, Jas. H........Ass't S.....Harveysburgh, Ind.........To November, 1864.

98TH INFANTRY—Failed to complete its organization.

99TH INFANTRY—Mustered out June 5, 1865.

Butterworth, W. W..Surgeon...Mishawaka, Ind.............From February, 1863.
Poffenberger, Isaiah..Ass't S.....Walkerton, Ind..............From April, 1865.
Robinson, L. D....... " Coatesville, Ind.............To August, 1863.

100TH INFANTRY—Mustered out June 8, 1865.

France, Samuel........Surgeon.. Bourbon, Ind ................To August, 1863.
Leavitt, Philander C.. " Acton, Ind...................From November, 1863.
*McGee, Richard......Ass't S.....Edgar Co., Ill.................Dismissed May, 1863.
Swartz, David J...... " Auburn, Ind....................From October, 1862. G.

101ST INFANTRY—Mustered out June 24, 1865.

Bennett, Basil B......Ass't S.....Wabash, Ind....................From June, 1864.
Graham, Wm. B......Surgeon...Noblesville, Ind.............From March, 1864.
Lent, Cyrus V. N..... " Liberty Mills, Ind.........To February, 1863; also 138th Inf.
Whitesell, Philip P... " Clarksville, Ind..............Dismissed May, 1863.
Melsheimer, Chas. T..Ass't S.....Bluffton, Ind.....................To February, 1863.
Dewey, Annin W.....Surgeon.......................................Dismissed Dec., 1863.

From the 102D to the 114TH, inclusive—Failed to complete their organization.

115TH INFANTRY, (6 months)—Mustered out February 25, 1864.

Blackwell, John A...Surgeon...Foristell, Mo.................From Sept., 1863; also 1st Lt. 12th Inf.
Cooper, Joel S.........Ass't S.....Topeka, Kan....................From September, 1863.
Slavens, Zenas L...... " Parkville, Ind..................From September, 1863.

116TH INFANTRY—(6 months.)—Mustered out from February 29 to March 2, 1864.

Adams, M. M..........Ass't S.....Greenfield, Ind...............From September, 1863.
Bonnell, M. H..........Surgeon...Lebanon, Ind...................From September, 1863.
Messner, Sam'l F .....Ass't S.............................................To November, 1863.
Wright, Ivy E ......... " .............................................From November, 1863.

117TH INFANTRY—(6 months )—Mustered out from February 23 to 27, 1864.

Thomas, James H.....Ass't S.....Chenoa, Ill.......................From September, 1863.

118TH INFANTRY—(6 months.)—Mustered out from March 1 to 4, 1864.

Buck, Robert H.......Surgeon...418 Wash'n ave., St. Louis, Mo , or Indianapolis, Ind. From Sept., 1863; also 13th Cav. and 75th Inf.
Blount, Rufus F.......Ass't S.....Wabash, Ind.....................From September, 1863.

* Was at Adams Hospital, Memphis, in 1863.

## INDIANA—Continued.

119TH INFANTRY—(See 7th Cavalry.)

120TH INFANTRY—Mustered out January 8, 1866.

Barker, Wm. L........Surgeon...Boonville, Ind ................To July, 1864.
French, John S........Ass't S.....Alamo or Crawfordsville, Ind. From April, 1864, 2d Lt. Co. B.
Neely. John M.........Surgeon...Owensville, Ind...............From September, 1864.
Harrison, R. G.........Ass't S......................................To May, 1865.

121ST INFANTRY—(See 9th Cavalry.)

122D INFANTRY—Failed to complete its organization.

123D INFANTRY—Mustered out August 25, 1865.

Dutton, Daniel B .....Ass't S.....Clyde. Kans....................From March, 1864. H. R.
Leech, Elliott W...... " Shelbyville, Ind.............To 1864.
Spurrier, John H......Surgeon...Rushville, Ind...............A. W. M. Also 16th Inf.
Wilson, Jacob B ......Ass't S......................................From September, 1864.
Bogart, John M........H. Stew...Clinton, Ind.

124TH INFANTRY—Mustered out August 31, 1865.

Edwins, S. W.... .....Ass't S.....Frankton, Ind..............From October, 1864.
*Gregg, V. H...........Surgeon...Connersville, Ind... ........From March, 1864.
King, Wm. F...........Ass't S.....Centreville, Ind...... .....To Surg. 147 Inf. March, 1865.
Keiser, Alfred......... " ......................................To March, 1864.

125TH INFANTRY—(See 10th Cavalry.)

126TH INFANTRY—(See 11th Cavalry.)

127TH INFANTRY—(See 12th Cavalry.)

128TH INFANTRY—Mustered out April 10, 1866.

Meaker, Lysander....Ass't S.....La Porte, Ind.................To Dec., 1864. H. R.
Hoffman, M. F. A....Surgeon......................................From July, 1864; also 9th Inf.
Salisbury, David......Ass't S......................................From November, 1865.

129TH INFANTRY—Mustered out August 29, 1865.

Carr, Geo. W............Surgeon...Ligonier, Ind.....................Also Ass't S. 44th Inf., and Lt. Col. 93d Inf. Dead.
Tolerton, James....... " Rochester, Ind..............From July, 1865. Alleged dead.
Gorrell, Joseph R.....Ass't S......................................To March, 1865.
DeLong, D. D.........H Stew...Annville, Pa.

130TH INFANTRY—Mustered out December 2, 1865.

Baker. Braxton........Ass't S.....Alexandria, Ind ............From December, 1864.
Jones, Thos. N.........Surgeon...Anderson, Ind..............To July, 1864; also 2d Cav.
Pattison, Geo W..... " Kokomo, Ind.. ..............From December, 1864.
Williamson, E.........Ass't S.....Dead.......................................To March, 1865.

---

*In charge of hospital at Charlotte, and at Greensburgh, N. C., in 1865.

## INDIANA—Continued.

### 131st Infantry—(See 13th Cavalry.)

### 132d Infantry—(100 days )—Mustered out September 7, 1864.

Phipps, John M........Surgeon...Evansville or Indianapolis, Ind. From May, 1864. H. R.
Jones, Jas. T............Ass't S.....Franklin, Ind................From May, 1864.

### 133d Infantry—(100 days.)—Mustered out September 5, 1864.

Kuester, Chas. E......Ass't S.....Terre Haute, Ind...........From June, 1864; also 156th Inf.
Archer, Sam'l M...... " ..........................A. W. M.
Hitchcock, John W...Surgeon..................................A. W. M. Also 18th Inf.

### 134th Infantry—(100 days.)—Mustered out September 2, 1864.

Craig, John M.........Ass't S.....Baxter Springs, Kan., or Greensburgh, Ind........ From May, 1864, also 146 Inf.
Brazelton, John B.... " Fairmont, Neb..............From May, 1864.

### 135th Infantry—(100 days.)—Mustered out September 29, 1864.

Berryman, J. A........Ass't S.....Potato Creek, Ind.........From May, 1864. H. R.
Cresap, Wm. S........ " Lebanon, Ind..................Also Chap. 10th and Surg. 154th Inf.
McClelland, J. S......Surgeon....................................From May, 1864.

### 136th Infantry—(100 days,) Mustered out September 2, 1864

Spain, A. W...........Ass't S.....Vigo or Terre Haute, Ind. From May, 1864; also 80th Infantry.
Fullerton, Geo. W... " ..................................From May, 1864.
Garver, Jas. A.........Surgeon....................................From May, 1864; also 8th Cavalry.

### 137th Infantry—(100 days ) Mustered out September 21, 1864.

Roe, John L............Surgeon...North Madison, Ind.......From May, 1864. Died November, 1876.
Murray, Ralph V.....Ass't S....Zanesville, Ohio............From May, 1864.
Wilson, Isaac.......... " ..................................From July. 1864; also 1st Lieut. 60th Inf.

### 138th Infantry—(100 days,) Mustered out September 22, 1864.

Lent, Cyrus V. N....Surgeon...Liberty Mills, Ind..........From May, 1864; also 101st Infantry.
Gillum, Jas.............Ass't S.....Portland, Ind................From July, 1864.
Woods, Daniel L...... " Streator, Ill.......................From June, 1864; also 1st H. Art. and 153d Inf

### 139th Infantry—(100 days,) Mustered out September 29, 1864.

Bogart, Henry J......Ass't S.....Charlottesville, Ind........From June, 1864.
Champ, Geo. W....... " New Lisbon, Ind...........From June, 1864; also Capt. 37th Inf.
McCoy, John...........Surgeon....................................From June, 1864

### 140th Infantry—(1 year,) Mustered out July 11, 1865.

Piatt, Wm. C...........Ass't S.....Marion, Ind ..................From January, 1865.
Sweezey, Wm. C.....Surgeon...Olivet, Kans......................A. W. M.
Ballard, Micajah B...Ass't S.....Richmond, Ind..............From November, 1864

141st Infantry—Failed to complete its organization: recruits were assigned to the 140th Infantry.

## INDIANA—Continued.

### 142D INFANTRY—(1 year,) Mustered out July 14, 1865.

| Name | Rank | Residence | Remarks |
|---|---|---|---|
| Bruce, Geo. W | Surgeon | Winchester, Ind | From November, 1864; also 8th Inf. & 1st Cav. |
| St Clair, Owen | Ass't S. | Wakarusa, Ind | From November, 1864. Alleged dead. |
| Ferguson, Wm. T. | " | | From March, 1865. |

### 143D INFANTRY—(1 year,) Mustered out October 17, 1865.

| Name | Rank | Residence | Remarks |
|---|---|---|---|
| Allen, Wm. S. | Ass't S. | Auburn, Ind | From June, 1865. |
| Davidson Benj. F. | " | | A. W. M. Said to be I. |
| Pitcher, Stewart C. | Surgeon | Dead | From May, 1865. |

### 144TH INFANTRY—(1 year,) Mustered out August 5, 1865.

| Name | Rank | Residence | Remarks |
|---|---|---|---|
| Hawn, Emanuel R. | Surgeon | Indianapolis or Leavenworth, Ind. | From March, 1865; also 49th Inf. & 1st H Art. |
| Kay, Robert | Ass't S. | Salem or Livonia, Ind | From March, 1865; also 23d Inf. |
| Neat, Thos. C. | " | New Albany, Ind | From March, 1865. |

### 145TH INFANTRY—(1 year,) Mustered out January 21, 1866.

| Name | Rank | Residence | Remarks |
|---|---|---|---|
| Beck, Wm. H. | Surgeon | Hartsville, Ind | From May, 1865 |
| Davis, Jos. H. | Ass't S. | Reddington, Ind | From July, 1865. |
| Duffy, John S. | " | | From May, 1865. |

### 146TH INFANTRY—(1 year,) Mustered out August 31, 1865

| Name | Rank | Residence | Remarks |
|---|---|---|---|
| Carley, Rush | Ass't S. | Bethany, Ohio | From March, 1865. H. R. |
| Craig, John M. | " | Baxter Sprins or Greengsburgh, Ind. | From May, 1865; also 134th Inf. |
| Haines, Abraham B. | Surgeon | Aurora, Ind | From April, 1865; also 19th and 20th Inf. |

### 147TH INFANTRY—(1 year,) Mustered out August 4, 1865.

| Name | Rank | Residence | Remarks |
|---|---|---|---|
| King, Wm F. | Surgeon | Centreville, Ind | From June, 1865; also Ass't S 124th Inf. |
| Weddington, Sam C. | Ass't S. | Jonesborough, Ind | From March, 1865. H. R. |
| Reed, Albert S. | " | | From April, 1865. |

### 148TH INFANTRY—(1 year.) Mustered out September 5, 1865.

| Name | Rank | Residence | Remarks |
|---|---|---|---|
| Reagan, Jesse | Surgeon | Plainfield or Monrovia, Ind. | From May, 1865. |
| Beebe, James | Ass't S. | Whiteland, Ind | From May, 1865. |

### 149TH INFANTRY—(1 year,) Mustered out September 27, 1865.

| Name | Rank | Residence | Remarks |
|---|---|---|---|
| Gross, Jas. M. | Ass't S. | Freedom or Spencer, Ind. | A. W. M. |
| Hendricks, Wm. C. | Surgeon | Franklin or Ladoga, Ind. | To July, 1865; also 31st Inf. |
| Mullinnix, M. M. | Ass't S. | Spencer, Ind | From March, 1865. D. |
| Jones, Wm. B. | Surgeon | | A. W. M. |

### 150TH INFANTRY—(1 year) Mustered out August 5, 1865.

| Name | Rank | Residence | Remarks |
|---|---|---|---|
| Becks, Green C. | Surgeon | Battle Ground, Ind | From March, 1865. |
| Harrison, Thos. H. | Ass't S. | Lebanon, Ind | From March, 1865. |
| Wallace, Jas. P. | " | Animas City, Col | From March, 1865. |

INDIANA—Continued.

151ST INFANTRY—(1 year,) Mustered out September 19, 1865.

Moss, Gordon A.......Surgeon...Rensselaer, Ind..............From April, 1865. Alleged dead.
Elston, Wm. T.........Ass't S.....Francisville, Ind............From July, 1865.

152D INFANTRY (1 year)—Mustered out August 30, 1865.

Chamberlain, Jas. M..Surgeon...Waterloo, Ind ................From April, 1865.
Mercer, Wm. H.......Ass't S.....Corunna, Ind.................From March, 1865.
Sherwin, Heman H... " Rowan, Ind........................Died October, 1880.

153D INFANTRY (1 year)—Mustered out September 4, 1865.

Johnson, Isaac C......Ass't S.....Kokomo, Ind ..................From March, 1865.
O'Neal, Laughlin.....Surgeon...Somerset. Ind ................From March, 1865.
Woods, Daniel L......Ass't S....Streator, Ill.......................From April, 1865; also 138th Inf. and 1st H. Art.

154TH INFANTRY (1 year)—Mustered out August 4, 1865.

Cresap, Wm. G........Ass't S....Lebanon, Ind.................From April, 1865; also Chap. 10th and 135th Inf. Dead.
Gentry, Z. B...........Surgeon...Frankfort, Ky ..............From April. 1865. D.
Richardson, A. G.....Ass't S....Veedersburgh or Stone Bluff, Ind. From April, 1865.

155TH INFANTRY (1 year)—Mustered out August 4, 1865.

Arnold, Martin B.....Ass't S.....Merrillville, Ind ............From June, 1865.
Chandler, Jos. A...... " Yellow Creek or Warsaw, Ind. From April, 1865.
Smith, John W........Surgeon...Gosport, Ind.....................From May, 1865.

156TH INFANTRY (1 year)—Mustered out August 4, 1865.

Kuester, Chas. E......Surgeon...Terre Haute, Ind............From April, 1865; 133d Inf.
Guffin, John ............ " Vermillion, Co., Ill.........From May, 1865; also 20th Inf.

157TH and 158TH INFANTRY—Failed to complete their organization.

IOWA.

1ST CAVALRY—Mustered out February 15, 1866.

Allen, David B.........Ass't S....West Liberty, Ohio ........To 30th Inf. April, 1863.
Cochran, Milton B....Surgeon...Davenport, Iowa............To August, 1864.
Elder, Thos. H ........H. Stew...Albia, Iowa......................H. R. for 1861 and 1862. G.
Hervey, Jas ............Ass't S.....Dubuque, Iowa ..............From September, 1864.
Ladd, John A......... " Traer, Iowa........................To September, 1863.
Lathrop, Chas. H.....Surgeon...Lyons, Iowa........................From Aug., 1864. H. R.
Morgan, Asa............Ass't S.....Cedar Bayou, Tex .........To 12th Ill. Cav. June, 1865; also 7th Inf.
Sanders, John J....... " ........................................Dismissed Nov., 1864.

2D CAVALRY—Mustered out September 19, 1865.

Yulee, Erastus D .....Ass't S.....Marshalltown, Iowa.........To June, 1864.
Noyes, Geo. H.........Surgeon...Nashua, N. H ..................From June, 1862. Dead.
Burgess, Jesse R..... Ass't S.....Alleged dead......................From January, 1863.
Reeder, Geo ..........Surgeon............................................To June, 1862.

## IOWA—Continued.

### 3D CAVALRY—Mustered out August 9, 1865.

| Name | Rank | Residence | Remarks |
|---|---|---|---|
| Carter, Geo. W | Surgeon | Marshalltown, Iowa | From June, 1863; also 9th Inf. |
| Maxwell, Thos. J | Ass't S | Biggsville, Ill | To 138th U. S. C. T. July, 1865. |
| Orr, Wm. L | " | Ottumwa, Iowa | To 21st Inf. Dec., 1862. U. S. Ex. S. |
| Warford, F. W | " | Cicero, Ind | To 4th Ark. Cav. Jan., 1864. |
| Whitten, Samuel | " | Alleged dead | From April, 1864. |
| McGugin, David L | Surgeon | | To April, 1863. |
| Fuller, E. E | H. Stew | Keokuk, Iowa | From August, 1861, to September, 1862. |

### 4TH CAVALRY—Mustered out August 10, 1865.

| Name | Rank | Residence | Remarks |
|---|---|---|---|
| Bird, Wellington | Ass't S | Mt. Pleasant, Iowa | To March, 1862. |
| Cummings, Stephen | " | Sand Springs, Iowa | From July, 1863. |
| Findley, Wm. McK | " | Bloomfield, Iowa | To June, 1863. |
| * McClure, A. W | Surgeon | Mt. Pleasant, Iowa | To April, 1863. |
| Robinson, Wm | " | Cedar Falls, Iowa | From July, 1863. G. |
| Taylor, Robert R | Ass't S | Glasgow, Iowa | To October, 1862. |
| Taylor, Samuel W | " | | From June, 1864. |

### 5TH CAVALRY—(The 5th Infantry was consolidated with this regiment September 1, 1864)—Mustered out August 11, 1865.

| Name | Rank | Residence | Remarks |
|---|---|---|---|
| McDeWitt, Geo. S | Ass't S | Elliott, Iowa | To March, 1864. |
| Shelly, B. Y | " | Niobrara, Nebr | From January, 1863. |
| Wise, B. Taylor | Surgeon | Hannibal, Mo | From October, 1862. |
| Lewis, T. F | Ass't S | | To July, 1865. |
| Lowe, Enos | " | | To September, 1862. |

### 6TH CAVALRY—Mustered out October 17, 1865.

| Name | Rank | Residence | Remarks |
|---|---|---|---|
| Bardwell, Thos. S | Ass't S | Marion, Iowa | From February, 1863. I. |
| Camburn, Jacob H | Surgeon | Cedar Rapids, Iowa | From February, 1863. |
| Haynes, Samuel C | Ass't S | | A. W. M. Also 37th Inf. |

### 7TH CAVALRY—(The Sioux City Cavalry and three companies of 41st Infantry were transferred to this Regiment)—Mustered out May 17, and June 22, 1866.

| Name | Rank | Residence | Remarks |
|---|---|---|---|
| La Force, Jas. W | Ass't S | Floris, Iowa | To December, 1864. G. |
| Yeomans, S. P | " | Charles City, Iowa | From August, 1863. |
| Willey, Andrew J | Surgeon | Mt. Ayer, Iowa | From April, 1863. |

### 8TH CAVALRY—Mustered out August 13, 1865.

| Name | Rank | Residence | Remarks |
|---|---|---|---|
| Bird, H. T | H. Stew | Mt. Pleasant, Iowa. | |
| Carnahan, A. S | Surgeon | Andrew, Iowa | To November, 1864. |
| Finley, Wm. H | " | Hopkinton, Iowa | To April, 1864. |
| Smith, Jos. F | Ass't S | Gainville, or Clarinda, Iowa. | From June, 1864. |
| Warner, Daniel H | Surgeon | | From February, 1865. |

### 9TH CAVALRY—Mustered out from February 3, to March 23, 1866.

| Name | Rank | Residence | Remarks |
|---|---|---|---|
| Shollenbarger, J. B | H. Stew | Sigourney, Iowa. | |
| Bell, John | Surgeon | Dallas, Tex | From March, 1865. D. |
| Ward, Jesse A | Ass't S | Fairbanks, Iowa | From March, 1865. |
| Wassow, Jesse | Surgeon | La Porte City, Iowa | To Jan., 1865; also 32d Inf. |
| Kirkup, Edwin | Ass't S | Healdsburgh, Cal | To 18th Inf. Feb., 1865. |
| Sykes, Jas | | Beverly, Ill | Treated Co. E in summer of 1865–'6, at Helena, Ark. |

---

* Inspecting surgeon at enlistment.

## IOWA—Continued.

### 1st Infantry—(3-months.)

### 2d Infantry—(The veterans and recruits of the 3d Infantry were transferred to this Regiment November 4, 1864)—Mustered out July 12, 1865.

| Name | Rank | Residence | Remarks |
|---|---|---|---|
| Nassaw, W. W | Ass't S | Burlington, Iowa | To Brig. Surg. April, 1862. |
| Pyle, Elliott | " | Burlington, Ia.; or Butler, Mo | To 54th U. S. C. T. Oct., 1863. |
| Turner, Wm. H | " | Keokuk, Iowa | To January, 1865. |
| Marsh, Willis R | Surgeon | | From June, 1861. |
| Clark, Prentiss B | Ass't S | Tabor, Iowa | From April, 1865; also 8th Inf. |

### 3d Infantry—Consolidated with the 2d Infantry November 4, 1864.

| Name | Rank | Residence | Remarks |
|---|---|---|---|
| Cool, Daniel M | Surgeon | Council Bluffs, Iowa; or Chicago, Ill. | To September, 1862. |
| Keables, Benj. F | " | Pella, Iowa | To June, 1864. H. R. |
| Schooley, John W | Ass't S | Golden, Colo | To June, 1864. |
| Robinson, S. E | A. A. S | West Union, Iowa | Not in A. G. R. |
| Edwards, Thos. O | Surgeon | | To April, 1862. |
| Martin, David R | Ass't S | | To June, 1863. |

### 4th Infantry—Mustered out July 24, 1865.

| Name | Rank | Residence | Remarks |
|---|---|---|---|
| Greenleaf, D. C | Surgeon | Bloomfield, Iowa | From December, 1864. |
| Shaw, Alex | Ass't S | Denver, Colo | To 29th Inf. Aug., 1863. |
| Whitfield, Isaiah J | " | Grand Rapids, Mich | From December, 1864. |
| Robins, Myron W | Surgeon | Las Vegas, N. M | To September, 1864. |
| Grimes, W. S | Ass't S | Salt Lake, U. T | To September, 1862. |
| Baley, Lewis | " | | To March, 1863. |

### 5th Infantry—Consolidated with 5th Cavalry September 1, 1864.

| Name | Rank | Residence | Remarks |
|---|---|---|---|
| Darrow, W. H | Ass't S | Columbus Junction, Ia | From September, 1862, to Sept., 1864. |
| Rawson, Chas. H | Surgeon | Des Moines, Iowa | To Brig. Surg. April, 1862. |
| Huntsman, H. C | Ass't S | Oskaloosa, Iowa | To 50th U. S. C. T. Aug., 1863. |
| Carpenter, P. A | " | Alleged dead | To Sept., 1864. A. W. M. |

### 6th Infantry—Mustered out July 21, 1865.

| Name | Rank | Residence | Remarks |
|---|---|---|---|
| Lambert, Wm. S | Surgeon | Albia, Iowa | From January, 1865. |
| Smith, Norman M | Ass't S | Monticello, Iowa | From October, 1862. |
| Lake, John E | " | | To September, 1862. |
| Shaw, Albert T | Surgeon | Osceola, Iowa | Missing since Dec., 1864. |

### 7th Infantry—Mustered out July 12, 1865.

| Name | Rank | Residence | Remarks |
|---|---|---|---|
| Everingham, Jas | Surgeon | Butler, Mo | From October, 1863. |
| Lake, Calvin B | " | Ames, or Indianola Iowa | To September, 1863. |
| Morgan, Asa | Ass't S | Cedar Bayou, Tex | To June, 1862; also 1st Cavalry. |
| Ashton, John | " | | From September, 1862. |

### 8th Infantry—Mustered out April 20, 1866.

| Name | Rank | Residence | Remarks |
|---|---|---|---|
| Cook, Sam'l D | Surgeon | Sigourney, Iowa | From Sept., 1864; U. S. Ex. S. |
| Hoffmeister, A. W | " | Ft. Madison, Iowa | To August, 1864. |
| Horton, C. F | Act'g S | Shellsburgh, Iowa | A. G. reports him Act'g Surg. from Nov., 1861, to June, 1862. |
| Huston, Isaac M | Ass't S | Victor, Iowa | From October, 1864. |
| Irwin, James | Surgeon | Fort Collins, Colo | To April, 1863. |
| McGovern, Chas | Ass't S | | To August, 1863. |
| Clark, Prentis B | " | | To Jan., 1862; also 2d Inf. |
| McConnell, Jas | H. Stew | Rush Centre, Kan. | |

## IOWA—Continued.

### 9TH INFANTRY—Mustered out July 18, 1865

| Name | Rank | Residence | Remarks |
|---|---|---|---|
| Hart, Henry W | Ass't S | Council Bluffs, Iowa | To 38th Inf. Oct., 1862. G. |
| McGorrick, E. J | Surgeon | Des Moines, Iowa | From Jan., 1863; also 17th Inf. (S. G. of Iowa.) |
| McClure, Benj | " | Dubuque, Iowa | To January, 1863. |
| Carter, Geo. W | Ass't S | Marshalltown, Iowa | To 3d Cav. June, 1863. |
| Reed, Chas. A | " | | A. W. M. |

### 10TH INFANTRY—Mustered out August 15, 1865.

| Name | Rank | Residence | Remarks |
|---|---|---|---|
| Mohr, R. J | Surgeon | Los Angeles, Cal., or Fairfield, Iowa. | From April, 1862, U. S. Ex. S. |
| Skinner, John O | Ass't S | Polk City, Iowa | To June, 1865. |
| Willey, And'w J | " | Mount, Ayr, Iowa. | To February, 1862. |
| Everett, Wm | " | | To September, 1864. |
| Davis, Wm. P | Surgeon | | To April, 1862. |
| Cummings, Wm. C | Ass't S | | To October, 1862. |
| Folger, John M | H. Stew | Indianola, Iowa. | |

### 11TH INFANTRY—Mustered out July 15, 1865.

| Name | Rank | Residence | Remarks |
|---|---|---|---|
| Batdorf, J C | Ass't S | Mechanicsville, Iowa | To June, 1863. |
| Lloyd, Fred'k | " | Care of A. G. U. S. A. | To 16th Inf. June, 1862. |
| Miles, Jas D | " | Crawfordsville or Washington, Iowa. | From July, 1863. H. R. |
| Watson, Wm | Surgeon | Dubuque, Iowa | To U. S. V. March, 1863. |
| Miller, John G | " | Lead City or Deadwood, Dak. Ter. | To July, 1865. |
| Meyer, Frederick | Ass't S | | To June, 1863. |
| Johnson, D. P | " | | To September, 1862. |

### 12TH INFANTRY—Mustered out January 20, 1866.

| Name | Rank | Residence | Remarks |
|---|---|---|---|
| Barr, James | Ass't S | Algona, Iowa | From November, 1865. U. S. Ex. S. |
| Finley, Wm. H | " | Hopkinton, Iowa | To August, 1863. |
| Huff, Sanford W | Surgeon | Sigourney, Iowa | From Jan., 1864. Dead. |
| Parker, Chas. C | " | Fayette, Iowa | To April, 1862. |
| Underwood, Myron | Ass't S | Eldora, Iowa | To September, 1865. U. S. Ex. S. |

### 13TH INFANTRY—Mustered out July 21, 1865.

| Name | Rank | Residence | Remarks |
|---|---|---|---|
| McKee, Jos. M | Surgeon | Rock Island, Ill | To November, 1862. |
| Thrall, Seneca B | Ass't S | Ottumwa, Iowa | To April, 1864. |
| Thomas, Moses W | Surgeon | Des Moines, Iowa | A. W. M. |
| Morrison, John C | Ass't S | | To November, 1864. |
| Boucher, Jas. H | " | | To U. S. V. August, 1862. |

### 14TH INFANTRY—Mustered out August 8, 1865.

| Name | Rank | Residence | Remarks |
|---|---|---|---|
| Staples, Geo. M | Surgeon | Dubuque, Iowa | To November, 1864. |
| Pierce, Sam N | Ass't S | Cedar Falls, Iowa | To April, 1863. U. S. Ex. S. |
| Haskins, Shadrack | " | Earlville, Iowa | To November, 1864. |
| Stevens, John H | " | | To November, 1864. |

### 15TH INFANTRY—Mustered out July 24, 1865.

| Name | Rank | Residence | Remarks |
|---|---|---|---|
| Gibbon, Wm. H | Surgeon | Chariton, Iowa | To December, 1864. |
| Nelson, Wm. W | Ass't S | Birmingham, Iowa | A. W. M. |
| Davis, Samuel B | Surgeon | | To U. S. V. March, 1863. |

## IOWA—Continued.

### 16TH INFANTRY—Mustered out July 19, 1865.

| | | | |
|---|---|---|---|
| Lloyd, Frederick | Surgeon | Care A. G. U. S. A. | To September, 1863; also 11th Inf. |
| McNeil, D. C. | Ass't S. | Oceola, Mo | To April, 1863; U. S. Ex. S. |
| McClelland, F. | " | Wall Lake, Iowa | To U. S. V. August, 1864. |
| Phillips, Josiah L. | Surgeon | Sioux Falls, Dak | From Oct., 1863. Dead. |
| Alexander, Dixon | Ass't S. | | A. W. M. |
| Camburn, Jacob H. | Surgeon | | To June, 1862. |

### 17TH INFANTRY—Mustered out July 25, 1865.

| | | | |
|---|---|---|---|
| Coleman, W. F. | Ass't S. | Decorah, Iowa | To February, 1864. U. S. Ex. S. |
| Early, J. H. | Surgeon | Palmyra, Mo | To May, 1865. U. S. Ex. S. |
| McGorrisk, E. J. | Ass't S. | Des Moines, Iowa | To November, 1862; also 9th Inf. |
| Udell, Nathan | Surgeon | Centreville, Iowa | Dismissed July, 1862. |
| Biser, C. C. | Surgeon | | From July, 1865. |
| Barclay, Wm D. | Ass't S | | To October, 1862. |

### 18TH INFANTRY—Mustered out July 20, 1865.

| | | | |
|---|---|---|---|
| Allen, Jno. H. | Surgeon | Maquoketa, Iowa | To March, 1864. |
| Kirkup, Edwin | " | Healdsburgh, Cal | To May, 1865; also 9th Cav. |
| Maynard, H. H. | Ass't S. | Santa Ana, Cal | To 2d Ark Cav. March, 1864. |
| Harvey, James | " | | To June, 1862. |
| Sanford, H. C. | " | Dead | From August, 1864. |

### 19TH INFANTRY—Mustered out July 10, 1865.

| | | | |
|---|---|---|---|
| Bell, Thos. S | Ass't S. | Wapello, Iowa | G. Was Hosp. Steward of Regt. prior to date of com. |
| Harvey, Philip | Surgeon | Portland, Oregon, or Burlington, Iowa. | To May, 1863. |
| Sloanaker, Lewis M. | " | Montrose, Iowa | From July, 1863. Dead. |
| Balch, S. F. | Ass't S. | | To July, 1863. |
| Hurst, Denison A. | " | | To February, 1863. |
| Lathrop, Moses C. | " | | To 98th U. S. C. T. October, 1863. |

### 20TH INFANTRY—Mustered out July 8, 1865.

| | | | |
|---|---|---|---|
| Blanding, Abram O. | Surgeon | Battonville, Fla | From April, 1865. H. R. for May, 1865. |
| Howey, Harris | " | Wapello, Iowa | To January, 1865. |
| Ristine, Henry | " | Cedar Rapids, Iowa | To May, 1863. U. S. Ex. S. |
| Marlin, Kusey S. | Ass't S. | Dakota, Ill | From December, 1862. |
| Jennings, Jno. A. | H. Stew | Chicago, Ill. | |

### 21ST INFANTRY—Mustered out June 10, and July 15, 1865.

| | | | |
|---|---|---|---|
| Benham, Lucius | Ass't S. | St. Charles, Mo | To July, 1863. |
| Chase, Dwight W. | Surgeon | Delphos, Kan | To May, 1865. |
| Hunt, H. H. | " | Independence, Iowa | From June, 1863. |
| Orr, Wm. L. | " | Ottumwa, Iowa | To October, 1864; also 3d Cav. U. S. Ex. S. |
| Barnes, Rich'd A. | Ass't S. | | To March, 1863. |
| Hyde, Wm. A. | Surgeon | | To November, 1862. |

IOWA—Continued.

22D INFANTRY—Mustered out July 25, 1865.

| Name | Rank | Address | Service |
|---|---|---|---|
| Dinwiddie, Wm. A | Ass't S | Care of A. G. U. S. A | To Feb., 1865; also H. Stew. 40th Inf. |
| Shrader, John C | Surgeon | Iowa City, Iowa | From July, 1864. Formerly Capt. Co. H. |
| White, Wm. H | " | Atlanta, Ga | To January, 1864. Dead. |
| Peabody, Oren | Ass't S | | To 23d Inf. May, 1863. |

23D INFANTRY—Mustered out July 26, 1865.

| Name | Rank | Address | Service |
|---|---|---|---|
| Bosbyshell, C. B | Ass't S | Glenwood, Iowa | To June, 1863. |
| Cornell, N. R | " | Gunnison Col. or Knoxville, Iowa. | To 40th Inf. Feb., 1864. |
| Campbell, Smith V | " | Marysville, Mo | To July, 1863. |
| *Owen, Henry | H. Stew | Wichita, Kan. | |
| Calwell, T. J | Ass't S | Dallas Centre, Iowa | From March, 1864 Alleged dead. |
| Peabody, Oren | Surgeon | | From May, 1863; also 22d Inf. |
| East, Alvis H | " | | To April, 1863. |

24TH INFANTRY—Mustered out July 17, 1865.

| Name | Rank | Address | Service |
|---|---|---|---|
| Eli, John F | Surgeon | Cedar Rapids, Iowa | To June, 1863. |
| Lyons, Henry M | " | 832 Jackson st., Chicago, Ill. | From December, 1864. |
| Lanning, J. M | Ass't S | Clay Centre, Kan | From February, 1865. |
| Witherwax, J. M | Surgeon | Alleged dead | To November, 1864. |

25TH INFANTRY—Mustered out June 6, 1865.

| Name | Rank | Address | Service |
|---|---|---|---|
| Farr, Henry M | Surgeon | Salem, Iowa | To September, 1864. |
| Gray, James D | Ass't S | Talleyrand, Iowa | To September, 1863. |
| Marsh, Wm. S | Surgeon | Mt Pleasant, Iowa | To February, 1863. |
| Marsh, Charles F | " | Mt. Pleasant, Iowa | From December, 1864. |

26TH INFANTRY—Mustered out June 6, 1865.

| Name | Rank | Address | Service |
|---|---|---|---|
| Hudson, Abijah T | Surgeon | Stockton, Cal | From September, 1862. |
| MacQuigg, Wm | Ass't S | Lyons, Iowa | To January, 1863. |
| Wetherell, Geo. F | " | Lyons, Iowa | From Sept., 1862. G. |
| Teal, Cornelius | " | | To May, 1864. |

27TH INFANTRY—Mustered out August 8, 1865.

| Name | Rank | Address | Service |
|---|---|---|---|
| Boomer, Albert | Ass't S | Delhi, Iowa | To August, 1864. |
| Hastings, David C | " | Quasqueton. Iowa | From October, 1862. |
| Sanborn, John E | Surgeon | Rockport, Mass | From October, 1862. |

28TH INFANTRY—Mustered out July 31, 1865.

| Name | Rank | Address | Service |
|---|---|---|---|
| Groves, Leroy S | Ass't S | Afton, Iowa | From March, 1865. |
| Statler, E. J. B | " | Marshalltown, Iowa | To January, 1864 |
| Stewart, David | " | North Liberty, Iowa | To May, 1863; also Capt. Co. E. to Feb., 1863. |
| Vest, John W. H | Surgeon | Montezuma, Iowa | To December, 1864. |
| Daniels, Wesley A | " | Traer, Iowa | From January, 1865. |
| Lathrop, Wm P | Ass't S | | To December, 1862. |
| Boynton, H. W | H. Stew | Plankinton, Dak. Ter. | |

29TH INFANTRY—Mustered out August 10, 1865.

| Name | Rank | Address | Service |
|---|---|---|---|
| Eakin, David F | Ass't S | Beloit, Kan | To February, 1865. |
| Grimes, W. S | Surgeon | Denver. Col | To June, 1863. |
| Nicholson, Wm. L | " | Ft. Dodge, Iowa | From September, 1864. |
| Rice, John H | Ass't S | Magnolia, Iowa | From December, 1864. |
| Shaw, Alex | " | Denver, Col | To Aug., 1864; also 4th Inf. |

* Frequently acted as Surgeon during entire service.

## IOWA—Continued.

### 30TH INFANTRY—Mustered out June 5, 1865.

| Name | Rank | Residence | Service |
|---|---|---|---|
| Allen, David B | Surgeon | West Liberty, Ohio | To Feb., 1864; also 1st Cav. |
| Lewis, Chas. G | Ass't S | Ottumwa, Iowa | To January, 1863. |
| Rogers, Sam'l C | Surgeon | 922 W. Washington, st., Boston, Mass. | From June 3, 1865. |
| Price, Nathan L | " | Exline, Iowa | To May, 1865. |
| Bond, John W | " | | To March, 1863. |
| Walker, Peter | Ass't S | | To December, 1862. |

### 31ST INFANTRY—Mustered out June 27, 1865.

| Name | Rank | Residence | Service |
|---|---|---|---|
| Carhart, G. L | Surgeon | Marion or Mount Vernon, Iowa. | To December, 1864. |
| French, Lucius | Ass't S | Davenport, Iowa | To June, 1863. U. S. Ex. S. |
| Gates, Horace H | Surgeon | Glidden, Iowa | From June 15, 1865. |
| Taylor, Elisha T | Ass't S | | To March, 1864. |
| Dawson, C. I | " | Dead | To April, 1863. |

### 32D INFANTRY—Mustered out August 24, 1865.

| Name | Rank | Residence | Service |
|---|---|---|---|
| Byam, Philander | Surgeon | Hopkinton, Iowa | From Feb., 1865. D. |
| Church, W. B | H. Stew | Marshall, Mich. | |
| Olney, Stephen B | Surgeon | Fort Dodge, Iowa | To October, 1864. |
| Smith, Newcomb S | H Stew | Yankton Agency, Dak. Ter. | Also Ass't S. 35th Inf. |
| Waters, Wm. B | Ass't S | Marshalltown, Iowa | To July, 1863. |
| Wasson, Jesse | " | Laporte City, Iowa | To March, 1863; also 9th Cav. |
| Huston, Wm. L | " | Marengo, Iowa | From August, 1863. |

### 33D INFANTRY—Mustered out July 17, 1865.

| Name | Rank | Residence | Service |
|---|---|---|---|
| *Craddick, W. W | A. H. S | Knoxville, Iowa | To March, 1863. |
| Franken, B | H. Stew | Sigourney, Iowa. | |
| Scott, Wm | Ass't S | Centreville, Iowa | To December, 1864. |
| Hopkins, Jno. Y | Surgeon | Alleged dead | From July, 1864. |
| Parks, Arad | " | | To June, 1864. |

### 34TH INFANTRY—Mustered out August 15, 1865.—(The 38th Infantry was consolidated with this Regiment January 1, 1865.)

| Name | Rank | Residence | Service |
|---|---|---|---|
| Coffman, Victor H | Surgeon | Omaha, Neb | From January, 1864. |
| Davis, Charles W | " | Indianola, Iowa | To November. 1863 |
| McCleary, Jno. D | Ass't S | | To June, 1863. |
| King, Ichabald | " | Alleged dead | From January, 1865. |
| Peebles. John M | " | | To May, 1865 |
| Jay, Henry W | " | | To February, 1863. |

### 35TH INFANTRY—Mustered out August 10, 1865.

| Name | Rank | Residence | Service |
|---|---|---|---|
| Chambers, Chas. L | Surgeon | Muscatine or Tipton, Iowa. | To August, 1863. |
| Cobb, Stephen M | " | Muscatine, Iowa | From January, 1864, U. S. Ex. S |
| Rigart, Emanuel H | Ass't S | Des Moines or Tipton, Iowa. | To September, 1863. |
| Smith, Newcomb S | " | Yankton Agency, Dakota Territory. | To May, 1865; also Hos. Steward 32d Inf. |

*Says he prepared all prescriptions.

## IOWA—Continued.

### 36TH INFANTRY—Mustered out August 24, 1865.

| Name | Rank | Residence | Service | |
|---|---|---|---|---|
| Sawyers, S. H. | Surgeon | Washington, D. C. | To December, 1864. | G. |
| Strong, C. G. | " | San Francisco, Cal | From January, 1865. | |
| Smyth, Patrick A. | Ass't S. | | A. W. M. | |
| Cousins, Moses | Surgeon | | To April, 1863. | |

### 37TH INFANTRY, (Graybeard Regiment)—Mustered out May 24, 1865.

| Name | Rank | Residence | Service | |
|---|---|---|---|---|
| Finley, John W. | Surgeon | Mt. Pleasant, Iowa | From March, 1862. Alleged dead. | |
| Orr, Joseph | Ass't S. | Mt. Pleasant, Iowa | From March, 1863. | |
| Dorn, Edward | " | | A. W. M. | |
| Haynes, Sam'l C. | " | | To March, 1863; also 6th Cav. | |
| De Witt, Geo. S. | " | | To February, 1863. | |

### 38TH INFANTRY—Consolidated with the 34th Infantry June 1, 1865.

| Name | Rank | Residence | Service | |
|---|---|---|---|---|
| Hart, Henry W. | Surgeon | Council Bluffs, Iowa | A. W. M.; also 9th Inf. | G. |
| McNutt, Robert | Ass't S. | East Des Moines, Iowa | Dismissed Sept., 1864. | |
| Duncan, Edward A. | " | | To July, 1863. | |

### 39TH INFANTRY—Mustered out June 5, 1865.

| Name | Rank | Residence | Service | |
|---|---|---|---|---|
| Davis. E. P. | Ass't S. | McCune, Kan | To January, 1865. | |
| Leonard, Wm. L. | " | Winterset, Iowa | To 7th Ill. Inf. December, 1863 | G. |
| Woods, Peter N. | Surgeon | Fairfield, Iowa | From September, 1862. | |

### 40TH INFANTRY—Mustered out August 2, 1865.

| Name | Rank | Residence | Service | |
|---|---|---|---|---|
| Cornell, N. R. | Surgeon | Knoxville, Iowa | From February, 1864; also 23d Inf | |
| Elwood, A. S. | Ass't S. | Monroe, Iowa | To October, 1863. | |
| Morgan, James W. | " | Port Byron, Ill. | From May, 1864. | |
| Scales, H. J. | " | Knoxville, Iowa | To February, 1864. H. R. | G. |
| Dinwiddie, Wm. A. | H. Stew. | Care A. G. U. S. A. | 1862; also Ass't Surgeon 22d Inf. | |
| Robinson, David W. | Surgeon | Mt. Pleasant, Iowa | To December, 1863. | |

There were no 41ST, 42D, or 43D Regiments.

### 44TH INFANTRY, (100 days)—Mustered out September 15, 1864.

| Name | Rank | Residence | Service | |
|---|---|---|---|---|
| Irwin, James | Surgeon | | From June, 1864. | |
| Russell John H. | Ass't S. | | From June, 1864. | |
| Thompson, Orrin B. | " | | From June, 1864. | |

### 45TH INFANTRY, (100 days)—Mustered out September 16, 1864.

| Name | Rank | Residence | Service | |
|---|---|---|---|---|
| Estabrook, Wm. W. | Surgeon | Winterset or Cedar Falls, Iowa. | From May, 1864. | |
| Hurley, John | Ass't S. | Toolsborough. Iowa | From May, 1864. | |
| Stutsman, Sam'l H. | " | Des Moines, Iowa | From May, 1864. | |

### 46TH INFANTRY, (100 days)—Mustered out September 23, 1864.

| Name | Rank | Residence | Service | |
|---|---|---|---|---|
| Duncan, Joseph R. | Surgeon | Crawfordsville, Ind. | From June, 1864. | G. |
| McCleary Jno. D. | Ass't S. | Indianola, Iowa | From June, 1864. | |
| Rosser, Wm. H. | " | Troy, Iowa | From June, 1864. | |

### 47TH INFANTRY, (100 days)—Mustered out September 28, 1864.

| Name | Rank | Residence | Service | |
|---|---|---|---|---|
| Cherry, S. B. | Ass't S. | Winterset, Iowa | From June, 1864. | |
| Fry John H. | " | Union Mills, Iowa | From June, 1864. | G. |
| Wright, James D. | Surgeon | Chariton, Iowa | From June, 1864. | |

IOWA—Continued.

48TH INFANTRY, (100 days)—Mustered out October 20, 1864.

Blanchard, Jno A.....Surgeon..........................................From June, 1864.
Wundt, Chas. L.......Ass't S..........................................From July, 1864.

## KANSAS.

2D CAVALRY—Also known as the 2d Infantry (3 months)—Mustered out June 22, 1865.

Adamson, V. V........Ass't S....Holton, Kan.................From September, 1864.
Root, Joseph P........ " Wyandotte, Kan.............To April, 1865 H. R.
Wood, Geo. B.......... " ..........................................To September, 1862.

5TH CAVALRY—Part mustered out August 11 to December 8, 1864; Companies L and M consolidated with 15th Cavalry August 22, 1865.

Carpenter, Wm. B...Surgeon...Leavenworth, Kan.........To September, 1864.
Huntoon, Andrew J.. " Topeka, Kan.................Dismissed March, 1863.
Porter, David R......Ass't S....Kansas City, Mo............To January, 1865.
Whitehorn, Sam'l..... " ..........................................To October, 1863.
Raiff, B. F..............A. A. S...Osceola, Iowa.

6TH CAVALRY—Mustered out November 18, 1864, to July 18, 1865.

Melick, Wesley........Surgeon...Metz, Mo........................From March, 1865.
Redfield, John S...... " ..........................................To February, 1865.

7TH CAVALRY—Mustered out September 29, 1865.

Lansing, J. W.........H. Stew...Lansing, Kan
Martin, Jos. S..........Surgeon...Highland or Iowa Point, Kan. A. A. Surg., U. S. A.
Weaver, Jos. L......... " Leavenworth, Kan.........To June 1864.
Crook, Joel J...........Ass't S....Leadville Colo..............From October, 1864.
Speer, Albert G.......H. Stew...Box 10, Hiawatha, Kan

9TH CAVALRY—Mustered out July 17, 1865

Bostwick, H. C........Surgeon...New Tacoma, Wash. T...To January, 1863.
Beach, Abijah I.......Ass't S....Seattle, Wash. Ter., or Council Grove, Kan. From January, 1864.
Hart, John A...........H. Stew...Iola, Kan..........................Also Surg. 16th Cavalry.
Phillips, A. J.......... " Lawrence, Kan.
Wakefield, Wm........Surgeon...Humboldt, Kan.............To May, 1865; U. S. Ex S
Winans, Norman D..Ass't S...Centreville, Kan............To November, 1864.

11TH CAVALRY—Mustered out from June 13, to September 26, 1865.

Ainsworth, R. M......Surgeon...Kansas City, Mo............Dismissed July, 1865.
Adams, Josiah D.....Ass't S....North Cedar or Independence, Kan. A. W. M.
Hogeboom, Geo. W...Surgeon...Topeka or Oskaloosa, Kan. To June, 1863, also 8th Inf
Taylor, G. C...........Ass't S....Louisville, Kan.............From April, 1864.
Johnson, D. H.........H. Stew...Paola, Kan.
Koentz, John P........H. Stew...Onaga, Kan.

14TH CAVALRY—Mustered out June 25, 1865.

Chenoweth, A. W.....Surgeon...Pineville, Mo.................From January, 1864; U. S Ex. S.
Peck, Willis J..........Ass't S..........................................From August, 1864.

KANSAS—Continued.

15TH CAVALRY—Mustered out October 19, 1865, except Co. H, mustered out December 7, 1865.

Twiss. Edward........Surgeon...Athens, Mich .................From April, 1864.
Ashmore, Samuel.....Ass't S.......................................Reported to be in penitentiary.

16TH CAVALRY—Co. I mustered out November 28, 1865; the rest December 6, 1865.

Hart, John A.. ........Surgeon...Iola, Kan......................To Nov., 1865. H. R.

1ST INFANTRY—Part mustered out June 16 and 17, 1864, the rest August 30, 1865.

Bailey, Mahlon ... ....Surgeon...Topeka Kan...................To June, 1864.
Budington, Geo. E... " Leavenworth, Kan.........Dead.
Speck, Jos:..............Ass't S.......................................From June, 1863.
King. Chas ........ ..... " ......................................To December, 1862.
Smith, Samuel D......Surgeon......................................To April, 1862.

1ST INDIAN HOME GUARD—Mustered out May 31, 1865.

Pattee, E. L......... ..Surgeon...Manhattan, Kan.... .......Missing since June, 1863. B.
Holliday, A. S ......... " ......................................Missing since August, 1862.

*2D INDIAN HOME GUARD—Mustered out May 31, 1865.

Ritchie, Andrew J...Surgeon......................................To April, 1865.
Hitchcock, D D ......Ass't S.......................................From March, 1863.
Campdoras, M. A..... " ......................................To October, 1863.

3D INDIAN HOME GUARD—Mustered out May 31, 1865.

Walgamott, Geo W...Surgeon......................................To 83d U. S. C. T. Oct., 1863.
Chandler, Dan'l L ...H Stew...Ogden, Kan.

4TH and 5TH REGIMENTS INDIAN HOME GUARD—Failed to complete.

8TH INFANTRY—Mustered out November 28, 1865.

Clark, Nathaniel C ..Surgeon...Doniphan, Kan..............From November, 1864. Alleged dead.
Chamberlain, O....... " Grassy Cove, Tenn.........To September, 1864.
Hageboom, Geo. W...Ass't S.....Topeka or Oskaloosa, Kan To Surg. 11th Cavalry, September, 1862.
Talcott, Edwin J..... " Spring Hill, Ill................To February, 1865. P M.
Woodward, J. B ......Surgeon...Lawrence, Kan., or Montpelier, Vt. To 10th Inf Feb., 1862.
Buterbaugh, John....Ass't S.......................................To March, 1864.

10TH INFANTRY—Part mustered out August 18 to 22, 1864; the rest August 30, 1865.

Scott, John W .........Surgeon...Iola. Kan.........................To May, 1863.
Woodward J. B...... " Montpelier, Vt., or Lawrence Kan. To May, 1864; also 8th Inf.
Miller, Geo. A .........Ass't S.......................................To June, 1863.
Parker. P. Gould..... " ......................................To July, 1864.
Tuttle, Henry D .....Surgeon......................................From June, 1864.

* Original Co. E (Osage Indians) deserted Sept., 1862. Second Co. E formed of Cherokee Indians.

## KANSAS—Continued.

12TH INFANTRY—Mustered out June 30, 1865; except Co. H, August 6, 1865.

*Lindsay, Thos........Ass't S.....Garnett, Kan..................From September, 1862; U. S. Ex. S.
Stuckslager, C. R..... " McKeesport, Pa.............From September, 1862.
Everhart, John F..... " ..................................To November, 1863.

13TH INFANTRY—Mustered out June 26, 1865.

Caffee, Amos H........Surgeon.. Carthage, Mo...................Also 1st Ark. Cav. U. S. Ex. S.
Grimes, Wm. H........ " Alleged dead...................To October, 1864.
Shipley, Richard W..Ass't S..........................................To October, 1863.
Becker, John........... " ..................................To February, 1864.

## KENTUCKY.

1ST CAVALRY—Mustered out September 20, 1865.

Brady, John A.........Surgeon...Louisville, Ky...................To December, 1862.
Brown, Hawkins...... " Hustonville, Ky..............To December, 1864.
Cambell, Andrew A..Ass't S.....Hustonville, Ky..............To December, 1864.
Huffman, A. G......... " Peabody, Kan..................To June, 1864.
Riffe, James C......... " .................................. To June, 1862.

2D CAVALRY—Mustered out from July 9, to 27, 1865.

Griffiths, D. J.........Ass't S.....Louisville, Ky...................U. M. Also 2d Inf.
Stuart, Robert......... " ..................................To June, 1863
Finley, John Y.........Surgeon..........................................To October, 1864.
Griffiths, Geo. W......H. Stew...Louisville, Ky...................U. S. Ex. S.

3D CAVALRY—Mustered out July 15, 1865.

Fairleigh, Robert M..Surgeon...1833 Franklin ave., St. Louis, Mo. To January, 1865.
McNary, Robert B...Ass't S....Holden, Mo.........................From April, 1863.
Singleton, Wm.........Surgeon...Hardensburgh, Ky.........To July, 1862.

4TH CAVALRY—Mustered out August 21, 1865.

Butler, Chas. H. .....Surgeon...Clifford, Ind.........................From November, 1863.
Middleton, D. P.......Ass't S....Louisville, Ky.................Missing since March, 1862.
Bachman, J. P......... " ..................................To December, 1864.
Adams, Sam'l L......Surgeon..........................................To September, 1862.
Mallory, Henry........ " Hamilton, Ohio...............To July, 1863.

5TH CAVALRY—Part mustered out May 3, 1865; veterans and recruits transferred to 3d Cavalry.

Forrester, William...Surgeon...Louisville, Ky...................From April, 1863.
Mitchell, Jacob B.....Ass't S.....Colorado Springs, Colo...To 12th Tenn. Cav. Mar., 1864.
Alexander, Rob't M.. " Burksville, Ky...................To March, 1862.
Owsley, Wm. T....... " 24 I st N. E., Washington, D. C. From June, 1864
Walker, Tuntsall Q..Surgeon..........................................To February, 1862
Mulholland, Hugh ... " .................................. To April, 1863; also 16th Cav.

6TH CAVALRY—Mustered out September 6, 1865.

Chapman, Chas. B...Ass't S.....803 Montgomery st., San Francisco, Cal. Dismissed September 23, 1865. Alleged dead.
Keeler, Leavens J....Surgeon...977 State st., Chicago, Ill. Dismissed Aug. 14, 1864.
Drye, John............ " ..................................From September, 1864.
McMillan, Geo. A.... " ..................................To December, 1861.
Newman, Wm. H.... " ..................................To May, 1863.

---

*On duty in charge of 18th Illinois Infantry at Little Rock, Ark., in June, 1865.

## KENTUCKY—Continued.

### 7TH CAVALRY—Mustered out July 10, 1865.

| Name | Rank | Residence | Service |
|---|---|---|---|
| Spilman, Chas. T. | Surgeon | Paint Lick, Ky. | From May, 1863. |
| Burnam, Andrew T. | Ass't S. | | From June, 1864. |
| Sharp, William S. | Surgeon | Paris, Ky. | To May, 1863. |
| Wolff, Solomon S. | Ass't S. | | To December, 1864. |
| Peters, Preston. | A. A. S. | Louisville, Ky. | |

### 8TH CAVALRY—(1 year)—Mustered out September 23, 1863.

| Name | Rank | Residence | Service |
|---|---|---|---|
| Bennett, La Fayette. | Surgeon | Middleton, Ky. | From June, 1863; also 13th Cav and 26th Inf. |
| Ross, W. S. | " | Madisonville, Ky. | To May, 1863. |
| Whittington R. W. | Ass't S. | 463 W. Jefferson st., Louisville, Ky. | From November, 1862. |

### 9TH CAVALRY—(1 year)—Mustered out September 11, 1863.

| Name | Rank | Residence | Service |
|---|---|---|---|
| Bailey, William. | Surgeon | Louisville, Ky. | A. W. M. |
| Botts, W. H. | Ass't S. | Clay Village, Ky. | From September, 1862. |
| Hawkins, F. A. | H. Stew. | Clay Village, Ky. | |

### 10TH CAVALRY—(1 year)—Mustered out September 16 and 17, 1863.

| Name | Rank | Residence | Service |
|---|---|---|---|
| Fleming, John F. | Surgeon | Elizaville, Ky. | From September, 1862. |
| Maguire, Samuel. | Ass't S. | Greensburgh, Ind. | From Sept., 1862; also 45th Inf. |

### 11TH CAVALRY—Part mustered out July 12 to 17, 1865; veterans and recruits transferred to 12th Cavalry.

| Name | Rank | Residence | Service |
|---|---|---|---|
| Peyton, James F. | Surgeon | Stanford, Ky. | A. W. M.; also 19th Inf. |
| Peyton, James H. | " | Terre Haute, Ind. | To March, 1863. |
| Hewitt, Thos. W. | Ass't S. | | A. W. M. |
| Rogers, John F. | " | Trimble Co., Ky. | To January, 1863. |
| Pinkerton, Lewis F. | Surgeon | | To February, 1863. |

### 12TH CAVALRY—Mustered out August 23, 1865.

| Name | Rank | Residence | Service |
|---|---|---|---|
| Brown, E. O. | Surgeon | 331 Washington street, Louisville, Ky. | To Sept., 1863; also 26th Inf. |
| Littlepage, S. B. | Ass't S. | Rockport, Ind. | A. W. M. |
| Fletcher, Horace. | " | | A. W. M. |
| Swan, Thos. J. | Surgeon | | To May, 1865. |

### 13TH CAVALRY—(1 year)—Mustered out January 10, 1865.

| Name | Rank | Residence | Service |
|---|---|---|---|
| Bennett, La Fayette. | Surgeon | Middleton, Ky. | From Dec., 1863; also 8th Cav. and 26th Inf. |
| Stone, Wm. D. | Ass't S. | | From December, 1863. |
| Harper, Jos. T. | " | | From April, 1864. |
| Perryman, R. H. | H. Stew. | Neetsville, Ky. | |

### 14TH CAVALRY—(1 year)—Mustered out from September 16, 1863, to March 24, 1864.

| Name | Rank | Residence | Service |
|---|---|---|---|
| Daniels, John M. | Con't S. | Proctor, or Pleasant Hill, Ky. | From May to Aug., 1863. Not in A. G. R. |
| Fithian, Wash | Surgeon | Paris, Ky. | To March, 1863; also 18th Inf. |
| Turner, James P. | " | Mount Sterling, Ky. | From March, 1863. |
| Jones, Matthew G. | Ass't S. | Hillsborough, Ky. | From July, 1863. |
| Hensley, Jas. W. | " | Kiddville, Ky. | A. W. M. |

KENTUCKY—Continued.

15TH CAVALRY—(1 year)—Mustered out from October 6 to 29, 1863.

Medairis, Salathiel...Ass't S.......................................To April, 1863.

16TH CAVALRY—Consolidated with 12th Cavalry October 15, 1864.

Mulholland, Hugh....Surgeon.......................................To Dec., 1863; also 5th Cav.

17TH CAVALRY—(1 year)—Mustered out September 20, 1865.

Hart, Chas. F.........Surgeon.......................................From August, 1865.

1ST INFANTRY—Mustered out June 18, 1864.

Menzies, Samuel G...Surgeon...137 W. 6th street, Cincinnati, O. From June, 1861.
White, W. Lee.........Ass't S.....U. S. Pension Office.......To January, 1862.
Dickson, John......... " ..................................From January, 1862.

2D INFANTRY—Part mustered out June 19, 1864; veterans and recruits transferred to the 17th Infantry.

Russell, Leonidas.....Ass't S ....Murfreesborough, Tenn..To May, 1862.
White, John F.........Surgeon...Avondale, Ohio..............To Jan., 1862. Died May, 1881.
Bonner, S. P..........Ass't S.....Dead................................To February, 1862.
Griffiths, David J.....Surgeon...Louisville, Ky ...............From Feb., 1862; also 2d Cav. U. M.
Rectannus, F...........Ass't S.......................................From March, 1864.
Reed, Wm. L.......... " ..................................To March, 1863.
Cox, Jas. E............ " ..................................To December, 1863.

3D INFANTRY—(formerly 1st Infantry)—Mustered out from October 13, 1864, to January 10, 1865.

Rhover, Samuel K ...Ass't S.....Bloomington, Ind...........A. W. M.
Scott, James R.........Surgeon...Edgewood, Ill ..................From March, 1863.
Foreman, Joseph...... " Port Royal, Ky..............To Sept., 1863; also 34th Inf.
Burns, John B......... " ..................................From November, 1863.
Owens, Hector......... " Dead..............................To January, 1863.
Turk, James G.........Ass't S.......................................To August, 1862.
Storts, C. H............A. A. S....Rolla Mo.

4TH INFANTRY—(Mounted)—Mustered out August 17, 1865.

Young, Matthew H...Surgeon...Ashland, Ky.....................From December, 1864.
KcKellup, John W...H. Stew...Vanceburgh, Ky.
Burdett, Stephen L .Surgeon...Lancaster, Ky..................To Otober, 1864.
Phillips, Harrison.....Ass't S.......................................From June, 1865.

5TH INFANTRY—(Formerly 3d Infantry, Louisville Legion)—Mustered out September 14, 1864.

Miller, Sam'l J. F.....Ass't S.....202 W. 4th street, Cincinnati, Ohio. From May, 1862.
Myatt, John............H. Stew...Louisville, Ky.
Swain, Enos S.........Surgeon...Smithfield, Ky.................From October, 1862.
Matthews, John....... " ..................................To January, 1862.
Gilpin, Wm. E.........Ass't S.......................................To November, 1861.

6TH INFANTRY—Mustered out from September 23, 1864, to January 2, 1865.

Long, E. T..............Ass't S ....Bethlehem, Ky ..............A. W. M.
Drane, Joseph S......Surgeon.......................................From December, 1861.

KENTUCKY—Continued.

### 7TH INFANTRY—Mustered out March 11, 1866.

| Name | Rank | Residence | Service |
|---|---|---|---|
| Berry, William | Surgeon | Louisville, Ky | To May, 1864. |
| Davidson, Wm. R. | Ass't S. | Evansville, Ind | To August, 1865; also 22d Inf. |
| Herndon, C. L. C. | " | Louisville, Ky | To Oct., 1864. Dead. |
| Tammadge, Henry | " | Louisville, Ky | To April, 1862; also 34th Inf |
| Hogan, H. W. | Act. S | Maco, Ky | Served winter of 1861 and 1862. Not in A. G. R. |
| Conant, Abel C. | Surgeon | Dead | To September, 1864. |

### 8TH INFANTRY—Mustered out November 17, 1864.

| Name | Rank | Residence | Service |
|---|---|---|---|
| Mills, John A. | Surgeon | Winchester, Ky | A. W. M. |
| Pirtle, John R. | " | 332 W. Walnut st.. Louisville, Ky. | To December, 1862. |
| Morton, C. H. | Ass't S. | | From May, 1863. |
| Robinson, Wm | " | | Dismissed August, 1863. |
| Daniels, Ansil | A. Ass't S. | Irvine, Ky | Nov. and Dec., 1861; also 47th Inf. |

### 9TH INFANTRY—Mustered out December 15, 1864.

| Name | Rank | Residence | Service |
|---|---|---|---|
| Duncan, James R. | Surgeon | Newton, Kan. | To January, 1862; also 37th Inf. |
| Lindsay, John A. | Ass't S. | Salineville, Ohio | A. W. M. |
| Stone, Barton W. | Con't S. | Fountain Run, Ky | Not in A. G. R. |
| Jeffray, T. R. W. | Surgeon | | A. W. M. |
| Chamberlain, J. B. | Ass't S. | | To April, 1863. |
| Clemens, A. J | A. Ass't S. | Clay Co., Tenn. | |

### 10TH INFANTRY—Mustered out December 6, 1864.

| Name | Rank | Residence | Service |
|---|---|---|---|
| Stocking, C. H | Surgeon | Freeport, Ill | From April, 1864. Dead. |
| Hatchitt, Jas. G. | " | Frankfort, Ky | To U. S. Vols. Apr., 1862. |
| Perkins, Jabez | Ass't S. | | To U. S Vols. Nov., 1863. |

### 11TH INFANTRY—Mustered out December, 1864.

| Name | Rank | Residence | Service |
|---|---|---|---|
| Eller, Wm. Y. | H. Stew. | Woodbury, Ky. | |
| Kimbly, J. T. | Surgeon | Owensborough, Ky | From December, 1861. |
| Simpson, Samuel | Ass't S. | Union City, Tenn. | To January, 1864. |
| Still, E. C | " | Macon City, Mo | Not in A. G. R. |
| Higgins, Jas. T. | " | Owensboro, Ky | From April, 1863. |

### 12TH INFANTRY—Mustered out July 11, 1865.

| Name | Rank | Residence | Service |
|---|---|---|---|
| Winfrey, A. V | Ass't S. | Wathena, Kan | To December, 1863. |
| Richardson, E | Surgeon | Louisville, Ky | To June, 1862. |
| Rodman, Wm. B. | " | | From May, 1865. |
| Pollitt, Wm M. | Ass't S. | | To September, 1864. |
| Bishop, John W. | " | | To July, 1865. |
| Mullins, Wm. H. | Surgeon | | To March, 1865. |

### 13TH INFANTRY—Mustered out January 12, 1865.

| Name | Rank | Residence | Service |
|---|---|---|---|
| Moore, C. D | Surgeon | Columbia or Camp Knox, Ky. | From January, 1862. |
| Taylor, Flavius J. | Ass't S. | Seymour, Ky | From January, 1863. |
| Cooper, Edward S. | " | Baldwin, Mo. | A. W. M |
| Ingram, Isaac G | " | | To April, 1862. |

KENTUCKY—Continued.

### 14TH INFANTRY—Mustered out September 15, 1865.

Miller, A. C .............Surgeon...Cleveland, Ohio.................To May, 1863.
Yates, Strother J...... " Louisa, Ky .........................To January, 1865.
Meacham, Franklin...Ass't S.....Care A. G. U. S. A.........To November, 1862.
Stubbins, Benj. A.....Surgeon.........................................From August, 1865.
Richards, S. D.. .......Ass't S.............................................To June, 1863.
Mobley, Cyrus L...... " .........................................To January, 1865.
Hereford, B. W........H. Stew...Prestonburgh, Ky.

### 15TH INFANTRY—Mustered out January 14, 1865

Dunn, Edward H.....Surgeon...Mt. Washington, Md.......From February, 1863.
Logan, Richard F..... " Southville, Ky...............To November, 1862. U. S. Ex. S.
Woodruff, Ezra........Ass't S.....Care A. G. U. S. A.........To November, 1863.
Whitaker, Eli D........ " ..........................................To November, 1864.
Weatherby, L. P......Surgeon.........................................To July, 1862.

### 16TH INFANTRY—Mustered out July 15, 1865.

Taylor, Fred'k M......Surgeon...Alleged dead..................From January, 1865.
Jones, Lewis J.........Ass't S.....Hillsborough, Ky...........From April, 1863.
Cartwell, Simon M...Surgeon...Maysville, Ky ................To Nov., 1864. Ex. S.

### 17TH INFANTRY—Mustered out January 23, 1865; veterans and recruits transferred to the 21st Infantry.

Burgess, Warren J...Surgeon...Du Quoin, Ill....................From February, 1862.
Hubbard, Stewart.....Ass't S.....Archibald, Ohio or A. W. M. Woodlawn, Neb.
Cloak, Burkitt.........Surgeon.........................................To April, 1862; also 25th Inf.
Shackelford, A. P.....Ass't S.....Madisonville, Ky............To March, 1862; also 25th Inf.
Warmoth, Geo. W.... " ..........................................To April, 1862.
Cosby, Albert D....... " ..........................................To Dec., 1862; also 35th Inf.
Compton, John W.... " ..........................................To March, 1863.

### 18TH INFANTRY—Mustered out July 18, 1865.

Fithian, Joseph....... Surgeon...Paris, Ky...........................To March, 1865.
Elliott, Justin C...... " Titusville, Pa.....................To 100th U. S. C. T. June, 1864.
Dinwiddie, Robert... " ..........................................From June, 1865; also 27th Inf.

### *19TH INFANTRY—Mustered out January 26, 1865.

Peyton, James F......Ass't S.....Stanford, Ky.....................To April, 1863; also 11th Cav.
Sparks, Jas. B.........Surgeon...Charlottesville, Ind........To January, 1863.
Semlere, A. H.........Ass't S.....Hopkinsville, Ohio.........To June, 1864 Dead.
Logan, Pleasant W... " Stanford, Ky .................To July, 1862; also 1st Tenn. Cavalry.
Forbes, William N... " ..........................................To July, 1864.

### 20TH INFANTRY—Mustered out January 17, 1865.

Curran, Wm. H.......Ass't S.....Claysville, Ky .................To August, 1862.
Noel, W. C............... " Evening Shade, Ark.....To December, 1861.
Welch, John C.........Surgeon...Nicholasville, Ky...........From January, 1862.
Norton, Prior N......Ass't S.............................................From August, 1862.

---

*The Hospital Register of the 97th Illinois Volunteers on file in A. G. Office is said to contain names of the sick and wounded of this regiment from December 5, 1862, to March 4, 1863.

KENTUCKY—Continued.

21ST INFANTRY—Mustered out December 9, 1865.

Walton, C. J............Surgeon...Munfordville, Ky..........To February, 1865.
Herndon, C. L. C......    "    ..................................From March, 1865.
Todd, Orrin D.........Ass't S.......................................From May, 1865.
Fitzhugh, T. C.........    "    ..................................To June, 1864.
Wheat, J. O...........    "    ..................................Missing since April, 1862.

22D INFANTRY—Mustered out January 20, 1865.

Davidson, Wm. R.....Ass't S.....Evansville, Ind.............To 7th Inf. Dec., 1861.
Manfred, Henry......Surgeon...2 Hopkins street, Cincinnati, Ohio. From May, 1864.
Stevenson, Benj. F...    "    Visalia, Ky....................To February, 1864; also 23d Inf.
Bullock, G. R..........A. Ass't S.Orangeburg, Ky.

23D INFANTRY—Mustered out December 27, 1865.

Hasbrouck, Wm. L...Ass't S....Greensburgh, Ind..........From March, 1863.
Strothotte, Arnold...Surgeon...Newport, Ky.................To November, 1862.
Stevenson, Benj. F...Ass't S.....Visalia, Ky....................To January, 1862; also 22d Inf.
Morrison, Alonzo M..Surgeon...Goshen, Ky.....................From December, 1862.

24TH INFANTRY—Mustered out January 31, 1865.

Sympson, James......Surgeon...Winchester, Ky..............From January, 1862.
Moss, Wm. H. I.......Ass't S........................................A. W. M.
Gardner, Joseph......    "    ..................................A. W. M.
White, Wm. S..........    "    ..................................To May, 1862.
Paynter, Marcus E...    "    ..................................To February, 1863.

25TH INFANTRY—Consolidated with 17th Infantry March, 1862.

Shackelford, A. P....Ass't S.....Madisonville, Ky............From January, 1862; also 17th Inf.
Cloak, Burkitt.........Surgeon.........................................From January, 1862; also 17th Inf.

26TH INFANTRY—Mustered out July 10, 1865.

Brown, E. O............Ass't S.....331 Washington street, Louisville, Ky. To May, 1865; also 12th Cav.
Bennett, La Fayette..    "    Middleton, Ky...............To 8th Cav. June, 1863; also 13th Cav.
Jett, Wm. H............Surgeon...Rowlett's Depot, Ky......From April, 1865; also 33d Inf.
Bailey, Jonathan R...    "    Ferguson's Station, Ky...To April, 1862 Ex. S.
Bailey, James M......    "    Ferguson's Station, Ky...To December, 1864.
Walshe, James.........Ass't S........................................To April, 1864.
Foster, Isaac............H. Stew...Beda, Ky.

27TH INFANTRY—Mustered out March 29, 1865.

Heston, Robert L.....Surgeon...Litchfield, Ky................From March, 1862.
Dinwiddie, Robert...Ass't S........................................From August, 1863; also 18th Inf.
Sanders, Thomas.....    "    ..................................To March, 1863.

28TH INFANTRY—Mustered out December 14, 1865.

Marquis, Wm. V......Ass't S....Glade Mills, Pa..............To September, 1864.
Post, Jas. A............Surgeon...Birmingham, Mich.........To July, 1865.
Anderson, Turner...    "    Louisville, Ky.................From August, 1865.
Habermehl, Jos.......Ass't S........................................To November, 1862.
Hynes, Alfred M......Surgeon.........................................To November, 1864.
Stocking, Charles.....Ass't S........................................To August, 1865.

KENTUCKY—Continued.

29TH INFANTRY—Failed to complete its organization.

30TH INFANTRY—(1 year)—Mustered out April 18, 1865.

Cox, Columbus A.....Ass't S.....Stanford, Ky..................From April, 1864.
Gardner, Wm. H......Surgeon...Alleged dead..................From February, 1864.

31ST INFANTRY—Failed to complete its organization.

32D INFANTRY, (9 months)—Mustered out from May 28 to August 12, 1863.

Davidson, Benj. F....Ass't S.....Mouth of Wolf, Tenn.....From April, 1863.
Scott, Wm. F..........Surgeon...Somerset, Ky..................From April, 1863.

33D INFANTRY—Consolidated with the 26th Infantry April 1, 1864.

Jett, Wm. H............Ass't S.....Rowlett's Depot, Ky......A. W. M.; also 26th Inf.

34TH INFANTRY—Mustered out June 24, 1865.

Foreman, Joseph......Ass't S.....Port Royal, Ky..............From Nov., 1864; also 3d Inf.
Ronald, Geo. W.......Surgeon...344 W. Jefferson street, Louisville, Ky. To April, 1863.
Ryan, Hugh ............Ass't S.....Old Deposit or 433 Market st., Louisville, Ky. To March, 1864. B.
Tammage, Henry.....Surgeon...Louisville, Ky ..............From May, 1863; also 7th Inf.

35TH INFANTRY (1 year)—Mustered out December 29, 1864.

Letcher, Benj..........Ass't S.....Henderson, Ky ..............From November, 1863.
Stage, Wm. B.......... " Vienna, Ind .....................From November, 1863.
Cosby, Albert D ......Surgeon..........................................From October, 1863; also 17th Inf.

36TH INFANTRY—Failed to complete its organization.

37TH INFANTRY (1 year)—Mustered out December 29, 1864.

Duncan, James R.....Surgeon...Newton, Kan.................From Nov., 1863; also 9th Inf.
Haselwood, R. W .....Ass't S.....Pitman, Ky ..................From November, 1863.

38TH INFANTRY—Failed to complete its organization.

39TH INFANTRY—Mustered out September 15, 1865.

*Draper, James N ...Ass't S.....Pikeville, Ky ..................From September, 1863.
Herford, J. H..........Surgeon...Pikeville, Ky ..................Dismissed Dec., 1863.
Phillips, Wm. E ...... " ..................................................From February, 1864.
Phillips, Jas. H........Ass't S..............................................From April, 1865; also 40th Inf.
Rice, Isaac ..............H. Stew...Painterville, Ky.

40TH INFANTRY (1 year)—Mustered out December 30, 1864.

Loy, Sam'l N.........H. Stew...Aberdeen, Ohio.
Bland, Wm. B.........Surgeon..............................................From May, 1864; also 53d Inf.
Holloway, Oscar E...Ass't S..............................................From May, 1864.
Phillips, Jas. H....... " ......................................................To May, 1864; also 39th Inf.
Roberts, Joseph G ...Surgeon..............................................To April, 1864.

* On duty as Acting Assistant Surgeon from July 6 to September 6, 1863.

## KENTUCKY—Continued.

41ST, 42D, 43D and 44TH INFANTRY—Failed to complete.

45TH INFANTRY (1 year)—Mustered out Dec. 24, 1864, and Feb. 14, 1865.

Rowland, Joseph L..Ass't S.....Hazle Green, Ky............From April, 1864.
Scobey, Wm. E........ " Kankakee, Ill................From January, 1864.
Maguire, Samuel......Surgeon...Greensburg, Ind............From November, 1863; also 10th Cav.

46TH INFANTRY—Failed to complete.

47TH INFANTRY (1 year)—Mustered out from Dec. 26, 1864, to April 12, 1865.

Daniels, Ansil.........Con't S....Irvine, Ky.....................Not in A. G. R.; also 8th Inf.
Daniels, John M......Surgeon...Proctor, Ky.....................From Nov., 1863. Dead.
Glass, Wilson H.......Ass't S.....Bunch Creek, Ky..........From December, 1863.
Sumner, Geo............ " .....................................To January, 1864.

48TH INFANTRY (1 year)—Mustered out December, 1864.

Mott, John D..........Ass't S.....Princeton, Ky..............From November, 1863.
Randolph, Wm........Surgeon.............................................From October, 1863.
Bush, Reuben R......Ass't S.............................................From October, 1863.

49TH INFANTRY (1 year)—Mustered out December 26, 1864.

Hogan, H. W..........Ass't S.....Waco, Ky.....................From June, 1864.
Miller, H. C...........Surgeon...Louisville, Ky.................From June, 1864; also 53d Inf.
Swisher, W. B.........Ass't S.....Unadilla, Nebr.............From November, 1863.

50TH and 51ST INFANTRY—Failed to complete.

52D INFANTRY (1 year)—Mustered out January 17, 1865.

Weyer, Geo. W........Surgeon...St. Louis, Mo.................From October, 1863.
Hawthorne, Rob't D..Ass't S.............................................From February, 1864.
Alter, Henry H........ " .....................................From May, 1864.

53D INFANTRY (1 year)—Mustered out September 17, 1865.

*Montmollin, J. M...Ass't S.....Ashland, Ky.................From July, 1865.
Bland, Wm. B.........Surgeon.............................................From Feb., 1863; also 40th Inf.
Miller, Henry C........Ass't S.....Louisville, Ky...............From Feb., 1865; also 49th Inf.

54TH INFANTRY (1 year)—Mustered out September 1, 1865.

Hunt, Thomas B......Ass't S.....Warsaw, Ill.....................From October, 1864.
Leber, Fred. C.........Surgeon...Louisville, Ky...............From September, 1864.
McMahon, James.....Ass't S.............................................From September, 1864.

55TH INFANTRY (1 year)—Mustered out September 19, 1865.

Slaughter, B. F........Surgeon.............................................From April, 1865.
Parmer, E. R..........Ass't S.....Louisville, Ky...............To August, 1865.

* Was on duty as A. A. Surg. in charge of hospital at Ashland, Ky., from May 20, 1863, to August 11, 1864; and at Lexington, Ky., from September 15, 1864, to June 1, 1865, and at small-pox hospital at Lexington from June 2 to 10, 1865.

## LOUISIANA.

1ST CAVALRY—Mustered out December 18, 1865.

Smith, Hosea H.......Surgeon..............................................From August, 1863; also 8th N. H. Inf.

2D CAVALRY (formerly 3d Infantry)—Consolidated with the 1st Cavalry September 7, 1864.

Cooper, John............Surgeon...Painted Post, N. Y........A. W. M.
Williamson Wm. L...Ass't S.........................................Dismissed Sept., 1864.
Gilbert, Philip I.......      "     ..........................................Dismissed May, 1864.

1ST INFANTRY—Mustered out July 12, 1865.

Meserve, Richard H..Ass't S.....Limerick, Me..................To November, 1864.
Gordon, Seth C.......Surgeon...Portland, Me..................From October, 1863; also 13th Maine Infantry.
Black, Wm. T..........      "     Calais, Me............................To July, 1863; also 12th Maine Infantry.
Green, J. Dunham...Ass't S...........................................To 91st U. S. C. T. October, 1863.

2D INFANTRY—Mustered out September 11, 1865.

Dean Chas. A..........Surgeon...Baton Rouge, La............From March, 1864; also 89th U. S. C. T.
Gosson, Gustavus.....Ass't S.....St. Peters, Mo...............To February, 1864.
Vandergriff, J. B......      "     ..........................................To 1st N. O. Sept., 1864.
Kellogg, Geo............Surgeon...30 St. Charles st., N. O...To March, 1864.

1ST NEW ORLEANS—Mustered out May, 1866.

Paine, J. T..............Ass't S.....242 Esplanade st., New Orleans, La. From January, 1866.
Avery, Geo. W.........Surgeon...Hartford, Conn .............From December, 1863; also 9th Conn. Inf.
Vandergriff, Jas. B...Ass't S...........................................To December, 1865; also 2d Inf.

2D NEW ORLEANS—Failed to complete; enlisted men were assigned to the 1st New Orleans.

## MAINE.

1ST CAVALRY—Mustered out August 1, 1865.

Haley, Geo. W.........Ass't S.....Peabody, Mass................Dismissed Nov., 1862.
Northrup, Geo. J.....      "     Marquette, Mich.............From April, 1864; also 1st D. C. Cav.
Stevens, Horace.......Surgeon...Skowhegan, Me.............From Dec., 1864. H. R.
Parker. Alex. M......Ass't S.....Stevens, Me...................To September, 1864.
Getchell, Emory T...H. Stew...Brunswick, Me.
Colby, Geo. W .........Surgeon...Dead..............................To November, 1864.
Bodfish, Frank.........Ass't S...........................................From May, 1865.

2D CAVALRY—In service August 31, 1865.

Norris, Louis E.......Ass't S.....Hampden, Me..................To June, 1865; also 17th Inf.
Eaton, John R.........      "     Wilton, Me.........................A. W. M. H. R. From May, 1864.
Martin, Geo. W........Surgeon...Augusta, Me......................From Nov., 1863; also 4th and 6th Inf.
Smith, Andrew R. G..H Stew...N. Whitefield, Me..........M. D.

MAINE—Continued.

1ST HEAVY ARTILLERY—Organized as the 18th Infantry; changed to Heavy Artillery December, 1862; a portion of the 17th and 19th Infantry were transferred to this regiment. Mustered out September 11, 1865.

| Name | Rank | Address | Service |
|---|---|---|---|
| Paine, R. E. | Surgeon | Camden, Me | To February, 1864. |
| Elkins, Jerome B. | " | Oldtown, Me. | From March, 1864. |
| Lincoln, Albert | Ass't S. | Denneysville, Me | From December, 1862; U. S. Ex. S. |
| Reynolds, Henry A. | " | Americus or Grand Fork, D. T. | From May, 1864. |

The following Surgeons were on duty with the 1st Battery and Batteries 1st Division, 19th Army Corps, and Artillery Brigade, 19th Army Corps, to which the Battery was attached in 1863-'64, as per report of Surgeon-General U. S. A.

| Name | Rank | Address | Service |
|---|---|---|---|
| Blaisdell, W | Ass't S. | (75th N. Y. V.) Dead. | 1st Battery, May, June, 1863, Batteries 1-19, August, 1863. |
| Stubb, Arnold | " | 136 Dean st., Brooklyn, N.Y. (90th N. Y. V.) | Batteries 1-19, September, 1863, January, '64; 19th Art. Corps Nov. 16 to Dec. 31, 1864. |
| Fordyce, B. A. | " | Union Springs, N. Y. (160th N. Y. V.) | Batteries 1-19, February, 1864. |
| Dodge, L. | " | (15th Me. V.) Dead. | Batteries 1-19, March and April, 1864. |
| Hasbrouck, S. E. | " | (133d N. Y. V.) Dead. | Aug. to Nov. 16, 1864. |

1ST INFANTRY, (veteran)—Formed by the consolidation of the 5th, 6th, and 7th Infantry September 20, 1864. Mustered out June 28, 1865.

| Name | Rank | Address | Service |
|---|---|---|---|
| Getchell, S. P. | Ass't S. | Portland, Me. | From May, 1864; also 7th Inf. |
| Everleth, Francis M. | Surgeon | Waldoboro', Me. | From February, 1863; also 7th Inf |
| Packard, Alpheus S. | Ass't S. | Providence, R. I. | From October, 1864. |

2D INFANTRY—Part mustered out June 9, 1863; the rest transferred to 20th Infantry.

| Name | Rank | Address | Service |
|---|---|---|---|
| Morrison, Samuel B. | Surgeon | Bangor, Me. | From August, 1861, U. S. Ex. S. |
| Main, John T. | Ass't S. | Unity, Me | To April, 1863. |
| Hamlin, A. C. | " | Bangor, Me. | To Brig. Surg. April, '62. |
| Palmer, A. D. | " | Dead. | |
| Allen, Wm. H. | Surgeon | | To October, 1861. |
| Benson, W. R. | Ass't S. | | A. W. M. From April, '63. |
| Edgerly, Daniel W. | H. Stew. | U. S. Pension Office. | |

3D INFANTRY—Part mustered out June 28, 1864; the rest transferred to 17th Infantry.

| Name | Rank | Address | Service |
|---|---|---|---|
| Brickett, Geo. E. | Ass't S. | Augusta, Maine. | To August, 1861; also 21st Inf. U. S. Ex. S. |
| Getchell, Frank H. | " | 1413 Spruce street, Philadelphia. | To October, 1862. |
| Palmer, Gideon S. | Surgeon | Washington, D. C. | To Brig. Surg. Oct. 1861. |
| Watson, James D. | Ass't S. | Avoca, Iowa | From December, 1862. |
| Hildreth, Thaddeus | Surgeon | Dead. | |
| Jewett, Wm. H. | Ass't S. | Dead. | |

MAINE—Continued.

4TH INFANTRY—Part mustered out July 19, 1864; the rest transferred to 19th Infantry.

Cobb, Albion..........Ass't S....Casco, Maine.....................A. W. M.
Libby, Abial.............Surgeon...Richmond, Maine..........To July, 1862.
Martin, Geo. W........Ass't S....Augusta, Maine..............From July, 1862, to May, 1863; also 2d Cav. and 6th Inf.
Banks, Wm. A.........Surgeon...Rockland, Maine............To July, 1861. U. S. Ex. S.
Hopkins, Elisha.......Ass't S.....Seaport, Maine..............Dismissed July, 1861; also 14th Inf. H. R.
Benson, Wm. R....... " ..........................................To September, 1862.
Hunkins, Seth C .....Surgeon...Dead.....................................A. W. M.

5TH INFANTRY—Part mustered out July 27, 1864; the rest transferred to 6th Infantry.

Warren, Francis G...Surgeon...Biddeford, Maine..........From January, 1863.
Buxton, Benj. F...... " Warren, Maine................To January, 1863.
Manson, Melville H..Ass't S....Shakopee, Minn.............From May, 1863, U. S. Ex. S.
Walker, Jas. E........A. A. S ...1776 Washington street, Boston, Mass. Not in A. G. R.
Brickett, Geo. E......Con't S....Augusta, Maine..............August and September, 1861. Not in A. G. R. U. S. Ex. S.
Noyes, Wm. S.........Ass't S...............................................To March, 1863.

6TH INFANTRY—Part mustered out August 15, 1864; the rest transferred to 7th Infantry.

Buck, Wm................Surgeon...Foxcroft, Maine ............From August, 1863, U. S. Ex. S.
Straw, Sam'l B........Ass't S.....Lock box 119, Newburgh, N. Y. From October, 1862; also Capt. 11th Inf.
Sanger, Eugene F... " Bangor, Maine .................To March, 1862.
Martin, Geo. W....... " Augusta, Maine................To July, 1862; also 2d Cav. and 4th Inf.
Blossom, Alden........ " Boothbay, Maine...........To April, 1863.
Baker, John............ " Biddeford, Maine...........To October, 1861.

7TH INFANTRY—Original members mustered out September, 1864; veterans and recruits transferred to 5th and 6th Infantry to form the 1st Veteran Infantry.

Everleth, Francis M..Surgeon...Waldoboro', Maine.........From February, 1863; also 1st Inf.
Hunter, Sam'l B...... " Machias, Maine...............To February, 1863; also 15th Inf. U. S. Ex. S.
Getchell, Stillman P..Ass't S....Portland, Maine ............Also 1st Inf. Not in A. G. R.
Watterhouse, Ai...... " Jamestown, N. Y..........To Surg. 43d U. S. C. T. March, 1864. Ex. S.
Baker, Thos. C........Surgeon...Dead .................................To December, 1861.

8TH INFANTRY—In service August 31, 1865.

Levensaler, H. C......Surgeon...Thomaston, Maine.........From Sept., 1863; also 19th Inf.
Williams, Benj.........Ass't S....Rockland, Maine............From August, 1864.
Houghton, J. S ........ " Goldendale, Wash. Ter...To June, 1862.
Mitchell, Jos D.......Surgeon ..Jacksonville, Fla...........To April, 1863.
White, Horace C......Ass't S....Somerville, Mass............To May, 1863.
Richardson, I. G...... " Augusta, Maine...............To June, 1864.
Fisher, Paul M........Surgeon...Dead....................................To July, 1862.
Benson, Wm. R.......Ass't S....Died in 1866...................To January, 1865.

## MAINE—Continued.

### 9TH INFANTRY—Mustered out July 13, 1865.

Richardson, Joel......Surgeon...Arrow Rock, Mo............To December, 1862.
Mitchell, Alfred.......Ass't S....Brunswick, Maine...........To September. 1864.
Abbott, Delon H......Surgeon...Vandemere, N. C.. ........From June, 1865.
Rice, Otis P............Ass't S....Malden, Mass..................From January, 1865. H. R. D.
Spooner, S. G.........H. Stew...Princeton, Maine.
Hill, Luke...............Ass't S..........................................To October, 1863.

### 10TH INFANTRY—Part mustered out May 7 and 8, 1863; the rest transferred to 29th Infantry November 1, 1863.

Howard, H. N.........Ass't S.....Washington, D. C.........From Sept., 1862; also 29th and 30th Inf.
Perry, Daniel O......Surgeon...Portland, Maine............To October, 1862. Dead.
Sawyer, Jas...........Ass't S.....Biddeford, Maine..........To January, 1863. U. S. Ex. S.
Day, Josiah F., jr.....Surgeon...Alfred, Maine.................To May, 1863; also 29th Inf.

### 11TH INFANTRY—In service August 31, 1865.

Wilbur, G. A...........Surgeon...Skowhegan, Maine.........To May, 1862. U. S. Ex. S.
Wedgewood, M. C...Act'g S....Lewiston, Maine............Not in A. G. R.
Cook, Richard L.......Ass't S....Omro. Wis........................From Dec., 1862. H. R.
Royal, Woodman W.. " San Diego, Cal.............From March, 1864.
Gordon, Wm. C....... " Dead.
Blunt, Nathan F......Surgeon...Dead..................................To June, 1865.
Clark, Albert S....... " ..........................................To January, 1862.

### 12TH INFANTRY—In service August 31, 1865.

Thompson, Jas. H ...Surgeon...Milwaukee, Wis............To December, 1864.
Black, Wm. T.........Ass't S.....Calais, Me..........................To August, 1862. H. R; also 1st La. Inf.
Thompson, E. A......Surgeon...Dover, Me..........................To November, 1863.
Towle, Wm. C.........Ass't S.....Fryeburgh, Me..............To November, 1863; also 23d Inf.
Collins, Geo ............Surgeon...Dead....................................From May, 1865.

### 13TH INFANTRY—Part mustered out January 6, 1865, the rest transferred to 30th Infantry.

Bates, Jas. M..........Surgeon...Yarmouth, Me.................From November, 1861. H. R. for 3 years.
Gordon, Seth C........Ass't S....Portland, Me....................To 1st La. Inf., October, 1863.
Files, Jas. R............ " Dead.....................................From December, 1862.

### 14TH INFANTRY—Mustered out August 28, 1865.

Adams, Enoch.........Surgeon...Litchfield, Me...............To May, 1864. H. R.
Hopkins, Elisha....... " Seaport, Me.........................To Jan., 1865; also 4th Inf. H. R.
Evans, Simeon A......Ass't S.....Conway, N. H.................To January, 1865.
Sweat, Jesse P ........Surgeon...Brownfield, Me..............From April, 1865; also 23d Inf. H. R.
Costelloe, Peter........Ass't S ...Crescent City, Cal .........From June, 1865.
Wescott, Wm. W...... " Dead......................................To June, 1862.

## MAINE—Continued.

### 15TH INFANTRY—In service August 31, 1865.

| | | | |
|---|---|---|---|
| Higgins, Geo. Z | Surgeon | Strong, Me | From March, 1865. |
| Holmes, Arthur A | Ass't S | Bridgeport, Conn | From May, 1865. |
| Kimball, J. H | " | Bridgeton, Me | To May, 1863. H. R. Also 31th and 32d Inf. |
| Donnell, Jotham | Surgeon | Holton, Me | To Dec., 1864 H. R. |
| Hunter, Sam'l B | Ass't S | Machias, Me | To Dec., 1861; also 7th Inf. U. S. Ex. S. |
| Dodge, Lorenzo | " | Dead | To February, 1865. |

### 16TH INFANTRY—Part mustered out June 5, 1865, the rest transferred to 20th Infantry.

| | | | |
|---|---|---|---|
| Alexander, Chas | Surgeon | Eau Claire, Wis | To November, 1864. |
| Eaton, Wm. W | " | Danvers, Mass | From Nov., 1864. H. R. |
| Bolster, David P | Ass't S | Augusta or Weeks' Mills, Me. | From Feb., 1865; also 21st Inf. |
| Baxter, Joseph B | " | Dead. | |
| Hunter, Warren | " | | To January, 1863. |

### 17TH INFANTRY—Mustered out June 4, 1865, the rest transferred to 1st Infantry.

| | | | |
|---|---|---|---|
| Norris, L. E | Ass't S | Hampden, Me | To Oct., 1863; also 2d Cav. |
| Wescott, Wm | " | Gorham, Me | To December, 1863. |
| Hersom, Nahum A | Surgeon | Portland, Me | From April 1863; also 20th Inf. Dead. |
| Sturgis, Jas. G | | Standish, Me | From November, 1864. |
| Wiggins, H. L. K | Surgeon | Dead. | |
| Coleman, N. B | Ass't S | 204 Sutter st., San Francisco, Cal. | From November, 1863. |
| Ingalls, Pascal P | " | 285 West Broadway, Boston, Mass. | To March, 1863. |

### 18TH INFANTRY—See 1st Heavy Artillery.

### 19TH INFANTRY—Part mustered out May 31, 1865, the rest transferred to 1st Heavy Artillery.

| | | | |
|---|---|---|---|
| Billings, A. J | Surgeon | Freedom, Me | To January, 1864. H. R. |
| Hawes, J. Q. A | " | Hallowell, Me | To November, 1864. |
| Bolan, Wallace | Ass't S | Augusta, Me. | To March, 1864. |
| Sturgis, Benj. F | " | Auburn, Me | To Oct., 1864. U. S. Ex. S. |
| Levensaller, H. C | " | Thomaston, Me | To Aug., 1863; also 8th Inf |
| Parker, Fred. G | " | Presque Isle, Me | To March, 1864. |
| Bussey, B. B., jr | " | Bismarck, Dak | From November, 1864. |
| Randall, Wm. H | Surgeon | | From November, 1864. |

### 20TH INFANTRY—Mustered out July 16, 1865.

| | | | |
|---|---|---|---|
| Monroe, Nathan P | Surgeon | Belfast, Me | To May, 1863 Dead. |
| Benson, John | " | Newport, Me | To August, 1863. |
| Shaw, Abner O | " | Portland, Me | To February, 1865. |
| True, Wm. H | " | Portland, Me | From March, 1865; also 25th Inf. |
| Pendleton, L. W | H. Stew | Portland, Me. | |
| Hersom, N. A | Ass't S | Portland, Me | To Surg. 17th Inf. April, 1863. |
| Bennett, S. A | " | New Portland, Me | Dismissed March, 1863. |
| Barker, G. M | " | | To June, 1865. |
| Stevens, Chas G | " | | From July, 1865. |

MAINE—Continued.

21ST INFANTRY—(9 months.)—Mustered out August 25, 1863.

Brickett, Geo. E......Surgeon...Augusta, Me..................From Sept. 1862; also 3d Inf. U. S. Ex. S.
Bolster, David P......Ass't S......Augusta or Weeks' Mills, Me. From Sept., 1862; also 16th Inf.
Thomas, Silas C...... " Thomaston, Me.............A. W. M. D.
Cushing, John S....... " Skowhegan, Me.............To Nov., 1862. U. S. Ex. S.

22D INFANTRY—(9 months)—Mustered out August 14, 1863.

Huckins, Jason........Ass't S.....East Corinth, Me...........From October, 1862.
Cook, John W......... " Iowa City, Iowa............To December, 1862.
Jordon, Josiah.........Surgeon...Dead.

23D INFANTRY—(9 months)—Mustered out July 15, 1863.

Sweat, Jesse P.........Surgeon...Brownfield, Me.............From Oct., 1862. H. R. Also 14th Infantry.
Towle, Wm. C.........Ass't S.... Fryeburgh, Me.............To Jan., 1863; also 12th Inf.
Ricker, Richard R... " Lewiston, Me................To Jan., 1863; also 31st Inf.

24TH INFANTRY—(9 months)—Mustered out August 25, 1863.

Harlow, Roscoe L.....Surgeon...Lewistown and Auburn, Me. From Nov., 1862. H. R.
Morton, John A........Ass't S.....Bethel, Me...................From December, 1862.
Manson, John C ......Surgeon...Pittsfield, Me................To November, 1862.

25TH INFANTRY—(9 months)—Mustered out July 10, 1863.

True, Wm. H..........Ass't S.....Portland, Me................From Sept. 1862; also 20th Inf.
Carr, Josiah ............Surgeon...Dead...................................Also 30th Infantry.
Bowker, Cyrus K.....Ass't S................................................From September, 1862.

26TH INFANTRY—(9 months)—Mustered out August 17, 1863.

Abbott, Chas............Surgeon ..Winterport, Me.............Died 1879.
Collins, Willard C....Ass't S.....Bucksport, Me...............From October, 1862.
Williams, Benj.........H. Stew...Rockland, Me.

27TH INFANTRY—(9 months)—Mustered out July 17, 1863.

Kimball, J. E. L.......Surgeon...Saco, Me.......................From September, 1862.
Hall, Freeman..........Ass't S.....Biddleford, Me..............From September, 1862.
Cross, Chas. M......... " ........................................From February, 1863.

28TH INFANTRY—(9 months)—Mustered out August 31, 1863.

Jennings, Reuben B..H Stew...Farmington, Me............To Feb., 1863. Died 1882.
Plaisted, Elijah F.....Surgeon...Dead.
Lake, Elias H..........Ass't S.....Dead.

29TH INFANTRY—In service August 31, 1865.

Howard, Horatio N..Ass't S.....Washington, D. C..........To March, 1865; also 10th and 30th Infantry.
Day, Josiah F., Jr....Surgeon...Alfred, Me....................From Sept., 1863; also 10th Inf.
Cotton, Henry C......Ass't S.....Prescott, Wis.................From January, 1864.
Sweet, Atwell W...... " Winterport, Me. ............From April, 1865.

## MAINE—Continued.

### 30TH INFANTRY—Mustered out August 20, 1865.

| | | | |
|---|---|---|---|
| Howard, Horatio N. | Surgeon | Washington, D. C. | From May, 1865; also 10th and 29th Inf. |
| Currier, Geo. W | H. Stew | Mechanics Falls, Me. | |
| Carr, Josiah | Surgeon | Dead. | Also 25th Infantry. |
| Packard, Chas. K | Ass't S | Dead. | |

### 31ST INFANTRY—Mustered out July 15, 1865.

| | | | |
|---|---|---|---|
| Fisher, Preston | Surgeon | Santa Cruz, Cal | To November, 1864. D. |
| French, Albert G | Ass't S | Lewiston, Me | To July, 1864. |
| Ricker, Richard R | " | Lewiston, Me | To Dec., 1864; also 23d Inf. |
| Kimball, John H | Surgeon | Bridgeton, Me. | From Sept., 1864; also 15th and 32d Inf. |
| Smith, Henry S. B | Ass't S | Bowdoinham, Me | From May, 1864; also 32d Inf |
| Wiggin, S. D | " | Ellsworth, Me | From February, 1865. |
| Mitchell, John D | Surgeon | | To September, 1864. |

### 32D INFANTRY—Consolidated with the 31st Infantry December 12, 1864.

| | | | |
|---|---|---|---|
| Kimball, John H | Surgeon | Bridgeton, Me | From Sept., 1864; also 15th and 31st Inf. |
| Smith, Henry S. B | Ass't S | Bowdoinham, Me | From May, 1864; also 31st Inf. |

### COAST GUARD BATTALION.

The following medical officers were on duty with this Battalion from March, 1864, to August, 1865.

| | | | |
|---|---|---|---|
| Bayne, J. H | Surgeon | Dead. | |
| Potter, Z. H. | A. A. S. | Pension Office, Washington, D. C. | From June, 1864, to May, 1865. |
| Fessenden, H. C | " | Eastport, Me. | From Aug., 1864, to Aug., 1865. |
| Stephens, J. L | " | 1300 Ross street, Richmond, Va | From March to May, 1865. |
| Page, A. F | " | Bucksport, Me | From June to Aug. 1865. |
| Brickett, G. E | " | Augusta, Me | June and July, 1865. |
| Toward, J. W | " | Augusta, Me | From May to July, 1865. |
| Bradbury, O. N | " | Norway. Me | From May to July, 1865. |
| Merrill, S. H | " | Portland, Me. | In May. 1864. |
| Porter, P. C | " | 140 Kinzie st., Chicago, Ill. | From May to July, 1865. |
| Fry, Thos | " | Dead. | |
| Monroe, N. P | " | Dead. | |

## MARYLAND.

### 1ST CAVALRY—Mustered out August 8, 1865.

| | | | |
|---|---|---|---|
| Dodson, Robt. A | Surgeon | St. Michael's, Md. | From September, 1863. |
| Dunnott, Thos. J | " | 317 N. 2d st., Harrisburg, Pa. | To September, 1863. |
| Warner, John E | " | 66 N. Greene st., Baltimore, Md. | To March, 1862. |
| Burleigh, Wm. E | Ass't S | | From June, 1865. |
| Lee, Chas. E | " | | To March, 1862 |
| Ensor, J. F | " | | To January, 1865. |

## MARYLAND—Continued.

### 1st Cavalry—(P. H. B.)—Mustered out June 28, 1865.

| Name | Rank | Address | Service |
|---|---|---|---|
| McIlvain, John | Ass't S. | | From May, 1865. |
| Onderdonk, D. W. | Surgeon | | From January, 1865. |
| Way, W. R. | " | 3 S. Broadway, Baltimore, Md. | To December, 1864. |

### 2d Cavalry was a 6-months' organization.

### 3d Cavalry—Mustered out September 7, 1865.

| Name | Rank | Address | Service |
|---|---|---|---|
| Borck, Edward, jr | Ass't S. | 3613 N. 9th st., St. Louis, Mo. | To December, 1864 |
| Stevenson, John M. | Surgeon | Baltimore, Md | Alleged dead. |
| Claridge, Jos. S. | Ass't S. | | From March, 1864. |

### 1st Infantry—Mustered out July 2, 1865.

| Name | Rank | Address | Service |
|---|---|---|---|
| Baer, Edward R | Surgeon | 142 Bolton street, Baltimore, Md | From May, 1864. |
| Mitchell, Thos E | Surgeon | Columbus, Neb | To April, 1864. |
| Ansell, Aaron | Ass't S. | | From February, 1865. |
| Bagley, Jos. H | " | | To May, 1864. |

### 1st Infantry (E. S.)—Consolidated with 11th Infantry February 23, 1865.

| Name | Rank | Address | Service |
|---|---|---|---|
| Kemp, J. McK | Ass't S. | Reisterstown, Md. | From April, 1863; also 11th Inf |
| Phelips, Francis P | Surgeon | Cambridge, Md | To November, 1862. |
| Lecompte, G. B. | " | Dead. | |
| Manning, A. L. | Ass't S. | | To December, 1864. |

### 2d Infantry—Mustered out July 17, 1865.

| Name | Rank | Address | Service |
|---|---|---|---|
| Beatty, Jos. E | Surgeon | Middletown, Md | To March, 1865. |
| McCullough, J. H. | " | Harrisburg, Pa | From April, 1865. |
| Scarboro, Silas | Ass't S. | Dublin, Md | To July, 1864. |
| Morony, E. P. | Surgeon | | To March, 1863. |

### 2d Infantry (P. H. B.)—Mustered out May 29, 1865.

| Name | Rank | Address | Service |
|---|---|---|---|
| Healey, Patrick A. | Ass't S. | Dead | To October, 1864. |
| Smith, Samuel P. | Surgeon | Dead | To October, 1864. |
| Crain, Wm. B. | " | | From, May, 1865. |

### 2d Infantry (E. S.)—Consolidated with 1st E. S. January 23, 1865.

| Name | Rank | Address | Service |
|---|---|---|---|
| Cooper, E. W. | Ass't S. | Camden, Del | From Nov., 1862. H. R. |
| Owings, H. W. | Surgeon | 274 Madison ave., Baltimore, Md. | To Oct., 1864; also 4th Inf. |
| Valk, Wm. W | " | Dead | To Oct., 1862; also 4th Inf. |
| Robinson, Rob't K. | Ass't S. | | To September, 1862. |
| Atkinson, Edw'd E. | Surgeon | Ridgely, Md | To May, 1863. |

### 3d Infantry—Mustered out July 31, 1865.

| Name | Rank | Address | Service |
|---|---|---|---|
| Currey, Jas. H. | Ass't S. | 76 S. Paca street, Baltimore, Md. | To July, 1862. |
| Hutchinson, Edwin | " | Utica, N. Y | To 137th N. Y. Sept., 1863. |
| Anderson, W. A. | Surgeon | La Crosse, Wis | From March, 1864. |
| Stevenson, John M. | " | Baltimore, Md | Alleged dead. |
| White, Alphonso A. | " | U. S. custom house, Baltimore, Md. | To July, 1862. |
| Dunlap, Albert | Ass't S. | | From March, 1864. |

MARYLAND—Continued.

3D INFANTRY (P. H. B.)—Mustered out May 29, 1865.

| | | | |
|---|---|---|---|
| McKee, C. E. S. | Surgeon | Hagerstown, Md | From September, 1862. |
| Stewart, Henry C | Ass't S. | Jacksonville, Ill | To December, 1862. |
| Beerbower, Jesse | " | | To May, 1864. |
| Inloes, H. A., jr | " | | From September, 1864. |

4TH INFANTRY—Mustered out May 31, 1865.

| | | | |
|---|---|---|---|
| Cadden, Chas. W | Surgeon | 130 Arlington ave., Baltimore, Md. | Also Purnell Legion. Dead. |
| Dodge, A. W. | Ass't S. | 201 Hanover st., Baltimore, Md. | From May, 1864. Ex. S. |
| Owings, H. W | " | 48 McCullough st., Baltimore, Md. | To 2d Inf. June, 1863. |
| Valk, Wm. W. | Surgeon | Dead | Also 2d (E. S.) Inf. |
| Carter, John C. | Ass't S. | | To April, 1864. |

5TH INFANTRY—Mustered out September 1, 1865.

| | | | |
|---|---|---|---|
| Goldsborough, C. H. | Ass't S. | Hunterstown, Pa | To November, 1864. |
| Norris, Wm. H | Surgeon | 65 N. Charles st., Baltimore, Md. | To October, 1864. |
| Roop, Francis A | Ass't S. | Seaford, Del | To May, 1865. |
| Uhler, John R | Surgeon | 34 Fayette street, Baltimore, Md. | From November, 1864. |

6TH INFANTRY—Mustered out June 20, 1865.

| | | | |
|---|---|---|---|
| Foreman, Edwin K | Surgeon | Littlestown, Pa | From December, 1864. |
| Simpers, Chas. T | " | 1841 N. 23d st., Philadelphia, Pa. | To October, 1864. |
| Nelson, C. F. H. | " | | To November, 1863. |
| Maughlin, Hugh A | Ass't S. | | From February, 1865. |

7TH INFANTRY—Mustered out May 31, 1865; except Company K, transferred to 1st Veterans.

| | | | |
|---|---|---|---|
| Bolton, J. H | Ass't S. | Bond and Gay sts., Baltimore, Md. | To October, 1864. |
| Jarrett, Jas. H | Surgeon | Towsontown. Md. | To March, 1864; also Purnell Leg. Ex. S. |
| Robinson, Robert H. | " | 120 N. Calvert st., Baltimore, Md. | From August, 1864. |
| Buhrman, Harvey | Ass't S. | Foxville, Md | From March, 1865. |

8TH INFANTRY—Company K mustered out March 11, 1864; the rest mustered out May 31, 1865.

| | | | |
|---|---|---|---|
| White, A. A | Ass't S. | U. S. Custom House, Baltimore, Md. | A. W. M. |
| Wheeler, Wm. B | " | Boonsboro', Md | To December, 1864. |

9TH and 10TH INFANTRY were six-months' organizations.

11TH INFANTRY—Mustered out June 15, 1865; veterans transferred to 2d Infantry.

| | | | |
|---|---|---|---|
| Kemp, J. McK | Surgeon | Delaware City, Del. | From February, 1865; also 1st E. S. |

12TH INFANTRY—(100 days)—Mustered out May 29, 1865.

## MARYLAND—Continued.

13TH INFANTRY—Mustered out May 29, 1865. (This regiment was organized as the 1st P. H. B )

| Name | Rank | Address | Remarks |
|---|---|---|---|
| Boone, Jerningham | Surgeon | Buckeystown, Md. | To June, 1865. |
| Willard, James | Ass't S | Lovettsville, Va. | To February, 1865. |
| O'Donnell, Jas S. | Surgeon | Stockton, Kan | A. W. M Also Purnell Legion. |
| O'Donnell, E. J | Ass't S. | | From April, 1865. |
| Farish, Jas | " | | From April, 1865. |

PURNELL LEGION MARYLAND INFANTRY.

| Name | Rank | Address | Remarks |
|---|---|---|---|
| O'Donnell, Jas. S. | Surgeon | Stockton, Kans. | A. W. M. Also 13th Inf. |
| Rippard, W. H | Ass't S. | | From May, 1863. |
| Bowen, H. F. | " | | To June, 1862. |
| Hall, John T. | " | | To January, 1862. |
| Jarrett, Jas. H | " | Towsontown, Md. | To March, 1862; also 7th Inf. Ex. S. |
| Cadden, Chas. W. | " | Dead | To 4th Inf. |

MISCELLANEOUS.

| Name | Rank | Address | Remarks |
|---|---|---|---|
| Colburn, A. W. | A. A. S | 335 W. Lombard st., Baltimore, Md. | |

## MASSACHUSETTS.

1ST CAVALRY—Mustered out June 29, 1865.

| Name | Rank | Address | Remarks |
|---|---|---|---|
| De Wolf, Oscar C. | Ass't S. | Chicago, Ill., (Board of Health.) | To December, 1862; also 2d Cav. |
| Wood, Albert | Surgeon | Worcester, Mass. | To November, 1864; also 29th Inf. U. S. Ex. S. |
| Abbott, Samuel W. | " | Wakefield, Mass. | From December, 1864. H R. |
| Munn, Curtis B. | H. Stew | Care A. G. U. S. A | Also 2d Inf. Surg. U. S. A. |
| Copeland, Chas. R. | " | Springfield, Mass. | From September, 1861, to March, 1863. |
| Holland, Jas. | Surgeon | Dead. | |
| Durgin, Samuel H. | Ass't S. | | From August, 1864. |
| Osborne, Geo. S. | " | | To January, 1864. Also 5th Cav. |
| Warner, Homer H. | " | | To August, 1864. |

2D CAVALRY—Mustered out July 20, 1865.

| Name | Rank | Address | Remarks |
|---|---|---|---|
| De Wolf, Oscar C. | Surgeon | Chicago, Ill., (Board of Health.) | To February, 1865; also 1st Cav. |
| Gamwell, Harlow | Ass't S. | Westfield, Mass. | To April, 1864; also 5th Cav. |
| Johnson, E. M | Surgeon | Dead | |
| Bucknam, Alvan F. | Ass't S. | Warren, Ill | From August, 1864. |

3D CAVALRY, (41st Volunteers)—Mustered out September 28, 1865. No H. R. with A. G. of Massachusetts.

| Name | Rank | Address | Remarks |
|---|---|---|---|
| Blanchard, A. H | Surgeon | Sherborn, Mass. | To February, 1864. |
| Leavit, Daniel F. | " | 151 E. 51st st., N. Y. City. | To July, 1865 |
| Tarbell, Geo. G. | Ass't S. | 105 Boylston st., Boston. | From April, 1865; U. S. Ex. S. |
| Allen, Daniel S. | " | Sangus, Mass. | To Surg. 17th Inf. March, 1865. |
| Ambrose, David | H. Stew | Lawrence, Mass. | From June, 1863, to May, 1865. |
| Blackmer, John | Ass't S. | Springfield, Mass. | To 47th Inf. Nov., 1862. (Not in A. G. R. for 3d Cav. |

## MASSACHUSETTS—Continued.

### 4TH CAVALRY—In service August 31, 1865.

| Name | Rank | Address | Remarks |
|---|---|---|---|
| Mercer, Fred'k W | Surgeon | 2600 Calumet ave., Chicago, Ill. | To April, 1864; also 20th and 47th Inf. |
| Garvin, Paul C | " | Frankfort, Kans | From May, 1864. H. R. Also 40th and 51st Inf. |
| Russell, Edward | Ass't S. | Dead. | |
| Hill, E. K | " | | To December, 1864. |
| McGregor, Jno | " | | To April, 1864. |
| Weber, Julius | " | | To June, 1865. |

### 5TH CAVALRY, (colored)—Mustered out October 31, 1865.

| Name | Rank | Address | Remarks |
|---|---|---|---|
| Wadsworth, O F | Surgeon | 139 Boylston st., Boston | From April, 1865. |
| Parker, Fred'k G | " | Prescott, Ia., or Presque Isle, Me. | From February, 1865. |
| Gamwell, Harlow | " | Westfield, Mass | From January, 1864, to February, 1865; also 2d Cav. |
| King, J. H. F | " | 3716 Chestnut Hill, Philadelphia, Pa. | Not in A. G. R. |
| Cushman, Isaac S | " | Dead. | |
| Ingalls, Samuel | Ass't S. | | To April, 1864. |
| Osborne, Geo. S | Surgeon | | To May, 1864. Also 1st Cav. |

### 1ST HEAVY ARTILLERY (14th Infantry) Mustered out August 16, 1865.

| Name | Rank | Address | Remarks |
|---|---|---|---|
| Dana, David | Surgeon | Lawrence, Mass | To October, 1862. |
| Larabee, Geo. H | Ass't S. | Pembroke, N H | To March, 1865. |
| Cutler, Edward R | Surgeon | Waltham, Mass | To July, 1865. |
| Towle, Samuel K | Ass't S. | Haverhill, Mass | To 30th Inf Feb., 1862. |
| Dutton, Samuel L | " | 32 Dartmouth st., Boston | To 40th Inf. March, 1864. |
| Willard, Josiah N | Surgeon | Dead. | |
| Mason, Geo E | Ass't S. | | From April, 1865. |
| Mason, Edw'd B | " | | To June, 1863. |

### 2D HEAVY ARTILLERY—Mustered out September 3 and 15, 1865.

| Name | Rank | Address | Remarks |
|---|---|---|---|
| Curtis, Hall | Surgeon | 2 Spruce street, Boston, Mass. | From June, 1863, to May, 1864; also 24th Inf. |
| Emmerton, Jas. A | " | Salem, Mass | From June, 1865. H. R. Also 23d Inf |
| Denny, Jas. H | Ass't S. | Boston, Mass | From Dec., 1863. H. R. |
| Barrington, Jno. C | " | Dead. | From Jan., 1865; also 28th Inf. |

### 3D HEAVY ARTILLERY—Mustered out September 18, 1865.

| Name | Rank | Address | Remarks |
|---|---|---|---|
| Pinkham, Geo. E | Ass't S. | Lowell, Mass | To August, 1865; also 6th Infantry. |
| Nichols, Wm., Jr | Surgeon | 62 Temple st., Boston, Mass. | From Feb., 1865; also 2d Infantry. |

### 4TH HEAVY ARTILLERY—No H. R., and none S. G. of Massachusetts.

| Name | Rank | Address | Remarks |
|---|---|---|---|
| Stearns, John | Surgeon | 200 Dartmouth st., Boston | From December, 1864. |
| Saville, J. Frank | Ass't S. | 137 W. 15th st., N. Y. City. | From December, 1864. |

## MASSACHUSETTS—Continued.

### 16TH INDEPENDENT BATTERY—(Light Artillery.)

| Name | Rank | Address | Remarks |
|---|---|---|---|
| Ordway, John P | Surgeon | 168 Tremont st., Boston, Mass. | From May to Aug., 1861. Battery A not in A. G. R. |
| Steiger, Emil | " | Prarie du Chien, Wis | From Oct., 1862, to Feb., 1863. 9th Battery not in A. G. R. |

### 1ST INFANTRY—Mustered out May 25, 1864.

| Name | Rank | Address | Remarks |
|---|---|---|---|
| Whiston, E. A | Surgeon | 34 Broomfield st., Boston, Mass. | From March, 1863; also 16th Inf. |
| Salter, Richard H | " | 1 Stanford st., Boston, Mass. | To Feb., 1863. H. R. |
| Green, Sam'l A | Ass't S | Boston, Mass., (Board of Health) | To 24th Inf. Aug., 1861. |
| Monroe, F. Le B | " | 101 Fulton street, Brooklyn N. Y. | To 15th Inf. Jan., 1863. H. R. |
| Soward, John E | H. Attd't | Mattapan, (Boston,) Mass. | |
| Dana, Alfred C. | H. Stew | Franklin, Mass | 3 years. |
| Pickard, Isaiah L | Ass't S | Alleged dead. | |
| Oakes, T. Fletcher | " | Alleged dead | To 56th Inf. Aug., 1863. |
| Garvie, Jno. B | " | | Deserted Dec., 1863. |

### 2D INFANTRY—Mustered out July 11, 1865.

| Name | Rank | Address | Remarks |
|---|---|---|---|
| Stone, Lincoln R | Surgeon | Newton, Mass | To April, 1863; also 54th (colored) Inf. |
| Nichols, Wm., Jr | Ass't S | 62 Temple st., Boston | To 3d Art Feb., 1865. |
| Munn, Curtis E | Surgeon | Care A. G. U. S. A | From Jan., 1865; also 27th Inf. and 1st Cav. |
| Kinsman, Fred. G. | H. Stew | Fitchburg, Mass. | |
| Leland, Francis | Surgeon | Dead | To November, 1862. |
| Sargent, L. M. | " | Dead | To September, 1861. |

### 3D INFANTRY—(9 months)—Mustered out June 26, 1863.

| Name | Rank | Address | Remarks |
|---|---|---|---|
| Stocker, Alfred A | Surgeon | 84 Prospect street, Cambridgeport, Mass. | From October, 1862; also 58th Inf. |
| Howes, W. R | Ass't S | Hanover, or Lakeville, Mass. | A. W. M. H. R. |

### 4TH INFANTRY—(9 months)—Mustered out August 28, 1863.

| Name | Rank | Address | Remarks |
|---|---|---|---|
| Waldock, Jas | Surgeon | 48 Alleghany st., Boston, Mass. | From December, 1862. |
| Gould, Jas. F | Ass't S | 418 Broadway, So. Boston, Mass. | From Dec., 1862. H. R. |
| Howland, Chas | H. Stew | Rockland, Mass. | |
| Nortoni, E. W | Ass't S | | From December, 1862. |

### 5TH INFANTRY—(9 months)—Mustered out July 2, 1863.

| Name | Rank | Address | Remarks |
|---|---|---|---|
| Ingalls, Wm | Surgeon | 556 Tremont street, Boston, Mass. | From October, 1862; also 57th and 59th Inf. |
| Hoyt, Dixie C | Ass't S | Dead. | |

### 6TH INFANTRY—(9 months)—Mustered out July 3, 1863.

| Name | Rank | Address | Remarks |
|---|---|---|---|
| Burnham, Walter | Surgeon | Lowell, Mass | From September, 1862. |
| Pinkham, Geo. E | Ass't S | Lowell, Mass | From Dec., 1862; also 3d H. Art. |
| Humphrey, O. M | " | Minneapolis, Minn | From September, 1862. |

MASSACHUSETTS—Continued.

7TH INFANTRY—Mustered out June 27, 1864.

| Name | Rank | Residence | Service |
|---|---|---|---|
| Lincoln, Wm. H | Surgeon | Millbury, Mass | From Feb., to Sept., 1863. H. R. |
| Holman, Silas A | " | 119 Olive st., St. Louis, Mo. | To U. S. V. Sept., 1863. H. R. |
| Adams, Zabdiel B | Ass't S | Framingham, Mass | To 32d Inf. May, 1862. |
| Cowdrey, A. H | " | Stoneham, Mass | To 37th U. S. C. T. Oct., 1863. |

8TH INFANTRY—(9 months)—Mustered out August 7, 1873.

| Name | Rank | Residence | Service |
|---|---|---|---|
| Haddock, Chas | Surgeon | Beverly, Mass | From November, 1862. |
| Robinson, J. L | Ass't S | Wenham, Mass | From November, 1862. |

9TH INFANTRY—Mustered out June 21, 1864.

| Name | Rank | Residence | Service |
|---|---|---|---|
| Sullivan, J. F | Surgeon | 7 Van Ness ave., San Francisco, Cal. | From December, 1862. |
| Pineo, Peter | " | Hyannis, Mass | To August, 1861. |
| Ryan, John | Ass't S | Dead. | |
| Drew, S. Watson | Surgeon | Dead. | |
| O'Connell, Patrick | Ass't S | Dead | To September, 1861. |
| Lincoln, F. M | " | Dead | To 35th Inf. July, 1862. |
| Fitzpatrick, J. W | " | | To Surg. U. S. V. March, 1863. |

10TH INFANTRY—Mustered out July 6, 1864.—Records with Colonel Joseph B. Parsons, Northampton, Mass.

| Name | Rank | Residence | Service |
|---|---|---|---|
| Chamberlain, C. N | Surgeon | Lawrence, Mass | To May, 1863. |
| Holbrook, Wm | Ass't S | Palmer, Mass | To 18th Inf. Jan., 1862. U. S. Ex. S. |
| Jewett, Geo | " | Fitchburgh, Mass | To Surg. 51st Inf. Nov., 1862. |
| Robinson, A. B | Surgeon | Boston Highlands, Mass | From May, 1863. |
| Wells, Chas. C | H. Stew | Saratoga Springs, N. Y | June, 1861, to Oct., 1862. |
| Gilman, John H | Ass't S | | From March, 1863. |

11TH INFANTRY—Mustered out July 14, 1865.—Veterans and recruits of the 16th transferred to this Regiment.

| Name | Rank | Residence | Service |
|---|---|---|---|
| Douglass, John A | Surgeon | Amesbury, Mass | To October, 1864. H. R. |
| Whittier, Sam'l C | Ass't S | Portsmouth, N. H | To 23d Inf., June, 1864. |
| Crozier, Thos | " | Care 3 Dexter Row, Boston, Mass. | A. W. M.; also 16th Inf. |
| Foye, John W | Surgeon | 1209 Columbia st., San Francisco, Cal. | Missing since April, 1863. |
| Smith, Cyrus B | " | Dead. | |
| Bell, Luther V | " | | To Brig. Surg. August, 1861. |
| Russel, Ira | " | | To Surg. U. S. V. April, 1862. |
| Williams, A. G | Ass't S | | To August, 1862. |

12TH INFANTRY—Mustered out July 8, 1864.

| Name | Rank | Residence | Service |
|---|---|---|---|
| Hinds, Wm. H. W | Surgeon | Milford, N. H | From July, 1863; also 17th Inf. |
| Wheeler, Chas. A | Ass't S | Leominster, Mass | From December, 1862. |
| Hayward, J. McL | Surgeon | Boston or So. Weymouth, Mass. | To April, 22, 1863. |
| BAXTER, J. H | " | Chief Medical Purveyor, care A. G. U. S. A. | To Brig. Surg. April, 1862. |
| McGregor, Jno. H | Ass't S | | To September, 1863. |

## MASSACHUSETTS—Continued.

### 13TH INFANTRY—Mustered out August 1, 1864.

| | | | |
|---|---|---|---|
| Whitney, A. W | Surgeon | West Newton, Mass | From July, 1861. Dead. |
| Heard, J. T | Ass't S | Bloomsbury Sq., Boston | To May, 1862. |
| Claffin, Wm. W | Ass't S | | To December, 1862. |
| Harriman, Jas. L | " | | To January, 1863. |
| Hixon, Lloyd W | " | | From March, 1863. |
| Parker, Edgar | " | | To September, 1863. |

### 14TH INFANTRY—(See 1st Heavy Artillery.)

### 15TH INFANTRY—Mustered out July 28, 1864.—Veterans and recruits transferred to the 20th Infantry.

| | | | |
|---|---|---|---|
| Bates, Jos. F | Surgeon | Worchester. Mass | Dismissed July, 1862. B. |
| Rockwood, Henry | Ass't S | South Weymouth, Mass | Dismissed Sept., 1863. |
| Munroe, F. Le B | Surgeon | 101 Fulton st., Brooklyn, N. Y. | From Jan., 1863; also 1st Inf. |
| Cornish, Theo. O | Ass't S | 404 4th st., Boston, Mass | From August, 1862. |

### 16TH INFANTRY—Mustered out July 27, 1864.

| | | | |
|---|---|---|---|
| Jewett, Chas. C | Surgeon | 101 Hicks st., Brooklyn, N. Y. | From Aug., 1862. H. R. |
| Whiston, E. A | Ass't S | 34 Broomfield st., Boston | To 1st Inf., March, 1863. |
| King, Geo | " | Franklin, Mass | To 29th Inf. March, 1864. |
| Crozier, Thos | " | Care 3 Dexter Row, Boston. | From May, 1863; also 11th Inf. |
| Wills, W. R | H. Stew | Waltham, Mass. | |

### 17TH INFANTRY—Mustered out July 11, 1865.

| | | | |
|---|---|---|---|
| Allen, Daniel S | Surgeon | Saugus, Mass | From March, 1865. H.R. Also 3d Cavalry. |
| Galloupe, Isaac F | " | Lynn, Mass | To Aug., 1864. U. S. Ex. S. |
| Eayrs, Chas. G. A | Ass't S | Nashua, N. H | To August, 1864. |
| Hinds, Wm. H. W | " | Milford, N. H | To 12th Inf. May, 1863. |
| *Walton John T | " | Buffalo, N. Y | Belonged to 103d Pa. Vols. Dead. |
| Clarke, Geo. W | " | | Dismissed Dec., 1864. |

### 18TH INFANTRY—Consolidated with the 32d Infantry October 21, 1864.

| | | | |
|---|---|---|---|
| Holbrook, Wm | Surgeon | Palmer, Mass | From Jan., 1862, to Sept., 1864; also 10th Inf. U. S. Ex. S. |
| Hastings, B. F | Ass't S | South Abington, Mass | To Sept., 1864. U. S. Ex. S. |
| †Smith, David P | Surgeon | Springfield, Mass | To January, 1862. Dead. |
| Brown, Orlando | Ass't S | Washington, Conn | To 29th Inf. Jan., 1862. |
| Nelson, Abial W | " | New London, Conn | To July, 1862. U. S. Ex. S. |
| Merriam, Jos. W | " | Iquique, Peru | To January, 1863 |
| Silcox, Edwin F | " | | Dismissed Jan., 1863. |
| Wilbur, Joshua G | " | | To November, 1863. |

---

* In charge of 17th Massachusetts from fall of 1864 to March, 1865.
† Avery J. Smith, of Springfield, Mass., has Surgeon Smith's records.

## MASSACHUSETTS—Continued.

### 19TH INFANTRY—Mustered out June 30, 1865.

| Name | Rank | Address | Remarks |
|---|---|---|---|
| Pratt, Gustavus P | Surgeon | Cohasset, Mass | From December, 1864. |
| Dyer, J. Franklin | " | Dead. | |
| Willard, Jos. N | Ass't S | Dead | To Surg. 14th Inf. Nov., 1862 |
| Fulton, David W | " | | From June, 1865. |
| Knapp, Wm. D | " | | Dismissed Dec., 1863. |
| Stone, Vestulan R | " | | To May, 1863. |
| Taft, Benj. F | " | Dead | To Mar., 1863; also 20th Inf. |

### 20TH INFANTRY—Mustered out June 16, 1865.

| Name | Rank | Address | Remarks |
|---|---|---|---|
| Perry, John G | Ass't S | 113 Madison ave., New York city. | To July, 1864. |
| Mercer, Fred'k W | Surgeon | 2600 Calumet ave., Chicago, Ill. | To April, 1865; also 4th Cav. and 47th Inf. |
| White, Elisha M | " | 99 Court street, Boston, Mass. | To June, 1865; also 37th Inf. |
| McGregor, Murdock | " | La Have, N. S | From May, 1865; also 33d Inf. |
| Hayward, Nathan | " | Dead. | |
| Bryant, Henry | " | Dead | To Brig. Surg. Sept., 1861. |
| Dinsmore, Geo. R | Ass't S | | From April, 1865. |
| Inches, Chas. E | " | 88 Charles street, Boston, Mass. | From April, 1865. |
| Taft, Benj. F | " | Dead | To 19th Inf. January, 1863. |

### 21ST INFANTRY—Consolidated with the 36th Infantry October 21, 1864.

| Name | Rank | Address | Remarks |
|---|---|---|---|
| Oliver, Jas | Surgeon | Athol, Mass | To August, 1864; also 61st Inf. |
| Carr, Edgar L | Ass't S | Pittsfield, N. H | To August, 1864; also 29th and 35th Inf. |
| Hastings, Jos. W | " | Warren, Mass | To 33d Inf. May, 1863. |
| Warren, Orrin | " | West Newbury, Mass | To 33d Inf. August, 1862. |
| Mitchell, John W | " | Palermo, Me | To 4th U. S. C. T. Sept., 1863. |
| Cutter, Calvin | Surgeon | Dead. | |

### 22D INFANTRY—Mustered out October 17, 1864.

| Name | Rank | Address | Remarks |
|---|---|---|---|
| Stearns, Isaac H | Surgeon | Soldiers' Home, Milwaukee, Wis. | From September, 1863. |
| Warren, E. L | " | Medford, Mass | To June 10, 1862. |
| Ainsworth, F. S | " | Dead. | |
| Perkins, Geo. T | Ass't S | Dead. | |
| Prince, Jas. P | " | 31 Kendall street, Boston, Mass. | To Surg. 36th Inf. Aug., 1862 |
| Simmons, M. E | Surgeon | | To August, 1863. |

### 23D INFANTRY—Mustered out June 25, 1865. No H. R., nor with A. G. of Massachusetts.

| Name | Rank | Address | Remarks |
|---|---|---|---|
| Whittier, Sam'l C | Surgeon | Portsmouth, N. H | From June, 1864; also 11th Inf. |
| Stone, Silas E | Ass't S | Walpole, Mass | To September, 1862. |
| Roberts, Jacob | " | 2033 Green street, Philadelphia, Pa. | To July, 1863. |
| Emmerton, Jas. A | " | Salem, Mass | To May, 1864; also in Co. F and 2d Heavy Artillery. |
| Cummings, E. P | " | Salem, Mass. | To September, 1864. |
| Derby, Geo | Surgeon | Dead. | |

## MASSACHUSETTS—Continued.

### 24TH INFANTRY—Mustered out from September to December, 1864. H. R. with A. G. of Massachusetts; none between July, 1863, and January 20, 1866.

| Name | Rank | Address | Remarks |
|---|---|---|---|
| Wheeler, Ed. R | Surgeon | Spencer, Mass | To December, 1864. H. R. |
| Briggs, Chas. E | Ass't S | 2735 Olive street, St. Louis, Mo. | To April, 1864; also 54th U. S. C. T. (Mass.) |
| Green, Sam'l A | Surgeon | Boston, Mass. (Board of Health) | To November, 1864; also 1st Inf. |
| Curtis, Hall | Ass't S | 2 Spruce street, Boston, Mass. | To 2d Heavy Artillery June, 1863. |
| Parsons, John W | " | Portsmouth, N. H | From April, 1865. |
| Tremaine, Wm. S | " | Care A. G. U. S. A | To Surg. 31st U. S. C. T. April, 1864. |

### 25TH INFANTRY—Mustered out July 13, 1865.

| Name | Rank | Address | Remarks |
|---|---|---|---|
| Bachelder, Jos. C | Ass't S | Templeton, Mass | To August, 1862. |
| Flagg, Samuel | " | Worcester, Mass | To August, 1863. |
| Hoyt, Alpheus E | " | Natick, Mass | Alleged dead. |
| Rice, J. Marcus | Surgeon | Worcester, Mass | To October, 1864. |
| Mecorney, Horace | Ass't S | | To August, 1863. |
| Shantz, Samuel E | " | | To December, 1863. |
| Temple, Theron | " | Amhurst, Mass | To March, 1862. |

### 26TH INFANTRY—Mustered out August 26, 1865.

| Name | Rank | Address | Remarks |
|---|---|---|---|
| Fox, Lorenzo S | Ass't S | Lowell, Mass | To June, 1864. |
| Smith, Isaac | " | Fall River, Mass | To October, 1864. |
| Willis, Lemuel M | " | Boston, Mass | To 74th U. S. C. T. Oct., 1862. |
| Perkins, Geo. T | Surgeon | Dead. | |
| Hooker, Anson P | " | Dead. | |
| Russell, Edward | Ass't S | Dead. | |
| Bradt, Jas. G | Surgeon | Dead. | |

### 27TH INFANTRY—Mustered out June 26, 1865.

| Name | Rank | Address | Remarks |
|---|---|---|---|
| Hubon, P. E | Ass't S | Worcester, Mass | To May, 1863; also 28th Inf. Dead. |
| Camp, Samuel | " | Great Barrington, Mass | To March, 1862. |
| Otis, Geo. A | Surgeon | U. S. A | Dead. |
| Munn, Curtis E | Ass't S | Care A. G. U. S. A | To 2d Inf. Dec., 1864; also 1st Cav. |
| Fish, Dyer B. N | Surgeon | Amherst, Mass | From Oct., 1864. H. R. |
| Sanderson, Wm. F | H. Stew | Springfield, Mass | Dead. |
| Fuller, Geo. E | " | Monson, Mass. | |

### 28TH INFANTRY—Mustered out June 30, 1865.

| Name | Rank | Address | Remarks |
|---|---|---|---|
| Hubon, Peter E | Surgeon | Worcester, Mass | From July, 1863; also 27th Inf. Dead. |
| Parsons, John E | Ass't S | Ayer, Mass | To July, 1863. |
| Snow, Geo. W | " | Newburyport, Mass | To Surg 35th Inf. March, 1863. U. S. Ex. S. |
| Chase, Albert A | " | Alleged dead. | |
| Barrington, Jno C | " | | To June, 1864; also 2d H. Art. Dead. |
| O'Connell, P. A | Surgeon | Dead | To Surg. U. S. V., June, 1863. |
| Rood, Jas. T | Ass't S | Holden, Mass | To November, 1862. |

MASSACHUSETTS—Continued.

29TH INFANTRY—Mustered out July 29, 1865.

Brown, Orlando ......Surgeon...Washington, Conn.........To July, 1862; also 18th Inf.
Cogswell, Geo. B ..... " North Easton, Mass........To March, 1864.
King, Geo ................ " Franklin, Mass ..............To May, 1865; also 16th Inf.
Carr, Edgar L.........Ass't S.....Pittsfield, N. H..............From Oct., 1864; also 21st and 35th Inf.
Jameson, Robert E .. " 23d Ward, Boston, Mass..A. W. M.
Wood, Albert.......... " Worcester, Mass ............To 1st Cav. August, 1863. U. S. Ex. S.
Bassett, Jas. C......... " ..................................To February, 1863.

30TH INFANTRY—In service August 31, 1865.

Davis, Samuel A.......Surgeon...Charlestown, Mass.........From Jan , 1865. H. R.
Greene, Francis C....Ass't S....Easthampton, Mass........To April, 1864.
Towle, Samuel K.....Surgeon...Haverhill, Mass..............To Nov., 1864; also 1st Heavy Artillery.
Holt, A. F................Ass't S.....Cambridgeport, Mass......To 1st Tex. Cav., Nov., 1862.
McCollen, John H ...H. Stew...Boston, Mass.
Jackson, Cornelius S..Ass't S.....Hudson, Mass.................From April, 1865.
Moore, Chas. W.......Surgeon.......................................To April, 1862.

31ST INFANTRY—Mustered out September 9, 1865.

Bidwell, Edwin C.....Surgeon...Vineland, N. J ...............A. W. M. H. R. U. S. Ex. S.
Clark, Elisha P........Ass't S.....Hopkinton, R. I ............From March, 1864.
Mann, Cyrus S......... " Newton, Mass ...............To March, 1864.
Payne, Jason T........ " 121 Toulouse st, New Orleans, La. To 73d U. S C. T. September, 1862.
Brown, Henry W..... " Dead.
Kittredge, F. D........ " Dead.
Train, Horace D...... " Dead.
Cady, Frank A ........Surgeon........................................ To February, 1862.

32D INFANTRY—Mustered out June 29, 1865.

Adams, Zabdiel B....Surgeon...Framingham, Mass.........From May, 1862, to Aug., 1863; also 7th Inf.
Faxon, W. Lyman ... " Supt. National Sailors' Home, Quincy, Mass. To June, 1865.
Fletcher, Sam'l W ... " Pepperell, Mass...............From June, 1865.
Morgan, Rich'd E....H. Stew...Holyoke, Mass.
Perkins, Geo. T.......Ass't S.....Dead..................................To 26th Infantry.
Bigelow, Windsor H. " .......................................To January, 1863.
McGregor, John H... " .......................................From March, 1865.
Young, Samuel S ..... " .......................................To April, 1863.

33D INFANTRY—Mustered out June 11, 1865.

Hastings, Jos. W......Surgeon...Warren, Mass.................From July, 1863; also 21st Inf.
Webb, Melville E .....Ass't S.....233 Boylston street and 1503 Washington st., Boston. From August, 1863.
Warren, Orrin .........Surgeon...West Newbury, Mass.....From August, 1862, to April, 1863; also 21st Inf.
Brown, W. S .......... Ass't S.....Stoneham, Mass..............To May, 1863; also 55th U. S. C. T. (Mass.)
McGregor, Murdock.. " La Have, N. S.................To 20th Inf. May, 1865.
Gage, Daniel P ........ " Lowell, Mass .................To February, 1863.

## MASSACHUSETTS—Continued.

### 34TH INFANTRY—Mustered out July 16, 1865.

| Name | Rank | Address | Remarks |
|---|---|---|---|
| Clark, Rouse | Surgeon | Whitinsville, Mass | From July, 1862. H. R. |
| Allen, Chas. G | Ass't S. | Barre, Mass | From April, 1864. |
| Millard, Henry J | " | North Adams, Mass | From February, 1865. |
| Thorndike, Wm | " | Milwaukee, Wis | To Surg. 39th Inf. Jan., 1864. |
| Fairbanks, Jos. R | H. Stew | Ashfield, Mass., or Amsterdam, N. Y. | |
| Smith, Cyrus B | Ass't S. | Dead | To 11th Inf. Feb., 1865. |

### 35TH INFANTRY—Mustered out June 9, 1865.

| Name | Rank | Address | Remarks |
|---|---|---|---|
| Snow, Geo. W | Surgeon | Newburyport, Mass | A. W. M.; also 28th Inf. U. S. Ex. S. |
| Munsell, Geo. N | Ass't S. | Harwich, Mass | To April, 1863. |
| Carr, Edgar L | " | Pittsfield, N. H | To 29th Inf. June, 1865; also 21st Inf. |
| Williams, Alfred | H. Stew | Roxbury, Mass. | |
| Lincoln, Francis M | Surgeon | Alleged dead. | |
| Clark, Albert W | Ass't S. | Alleged dead. | |
| Roche, Edw'd P | " | | From July, 1863. |

### 36TH INFANTRY—Mustered out June 8, 1865.

| Name | Rank | Address | Remarks |
|---|---|---|---|
| Tyler, Warren | Ass't S. | North Brookfield, Mass | To October, 1863; U. S. Ex. S. |
| Parrish, G. F | H. Stew | Fitchburgh, Mass. | |
| Prince, Jas. P | Surgeon | Said to be in West Indies | May, 1865, to Surg. U. S. V.; also 22d Inf. |
| Bryant, Albert H | " | Dead. | |

### 37TH INFANTRY—Mustered out June 21, 1865.

| Name | Rank | Address | Remarks |
|---|---|---|---|
| White, Elisha M | Surgeon | 99 Court st., Boston, Mass. | From January, 1865; also 20th Inf. |
| Crehore, Chas. F | " | Newton, Mass | To November, 1864. H. R. |
| Lawton, Thos. C | Ass't S. | Cranston, R. I | To February, 1864. |
| Champney, Wm. A | H. Stew | Hadley, Mass | Has Hospital Register. |
| Morgan, Richard | " | Holyoke, Mass. | |
| Ellis, J. Jas | Ass't S. | Dead | To March, 1863. |
| Inches, Jas E | " | | From April to June, 1865. |
| Mitchell, Albert L | " | | Dismissed December, '63. |

### 38TH INFANTRY—Mustered out June 30, 1865.

| Name | Rank | Address | Remarks |
|---|---|---|---|
| Ward, Edwin F | Surgeon | 33 W. 36th st., N.Y. City | From April, 1864. H. R. |
| Hartwell, Sam'l C | " | Southbridge, Mass | To March, 1864. |
| Thompson, Geo. F | Ass't S. | Belchertown, Mass | To Oct., 1864; also 1st Lieut. 21st Inf. |
| *Dinwiddie, Wm. A | Lt U.S A | Care A. G., U. S. A. | |

### 39TH INFANTRY—Mustered out June 1, 1865. H. R. with S. G. beginning February 18, 1864; A. G. has balance of records.

| Name | Rank | Address | Remarks |
|---|---|---|---|
| Thorndike, Wm | Surgeon | Milwaukee, Wis | From January, 1864; also 34th Inf. |
| Chipman, Jas. L | Ass't S. | Providence, R. I | To May, 1864. |
| Butler, Jno. F | " | †San Francisco, Cal | From June, 1864. |
| Mitchell, Henry H | " | | To S. 30th U. S. C. T. November, 1863. |
| Page, Calvin G | Surgeon | Dead | To November, 1863. |

* Was Assistant Surgeon 22d Iowa, and in charge of 38th Infantry December, 1864.
† Care J. A. Sampson, Custom House.

## MASSACHUSETTS—Continued.

### 40TH INFANTRY—Mustered out June 16, 1865.

| Name | Rank | Residence | Remarks |
|---|---|---|---|
| Hildreth, Chas. F | Ass't S | Suncook, N. H | From September, 1864. |
| Smith, Andrew M | Surgeon | Williamstown, Mass | To March, 1864. |
| Dutton, Sam'l L | " | 32 Dartmouth street, Boston | To May, '65; also 1st H. Art. |
| Cass Jonathan | Ass't S | Great Barrington, Mass | To July, 1863. |
| Merriam, Ephraim C | " | Washington, D. C | To July, 1864 |
| Garvin, Paul C | " | Frankfort, Kans | To 4th Cavalry May, '64; also 51st Inf. |
| Brewster, Oliver E | Surgeon | Dead. | |

### 41ST INFANTRY—(See 3d Cavalry.)

### 42D INFANTRY—(Militia, 9-months)—Mustered out August 20, 1863.

| Name | Rank | Residence | Remarks |
|---|---|---|---|
| Hitchcock, Thos B | Ass't S | Dead. | |
| Heintzelman, R. B | " | Alleged dead. | |
| Cummings, Arial I | Surgeon | | From November, 1862. |

### 43D INFANTRY—(Militia, 9-months)—Mustered out July 30, 1863.

| Name | Rank | Residence | Remarks |
|---|---|---|---|
| Webber, A. Carter | Surgeon | Cambridge, Mass | From Oct., 1862. H. R. |
| Marcy, Henry O | Ass't S | No. 116 Boylston st., Boston, Mass | From May, 1863; also 35th U. S. C. T. |
| Mason, Augustus | " | Brighton, Mass | To March, 1863. |

### 44TH INFANTRY—(Militia, 9-months)—Mustered out June 18, 1863.

| Name | Rank | Residence | Remarks |
|---|---|---|---|
| Fisher, Theo. W | Surgeon | 171 Warren ave., Boston | From April, 1863; also 1st Lt. 62d Inf. |
| McPhee, Daniel | Ass't S | | From March, 1863. |

### 45TH INFANTRY—(Militia, 9-months)—Mustered out July 7, 1863.

| Name | Rank | Residence | Remarks |
|---|---|---|---|
| Kneeland, Samuel | Surgeon | 61 Court st., Boston, Mass. | From October, 1862. |
| Treadwell, J. B | Ass't S | 420 Columbia ave., Boston. | From Oct., '62; also 62d and 54th Inf. (colored) |
| McLean, Daniel | " | Alleged dead. | |

### 46TH INFANTRY—(Militia, 9-months)—Mustered out July 29, 1863.

| Name | Rank | Residence | Remarks |
|---|---|---|---|
| Waterman, Jas. H | Surgeon | Westfield, Mass | From Oct., 1862. H. R. |
| Gilfillan, Thos | Ass't S | Northampton, Mass | From October, 1862; also 59th Inf. |

### 47TH INFANTRY—(Militia, 9-months)—Mustered out September 1, 1863

| Name | Rank | Residence | Remarks |
|---|---|---|---|
| Blackmer, John | Surgeon | No. 45 Pearl st., Springfield, Mass. | From November, 1862; also 3d Cav. |
| Mercer, Fred'k W | Ass't S | 2600 Calumet ave., Chicago, Ill. | From November, 1862; also 4th Cav. & 20th Inf. |

### 48TH INFANTRY—(Militia, 9-months)—Mustered out September 3, 1863.

| Name | Rank | Residence | Remarks |
|---|---|---|---|
| Hurd, Yorick G | Surgeon | Ipswich, Mass | From December, 1862. |
| Brown, Francis F | Ass't S | Reading, Mass | From December, 1862. |

### 49TH INFANTRY—(Militia, 9-months)—Mustered out September 1, 1863.

| Name | Rank | Residence | Remarks |
|---|---|---|---|
| Winsor, Frederick | Surgeon | Winchester, Mass | A. W. M. H. R. |
| Rice, Albert R | Ass't S | Springfield, Mass | A. W. M. |
| Reynolds, Jos. B | " | Dead | From July, 1863. |

## MASSACHUSETTS—Continued.

### 50TH INFANTRY (9 months)—Mustered out August 24, 1863.

| | | | |
|---|---|---|---|
| Cogswell, Wm | Surgeon | Bradford, Mass | From Nov., 1862. H. R. |
| Hancock, John | Ass't S. | Barre, Mass | From July, 1863. |

### 51ST INFANTRY (9 months)—Mustered out July 27, 1863.

| | | | |
|---|---|---|---|
| Jewett, Geo. | Surgeon | Fitchburgh, Mass | From Nov., 1862; also 10th Inf. |
| Darling. J. Horner | Ass't S. | Keene, N. H | From November, 1862. |
| Garvin, Paul C. | " | Frankfort, Kan | A. W. M.; also 4th Cav. and 40th Inf. |

### 52D INFANTRY (Militia, 9 months)—Mustered out August 14, 1863.

| | | | |
|---|---|---|---|
| Sawyer, Fred'k A. | Surgeon | Wareham, Mass | From Nov., 1862. H. R. U. S. Ex. S. |
| Richardson, John H. | Ass't S. | Medford or Medfield, Mass. | From November, 1862. |
| Sabin, Henry M. | " | Edwardsville, Ill | From May, 1863. |
| Coad, Mathias | P. Co. F. | Williamstown, Mich | Acted as Ass't Surg. |

### 53D INFANTRY (Militia, 9 months)—Mustered out September 2, 1863.

| | | | |
|---|---|---|---|
| McCollister, J. Q. A. | Surgeon | Harvard, Mass | From Dec., 1862. H. R. |
| Bond, Wm. L. | Ass't S. | Charlestown, Mass | From Dec., 1862. H. R. |
| Barrett, Wm. M. | " | 385 Shumet, ave., Boston, Mass. | From December, 1862. |

### 54TH INFANTRY (U. S. Colored)—Mustered out August 20, 1865.

| | | | |
|---|---|---|---|
| Briggs, Chas. E. | Surgeon | 2735 Olive st., St. Louis, Mo. | A. W. M. H. R. Also 24th Inf. |
| Treadwell, Joshua B. | Ass't S. | 420 Columbia ave., Boston. Mass. | From July, 1865; also 45th and 62d Inf. |
| Bridgham, Chas. B. | " | Bucksfield. Maine | To July, 1864. |
| Stone, Lincoln R. | Surgeon | Newton, Mass | To Ass't S U. S. V. Nov., 1865; also 2d Inf. |
| Pease, Giles M. | Ass't S. | 9 Hanson street, Boston, Mass. | To May, 1864. |
| Radzinsky, L. D. | " | McKeesport, Pa | To Surg. 104 U. S. C. T. June, 1865. |

### 55TH INFANTRY (U. S. Colored)—Mustered out August 29, 1865.

| | | | |
|---|---|---|---|
| Brown, Wm S | Surgeon | Stoneham, Mass | To July, 1865; also 33d Inf. |
| Wilder, Burt G | " | Cornell Univ'ty, Ithaca, N. Y. | From August, 1865. |
| Babbett, Warren M | Ass't S. | Randolph, Mass | To 103d U. S C. T., March. 1865. |
| Lathrop, Wm. H. | " | | From July, 1865. |

### 56TH INFANTRY—Mustered out July 12, 1865.

| | | | |
|---|---|---|---|
| Soule, Horatio S | Ass't S. | Winthrop, Mass | From Dec., 1863. H. R. |
| Oakes, T. Fletcher | Surgeon | Dead | Also 1st Infantry. |
| Roberts, Jerome E. | Ass't S. | | To September, 1864. |

## MASSACHUSETTS—Continued.

### 57TH INFANTRY—Mustered out July 31, 1865.

Carpenter, Chas. O ..Ass't S.....Holyoke, Mass................To January, 1865.
Heath, Chas. E....... " Lee, Mass......................Dismissed Nov., 1864.
White, Whitman V...Surgeon...1321 4th ave., N. Y. city...From December, 1863.
Ingalls, Wm............ " 556 Tremont st., Boston..Not in A. G. R.; also 5th and 59th Inf.
Clark, David S.........Ass't S.......................................From May, 1865; also 59th Inf.
Gavin, Michael F...... " 99 W. Broadway, Boston, Mass. From May, 1865.

### 58TH INFANTRY—Mustered out July 14, 1865.

Whitman, Frank......Surgeon...Bellows Falls, Vt..........From April, 1865.
Dawson, Thos .........Ass't S.....Charlottestown, P. E. I..From April, 1864.
Stoeker, Alfred A.....Surgeon...84 Prospect street, Cambridgeport, Mass. To Aug., 1864; also 3d Inf.

### 59TH INFANTRY—Consolidated with the 57th Infantry May 26, 1865. S. G. of Massachusetts has records.

Ingalls, Wm ............Surgeon...556 Tremont st., Boston..From October, 1863; also 5th and 57th Inf.
Gilfillan, Thos .........Ass't S.....Northampton, Mass........To September, 1864; also 46th Inf.
Nortoni, Edward W.. " New Cambria, Mo ........To January, 1865.
Dorman, Wm. B......H. Stew...Georgetown, Mass .........Dec. 10, 1863, to June 13, 1865.
Clark, David S.........Ass't S........................................March to May, 1865; transferred to 57th Inf.

### 60TH INFANTRY—One hundred days.

Mercer, F. W ...........Surgeon...2600 Calumet ave., Chicago, Ill.

### 61ST INFANTRY (1 year)—Mustered out July 16, 1865.

Oliver, James...........Surgeon...Athol, Mass.....................From Nov., 1864; also 21st Inf.
Olloqui, Rufus A......Ass't S.....Kingston, N. B .............From February, 1865.

### 62D INFANTRY (1 year)—Mustered out May 5, 1865.

Treadwell, J. B........Surgeon...420 Columbia avenue, Boston. To April, 1865; also 45th and 54th (colored) Inf.

## MICHIGAN.

### 1ST CAVALRY—Mustered out March 10 and 25, 1866.

Cox, Henry S....... ..Ass't S.....Franklin, Mich......... .... To June, 1865.
Johnson, Geo. K......Surgeon...Grand Rapids, Mich........To February, 1863.
Nash, Alfred...........Ass't S.....Joliet, Ill..........................To Dec., 1862; also 9th Cav.
Richards, Geo. B...... " 167 Congress st., East Detroit, Mich. From Jan., 1863; also 7th Cavalry.
Smith, Amos K........Surgeon...Salt Lake City, Utah Territory. From November, 1864.
Wilson, David G......Ass't S....Port Huron, Mich...........From April, 1865, to May, 1866; also 5th Cav.
Wooster, S. R..........Surgeon...Grand Rapids, Mich.......To Oct., 1864; also 8th Inf.
Eastman, Henry......Ass't S....Franklin, Mich................To November, 1865.
St. Clair, A. K......... " Detroit, or Port Huron, Mich. To 5th Cav. Nov., 1864.

## MICHIGAN—Continued.

### 2D CAVALRY—Mustered out August 17, 1865.

| Name | Rank | Residence | Remarks |
|---|---|---|---|
| Brownell, William | Surgeon | Utica, Mich | To November, 1864. |
| Dunlap, Jas. A | Ass't S. | Fenton, Mich. | From March, 1864. |
| Green, Wm. F | " | Clarksville, Tenn | To 1st Tenn. Cav. Sept., 1863. |
| Henderson, C. L | Surgeon | Grand Rapids, Mich. | To October, 1862. |
| Ranney, Geo. E | " | Lansing, Mich | From November, 1864. |

### 3D CAVALRY—Mustered out February 12, 1866.

| Name | Rank | Residence | Remarks |
|---|---|---|---|
| Andrews, Josiah | Surgeon | Paw Paw, Mice | To October, 1864. |
| Johnson, Col. D | Ass't S. | Lansing, Mich | To January, 1866. |
| O'Toole, P. W | " | Ann Arbor, Mich | To January, 1865. |
| Thompson, A | Surgeon | Colton, Cal | From March, 1865. |
| Woodman, L. C | Ass't S. | Paw Paw, Mich. | To Oct., 1863; also 11th Cav. |

### 4TH CAVALRY—Mustered out July 1, 1865.

| Name | Rank | Residence | Remarks |
|---|---|---|---|
| Armstrong, C. T | Ass't S. | Corunna, Mich. | From March, 1863. |
| Bacon, John H | " | Lansing, Mich | To 16th Inf. Jan., 1865. |
| Fish, Geo. W | Surgeon | U. S. Consul, Tunis, Africa. | From August, 1862. |

### 5TH CAVALRY—Part mustered out from 19th to 23d June, 1865; the rest transferred to 1st Cavalry.

| Name | Rank | Residence | Remarks |
|---|---|---|---|
| Beach, Byron B | Ass't S. | Care of Dr. Kermott, Detroit, Mich. | From December, 1863. |
| Morris, S. L | Surgeon | Holland, Mich | To July, 1864. |
| Stone, Addison | Ass't S. | Almont, Mich. | To September, 1863. |
| Wilson, David G | " | Port Huron, Mich | To 1st Cav. June, 1865. |
| Wilson, John P | Surgeon | Pontiac, Mich. | To October, 1863. |
| St. Clair, A. K | " | Detroit, or Port Huron, Mich. | From Nov., 1864; also 1st Cav. |

### 6TH CAVALRY—Part mustered out November 24, 1865; the rest transferred to 1st Cavalry.

| Name | Rank | Residence | Remarks |
|---|---|---|---|
| Johnson, Henry | Ass't S. | Jackson, Mich. | To November, 1865. |
| Spaulding, D. C | " | Lyons, Mich | To Oct., 1863; also 10th Cav. |
| Sleeth, Jas | " | Byron, Mich | To November, 1865. |
| Weare, Daniel G | Surgeon | Lockport, N. Y | Dead. |

### 7TH CAVALRY—Part mustered out December 15, 1865; the rest transferred to 1st Cavalry.

| Name | Rank | Residence | Remarks |
|---|---|---|---|
| Richards, Geo. R | Ass't S. | 167 Congress st., East Detroit, Mich. | To 1st Cav. Nov., 1865. |
| Sherman, Adna | " | Lamont, Mich | To April, 1863. |
| Upjohn, Wm | Surgeon | Nora, or Hastings, Mich. | To November, 1865. |

### 8TH CAVALRY—Mustered out September 22, 1865.

| Name | Rank | Residence | Remarks |
|---|---|---|---|
| Mignault, J. B. K | Surgeon | Sandwich, Ont | To September, 1864. |
| Mills, Hiram | Ass't S. | Port Huron, Mich. | From May, 1865. |
| Robertson, C. G | Surgeon | St. Clair, Mich | From November, 1864. |
| Wrmstrong, W. L | Ass't S. | | A. W. M. |
| Tobey, Sam'l D | " | | To July, 1865. |

## MICHIGAN—Continued.

### 9TH CAVALRY—Mustered out July 21, 1865.

| | | | |
|---|---|---|---|
| Nash, Alfred | Surgeon | Joliet, Ill | To Dec., 1864; also 1st Cav. |
| Young, Wm. H | " | Cor. Broadway and 43d st., N. Y. City. | From March, 1865. |
| Leach, Morgan L | Ass't S | Du Plain, Mich | To July, 1864. |
| Lathrop, C. C | " | | To June, 1865. |

### 10TH CAVALRY—Mustered out November 11, 1865.

| | | | |
|---|---|---|---|
| Leonard, C. W | Ass't S | Muskegon, Mich | To May. 1865. |
| Scott, Wm. D | " | Lamont, or Ithaca, Mich | From November, 1863. |
| Shaw, Thos | " | Hanover, Mich | From August, 1865. |
| Spaulding, D. C | Surgeon | Lyons, Mich | From Nov., 1863; also 6th Cav. |

### 11TH CAVALRY—Consolidated with 8th Cavalry July 20, 1865.

| | | | |
|---|---|---|---|
| Bissell, O. J | Ass't S | Grand Rapids, Mich | To December, 1863. |
| Osborn, Chas. A | " | Owasso Mich | To November, 1864. |
| Thompson, A. A | " | Flint, Mich | From Dec., 1863 to Aug., 1865; also 12th Inf. |
| Woodman, L. C | Surgeon | Paw Paw, Mich | From Oct. 1863 to Sept., 1865; also 3d Cav. |

### 1ST HEAVY ARTILLERY—(6th Infantry)—Mustered out August, 20, 1865.

| | | | |
|---|---|---|---|
| Chase, Milton | Ass't S | Otsego, Mich | To July, 1864. H. R. |
| French, Simeon ..S... | " | Battle Creek, Mich | To 20th Inf, July 1862. |
| Mason, John W | Surgeon | Dundee, Mich | From March, 1865 |
| Mottram, Chas V | " | Lawrence, Kans | To December, 1864. |
| Powers, David C | A. A. S | Coldwater, Mich | A. A. S. 1st Light Art in March and April, 1864. |

### 1ST ENGINEER INFANTRY—Mustered out September 22, 1865.

| | | | |
|---|---|---|---|
| De Camp. Wm. H | Surgeon | Grand Rapids, Mich | To November. 1864. |
| King, Robert H | Ass't S | Albion, Mich | From February. 1865 |
| O'Donoughue, W | Surgeon | Albion, Mich | To November, 1864. Re-commissioned January, 1865. H R. |
| Van Ostrand, H | Ass't S | Albion, Mich | From November. 1863. |
| Smith, Willard B | " | Ann Arbor, Mich | To May, 1863. |

### 1ST SHARPSHOOTERS—Mustered out July 28, 1865.

| | | | |
|---|---|---|---|
| Cornell, Geo. L | Ass't S | St. Clair. Mich | To December, 1863. |
| Eagleson, Thos | " | Parkersburgh, Ill | From August, 1864. |
| McNett. Jacob B | " | Grand Haven. Mich | To April, 1864. |
| Strong, Asahel B | " | Reading, Mich | To July, 1864. |
| Whelan, Arvin F | Surgeon | Hillsdale, Mich | From January, 1863; also 11th Inf. |

### 1ST INFANTRY—Mustered out July 9, 1865.

| | | | |
|---|---|---|---|
| Clapham, Edward | Ass't S | Kalamazoo, Mich | To 7th Inf., April, 1865. |
| Hobart, Andrew J | Surgeon | Clinton, Iowa | To September, 1864. |
| Fuller, William | " | Indianola, Iowa | From November, 1864. |
| Tunnicliffe, J. W | " | Jackson, Mich | To December, 1862; also 4th Inf. |
| Brodie, Wm | " | Detroit, Mich | Three months' service. |
| Smith, Cyrus | Ass't S | Jackson, Mich | Three months' service. |

## MICHIGAN—Continued.

### 2D INFANTRY—Mustered out July 28, 1865.

| Name | Rank | Residence | Service |
|---|---|---|---|
| Bonnine, Evan J | Surgeon | Niles, Mich | To September, 1864. |
| Clellan, Henry A | Ass't S. | Detroit, Mich | To April, 1864. |
| Lyster, Henry F | " | Detroit, Mich | To 5th Inf. July, 1862. |
| Palmer, Alonzo B | Surgeon | Ann Arbor, Mich | To September, 1861. |
| Robbins, Jerome | Ass't S. | Hubbardston Mich | From April 1865. |
| Vickery, R. S. | " | Fort D. A. Russell, Cheyenne, Wyo. Ter. | To March, 1865 In U. S. A. |
| Holton, Sam'l M | Surgeon | | From April, 1865. |

### 3D INFANTRY—Mustered out June 10, 1864; veterans and recruits transferred to 5th Infantry.

| Name | Rank | Residence | Service |
|---|---|---|---|
| Bliss, Zenos E | Surgeon | Grand Rapids. Mich | To U. S. V. Sept., 1862. Dead. |
| *Bliss, D. Willard* | " | Washington D. C | To U. S. V. Sept., 1861. |
| Grove, James | " | Grand Rapids, Mich | From Sept., 1862. |
| Morrison, W. B | Ass't S. | Grand Rapids, Mich | From June, 1862. |
| Wilson, Geo. B | " | | To June, 1862. |

### 3D INFANTRY—Mustered out May 25, 1866.

| Name | Rank | Residence | Service |
|---|---|---|---|
| Howard, L. A | | Hillsdale, Mich | Not in A. G. R. |
| Drake, Philo A | Ass't S | Hastings, Mich | To June, 1865. |
| Powers, H. H | Surgeon | Saranac, Mich | To May, 1865; also 27th Inf. |
| Slawson, C. M | " | Maple Grove, Mich | From October, 1865. |
| Winegar, Ira P | Ass't S | | To March, 1865. |

### 4TH INFANTRY—Mustered out from June 20 to July 18, 1864; veterans and recruits transferred to 1st Infantry.

| Name | Rank | Residence | Service |
|---|---|---|---|
| Clark, Wm. E | Surgeon | Centreville, Mich., or 411 W Monroe st., Chicago, Ill | To 19th Inf., Aug., 1862. |
| Chamberlin, D. P | " | Toledo Ohio | To March, 1863. |
| French, L. C | " | Hudson, Mich | To May, 1863 |
| Le Baron, Robert | Ass't S. | Pontiac, Mich | From May, 1863. |
| Tunnicliffe, J W | Surgeon | Jackson, Mich | To 1st Inf., Aug., 1861. |
| Watts, John S | Ass't S. | Dayton, Ohio | From August, 1862. |
| Doty, Edwin | H. Stew | Maple Rapids, Mich. | |

### 4TH INFANTRY—Company C mustered out February 26, the rest May 26, 1866.

| Name | Rank | Residence | Service |
|---|---|---|---|
| Griswold, Jos. B | Ass't S. | Grand Rapids, Mich | From December, 1864 U. S. Ex. S. |
| Hampton, C. D | " | Harbor Springs or Muir, Mich. | From October, 1864. |
| Spicer, Daniel A | Surgeon | King City, Mo | To Jan., 1866; also 10th Inf |
| Chamberlin, D. P | | Toledo, Ohio | Not in A. G. R. |

### 5TH INFANTRY—Mustered out July 5, 1865.

| Name | Rank | Residence | Service |
|---|---|---|---|
| Everett, Robert A | Ass't S. | Hillsdale Mich | To 16th Inf., May, 1863. |
| Lyster, Henry F | Surgeon | Detroit, Mich | To May, 1865; also 2d Inf |
| Rose, Preston B | Ass't S. | Ann Arbor, Mich | To March, 1865. |
| Adams, Jas. L | " | | Dismissed Jan., 1863. |
| Gunn, Moses | Surgeon | | To July, 1862. |

### 6TH INFANTRY—(See 1st Heavy Artillery.)

MICHIGAN—Continued.

7TH INFANTRY—Mustered out July 5, 1865.

| Name | Rank | Residence | Remarks |
|---|---|---|---|
| Barnum, Bolivar | Surgeon | Schoolcraft, Mich | To December, 1861; also 25th Inf. Dead. |
| Clapham, Edward | " | Kalamazoo, Mich | From April, 1865; also 1st Inf. |
| Dyer, Newell | Ass't S | Bath, Mich | From May, 1865. |
| Chaddock, Gilbert | Surgeon | Muskegon, Mich | To January, 1865. |
| Landon, Henry B | Ass't S | Bay City, Mich | To April, 1864. |
| Allen, Marvin A | " | | To July, 1863. |
| Bacon, Cyrus | " | Niles, Mich | To May, 1862. Dead. |

8TH INFANTRY—Mustered out July 30, 1865.

| Name | Rank | Residence | Remarks |
|---|---|---|---|
| Fox, Wells B | Surgeon | Bancroft, Mich | From July, 1863; also 22d Inf. H. R. |
| Shank, Hurlbut B | " | Lansing, Mich | To January, 1862. |
| Vanderveen, Aaron | Ass't S | Grand Haven, Mich | From June, 1863. |
| Wooster, Sam'l R | " | Grand Rapids, Mich | To 1st Cav. April, 1863. |
| Willett, John | " | Flint, Mich | To 30th Inf. December, 1864. Died June, 1881. |
| Wilson, James C | Surgeon | Flint, Mich | To March, 1863. |

9TH INFANTRY—Mustered out September 15, 1865.

| Name | Rank | Residence | Remarks |
|---|---|---|---|
| Barnes, Geo | Ass't S | Kalamazoo, Mich | From March, 1865. |
| King, Hawkins A | " | Quincy, Mich | To August, 1865. |
| Palmer, Wm H | " | Jackson, Mich | Dismissed January, 1864. |
| Smith, Cyrus | Surgeon | Jackson, Mich | To October, 1864. |
| Smith, Geo. G | " | Alliance, Ohio | From January, 1865. |

10TH INFANTRY—Mustered out July 19, 1865.

| Name | Rank | Residence | Remarks |
|---|---|---|---|
| Galbraith, F. B | Ass't S | Pontiac, Mich | To February, 1863. |
| Rouse, Jonathan S | Surgeon | South Seymour, Mich | From July, 1865; also 14th Inf. |
| Spicer, Daniel A | Ass't S | King City, Mo | To 4th Inf. Nov., 1864. |
| Vanderburg, D. W | " | Fall River, Mass | From May, 1863. |
| Wilson, John C | Surgeon | Flint, Mich | To March, 1862. |
| Sparling, Fred. W | " | | To May, 1865; also 14th Inf. |

11TH INFANTRY—Transferred to new 11th April, 1865.

| Name | Rank | Residence | Remarks |
|---|---|---|---|
| Elliott, Wm. N | Surgeon | White Pigeon, Mich | From September, 1861. |
| Packard, Nelson I | Ass't S | Sturgis, Mich | From October, 1862. |
| Vincent, Wesley | " | 181 W. Madison street, Chicago, Ill., or Lapeer, Mich | To April, 1863; also 102d U. S. C. T. |
| Whelan, Arvin T | " | Hillsdale, Mich | To October, 1862; also 1st Michigan Sharpshooters. |
| Griswold, Hiram S | " | Grand Blanc, Mich | From June, 1863. |

11TH INFANTRY—Mustered out September 16, 1865.

| Name | Rank | Residence | Remarks |
|---|---|---|---|
| Elliott, J. C | Ass't S | Buffalo, N. Y | Not in A. G. R. Dead. |
| Goodale, Henry A | Surgeon | East Tawas or Bay City, Mich. | From June, 1865; also 21st Inf. |
| Jones, Sam'l L | Ass't S | Petersburg or Wixom, Mich. | From May, 1865. |
| Nelson, Wm H. | Surgeon | Northport, Mich | From August, 1865. |
| Andrews, Luther A | Ass't S | | To July, 1863. |

## MICHIGAN—Continued.

### 12TH INFANTRY—Mustered out February 15, 1866.

| Name | Rank | Residence | Remarks |
|---|---|---|---|
| Coller, Eli H. | Surgeon | Athens, Mich. | From January, 1866. |
| Redzie, Robt. C. | " | Argyle College, Lansing, Mich. | To October, 1862. |
| Scott, Alex. H. | Ass't S. | St. Joseph, Mich. | From December, 1864. |
| Thompson, A. A. | " | Flint, Mich. | To Jan., 1863; also 11th Cav. |
| Bennschweiler, G. L. | Surgeon | | To April, 1862. |
| Marvin, Henry M. | Ass't S. | | To September, 1864. |
| Rundell, Jas. S. | Surgeon | | To October, 1865. |

### 13TH INFANTRY—Mustered out January 16 and July 25, 1865.

| Name | Rank | Residence | Remarks |
|---|---|---|---|
| Ewing, Alex. | Surgeon | Dexter, Mich. | Dead. (September, 1879.) |
| Howell, Chas. | Ass't S. | Dexter, Mich. | To June, 1865. |
| Pratt, Foster | " | Kalamazoo, Mich. | To Jan., 1865; recommissioned May, 1865. |
| Brestol, Smith H. | " | | To December, 1862. |
| Remmington, C. W. | " | | To January, 1664. |

### 14TH INFANTRY—Mustered out July 18, 1865.

| Name | Rank | Residence | Remarks |
|---|---|---|---|
| Batwell, Edward | Surgeon | Ypsilanti, Mich. | From December, 1861. |
| Rouse, Jonathan S. | Ass't S. | South Saginaw, Mich. | To 10th Inf. June, 1865. |
| Cole, Alvin J. | " | Fort Madison, Iowa | To March, 1865. |
| Sparling, Fred. W. | " | | To 10th Inf. May, 1862. |
| Wyker, Alfred | " | | To June, 1863. |

### 15TH INFANTRY—Mustered out August 13, 1865.

| Name | Rank | Residence | Remarks |
|---|---|---|---|
| Frazer, Wm. E. | Ass't S. | Washington, Iowa | To June, 1865. |
| Kibbee, Rufus | Surgeon | Port Huron, Mich. | To October, 1862. |
| Woodward, H. P. | Ass't S. | Wamego, Kan. | Dismissed May, 1862; also 18th Inf. |
| Hutchinson, John H. | Surgeon | | From February, 1864. |
| Murdock, Geo. W. | Ass't S. | | From June, 1865. |

### 16TH INFANTRY—(Stockton's Regiment)—Mustered out July 8, 1865.

| Name | Rank | Residence | Remarks |
|---|---|---|---|
| Breakey, Wm. F. | Ass't S. | Ann Arbor, Mich. | To April, 1864. |
| Everett, Robt. A. | Surgeon | Hillsdale, Mich. | To October, 1864; also 5th Inf. |
| Wixham, Isaac | " | Fentonville, Mich. | Dead. |
| Bacon, John H. | " | Lansing, Mich. | From January, 1865; also 4th Cav. |
| Butler, Wm. H. | Ass't S. | | To June, 1862. |
| Berry, Wm. L. | " | | From April, 1865. |
| Bowen, Geo. W. | " | | To May, 1863. |

### 17TH INFANTRY—Part mustered out June 3, 1865; the rest transferred to 2d Infantry.

| Name | Rank | Residence | Remarks |
|---|---|---|---|
| Cliff, Horatio T. | Ass't S. | Detroit, Mich. | From January, 1863. |
| Calkins, Abram R. | Surgeon | Allegan, Mich. | To October, 1862. |
| Crosby, Freeman R. | Ass't S. | Napoleon, Mich. | To April, 1864. |
| Cooper, Luke H. | " | Monroe, Mich. | To October, 1864. |
| Daniels, Albert H. | " | Galesburgh, Mich. | To October, 1862. |
| Bevier, Jonathan D. | Surgeon | Loda, Ill. | From October, 1862. |
| Heath, Delos L. | Ass't S. | | To 23d Inf. July, 1863. |

## MICHIGAN—Continued.

18TH INFANTRY—Part mustered out June 26, 1865; the rest transferred to 9th Infantry.

| | | | |
|---|---|---|---|
| Littlefield, John J | Ass't S | Auburn, Ind | From November, 1864. |
| Root, Simeon P | Surgeon | Somerset, Mich | To February, 1863. |
| Southworth, Chas T. | " | Monroe, Mich | To June, 1864 |
| Stevens, David S | " | Vassar or Caro, Mich | From July, 1864. |
| Woodward, H. P | Ass't S | Wamego, Kan | To May, 1863; also 15th Inf. |
| Baldwin, Garrett R. | " | | From May, 1863. |

19TH INFANTRY—Mustered out June 10, 1865; recruits transferred to 10th Infantry.

| | | | |
|---|---|---|---|
| Bennett, John | Surgeon | 332 Euclid ave., Cleveland, Ohio. | From August, 1863. |
| Clark, Wm. E | " | 411 W. Monroe st., Chicago, Ill., or Centreville, Mich. | To July, 1863; also 4th Inf. |
| Tompkins, L D | Ass't S | Cassopolis, Mich | To September, 1863. |
| Trowbridge, Geo. M. | " | Centreville, Mich | From October, 1863. |

20TH INFANTRY—Mustered out May 30, 1865.

| | | | |
|---|---|---|---|
| Baker, Henry B | Ass't S | Lansing, Mich | From August, 1864. |
| Chubb, Orville P | Surgeon | Omaha, Nebr. | From August, 1864. |
| French, Simon S | " | Battle Creek, Mich | To July, 1864; also 1st H. Art. |
| Rider, Ormail L | Ass't S | Burton, Ohio | To May, 1863. |

21ST INFANTRY—Part mustered out June 8, 1865; the rest transferred to 14th Infantry.

| | | | |
|---|---|---|---|
| Avery, John | Surgeon | Greenville, Mich | From March, 1863. Ex. S. |
| Goodale, Henry A | Ass't S | East Tawas or Bay City, Mich. | To 11th Inf., June, 1865. |
| Lee, Francis G | Surgeon | Portland, Mich | To January, 1863. |
| Thomas, Wm. B | " | Ionia, Mich | To December, 1862. U. S. Ex. S. |
| Blaker, Gilbert H. | Ass't S | Dead | To May, 1865; also 23d Inf. |
| Perry, Chas. R | " | | To February, 1863. |

22D INFANTRY—Mustered out June 26, 1865.

| | | | |
|---|---|---|---|
| Fox, Wells B | Ass't S | Bancroft, Mich | To 8th Inf. June, 1863. H. R. |
| McConnell, A. P | Surgeon | Ludington, Mich | From August, 1862. U. S. Ex. S. |
| Geismar, Henry | Ass't S | | To January, 1863; also 29th Inf. |
| Hammond, S. W | " | | From November, 1864. |
| Lawrence, Chas. W. | " | | To May, 1865. |

23D INFANTRY—Mustered out June 28, 1865.

| | | | |
|---|---|---|---|
| Bachelor, Jos. H | Ass't S | Hubbardston, Mich | From March, 1865, |
| Bogart, Gilbert E | " | Laporte City, Iowa | To April, 1864. |
| Cummings, R. W | " | San Francisco, Cal | To 1st U. S C. Art. March, 1864. Dead. |
| Fasquelle, Lewis W. | Surgeon | St. John's Mich | To November, 1862. |
| Hubbard, Theron T. | " | Deadwood, Dakota Ter | From May, 1865; also 30th Inf. |
| Leeder, Jas. R | Ass't S | South Saginaw, Mich | From June, 1864. |
| Heath, Delos L | Surgeon | | To December, 1864; also 17th Inf. |
| Blaker, Gilbert H | " | Dead | To December, 1862; also 21st Inf. |

## MICHIGAN—Continued.

### 24TH INFANTRY—Mustered out June 30, 1865.

| Name | Rank | Residence | Service |
|---|---|---|---|
| Beech, John H | Surgeon | Coldwater, Mich | Died October, 1878. |
| Collar, Alex | Ass't S | Wayne or Ishpemig, Mich. | To September, 1863. |
| Lauderdale, E | “ | Detroit, Mich. | From April, 1865. |
| Smith, Chas. C | “ | Belle Branch, Mich | To February, 1863. |
| Towar, Geo. W., Jr. | “ | Trenton, Mich | From April, 1863. |

### 25TH INFANTRY—Mustered out June 24, 1865.

| Name | Rank | Residence | Service |
|---|---|---|---|
| Barnum, Bolivar | Surgeon | Schoolcraft, Mich | From September, 1862; also 7th Inf. H. R. Dead. |
| Gregg, John M | Ass't S | Landon, (Oakville P. O.,) Mich. | To October, 1864. |
| Oakley, Francis M | “ | York, Mich | To February, 1864. |
| Miller, Philip D | “ | Schoolcraft, Mich | From March, 1865 |

### 26TH INFANTRY—Mustered out June 4, 1865.

| Name | Rank | Residence | Service |
|---|---|---|---|
| Marvin, Chas. W | Ass't S | Ithaca, Mich | From July, 1864. |
| Raymond, M. H | Surgeon | Grass Lake, Mich | From September, 1863. |
| Brooks, Odney D | Ass't S | | To April, 1864. |

### 27TH INFANTRY—Mustered out July 26, 1865.

| Name | Rank | Residence | Service |
|---|---|---|---|
| Davis, Jonathan E | Ass't S | Macomb, Mich | To January, 1864. |
| Niblack, Jas. W | “ | Cambria or Hillsdale, Mich. | From January, 1864. |
| Powers, H. H | “ | Saranac, Mich | To 3d Inf. Sept., 1864. |
| Stockwell, Cyrus M. | Surgeon | Port Huron, Mich | To Nov., 1863; U. S. Ex. S. |
| Smith, Hamilton E | “ | Detroit, Mich | From December, 1863. |
| Yarnold, Benj. E | Ass't S | | From September, 1864. |

### 28TH INFANTRY—Mustered out June 5, 1866.

| Name | Rank | Residence | Service |
|---|---|---|---|
| Cessna, Jos. P | Ass't S | Avilla, Indiana | To May, 1865. |
| Garwood, Alonzo | Surgeon | Cassopolis, Mich | From Aug., 1864; U. S. Ex. S |
| Green, Geo. W | Ass't S | Grand Crossing, Ill., or Three Rivers, Mich. | From October, 1864. |

### 29TH INFANTRY—Mustered out September 6, 1865.—(Many unsound men were mustered in this regiment.)

| Name | Rank | Residence | Service |
|---|---|---|---|
| Duncan, Titus | Surgeon | East Saginaw, Mich | To March, 1865. |
| Garrigues, Sam'l S | Ass't S | East Saginaw, Mich | To May, 1865. |
| Palmer, Elmore | Surgeon | Hubbardstown, Mich | From June, 1865. |
| Geismar, Henry | Ass't S | | From June, 1865; also 22d Inf. |

### 30TH INFANTRY—Mustered out June 17 to 30, 1865.

| Name | Rank | Residence | Service |
|---|---|---|---|
| Hubbard, Theron T. | Ass't S | Deadwood, Dak. T | To 23d Inf., May, 1865. |
| Willett, John | Surgeon | Flint, Mich | From Jan., 1865; also 8th Inf. Dead. |
| Ellison, Owen, Jr. | Ass't S | | From January, 1865. |

## MINNESOTA.

1ST CAVALRY (1-year Mounted Rangers)—Mustered out at different dates from October 20 to December 7, 1863.

Bingham, R. H. ......Ass't S.....Oshkosh, Wis................To 9th Inf. May, 1863; also 2d Inf.
Rhodes, Jas. C........ " Stillwater, Minn...........From Nov., 1862; also 1st H. Art.
Essler, Henry.........H. Stew...St. Peter, Minn.

2D CAVALRY—Companies B, C, D, E, F, G, I and M mustered out from November 17 to December 29, 1865; the rest April 2, 28, and May 4, 1866.

Farley, Chas. J.......Ass't S.....Fort Edwards, N. Y......From January, 1864.
McDonald, John A... " Chaska, Minn................To December, 1865
Daniels, Jared W .....Surgeon.........................................To November, 1865.
Vervais, Jos. A .......Ass't S...........................................Dismissed Nov., 1864; also 5th Inf.

BRACKETT'S BATTALION CAVALRY—Mustered out May 16, to June 1, 1866.

Johnson, C. O ........ Ass't S..........................................To November, 1864.
Le Dow, James....... " ..........................................To June, 1865.

HATCH'S INDEPENDENT BATTALION CAVALRY—Mustered out from April 26 to June 22, 1866.

Armington, J. L......Ass't S.....Cannon River Falls or Stillwater, Minn. To February, 1866; also 2d Inf.
Stees, Clinton G ...... " ..........................................To 1st H. Art. May, 1865.
Seigneuret, H. J...... " Henderson, Minn.. ...... From June, 1865, to June, 1866.

1ST HEAVY ARTILLERY—Mustered out September 27, 1865.

Mead, Milo M..........Surgeon...Oasis, Iowa...................From July, 1865 Alleged dead.
Rhodes, Jas. C.........Ass't S.....Stillwater, Minn ............To July, 1865; also 1st Cav.
Stone, J. Jerome......H. Stew...Wabasha, Minn.
Stees, Clinton G ......Surgeon..........................................To June, 1865; also Hatch's Cav.

1ST INFANTRY—Mustered out July 14, 1865.

Gabrielson, Peter....Ass't S....St. Paul, Minn..............To May, 1864; also 11th Inf.
Le Blond, John B.....Surgeon...Sioux Falls, Dak. Ter., or Brownsville, Minn. To May, 1864; recommissioned May 17, 1865.
*Stewart, Jacob H*..... " St. Paul, Minn..................To October, 1862 Ex. M. C.
Pugsley, E. G .. .....Ass't S..........................................To Aug., 1863; also 9th Inf.
Spear, Chas. H ....... " ..........................................From July, 1865.
Morton, Wm. H.......Surgeon...Dead..............................To June, 1863.
Le Boutillier, C. W ..Ass't S..........................................To October, 1862.

2D INFANTRY—Mustered out July 11, 1865.

Armington, Jno. L...Ass't S.....Cannon River Falls, Minn. To February, 1863; also Hatch's Cavalry.
Ayer, Otis............... " Le Sueur, Minn.............To Dec., 1863. U. S. Ex. S.
Bingham, R. H ........Surgeon...Oshkosh, Wis.............. To May 1862; also 1st Cav. and 9th Inf. Alleged dead.
Brown, Wm ........... " Chicago, Ill......................From March, 1865.
Bailey, Robert E......H. Stew...Rochester, Minn.
Tollman, M C.........Surgeon...Alleged Dead..................To December, 1864.

## MINNESOTA—Continued.

### 3D INFANTRY—Mustered out September 2, 1865.

| | | | |
|---|---|---|---|
| Bixby, Nahum | Ass't S. | Redwood Falls, Minn. | From June, 1864. |
| Gresley, Moses R. | " | South Weymouth, Mass. | A. W. M. |
| Milligan, F. H. | " | Wabasha, Minn. | To April, 1862. |
| Wedge, Albert C. | Surgeon | Albert Lea, Minn. | From November, 1863. |
| Butler, Levi | " | Dead. | |

### 4TH INFANTRY—Mustered out July 19, 1865.

| | | | |
|---|---|---|---|
| Cross, Elisha W. | Surgeon | Rochester, Minn. | To December, 1864. |
| Murphy, John H. | " | St. Paul, Minn. | To July, 1863; also 8th Inf. Board Exam. Surgeons. |
| Wedel, Henry R. | " | Winona, Minn. | To June, 1865. |
| Lambert, Geo. M. D. | Ass't S. | Cokato Lake, Minn. | From February, 1865. |

### 5TH INFANTRY—Mustered out September 6, 1865.

| | | | |
|---|---|---|---|
| Kennedy, V. P. | Surgeon | Litchfield, Minn. | To May, 1865. |
| Leonard, Wm. H. | " | Minneapolis, Minn. | From May, 1865. |
| Vervais, Jos. A. | Ass't S. | | To April, 1863; also 2d Cav. |
| Etheridge, F. B. | Surgeon | Alleged dead | To September, 1862. |

### 6TH INFANTRY—Mustered out August 19, 1865.

| | | | |
|---|---|---|---|
| Belden, Wallace P. | Surgeon | Spring Valley, Minn., or Canton, Iowa. | From September, 1864. |
| McMasters, Jas. M. | Ass't S. | Sauk Centre, Minn. | From May, 1864. U. S. Ex. S. |
| Wharton, Alfred | Surgeon | St. Paul, Minn. | To July, 1864. |
| Wilson, Henry | Ass't S. | St. Sophia, Kan., or Columbus, Neb. | From October, 1864. |
| Daniels, J. W. | " | | To Surgeon 2d Cav. April, 1864. |

### 7TH INFANTRY—Mustered out August 16, 1865.

| | | | |
|---|---|---|---|
| Ames, Albert A. | Surgeon | Minneapolis, Minn. | From August, 1865. |
| Mattock, E. B. | Ass't S. | St. Paul, Minn. | From July, 1863. |
| Burton, Percival | " | St. Paul, Minn. | From October, 1864. |
| Finch, Jeremiah E. | Surgeon | Hastings, Minn. | To May, 1863. |
| Folson, W. H. | H. Stew. | North Branch Station, Minn. | |

### 8TH INFANTRY—Mustered out July 10, 1865.

| | | | |
|---|---|---|---|
| Murphy, Jno. H. | Surgeon | St. Paul, Minn. | To March, 1865; also 4th Inf. Board Exam. Surgeons. |
| Rieger, Francis | " | 33 W. 3d street, St. Paul, Minn. | To April, 1864. |
| Rouse, Wm. H. | Ass't S. | Sioux City, Dak., or St. Anthony, Minn. | From September, 1862. |
| Thurston, Irvin H. | Surgeon | Garden City or Rapidan, Minn. | From June, 1865. |

### 9TH INFANTRY—Mustered out August 24, 1865.

| | | | |
|---|---|---|---|
| Bingham, R. H. | Surgeon | Oshkosh, Wis., or 1801 State st., Chicago, Ill. | From May, 1865; also 1st Cav. and 2d Inf. |
| Dewey, John | Ass't S. | St. Paul, Minn. | To September, 1863. |
| Twitchell, R. W. | " | Chatfield, Minn. | To 72d (old) and 119th U. S. C. T. July, 1864. U. S. Ex. S. |
| Pugsley, E. Y. | " | | From October, 1864; also 1st Inf. |
| Dixon, John C. | " | | To May, 1865. |

MINNESOTA—Continued.

10TH INFANTRY—Mustered out August 19, 1865.

Burnham, Alfred M..Ass't S.....Albert Lea, Minn...........Dismissed October, 1863.
Milligan, Francis H.. " Wabasha, Minn.............From September, 1864.
Sheardown, Sam'l B..Surgeon...Stockton, Minn................From October, 1862.
Brooks, Cyrus A......Ass't S.......................................From December, 1864.
Clark, Wm. W ........ " Alleged dead................To Sept., 1864.

11TH INFANTRY (1 year)—Mustered out June 26, 1865.

Gabrielson, Peter.....Ass't S....St. Paul, Minn..............From September, 1864; also 1st Inf.
McMahon, Henry.....Surgeon...Sauk Rapids, Minn.........From September, 1864.
Morris, R. L...........Ass't S.......................................From November, 1864.

## MISSISSIPPI.

1ST MOUNTED RIFLES—Mustered out June 26, 1865.

Bell, Samuel J.........Ass't S.......................................From April, 1864.

*1ST MISSISSIPPI MARINE BRIGADE—(Organized at St. Louis, Mo., from January 3 to April 4, 1863. The 1st Battalion Cavalry Mississippi Marine Brigade was consolidated with regiment August, 1864)—Mustered out from January 17 to February 1, 1865.

Robarts, James........Surgeon...Carbondale, Ill ..............A. W. M.
Meyers, Jas. S... .....Ass't S.....1516 N. 19th st., Philadelphia, Pa. A. W. M.
Cleaver, Israel......... " 137 S. 6th st , Reading, Pa. A. W. M.
Lawrence, J. W........ " Carbondale, Ill.
Booth, David S......... " Sparta, Ill.
Eldridge, C. R......... " Greenville, Ind.
McMahon, R. W...... " Quincy, Ill.
Jacobs, Theodore...... " Coal Valley, Ill.
Catley, Richard P.... " Dead...........................To January, 1864.
Malone, Alva J......... " Dead.

## MISSOURI.

1ST CAVALRY—(Five Companies of the 7th Cavalry were assigned to this regiment February, 1865)—Mustered out September, 1, 1865.

Bailey, Wm. W.........Surgeon...Fort Smith, Ark ............From March, 1865.
Foster, Wm. D.........Ass't S.....Hannibal, Mo.................To June, 1865: also 7th Cav. G.
Lynch, Jos. E.......... " ....................................To January, 1865.
McRae, Duncan.......Surgeon........................................To January, 1862.

1ST S. M. CAVALRY—Mustered out July 7, 11, and 12, 1865.

Carey, F. F.............H. Stew...Fremont Co , Iowa.
Trader, J. W...........Surgeon...Sedalia, Mo....................To April, 1865. Ex. S.
Osborn, Byron E...... " 54 State st., Auburn, N. Y. To October, 1863.
Hart, Jefferson G......Ass't S.....Unionville, Mo........ .....To April, 1865.

1ST BATTALION S. M. CAVALRY—Mustered out November 23 and December 2, 1862.

Bruere, John............Ass't S.........................................A. W. M.

*As reported by Surgeon-General U. S. A.

## MISSOURI—Continued.

### *2D CAVALRY—(Also Merrill's Horse)—Mustered out September 19. 1865.

Thomas, Abner D....Ass't S.....Harrison, Ark...............To Surg. 3d Ark. Cav., Dec., 1863.
Barrett, Wm. H....... " Harrisonville. Mo..........From August, 1865.
Thayer, S. B.............Surgeon...Battle Creek. Mich........To Oct., 1862; recommissioned Nov., 1862. Dead.
Knickerbocker, W.H..Ass't S.................................To April, 1863.
Douglass, Henry......Surgeon..................................To November, 1864.
Snyder, J. W. O......Ass't S....Pueblo, Col.................A. W. M.

### 2D S. M. CAVALRY—Mustered out February 28 to April, 1865.

Leffingwell, A. W....Ass't S.....Sullivan, Ill.....................To July, 1863; also 3d S. M. Cav. Dead.
Dickinson, E. C........Surgeon...1427 Grand ave., Kansas City, Mo.....................From May, 1862; also 11th S. M. Cav. Dead.
Kimmel Cyrus T......Ass't S.....Brunswick, Mo..............From June, 1862.
Lyon, Noah ............Surgeon...Hamilton, Ill...............To September, 1862.
Priest, Albert G......Ass't S.....Shelbyville, Mo............To June, 1862.
McDonnell, D. A...... " .......................................From September, 1863.

### 2D BATTALION S. M. CAVALRY—Mustered out March 31, 1863.

Cundiff, W. H. H.....Ass't S.....Pleasant Hill, Mo..........To 6th S. M. Cav. Sept., 1862; also 13th Cav. Ex. S.
Brown, John............ " St. Charles, Mo.............Not in A G. R.

### 3D CAVALRY—Mustered out June 14, 1865.

Smith, Jesse B.........H. Stew...Iberia, Mo.
Avery, La Fayette...Ass't S....La Grange, Mo ..............Dismissed Dec., 1864.
Granger, Wm. W...... " 1417 10 st., N.W., Washington, D. C. To March, 1864.
Taylor, John L.........Surgeon...Newark, Mo......................Dead.
Jones, Geo. C..........Ass't S......................................To September, 1862.

### 3D S. M CAVALRY—Disbanded February 4, 1863.

Bartlett, A. T..........Surgeon...Virden, Ill.......................A. W. M.
Leffingwell, A. W.....Ass't S.....Sullivan, Ill.....................A. W. M Also 2d S. M. Cav. Dead.

### 3D S. M. CAVALRY—(Was organized as 10th S. M. Cavalry)—Mustered out July 13. 1865.

Butman, Wm. C. P...Ass't S....Macon City, Mo.............To May, 1865.
Short, Wm L...........Surgeon.....................................To May, 1865.
Hollister, Jas..........Ass't S.......................................To June, 1864.
Jones, H. E............ " Louisiana, Mo..................To February, 1863.

### 4TH CAVALRY—Mustered out November 13, 1865.

Affolder, Jacob ........Ass't S....Westphalia, Kan............To Oct., 1864; also 5th Cav.
Nichols, H. W.........Surgeon...Canandaigua, N. Y........To July, 1863.
Wilcox, Wm. A........ " 802 Gamble st., St. Louis, Mo To June, 1864; also 1st S M. Inf.
Panabaker, John S...Ass't S.......................................To January, 1862.

---

* A. G. has hospital records.

## MISSOURI—Continued.

4TH S. M. CAVALRY—Mustered out at different dates from January 31 to April, 1865, and from July 5 to 8, 1865.

| Name | Rank | Residence | Service |
|---|---|---|---|
| Day, Wm. C | Surgeon | Peoria, Ill | To April, 1865; also 14th S. M. Cav. |
| Shoot, James H | " | Joslin, Mo | To April, 1865. |
| Whitney, D. V | " | | To June, 1863. |

5TH CAVALRY—Consolidated with the 4th Cavalry November, 1862.

| Name | Rank | Residence | Service |
|---|---|---|---|
| Affolder, Jacob | Ass't S. | Westphalia, Kan | A. W. M. Also 4th Cav. |
| Lingenfelder, P. T | Surgeon | 2601 N. 10th st., St. Louis, Mo. | A. W. M. |
| Reichenbach, H | " | | To January, 1862. |

5TH S. M. CAVALRY—Mustered out June 22, 1863.

| Name | Rank | Residence | Service |
|---|---|---|---|
| Warren, Joel H | Surgeon | Knobnoster, Mo | A. W. M. |
| Trasse, Henry | Ass't S. | | A. W. M. |

5TH S. M. CAVALRY—Mustered out July 8, 1865.

| Name | Rank | Residence | Service |
|---|---|---|---|
| Fetzer, John | Surgeon | Boonville, Mo. | To July, 1864. |
| Williams, John H | Ass't S. | Asheville, N. C | To April, 1865. |
| Feckete, Alex | " | | To April, 1865. |

6TH CAVALRY—Mustered out September 12, 1865.

| Name | Rank | Residence | Service |
|---|---|---|---|
| Gardner, N. M | Ass't S. | Ash Grove, Mo | To June, 1864. |
| Shurtleff, Benj. K | Surgeon | | From July, 1863 Dead. |
| Sperry, Harlow | Ass't S. | Olney, Mo | From October, 1864. |
| Tice, Douglas W | " | | To September, 1864. |
| Johnson, T. W | " | Bloomfield, Mo | To February, 1864. |
| Kiernan, J. L | Surgeon | | To May, 1863. |
| Bigelow, J. K | Ass't S. | | Dismissed Nov., 1862. |
| Decatur, Smith | A. A. S | Butler, Mo. | |

6TH S. M. CAVALRY—Mustered out July 18, 1865.

| Name | Rank | Residence | Service |
|---|---|---|---|
| Cundiff, W. H. H | Surgeon | Pleasant Hill, Mo | To 13th Cav. Sept., 1864; also 2d S. M. Cavalry. Ex S. |
| Weber, Casper A | Ass't S. | | From March, 1864. |
| Carter, Chas. L | " | Holden, Mo | To November, 1863. |
| Clanges, J. W. F | Surgeon | | To March, 1864. |
| Hughes, Benj. F | " | Georgetown, Mo | To Oct., 1862; also 7th S. M. Cavalry. |
| Bender, O. C | A. A. S | Heatville, Kan | From Aug. 26 to Sept. 26, 1862. |

7TH CAVALRY—Consolidated with the 1st Cavalry February 12, 1865.

| Name | Rank | Residence | Service |
|---|---|---|---|
| Bruner, J. F | Ass't S. | Sedalia, Mo | To February, 1863. |
| Foster, Wm. D | " | Hannibal, Mo | From July, 1863; also 1st Cav. G. |
| Murray, John | " | | To March, 1862. |
| Birch, Geo. B | Surgeon | Hannibal, Mo | To March, 1862. |

7TH S. M. CAVALRY—Mustered out by companies at different dates from March 20 to April 22, 1865, and July 11, 1865.

| Name | Rank | Residence | Service |
|---|---|---|---|
| Edwards, Jas. L | Ass't S. | Ennis, Texas | To April, 1865. Charges fee. |
| Montgomery, T. J | Surgeon | Sedalia, Mo | Died May, 1877. |
| Hughes, Benj. F | " | Georgetown, Mo | To 6th S. M. Cav. May, 1862. |
| Clapp, Fayette | Ass't S. | | To September, 1862 |
| Chastian, Mills T | " | Saline, Mo | To March, 1865. |

## MISSOURI—Continued.

### 8TH CAVALRY—Mustered out July 20, 1865.

| Name | Rank | Residence | Remarks |
|---|---|---|---|
| Robinson, E. T. | Surgeon | Springfield, Mo. | To February, 1863. |
| Van Eaton, F. H | " | Salma, Kan. | From February, 1865. |
| Soule, Isaac | Ass't S. | | From June 1863. |
| Clark, Elijah A | Surgeon | | To Surg. U. S. V. June, 1864; also 37th Ill. Inf. |
| Ebert, Edwin | Ass't S. | West Plains, Mo | Missing since Aug., 1862; also Phelps' Regt. |

### 8TH S. M. CAVALRY—Mustered out July 17, 1865.

| Name | Rank | Residence | Remarks |
|---|---|---|---|
| Brother, Ferdinand | Surgeon | Bunker Hill, Ill. | To January, 1865. |
| Evans, W. H. | Ass't S. | Sedalia Mo | To 13th Cav. Dec., 1864. |
| Suite, John S. | " | | To February, 1863. |
| Phelps, Fred'k R. | " | | To August, 1863. |

### 9TH S. M. CAVALRY—Mustered out July 13, 1865.

| Name | Rank | Residence | Remarks |
|---|---|---|---|
| Goodrich, C. F. | Ass't S. | New Haven, Mo. | To March, 1865. |
| Smith, Joseph D. | Surgeon | St. Joseph, Mo. | To November, 1864. |
| Castle, A. B. | Ass't S. | Lone Jack, or Pleasant Hill, Mo. | From June, 1862. |

### 10TH CAVALRY—(Six companies were organized as the 9th Cavalry)—Mustered out at different dates from August 5, 1864, to June 30, 1865; veterans and recruits were transferred to 2d Cavalry July 25, 1865.

| Name | Rank | Residence | Remarks |
|---|---|---|---|
| Feehan, Edward L. | Surgeon | 2129 Pine st., St. Louis, Mo. | Dismissed March, 1864; also 1st Light Artillery. |
| Raley, John N. | Ass't S. | Jameson, Mo | From Oct., 1864. U. S. Ex S. |
| Tolman, Wm L. | Surgeon | Farmington, Mo. | From September, 1864. |
| Law, David H. | Ass't S. | | To December, 1862. |

### 11TH CAVALRY—Mustered out July 27, 1865.

| Name | Rank | Residence | Remarks |
|---|---|---|---|
| Slade, John W. | Surgeon | New Hartford, Ill. | From September, 1863. |
| Lawrence, Thos. | Ass't S. | | To March, 1865. |
| Lawrence, Edward | " | Osceola, Iowa | From February, 1864. |

### 11TH S. M. CAVALRY—Consolidated with 2d S. M. Cavalry September, 1862.

| Name | Rank | Residence | Remarks |
|---|---|---|---|
| Dickinson, E. C. | Surgeon | 1427 Grand ave., Kansas City, Mo. | From May, 1862; also 2d and 14th S. M. Cav. Dead. |
| Still, E. C. | Ass't S. | Macon City, Mo. | A. W. M. Ex. S. |

### 12TH CAVALRY—Mustered out April, 1865.

| Name | Rank | Residence | Remarks |
|---|---|---|---|
| Corey, Geo. W. | Surgeon | Cheyenne, Wyoming Ter. | From February, 1864. |
| Jones, Wesley | Ass't S. | Assay Office, N. Y. City | To April, 1864. |
| Newman, G. W. | " | Albany, Mo. | To December, 1864. |
| Linn, Henry C. | " | St. Mary's, Kans. | From March, 1864. |
| Fordsham, Samuel | H. Stew. | Savannah, Mo. | |

### 12TH S. M. CAVALRY—Organization was broken up February 4, 1863, and companies A, B, and H transferred to 3d S. M. Cavalry, and companies C, D, E, F, and G to the 5th S. M. Cavalry.

| Name | Rank | Residence | Remarks |
|---|---|---|---|
| Douglass, Henry | Ass't S. | St. Louis, Mo. | A. W. M. Also 51st Inf. |
| Matthews, H. M. | Surgeon | | A. W. M. |

MISSOURI—Continued.

13TH CAVALRY—Mustered out at different dates from January 11 to July 3, 1866.

Crowley, J. W.........Surgeon...Salina, Kan.....................From December, 1865, to July, 1866.
Cundiff, W. H. H..... " Pleasant Hill, Mo..........To September, 1865; also 2d and 6th S. M. Cav.
Evans, Wm. H.........Ass't S....Sedalia, Mo....................To January, 1866; also 8th Cav.
Slaughter, P. M....... " Marionville, Mo.............To July, 1865.

14TH CAVALRY—Mustered out October 26 and November 17, 1865.

Rogers, Jas. S........ Ass't S........................................From May, 1865.

14TH S. M. CAVALRY—Disbanded March 3, 1863; and members transferred to the 4th and 8th S. M. Cavalry.

Day, W. C............. Ass't S.....Peoria, Ill.......................To 4th S. M. Cav.
Dickinson, E. C...... " 1427 Grand ave., Kansas City, Mo. To 11th S. M. Cav. May, 1862; also 2d S. M. Cav. Dead.
Watson, L. F..........Surgeon........................................From October, 1862; also 24th Inf.
Ashley, Andrew F.... " ........................................To September, 1862.

15TH CAVALRY—(20 months)—Formerly known as the 7th Missouri Militia—Mustered out July 1, 1865.

King, John........ .....Surgeon...Dead...............................From November, 1863.
Farmer, John W......Ass't S....Bolivar, Mo...................From September, 1864.

16TH CAVALRY—(20 months)—Formerly known as 6th Provisional Regiment. Mustered out July 1, 1865.

Pirtle, James T........Ass't S ...2608 Chateau ave., St. Louis, Mo. From February, 1865.
Young, Fenton, Jr....Surgeon...Sherman, Tex..............From August, 1864.

CASS COUNTY HOME GUARD—Mustered out February 28, 1862.

Holliday, Martin J...Surgeon........................................To December, 1861.
Warren, Jesse H......Ass't S....Knob Noster, Mo...........From June, 1861.

MAJOR BERRY'S BATTALION—Mustered out January 31 and February 1, 1862.

Ashley, A. F... ........Surgeon........................................A. W. M.

1ST LIGHT ARTILLERY—Mustered out at different dates from June 16 to August 23, 1865.

Feehan, Edw'd L....Ass't S.....2129 Pine st., St. Louis, Mo. To Surg. 10th Cavalry December, 1862
Hill, Wm.................Surgeon........................................To February, 1863.
Cornyn, Florence..... " ........................................To October, 1862.

2D ARTILLERY—(Formerly known as the 1st Missouri Artillery, U. S. Reserve Corps.) Mustered out at different dates from August 24 to December 20, 1865.

Seeman, Emil..........Surgeon...1821 Carondelet ave., St. Louis, Mo. To February, 1863.
Schulte, John J........Ass't S........................................Dismissed March, 1862.
Finlaw, Wm. C...... " ........................................To February, 1865
Pondrom, John B.....Surgeon........................................To September, 1864.

## MISSOURI—Continued.

BISSELL'S REGIMENT OF THE WEST, ENGINEERS—Consolidated February 17, 1864, with the 23d Missouri Infantry and designated as the 1st Missouri Engineers.

Book, John C..........Surgeon...Stewartsville, Mo..........From September, 1863. U. S. Ex. S.
Knower, Charles......Ass't S....St. Louis, Mo..............From October, 1861; also 1st Engineers. Dead.
Shelton, Chas. S......Surgeon...Jersey City, N. J..........To July, 1863. Dead.
Neal, Wm. A..........H. Stew...Elkhart, Ind..................H. R.

### 1ST BATTALION ENGINEERS.

Neal, Wm. A..........Ass't S.....Elkhart, Ind.................From April, 1864.
Book, John C.........Surgeon...Stewartsville, Mo..........From September, 1863; also Bissell's Engineers. U. S. Ex. S.
Knower, Charles......Ass't S....St. Louis, Mo...............To Oct., 1864; also Bissell's Engineers. Dead

1ST INFANTRY—(U. S. R. Corps)—Mustered out September 9 and October 6, 1862.

Ludwig, Charles..... Surgeon...1525 Choteau avenue, St. Louis, Mo. A. W. M.
Wyman, R. H......... " Keokuk, Iowa..............Also 21st Infantry. Died February 11, 1881.
Wolf, Joseph..........Ass't S..........................To March, 1862.
Theen, Gustav......... " ..........................To January, 1862.
Wilcox, Wm........... " ..........................From April, 1862.

1ST S. M. INFANTRY—Mustered out at different dates from December, 1864, to May, 1865.

Wilcox, Wm. A........Ass't S.....802 Gamble st., St. Louis, Mo. To Surg. 4th Cav October, 1863.
Hughes, C. H..........Surgeon...1218 St. Ange avenue, St. Louis, Mo. A. W. M.
Johnson, J. T.........Ass't S.....Leroy, Mo..................From January, 1864.
Jones, Henry W...... " ..........................To February, 1863.
Phelps, F. R.......... " ..........................To November, 1862.
McMartin, Thos. H...Surgeon..........................To June, 1862.
Lee, Allen M..........Ass't S..........................To June, 1863.

1ST INFANTRY (Northeast Regiment)—Consolidated with the 2d Northeast Infantry February 1, 1862, and designated the 21st Infantry.

Wyman, R. H .........Surgeon...Keokuk, Iowa ...............A. W. M. Dead.
Davis, Wm. H .........Ass't S..........................A. W. M.

2D INFANTRY (U. S. R. Corps)—Mustered out September 3, 1862.

Spinzig, Charles ......Surgeon...1302 South 5th st., St. Louis, Mo. From Sept., 1861; also 2d Inf. Dead, 1882.
Jahn, Ernst ...........Ass't S..........................From Sept., 1861; also 15th and 41st Inf.

2D INFANTRY—Mustered out at different dates from September 27 to October 1, 1864.

Bang, George..........Ass't S.....1314 North Market st., St. Louis, Mo. To September, 1862.
Spinzig, Charles ......Surgeon...1302 South 5th st., St. Louis, Mo. From Sept., 1862; also 2d U. S. R. Corps, Mo. Dead, 1882.
Stegman, Gustavus...A. A. S....St. Louis, Mo..............To Surg. 12th U. S. C. T. August, 1863.
Veeter, Richard.......Surgeon..........................To March, 1862.

MISSOURI—Continued.

**3D INFANTRY** (U. S. R. Corps)—Consolidated with Gasconade Battalion to form 4th Infantry January 18, 1862.

Boerner, Edmund.....Surgeon...Venedy, Ill....................A. W. M.
Steck, Francis ........Ass't S.........................................A. W. M.

**3D INFANTRY**—Mustered out at different dates from September 5 to November 22, 1864.

Haeussler, F...........Surgeon...St. Louis, Mo.................Three-months' service.
Stumberg, John H ...      "      St. Charles, Mo.............From June, 1864; also 29th Inf.
Spear, Geo. W.........H. Stew...135 Adams st., Toledo, Ohio.
Cooper, Howard A...Ass't S.........................................To Surg. 23d Inf. March, 1864.
Lyon, George G.......Surgeon.........................................To June, 1862.
Crow, A. T ........Ass't S.........................................To January, 1862.
Osborne, Henry.......Surgeon.........................................To March, 1864.
Reder, J. B.............      "      .........................................To February, 1862.
Krumsick, August....Ass't S.........................................Dismissed Jan., 1863.

**4TH INFANTRY** (U. S. R. Corps)—Mustered out January 13, 1862.

Roepke, Frederick ...Surgeon...1101 Madison st., St. Louis, Mo. From October, 1861.
Horn, Wm. E...........................................................To October, 1861.

**4TH INFANTRY**—Mustered out February 1, 1863.

Boerner, Edmund.... Surgeon...Venedy, Ill....................From January, 1862.
Feldmann, John......Ass't S.....Hermann, Mo...............From January, 1862.

**5TH INFANTRY**—Seven companies mustered out November 22, 1862, and the remaining companies transferred to the 27th and 35th Infantry Dec. 18, 1862.

Schoeneich, Henry...Ass't S.........................................A. W. M.; also 35th and 48th Inf.
Gemmer, Adalbert...Surgeon.........................................To September, 1862.

**6TH INFANTRY**—Mustered out August 17, 1865.

Joslyn, E. Milton.....Surgeon...Orange, Cal ..................To April, 1864.
Keller, Jacob..........      "      Steele's Mills, Ill.............From June, 1865
McChesney, W. F.....Ass't S.........................................To December, 1864.
Walker, Geo. S........Surgeon...2617 Washington ave., St. Louis, Mo To February, 1863.

**7TH INFANTRY**—Consolidated with the 11th Infantry December 14, 1864.

O'Reilly, P. S .........Ass't S.....703 N. 9th st., St. Louis, Mo. To November, 1864.
Powers, Edw'd M....Surgeon...523 Walnut st., St. Louis, Mo. To August, 1864.
Thayer, Benj. F ..... Ass't S.........................................To October, 1864.

**8TH INFANTRY**—Mustered out August 14, 1865.

Bailey, John R ........Surgeon...Mackinac, Mich.............To January, 1864. Ex. S.
Peterson, B. H.........      "      17 Prytana street New Orleans, La. To March, 1862.
Flint, Amos L .........Ass't S.....Nelson, Neb...................To August, 1864.
Brown, Troilus ........      "      St. Louis, Mo ................To July, 1861.
Nichols, H. W ........Surgeon...Canandaigua, N. Y........To August, 1861.

## MISSOURI—Continued.

### 9TH INFANTRY—(See 59th Illinois Infantry.)

### 10TH INFANTRY—Mustered out from August 24 to October 31, 1864.

| Name | Rank | Residence | Service |
|---|---|---|---|
| Payne, P. J | Surgeon | Keokuk, Iowa | From October, 1863. |
| Payne, Oliver B | " | Ferndale, Cal | To September, 1863. |
| Stewart, Absalom B | Ass't S | Santa Rosa, Cal | To 1st Ala. Cav. April, 1863. |
| Meredith, Hugh H | " | | To July, 1863; also 22d Inf. |
| Morgan, Thos. L | " | | Dismissed March, 1864. |

### 11TH INFANTRY—Mustered out January 15, 1866.

| Name | Rank | Residence | Service |
|---|---|---|---|
| Fish, M. W | Surgeon | 461 E. 14th st., Oakland, Cal | To May, 1865. |
| French, Z D | H. Stew | Sumner, Ill | Also 3d U. S. C. Cav. |
| Hawley, Thos. S | Surgeon | 3071 Easton avenue, St. Louis, Mo. | From June, 1865; also 111th Ill. Inf. |
| Hoffman, Ernest H | Ass't S | 909 N. Jefferson ave., St. Louis, Mo. | To June, 1863; also 24th U. S. C. T. |
| Smith, Thos | Surgeon | Fayette, Mo | To April, 1862. |

### 12TH INFANTRY—Mustered out at different dates from August 12 to November 14, 1864.

| Name | Rank | Residence | Service |
|---|---|---|---|
| Spiegelhalter, Jos | Surgeon | 1400 Chouteau ave., St. Louis, Mo. | From November, 1863. |
| Hohly, Frederick | Ass't S | Toledo, Ohio | To Surgeon 37th Ohio Inf. May, 1864. |
| Cook, Chas | Surgeon | | To September, 1862. |
| Fritz, Wm | Ass't S | | To March, 1862. |
| Junghanus, Louis H | Surgeon | | Dismissed Sept., 1863. |

### 13TH INFANTRY—(See 22d Ohio Infantry.)

### 14TH INFANTRY—Was in service but a few months.

### 15TH INFANTRY—Mustered out December 25, 1865.

| Name | Rank | Residence | Service |
|---|---|---|---|
| Chaffee, John B | Ass't S | 527 State st., Chicago, Ill. | A. W. M. |
| Rooch, August | Surgeon | 1305 Bremen street, St. Louis Mo. | To November, 1864. |
| Rutz, Gallus | Ass't S | Highland, Ill | Dismissed October, 1862. |
| Atkinson, E. L | Surgeon | | From Sept., 1865; also 23d Inf |
| Jahn, Ernst | " | | To October, 1863; also 2d U. S. R. C and 41st Inf. |
| Steiger, Wm | " | | To September, 1862. |

### 16TH INFANTRY—Did not complete organization.

### 17TH INFANTRY—Mustered out at different dates from September 15 to December 15, 1864.

| Name | Rank | Residence | Service |
|---|---|---|---|
| Bruckner, Chas | Ass't S | 493 Elm street, Cincinnati, Ohio. | From July, 1863. |
| McConoughby, J. B | Surgeon | 2334 Menard street, St. Louis, Mo. | A. W. M.; also Benton Cadets. |
| Adams, Andrew | Ass't S | | Dismissed May, 1863. |
| Hubrich, Hermann | Surgeon | | To March, 1862. |
| Rosch, Adolph | " | | To December, 1861. |

## MISSOURI—Continued.

### 18TH INFANTRY—Mustered out July 18, 1865.

Denslow, Oliver C...H. Stew...Milan, Mo....................To May, 1862.
Houts, S. B...............Surgeon...2624 or 810 Olive st., St. Louis, Mo. To November, 1864.
Torrey, Wm. O........Ass't S.....Hannibal, Mo.................To March, 1862.
Randolph, Frank F...Surgeon........................................From June, 1863.
Hamlin, Norman S.................. Yuba City, Cal................To September, 1862.

### 19TH and 20TH INFANTRY—Failed to complete.

### 21ST INFANTRY—(Formed by the consolidation of the 1st and 2d Northeast Infantry February 1, 1862)—Mustered out April 19, 1866.

Roberts, Abel C.......Surgeon...Fort Madison, Iowa........From July, 1863.
Stanley F. G..............Ass't S.....Buffalo, N. Y .............. To January, 1865.
Wyman, R. H.........Surgeon...Keokuk, Iowa...... ........Also 1st Inf. Died Feb., 1881.
Seaton, Jos. H......... " San Luis Obispo, Cal......To June, 1863.
Sisson, Harvey.........H. Stew...La Belle, Mo.
Crandall, Orson H...Ass't S........................................From April, 1863; also 24th Inf
Knickerbocker,W.H.. " ....................................From May, 1863.

### 22D INFANTRY—The members of this regiment were transferred to the 7th Cavalry and 10th and 24th Infantry February 20, 1862, and July 22, 1862.

Gates, Wm. M.........Surgeon...Carthage, Mo........ ........To March, 1862.
Meredith, Hugh H...Ass't S..........................................A. W. M.; also 10th Inf.

### 23D INFANTRY—Mustered out July 18, 1865.

Bluthardt, Theo. J...Surgeon...43 S. Poria st., Chicago, Ill. To January, 1864; also 1st Ill. Cav.
Cooper, Howard A...Ass't S.........................................To September, 1864; also 3d Inf.
Atkinson, E. L......... " ....................................From Feb., 1863; also 15th Inf.
Ellegood, Wm. T..... " ....................................To March, 1863.
Ralph, John B.........Surgeon.........................................To March, 1862.
Rolls, Jas. F............Ass't S..........................................To September, 1864.

### 24TH INFANTRY—Mustered out at different dates from October, 1864, to February 1, 1865, and recruits transferred to 21st Infantry.

Hocker, N. B...........Surgeon...Mt. Vernon, Mo.............Missing since Oct., 1862. U. S. Ex. S.
Little, John............ Ass't S.....Bloomington, Ill............From January, 1863; also 110th U. S. C. T.
Robberson, E. T......Surgeon...North Springfield, Mo....To January, 1862.
Baker, L. H............ " Payson, Ill.........................From April, 1862.
Crandall, Orson H...Ass't S.........................................From April, 1863; also 21st Inf.
Watson, L. T.......... " ....................................To Surgeon 14th Cav. (S. M.) October, 1862.

### 25TH INFANTRY—Organized as the 13th Infantry and changed to the 25th, afterwards consolidated with the 1st Infantry Engineers February 17, 1864.

Berghoff, John T.....Surgeon...St. Joseph, Mo.................A. W. M. U. S. Ex. S.
Egleston, John Q.....Ass't S...........................................From September, 1862: also 43d Inf.
Brey, Julius... ........ " ....................................To July, 1863.

MISSOURI—Continued.

26TH INFANTRY—Mustered out at different dates from November 4, 1864, to January 9, 1865, and August 13, 1865.

Barnett, Chas. F......Ass't S.....Bunker Hill, Mo.............To January, 1865.
Prout, J. S.............Surgeon.........................................To January, 1865.
Bryan, J. L.............Ass't S..........................................To July, 1863.

27TH INFANTRY—A portion of this regiment was mustered out September 17, November 3, 1864, and January 10, 1865, the balance was consolidated with the 31st and 32d Infantry June 13, 1865.

Bond, Benj. N.........Surgeon...Stanberry, Mo............... From August, 1862.
Bowman, John.........Ass't S..........................................From March, 1863.
Casey, E. A ............ " ..................................To January, 1863.
Murphy, J. S........... " ..................................To January, 1863.

27TH MOUNTED INFANTRY—(A portion of this regiment was three months' troops)—Mustered out at different dates from January 27 to February 28, 1862.

Clark, Logan...........Surgeon.........................................From September, 1861.
Hill, James H...........Ass't S..........................................To October, 1861.
Isaminger, A. E...... " ..................................From Sept., 1861.

28TH INFANTRY—Failed to complete.

29TH INFANTRY—A portion of this regiment was mustered out June 1865, the balance transferred to the 32d Infantry.

Stumberg, John H ...Ass't S....St. Charles, Mo..............To Surg. 3d Inf. June. 1864.
Morgan, John C.......Surgeon...1706 Green st., Phila., Pa. From August, 1862.
Carr, Cornelius B.....Ass't S..........................................From June, 1864.

30TH INFANTRY—Mustered out August 21, 1865.

Hill, James H...........Ass't S....Franklin, Ill .....................To September, 1863.
Sloan, Robert J........ " ..................................To 58th U. S. C. T. Aug., 1863.
Sargent, B. W .........Surgeon...Rochester, N. H.............To 6th U. S. C. T., H. Art'y. Nov., 1863.

31ST INFANTRY—Consolidated with the 32d Infantry November 12, 1864.

Ruge, Julius A.........Ass't S.....Washington, Mo.............To August, 1863.
*Reese, Alex. W......Surgeon...Warrensburgh, Mo.........From May to Nov., 1864.
Ellston, Addison......Ass't S.....Ellston, Mo........................From July, 1864; also 32d Inf.
Strother, C. G..........Surgeon.........................................To February, 1864.

32D INFANTRY—Mustered out July 18, 1865.

Newell, Horace........Ass't S.....Campbell Hill, Ill..........To Nov., 1864, also 42d Inf.
Watson, T. J............Surgeon...Freedom, Mo ..................A. W. M.
Hyde, Wm. A..........Ass't S..........................................To June, 1863.
Ellston, Addison...... " Ellston, Mo.......................To Apr., 1865; also 31st Inf.

33D INFANTRY—Mustered out August 10, 1865.

Smith, Thos ............Surgeon...Dayton, Ohio...................To March, 1863.
Bartlett, A. T.......... " Virden, Ill..........................A. W. M. H. R.
Sawyer, A. R..........Ass't S..........................................To December, 1862.
Kile, Milton ............ " ..................................Deserted October, 1864.

* Was also Post Surg. at Warrensburgh, Mo., from Nov. 22, 1864, to April 1, 1865.

## MISSOURI—Continued.

### 34TH INFANTRY—Failed to complete.

### 35TH INFANTRY—Mustered out June 28, 1865.

Lamb, J. B.............Surgeon...Parsons, Kan....................From August, 1862.
Schoenich, Henry.....Ass't S.........................................To 44th Inf. March, 1865; also 5th Inf.
Rooney, P. C. H......    "    ..........................................To July, 1863.

### 36TH, 37TH, AND 38TH INFANTRY—Failed to complete.

### 39TH MOUNTED INFANTRY—Mustered out March, 1865, and July 19, 1865.

Holman, John B......Surgeon...Boonville, Mo....................To April, 1865.

### 40TH INFANTRY—(1 year)—Mustered out August 8, 1865.

Judd, Homer............Surgeon..............................................From September, 1864.
Sneed, John F.........Ass't S................................................From September, 1864.
Rattinger, Rainer.....    "    1410 S. 7th st., St. Louis, Mo. From October, 1864.

### 41ST INFANTRY—(1 year)—Part mustered out July 11, 1865, the rest transferred to 51st Infantry.

Wieland, Gustavus...Ass't S.....Dutzow, Mo.......................From October, 1864.
Jahn, Ernst.............Surgeon..............................................From Sept., 1864; also 2d U. S. R. C., and 15th Inf.
Klueber, Hugo.........Ass't S................................................From October, 1864.

### 42D INFANTRY—(1 year)—Mustered out March 22 and June 28, 1865.

Gray, Abraham L....Ass't S.....Unionville, Mo...................From August, 1864.
Newell, Horace........Surgeon...Campbell Hill, Ill..........From Nov., 1864; also 32d Inf.
Smiley, Geo. P.........Ass't S................................................To March, 1865.

### 43D INFANTRY (1 year)—Part mustered out June 30, 1865; the rest transferred to 50th Infantry.

Dill, Edward W.......Ass't S.....Westport, Mo.....................From Nov., 1864. Dead.
Egleston, John Q.....Surgeon..............................................From Nov., 1864; also 25th Infantry.
Drace, W. F.............Ass't S................................................From October, 1864.

### 44TH INFANTRY—(1 year)—Mustered out March 22 and August 15, 1865.

Carez, F. F...............H. Stew...Bartlett, Iowa.
Wilson, L. A............Ass't S.....Newberg, Ark., or Rolla, Mo. From September, 1864.
Schoenich, Henry.....Surgeon..............................................A. W. M.; also 5th and 35th Infantry.
Schatz, Isaac...........Ass't S................................................To July, 1865.

### 45TH INFANTRY—(6 months and 1 year)—Part mustered out March 6, 1865; the rest transferred to 48th and 50th Infantry April 17, 1865.

Riddler, John G.......Surgeon...Jefferson City, Mo.........To March, 1865.
Rogers, Jas. G.........Ass't S.....Knobnoster, Mo.............From August, 1864.

### 46TH AND 47TH INFANTRY were 6 months' organizations.

MISSOURI—Continued.

48TH INFANTRY—(6 months and 1 year)—Part mustered out March 21, 23, and June, 29, 1865; the rest transferred to 50th Infantry.

Jackson, John W.....Surgeon...Washington, Mo.............From September, 1864.
Gibson, Wm. A........Ass't S.........................................From August, 1864.
Hooper, Wm............ " Otterville, Mo ...............From January, 1865.

49TH INFANTRY—(1 year)—Mustered out August 2 and December 20, 1865.

Rubey, Thos. S........Ass't S.....Macon, Mo ....................To August, 1865.
Monig, Oscar..........Surgeon...Americus, Mo...............To August, 1865.

50TH INFANTRY—(6 months and 1 year)—Mustered out from July 1 to August 11, 1865.

Bainbridge, P. A.......Ass't S.....Morley, Mo.................. From October, 1864.

51ST INFANTRY—(One year)—(The 52d, 54th, and 55th Infantry failed to complete, and were consolidated with this regiment May 1, 1865)—Mustered out August 31, 1865.

Matthews, H. M........Surgeon...St. Louis, Mo.................From May, 1865; also 12th S. M. Cav.
Spicer, C. W............Ass't S.....Fillmore, Mo ................From April, 1865.
Marcoot, John ........ " ...........................................From February, 1865.

MAJOR KREKEL'S BATTALION—(U. S. R. C.)—Mustered out January 10, 1862.

Bruere, John ...........Ass't S.....St. Charles, Mo..............From August, 1861.

BENTON CADETS—Mustered out January 8, 1862.

McConaughy, J. B...Ass't S.....2334 Menard street, St. Louis, Mo. Also 17th Infantry.
Cowan, Wm. V........Surgeon.

COLONEL PHELPS' MISSOURI INFANTRY—(Six months' service.)

Ebert, Edwin..........Ass't S.....West Plains, Mo............From Dec., 1861; also 8th Cav.
East, Alvish H.........Surgeon.........................................From October, 1861.

NEBRASKA.

1ST CAVALRY—(Veterans)—Organized as the 1st Infantry—Mustered out July 1, 1866.

Larsh, N. B..............Ass't S.....Nebraska City, Nebr......To November, 1864.
McClelland, Wm...... " Omaha, Nebr..................From October, 1862.
Wilkinson, G. W...... " Dakota City, Nebr.........To July, 1865.
Low, Enos ...............Surgeon...Omaha, Nebr.................To 5th Iowa Cav. Jan., 1862.

2D CAVALRY—(9 months)—Mustered out at different dates from September 4 to December 23, 1863.

Bowen, A ................Surgeon...Nebraska City, Nebr......From Dec., 1862; also Lt. Co. C. U. S. Ex. S.
Hanna, H. O............Ass't S.....Falls City, Nebr.............From April to Dec., 1863.
Latta, Wm. P.......... " Lincoln, Nebr................From Nov., 1862, to Dec., 1863.

## NEVADA.

1st Cavalry—Mustered out November 18, 1865, and July 12 and 21, 1866.

| | | | |
|---|---|---|---|
| Steel, Walcott | Ass't S. | Winnemuca, Nev | To October, 1863. |

## NEW HAMPSHIRE.

1st Cavalry—Mustered out July 15, 1865.

| | | | |
|---|---|---|---|
| Pierce, Geo. W | Surgeon | Winchester, N. H. | From March, 1865. H. R. |
| Eldredge, F. A | Ass't S. | Toledo, Ohio | From November, 1864. |

1st Heavy Artillery—Mustered out September 11, 1865.

| | | | |
|---|---|---|---|
| Morrill, Ezekiel | Surgeon | Concord, N. H | To June, 1865; also 13th Inf. |
| Bixby, Amos S | Ass't S. | Ludlow, Vt | To June, 1865. H. R. |
| Nims, Sam | H. Stew. | Keene, N. H. | |
| Price, Reuben W | Ass't S. | | To June, 1865. |

1st Infantry—(Three months.)

2d Infantry—Mustered out June 21, 1864.

| | | | |
|---|---|---|---|
| Worthly, Oscar | Ass't S. | Littleton, N. H | To September, 1862. |
| Kempton, Willard C. | " | Grantham, N. H | From August, 1865 |
| Bunton, Sylvanus | " | Mt. Vernon, N. H | To June, 1864. H. R. Also 7th Inf. |
| Woodward, Dan'l B. | H. Stew. | Ellenburgh, N. Y. | |
| Stone, Wm. P. | Surgeon | Dead. | |
| Hubbard, Geo. N | " | Dead | To September, 1861. |
| Merrow, Jas. M | " | Dead. | |
| Stark, Wm. G | Ass't S. | | Was Hosp. Stew. prior to July, 1864. Died Nov., 1880. |
| Moore, Jno. C. W. | Nurse | Concord, N. H | In 1863. Also Ass't S. 11th Inf. |

3d Infantry—Mustered out July 25, 1865.

| | | | |
|---|---|---|---|
| Kimball, F. B. | Surgeon | Andover, Mass | From May, 1865. |
| Eaton, Benj. F | Ass't S. | Hartford or Windsor, Vt. | To October, 1862. |
| Moulton, Albert A | Surgeon | Tilton, N. H | To November, 1862. |
| Burnham, Chas. A | Ass't S. | 327 Tremont st., Boston, Mass | From May, 1865. |
| Manter, Geo. W. | " | Manchester, N. H. | A. W. M. |
| Scovell, Albert D. | H. Stew. | Manchester, N. H. | 1863 and 1864. |
| Kittridge, Perry | Nurse | Merrimack, N. H | For awhile in 1863. |
| Farrar, Daniel | Ass't S. | | To May, 1863. |

4th Infantry—Mustered out August 23, 1865.

| | | | |
|---|---|---|---|
| Eastman, Josiah C. | Surgeon | Hampstead, N. H. | To October, 1862. |
| Walker, Jas. P. | Ass't S. | Manchester, N. H. | To November, 1864. |
| Greeley, Geo. P. | Surgeon | Nashua, N. H | To October, 1864. |
| *Dearborn, David P. | " | Brattleborough, Vt. | From December, 1864. |
| Wardwell, Henry F. | Ass't S. | Gorham, N. H | From May, 1865. |
| Beckley, Chas. C. | " | Plainfield, N. H. | To March, 1864. |

* Was private in Co. G from September 18, 1861, to March 22, 1862, and 2d Lieut. of same company from March 22 to November 4, 1862, and Assistant Surgeon from December 16, 1862.

## NEW HAMPSHIRE—Continued.

### 5TH INFANTRY—Mustered out June 28, 1865.

| Name | Rank | Residence | Remarks |
|---|---|---|---|
| Knight, Luther M. | Surgeon | Franklin, N. H | To May, 1863. U. S. Ex. S |
| Child, Wm | " | Bath, N. H | From Nov., 1862. U. S. Ex. S. |
| Trask, Chas. M | Ass't S. | No. 21 Pleasant st., Boston, Mass. | To October, 1864. |
| Robinson, Don A. | " | | From April, 1865. |
| Buckman, John H. | Surgeon | Dead. | |

### 6TH INFANTRY—Mustered out July 27, 1865.

| Name | Rank | Residence | Remarks |
|---|---|---|---|
| Cooper, Sherman | Surgeon | Westfield, N. J | To November, 1864. |
| Brown, Marshall L. | Ass't S. | Natick, Mass | From June, 1865. |
| Noyes, Jas. H | Surgeon | | From January, 1865. |
| Pierce, Elihu P. | Ass't S | | From March, 1864. |
| Tracey, Wm. A. | Surgeon | Dead | To March, 1863. |

### 7TH INFANTRY—Mustered out July 17, 1865.

| Name | Rank | Residence | Remarks |
|---|---|---|---|
| Smart, Wm. H | Ass't S. | Claremont, N. H. | To November, 1862. |
| Boynton, Henry | " | Woodstock, N. H | To January 1864. |
| Bunton, Sylvanus | Surgeon | Mt. Vernon, N. H. | From Sept., 1864. H. R. Also 2d Inf. |
| Perry, Geo. T. | Ass't S. | | From September, 1864. |
| Wilson, Moses S. | " | | To June, 1864. |
| Brown, Wm. W. | Surgeon | Dead. | |

### 8TH INFANTRY—In service August 31, 1865.

| Name | Rank | Residence | Remarks |
|---|---|---|---|
| Dearborn, Sam'l G. | Surgeon | Nashua, N H | To August, 1862. |
| Clark, Ellery C. | " | Norwalk, Conn | To August, 1864. |
| Stowell, David P. | Ass't S. | Waterville, Me | To June, 1864. |
| Chapman, Henry N. | H. Stew. | Washington, N. H | From Jan., 1864. H. R. |
| Thompson, A. J. | Surgeon | Dead. | |
| Smith, Hosea H. | Ass't S. | | To 1st La. Cav. Aug., 1863. |

### 9TH INFANTRY—Mustered out June 10, 1865; recruits transferred to 6th Infantry.

| Name | Rank | Residence | Remarks |
|---|---|---|---|
| Gibson, Francis N. | Surgeon | New Ipswich, N. H. | From Jan., 1865. H. R. for 1864. U. S. Ex. S. |
| Webster, Wm. A. | " | Manchester, N. H. | To Jan., 1865. U. S. Ex. S. |
| Emerson, John S | Ass't S. | 4 Washington Square, Lynn, Mass. | To 18th Inf April, 1865. |
| Shephard, A. W. | H. Stew. | Brookline, N. H | Also Ass't Surg. 18th Inf. |

### 10TH INFANTRY—Mustered out June 21, 1865; recruits transferred to 2d Infantry.

| Name | Rank | Residence | Remarks |
|---|---|---|---|
| Small, Horatio N. | Surgeon | Portland, Me. | From August, 1863; also 13th Inf. |
| Ferguson, John | " | Manchester, N. H. | To August, 1863. |
| Clement, Thos. R. | Ass't S. | Barnstable, Mass. | To September, 1864. |
| Wilkins, Wm. W. | " | Manchester, N. H. | To July, 1864. U. S. Ex. S. |
| Haynes, Jno | " | N. Londonderry, N. H. | To June, 1863. |
| Plummer, Albert. | " | | From January, 1865. |

### 11TH INFANTRY—Mustered out June 4, 1865; recruits transferred to 6th Infantry.

| Name | Rank | Residence | Remarks |
|---|---|---|---|
| Hayes, John A. | Surgeon | Great Falls, N. H. | From January, 1865. U. S. Ex. S. |
| Jones, Chas M. | Ass't S. | Great Falls, N. H. | From January, 1865. |
| Moore, Jno. C. W. | " | Concord, N. H | To October, 1864. |
| Ross, J. S. | Surgeon | Dead. | |
| Hutchins, E. R. | Ass't S. | | To December, 1862. |

## NEW HAMPSHIRE—Continued.

12TH INFANTRY—Mustered out June 21, 1865; recruits transferred to 2d Infantry.

Fowler, Hadley B....Surgeon...Bristol, N. H..................From August, 1862.
Carbee, Samuel P.....Ass't S.....Haverhill, N. H.............From November, 1863. U. S. Ex. S.
Higgins, Josiah B.....Chapl'n ...Alton, N. H....................Says he was H. Stew. and Assistant Surgeon.
Sanborn, John H..... Ass't S.....Franklin, N. H..............To July, 1864.

13TH INFANTRY—Original members mustered out June 21, 1865; the rest transferred to 2d Infantry.

Richardson. Sam A...Surgeon...Marlborough, N. H........From April, 1863.
Twitchell, Geo. B..... " Keene, N. H.....................To March, 1863.
Small, Horatio N......Ass't S.....Portland, Me..................To August, 1863; also 10th Inf.
Sullivan, John......... " No. 63 Tremont st., Boston. To August, 1864.
Morrill, Ezekiel....... " Concord, N. H...............To November, 1864; also 1st Heavy Artillery.
Emery, Jno. C......... " ..................................From April, 1865.

14TH INFANTRY—Mustered out July 8, 1865.

Thayer, Wm. H........Surgeon...171 Livingston st. Brooklyn, N. Y. From September, 1862.
Perkins, Marshall.....Ass't S.. .Marlow, N. H.................From September, 1862.

15TH INFANTRY—Mustered out August 13, 1865.

Hall, Jeremiah F......Surgeon...Portsmouth, N. H..........To January, 1863.
Kempton, Willard....H. Stew...Grantham, N. H.............Also Ass't S. 2d Inf.
Horsch, Carl H..........Surgeon...Dover, N. H....................From February, 1863.
Janvrin, Jos. E.......Ass't S.....5th Avenue Hotel, N. Y. City. From December, 1862.
Towle, Benj. N....... " ....................................From October, 1862.

16TH INFANTRY—Mustered out August 20, 1865.

Fisk, Cyrus M..... ....Ass't S.....Lowell, Mass.................From November, 1862. H. R.
*Sleeper, Hubert...... " Plainfield, N. H...... ......From March, 1863.
Adams, Paul S.........H. Stew...Newport, N. H.
Whittier, True P...... " Franklin, N. H.
Sanborn, Thos........ Surgeon...Dead...................................To June, 1863.

17TH INFANTRY—Two companies were organized and transferred to the 2d Infantry.

18TH INFANTRY—Mustered out July 29, 1865.

Emerson, John S......Surgeon...4 Washington Square, Lynn, Mass. From April, 1865. H. R. Also 9th Inf.
Shephard, Warner....Ass't S.....Brookline, N. H...........From December, 1864; also H. Stew. 9th Inf.

CAPTAIN JOEL H. TARBELL'S COMPANY MILITIA ARTILLERY—In service from August 1, 1864, to September 23, 1864.

Tarbell, Capt. J. H..................Lyndeborough, N. H.
Goodrich, John H....................N. Lyndeborough, N. H..Has full information.

---

* Was a prisoner of war at date of muster out of regiment.

## NEW JERSEY.

1st Cavalry—(Also called 16th Volunteers)—Mustered out July 24, 1865.

| Name | Rank | Residence | Remarks |
|---|---|---|---|
| Blackfan, J. W. | Ass't S. | Annandale, N. J. | Died June 10, 1881. |
| Phillips, Wm. W. L. | Surgeon | Trenton, N. J. | To September, 1864. U. S. Ex. S. |
| Dayton, F. V. | Ass't S. | Dead. | |
| Willis, Wm. S. | Surgeon | Dead. | |
| Baker, Benj. M. | Ass't S. | | To October, 1862. |
| Jones Samuel | " | | To June, 1865. |
| Van Duyn, S. W. | " | | From April, 1865. |

2d Cavalry—(Also called 32d Volunteers)—In service August 31, 1865.

| Name | Rank | Residence | Remarks |
|---|---|---|---|
| Bowlby, W. W. | Ass't S. | New York City | To Surg. 3d Cav. Dec., 1863; also 26th Inf. |
| Krauter, John L. | " | 734 Flushing ave. Brooklyn, N. Y. | A. W. M. |
| Todd, John R. | " | Lebanon, N. J. | Dead. |
| Dayton, F. V. | Surgeon | Dead. | |

3d Cavalry—(Also called 36th Volunteers)—Mustered out August 1, 1865.

| Name | Rank | Residence | Remarks |
|---|---|---|---|
| Bowlby, W. W. | Surgeon | New York city | From Dec., 1863; also 2d Cav. and 26th Inf. |
| Helm, John | Ass't S. | New Brunswick, N. J. | From Oct., 1864; also 3d Inf. |
| James, Douglas R. | " | | From February, 1865. |
| Morgan, L. O. | " | Box 127 S. Amboy, N. J. | To July, 1864. |
| Phillips, Sam'l A. | " | | Dismissed June, 1864. |

1st Infantry—Mustered out June 23, 1864.

| Name | Rank | Residence | Remarks |
|---|---|---|---|
| Miller, Levi D. | Ass't S. | Newton, N. J. | A. W. M. |
| Senderling, P. M. | " | 137 Wayne st., Jersey City, N. J. | To Surg. 8th Inf. May, 1864. |
| Gordon, Chas. C. | Surgeon | | To February, 1863. |
| Taylor, Edward F. | " | Middletown, N. J. | A. W. M. |

2d Infantry—Mustered out June 21, 1864.

| Name | Rank | Residence | Remarks |
|---|---|---|---|
| Clark, Henry C. | Ass't S. | Woodbury, N. J. | To 3d Inf. Feb., 1863. |
| Grant, Gabriel | Surgeon | 22 E. 30th st., New York, city. | To January, 1862. |
| Oakley, Lewis W. | " | Elizabeth, N. J. | From January, 1862. |
| Halsey, Luther F. | Ass't S. | Swedesborough, N. J. | To May, 1864; also 7th Inf. |
| Helm, John | " | New Brunswick, N. J. | From May, 1863; also 3d Cav. |

2d Infantry—(Veterans—1 year)—Mustered out July 11, 1865.

| Name | Rank | Residence | Remarks |
|---|---|---|---|
| Fitch, Geo. D. | Ass't S. | 3619 Powelton ave., Philadelphia, Pa. | From March, 1865; also 15th Inf. |

3d Infantry—Mustered out June 23, 1864.

| Name | Rank | Residence | Remarks |
|---|---|---|---|
| Clark, Henry C. | Surgeon | Woodbury, N. J. | A. W. M. Also 2d Inf. |
| Welling, E. L. | Ass't S. | Pennington, N. J. | To 11th Inf., July, 1862. |
| Coxe, L. Lewis | Surgeon | | To May, 1862. |
| Mattison, John V. | " | | To February, 1863. |
| Mattison, Wm. E. | Ass't S. | New Brunswick, N. J. | To March, 1863. |
| Trescott, J. C. | " | Dead | From March, 1863. |
| Terhune, Gilliam C. | " | Passaic, N. J. | A. W. M. Dead. |

## NEW JERSEY—Continued.

### 4TH INFANTRY—Mustered out July 9, 1865.

| Name | Rank | Address | Remarks |
|---|---|---|---|
| Bowlby, L. C. | Ass't S. | 1800 Market st., Phila., Pa. | To 23d Inf. March, 1863. Dead. |
| Dougherty, A. M. | Surgeon | Soldiers' Home, Newark, N. J. | To U. S. V. Oct., 1861. |
| Watson, Beriah A. | " | Jersey City, N. J. | From February, 1865. |
| Osborne, Jos. D. | " | Newark, N. J. | To Nov., 1864. Ex. S. |
| Blake, Duncan W. | Ass't S. | Gloucester, N. J. | From March, 1865. |
| Hendry, Bowman | " | 1525 Chestnut st., Phila., Pa. | To November, 1864; also 6th Inf. |
| Cloud, Albert J. | " | | From April, 1865. |

### 5TH INFANTRY—Mustered out November 6, 1864; veterans and recruits transferred to 7th Infantry.

| Name | Rank | Address | Remarks |
|---|---|---|---|
| *Beldon, O. S. | Ass't S. | Camden, N. J | Dismissed Dec., 1862. |
| Vanderveer, H. F. | Surgeon | Somerville, N. J. | To August, 1864. U. S. Ex. S. |
| Fisher, James C. | | New Brunswick, N. J. | To U. S. V. April, 1862. |
| Woodhull, A. W. | Ass't S. | Dead. | To 9th Inf. Feb., 1862. |
| Blundell, Wm. | " | Paterson, N. J. | To September, 1864. |

### 6TH INFANTRY—Mustered out September 7, 1864; veterans and recruits transferred to 8th Infantry.

| Name | Rank | Address | Remarks |
|---|---|---|---|
| Fagan, Henry M. | Ass't S. | Bloomfield, N. J. | To April, 1863. |
| Hendry, Bowman | " | 1800 Market st., Phila., Pa. | From Aug., 1862; also 4th Inf. |
| Wiley, John | Surgeon | Cape May, N. J. | From August, 1861. |
| Cooper, Wm. H. | Ass't S. | | Dismissed Nov., 1862. |
| Sharp, Redford | " | Dead. | To 15th Inf. Aug., 1862. |

### 7TH INFANTRY—Mustered out July 17, 1865.

| Name | Rank | Address | Remarks |
|---|---|---|---|
| Halsey, Luther F. | Ass't S. | Swedesborough, N. J. | Trsf'd to 2d Inf. April, 1863. |
| Hough, De Witt | Surgeon | Rahway, N. J | To September, 1864. |
| Lehlbach, Chas. | " | Newark, N. J | From November, 1864. |
| Satterthwaite, A. | Ass't S. | | To 12th Inf. July, 1862. |
| Jacques, Chas. B. | " | | To September, 1864. |
| Champion, C. S. | " | | From April 1865. |
| Paxson, Francis V. | " | | To May, 1863. |

### 8TH INFANTRY—Mustered out July 17, 1865.

| Name | Rank | Address | Remarks |
|---|---|---|---|
| McKelway, Alex. J. | Surgeon | Williamstown, N. J. | To April, 1864. |
| Ribble, Jas. I. B. | Ass't S. | Trenton, N. J. | To June, 1864; also 13th Inf. |
| Taylor, H. Genet | " | Camden, N. J. | To March, 1864. |
| Senderling, P. M. | Surgeon | 137 Wayne st., Jersey City, N. J. | From May, 1864; also 1st Inf. |
| Lamb, Wm. W. | Ass't S. | 1247 Hanover st., Phila., Pa. | From June, 1864. H. R. |

### 9TH INFANTRY—Mustered out July 12, 1865.

| Name | Rank | Address | Remarks |
|---|---|---|---|
| Brann, Lewis | Act'g S. | Elizabeth, N. J. | To March, 1862. |
| Gillette, Fidelio B. | Surgeon | 128 Colyer st., Brooklyn, N. Y. | From February, 1865. |
| Woodhull, A. W. | Ass't S. | Dead. | |
| Davies, John M. | " | | To May, 1865. |

* Claim agent.

## NEW JERSEY—Continued.

### 10TH INFANTRY—Mustered out July 1, 1865.

| Name | Rank | Address | Service |
|---|---|---|---|
| Fitch, Pelatiah | Ass't S. | 228 Pine st., Philadelphia, Pa. | From October, 1862. |
| Freeman, Otis R | Surgeon | Freehold, N. J | A. W. M. |
| Thomas, R., Jr | Ass't S. | Box 305, Trenton, N. J. | To 38th Inf. Sept., 1864. |
| Bryan, John W | Surgeon | | To March, 1862 |
| Stillo, Sam'l | Ass't S. | | To January, 1863. |
| Vansant, J. V | " | | From March, 1865. |

### 11TH INFANTRY—Mustered out July 5, 1865.

| Name | Rank | Address | Service |
|---|---|---|---|
| Heritage, John D | Ass't S. | Glassborough, N. J | A. W. M. |
| Ribble, Geo. T | " | Milford, N. J | From March, 1863. |
| Welling, Edward | Surgeon | Pennington, N. J | From Aug., 1862; also 3d Inf. |
| Young, Edwin B | " | New Brunswick, N. J. | To February, 1863. |
| Byington, E. L | Ass't S. | Died 1872. | |

### 12TH INFANTRY—Mustered out July 15, 1865.

| Name | Rank | Address | Service |
|---|---|---|---|
| Gillman, Uriah | Ass't S. | Woodstown, N. J | To June, 1865. H. R. |
| Miller, Samuel T | " | Paulsboro', N. J | To November, 1864. |
| Weideman, C. A | H. Stew. | Philadelphia, Pa. | |
| Satterwaite, Alvin | Surgeon | | To June, 1865; also 7th Inf. |

### 13TH INFANTRY—Mustered out June 8, 1865.

| Name | Rank | Address | Service |
|---|---|---|---|
| Brooks, Geo. L | Ass's S. | Jersey City, N. J | From April, 1865. |
| Lord, John J. H | Surgeon | Mt. Clair, N. J | To January, 1864. |
| Ribble, Jas. I. B | " | Trenton, N. J | From July, 1864; also 8th Inf. |
| Freeman, J. A | " | | To Ass't S. U. S. V. June, 1864. |
| Coriell, Wm. W | Ass's S. | New Market, N. J | To July, 1864. |

### 14TH INFANTRY—Mustered out June 18, 1865.

| Name | Rank | Address | Service |
|---|---|---|---|
| Disbrow, R L | Ass't S. | Tom's River, N. J | From Oct., 1863; U. S. Ex. S. |
| Treganowan, A | Surgeon | South Amboy, N. J | To November, 1863. |
| Woolverton, J | Ass't S. | Trenton, N. J | To October, 1862. |
| Martin, Joseph S | Surgeon | Elizabethport, N. J | From January, 1864. |
| Chambre, H. B | Ass't S. | Dover, N. J | To August, 1863. |

### 15TH INFANTRY—Mustered out June 22, 1865.

| Name | Rank | Address | Service |
|---|---|---|---|
| Fitch, Geo. D | Ass't S. | 3741 Lancaster ave., or 3619 Powelton ave., Philadelphia, Pa. | To the 2d Veterans June, 1865 |
| Hall, Chas. E | " | Freehold, N. J | To 40th Inf. Feb., 1865. |
| Sullivan, Geo. R | " | Flemington, N. J | To 39th Inf. Oct., 1864. |
| Sharp, Redford | Surgeon | Dead | |
| Dearborn, Geo. S | Ass't S. | Oxford, N. J | To November, 1862. |

### 16TH INFANTRY—(See 1st Cavalry.)

### 17TH, 18TH, 19TH, and 20TH INFANTRY—Failed to complete.

### 21ST INFANTRY—(9 months)—Mustered out June 19, 1863.

| Name | Rank | Address | Service |
|---|---|---|---|
| Janney, Wm. S | Ass't S. | 1535 N. Broad st., Philadelphia, Pa. | To Surg. 22d Inf. March, 1863. |
| McNeill, Daniel | Surgeon | 554 Palisade ave., Jersey City, N. J. | From September, 1862. |
| Conover, C | Ass't S. | | From June, 1863. |

NEW JERSEY—Continued.

22D INFANTRY—(9 months)—Mustered out June 25, 1863.

| | | | |
|---|---|---|---|
| Janney, Wm. S | Surgeon | 1535 N. Broad st., Philadelphia, Pa. | From April, 1863; also 21st Infantry. |
| Quick, Jacob | " | Philadelphia, Pa. | To March, 1863. |
| Jones, Sam'l A | Ass't S. | Englewood, N. J | From September, 1862. |
| Carey, John E | " | | From September, 1862. |

23D INFANTRY—(9 months)—Mustered out June 27, 1863.

| | | | |
|---|---|---|---|
| Hetzell, David G | Ass't S. | S.W. cor. 40th and Haverford sts., Philadelphia, Pa. | From September, 1862. |
| Bowlby, L. C | Surgeon | 1800 Market st., Philadelphia, Pa. | From March, 1863; also 4th Infantry. Dead. |
| Elmer, Robt. W | Ass't S. | Bridgeton, N. J | From September, 1862. |
| Cook, Wm | Surgeon | Alleged dead | To February, 1863. |

24TH INFANTRY—(9 months)—Mustered out June 29, 1863.

| | | | |
|---|---|---|---|
| Newell, Wm. L | Surgeon | Millville, N. J | From September, 1862. |
| Rowand, Thos. G | Ass't S. | Camden, N. J | From September, 1862. |
| Williams, Alvan | " | Phœnixville, Pa | From September, 1862. |

25TH INFANTRY—(9 months)—Mustered out June 20, 1863.

| | | | |
|---|---|---|---|
| Bateman, Robt. M | Ass't S. | Cedarville, N. J | From Oct., 1862. Said to be dead. |
| Dailey, Seffrine | " | Franklin, N. J | A. W. M. |
| Riley, James | Surgeon | Suckasunny, N. J | From October, 1862. |

26TH INFANTRY—(9 months)—Mustered out June 27, 1863.

| | | | |
|---|---|---|---|
| Bowlby, Wm. W | Ass't S. | New York city | To Dec., 1862; also 2d and 3d Cavalry. |
| Osborne, Thos. S | " | | To April, 1863. |
| Thomas, L. G | Surgeon | | From September, 1862. |

27TH INFANTRY—(9 months)—Mustered out July 2, 1863.

| | | | |
|---|---|---|---|
| Richmond, John B | Surgeon | Newark, N. J | From September, 1862. H. R. |
| Stiger, J. Henry | Ass't S. | Mendham, N. J | From October, 1862; also 33d Inf. |
| Suydam, Chas. H | " | | A. W. M.; also 34th Inf. |

28TH INFANTRY—(9 months)—Mustered out July 6, 1863.

| | | | |
|---|---|---|---|
| Baker, Benj. N | Ass't S. | Rhinebeck, N. Y | A. W. M. |
| Berg, J. Fred | " | North Branch, N. J | A. W. M. |
| Newell, Wm. D | Surgeon | | From September, 1862. |

29TH INFANTRY—(9 months)—Mustered out July 6, 1863.

| | | | |
|---|---|---|---|
| Cook, Henry G | Surgeon | Holmdel, N. J | From September, 1862. |
| Hunt, Ezra M | Ass't S. | Morristown or Metuchen, N. J. | To January, 1863. U. S. Ex. S. |
| Shackleton, J. G | " | Matawan, N. J. | From September, 1862. |
| Lawrence, E. W | " | Philadelphia, Penn | A. W. M. |

30TH INFANTRY—(9 months)—Mustered out June 27, 1863.

| | | | |
|---|---|---|---|
| Lanning, J. T | Ass't S. | Emporium, Pa | From April, 1863; also 35th Inf. |
| Wolverton, Jos. W | Surgeon | Monmouth Co., N. J | From November, 1862. |
| Cummings, Geo. G | Ass't S. | | From September, 1862. |
| Barclay, Alex | Surgeon | | To March, 1863. |

## NEW JERSEY—Continued.

### 31ST INFANTRY—(9 months)—Mustered out June 24, 1863.

| | | | |
|---|---|---|---|
| Brown, Robert B. | Surgeon | Jeansville, Pa. | From September, 1862. |
| Cook, Jos. S. | Ass't S. | Washington, N. J. | To April, 1863. |
| Jennings, Nathaniel. | " | Gunnison, Col. | From September, 1862. |
| Willis, Wm. S. | " | | From April, 1863. |

### 32D INFANTRY—(See 2d Cavalry.)

### 33D INFANTRY—Mustered out July 17, 1865.

| | | | |
|---|---|---|---|
| Stickney, Chas. W. | Ass't S. | 65 S. Orange st., Newark, N. J. | From September, 1863. H. R. |
| Stiger, J. Henry | " | Mendham, N. J. | From September, 1863; also 27th Inf. |
| Reily, James | Surgeon | | From September, 1863. Died 1872. |

### 34TH INFANTRY—Still in service August 31, 1865.

| | | | |
|---|---|---|---|
| Hetzell, David J. | Ass't S. | 4011 Haverford street, Philadelphia, Pa. | From October, 1863. |
| Badger, Con. C. | " | | From February, 1865. |
| Suydam, Chas. H. | Surgeon | | From July, 1864; also 27th Inf. |
| Bowen, John B. | " | Bridgeton, N. J. | To May, 1864. |

### *35TH INFANTRY—Mustered out July 20, 1865.

| | | | |
|---|---|---|---|
| Lanning, John T. | Ass't S. | Emporium, Pa. | To July, 1864; also 30th Inf. |
| Summers, Geo. E. | Surgeon | Columbus, Ohio. | To January, 1865. |
| Reed, Edward H. | Ass't S. | Dead | To March, 1865. |
| †Taylor, R. G. | Surgeon | | From April, 1865. |
| Wolverton, Samuel | Ass't S. | | From June, 1865. |

### 36TH INFANTRY—(See 3d Cavalry.)

### 37TH INFANTRY—Was 100 days' organization.

### 38TH INFANTRY—(1 year)—Mustered out June 30, 1865.

| | | | |
|---|---|---|---|
| Hart, Israel | Ass't S. | Pennington, N. J. | From September, 1864. |
| Thomas, Richard, Jr. | Surgeon | Box 305, Trenton, N. J. | From September, 1864; also 10th Inf. |
| Coombs, Wm. S. | | | From September, 1864. |

### 39TH INFANTRY—(1 year)—Mustered out June 17, 1865.

| | | | |
|---|---|---|---|
| Sullivan, George R. | Surgeon | Flemington, N. J. | From November, 1864; also 15th Inf. |
| Douglass, Geo. W. | Ass't S. | | From October, 1864. |

### 40TH INFANTRY—(1 year)—Mustered out July 13, 1865.

| | | | |
|---|---|---|---|
| Hall, Charles E. | Surgeon | Freehold, N. J. | From February, 1865; also 15th Inf. |
| Wildman, Elias N. | Ass't S. | Dead | From March, 1865. |
| Heed, Harmon | " | Amherst, Mass. | A. W. M. |

* Jas. H. White, Sergeant, Long Branch, N. J., has memorandum of all killed and wounded in Co. H.
† Assistant Surgeon to March, 1864.

## NEW MEXICO.

1ST CAVALRY—Part of the 1st, 2d, 4th, and 5th Infantry were consolidated with this regiment May 31, 1862. The original members were mustered out July 31, 1864. The regiment was consolidated with the 1st Battalion of Cavalry and Infantry August 31, 1866.

Shout, John H.........Ass't S.....Las Vegas, N. M............To 1st Inf. (new) Sept., 1864.
Brey, Julius C......... " ........................................To March, 1866.
Peck, Allen .............Surgeon........................................To July, 1864; also 3d Inf. and 1st Cav.
Gwyther, George ..... " ........................................A. W. M.

1ST INFANTRY—Part mustered out May 31, 1862; the rest transferred to the 1st Cavalry (new.)

Booth, L. E.............H. Stew...Trinidad, Col.
Shout, John H.........Ass't S.....Las Vegas, N. M............From August, 1861; also 1st Cav.
Whitlock, J. M.........Surgeon........................................To May, 1862.

1ST INFANTRY (New)—Part mustered out from September 12 to November 7, 1866; the rest transferred to the 1st Cavalry to date from August 31, 1866.

Shout, John H.........Surgeon...Las Vegas, N. M............From Sept , 1864; also 1st Cav. and 1st Inf.
Rankin, Sylvester.....Ass't S........................................To March, 1865.

2D INFANTRY—Part mustered out May 31, 1862; the rest transferred to the 1st (new) Cavalry.

Gray, A. L ..............Surgeon........................................From August, 1861.
Rankin, Sylvester.....Ass't S........................................From Aug., 1861; also 1st (new) Inf.

3D INFANTRY (Mounted)—Mustered out from March 9 to 20, 1862.

Peck, Allen F..........Surgeon........................................From Nov., 1861; also 4th Inf. and 1st Cav.

4TH INFANTRY—Part mustered out May 31, 1862; the rest transferred to 1st Cavalry.

Peck, Allen F..........Surgeon........................................From Nov., 1861; also 3d Inf. and 1st Cav.
Craine, Alfred A......Ass't S........................................From March, 1862.

## NEW YORK.

1ST CAVALRY (Lincoln Cavalry)—Mustered out June 27, 1865.

Beakes, George M.....Ass't S.....Bloomington, N. Y........To October, 1863.
Douglass, George C.. " Salt Lake City, Utah......To Surg. 134th Inf Jan, 1865.
Elliott, Frederick... .Surgeon...67 West 38th st., New York City. To November, 1864
Welch, Abraham...... " Maysville, Col ..............From Jan., 1865; also 21st Cav. Dead.
Powell, Thomas D ...Ass't S.....N. Java, N. Y..............From Jan., 1865. Dead.

1ST CAVALRY (Veteran)—Mustered out July 20, 1865.

Dickerson, D. E.......Surgeon...Kansas City, Mo ...........From July, 1863.
Alleman, Levi J ......Ass't S....Boone, Iowa.....................From November, 1863.
Rippey, John N....... " Lancaster, Ohio ............A. W. M.

## NEW YORK—Continued.

1ST CAVALRY (Provisional)—Formed June 17, 1865, by consolidating the 10th and 24th Cavalry—Mustered out July 19, 1865.

| | | | |
|---|---|---|---|
| Catlin, Charles A | Ass't S | Redwood, N. Y | From March, 1865; also 10th Cavalry. |
| George, Charles L | Surgeon | Auburn, N. Y | From September, 1864. |
| Lanning, Oliver | Ass't S | Dead. | |

2D CAVALRY (Harris' Light Cavalry)—Part mustered out September 10, 1864; the rest June 5, 1865.

Dr. Hackley says all the books were captured at Ream's Station.

| | | | |
|---|---|---|---|
| Hackley, Charles E | Surgeon | 47 W. 31st street, New York city. | To September, 1864. |
| Kingston, Samuel F | " | Oswego, N. Y | From November, 1864. |
| Trenor, John, Jr | Ass't S | Dead. | |
| Margiarotti, Regola | " | Dead | From January, 1865. |

2D VETERAN CAVALRY (Empire Light Cavalry)—Mustered out November 9, 1865.

| | | | |
|---|---|---|---|
| Balch, Galusha B | Ass't S | Yonkers, N. Y | From January, 1864; also 98th Inf. |
| Damainville, Lucien | Surgeon | 245 W. 52d street, New York city. | From August, 1864. |
| Perry, John L | " | Saratoga Springs, N. Y | To June, 1864. |

2D PROVISIONAL CAVALRY—Formed June 17, 1865, by consolidation of 6th and 15th Regiments New York Cavalry—Mustered out August 9, 1865.

| | | | |
|---|---|---|---|
| Clark, Augustus P | Surgeon | 693 Main street, Cambridge, Mass. | From May, 1863; also 6th Cav. |
| Halsted, Milton A | Ass't S | Jacksonville, Ill | From January, 1864; also 15th Cav. |
| Wall, John C | " | Dead. | |

2D MOUNTED RIFLES—Mustered out August 10, 1865.

| | | | |
|---|---|---|---|
| Paine, Rob't T., Jr | Surgeon | Lockport, N. Y | From August, 1863. |
| Woodworth, Eli D | Ass't S | Eagle Village, N. Y | From February, 1864. |
| Wilson, Hugh McG | " | 162 Randolph street, Detroit, Mich. | To May, 1865. |

3D CAVALRY (Van Allen Cavalry)—Consolidated with 7th Cavalry July 21, 1865.

| | | | |
|---|---|---|---|
| Palmer, William H | Surgeon | Providence, R. I | To August, 1864. |
| Van Alstyne, Jno. L | " | Binghamton, N. Y | To July, 1865. |
| Douglas, Frederick | Ass't S | Dead. | |
| Brown, Wm. R | " | Philadelphia, Pa | From April, 1865. |

3D PROVISIONAL CAVALRY—Formed June 23, 1865, by consolidation of 13th and 16th Cavalry—mustered out September 21, 1865.

| | | | |
|---|---|---|---|
| Burdick, James T | Ass't S | 459 Gates ave., Brooklyn, N. Y. | From July, 1864. |
| Horniston, James M | Surgeon | Brooklyn, N. Y | From October, 1863. |
| Terry, Charles H | Ass't S | 540 Washington street, Brooklyn, N. Y. | From January, 1865; also 13th Cav. |

NEW YORK—Continued.

4TH CAVALRY—(1st German; Dickel's Mounted Rifles)—Consolidated with 9th Cavalry February 27, 1865.

Beebe, DeWitt C......Surgeon...Sparta, Wis.......................From December, 1864.
Brown, Martin.........Ass't S.....Cape Vincent, N. Y.......To June, 1863.
Franklin, Morris J... " 77 7th ave., New York City. To October, 1862.
Streeter, Buel G......Surgeon...Warren, Pa.......................To September, 1863; also 9th Cav.
Meyer, Adolph......... " Dead.
Snow, Thos..............Ass't S.......................................To June, 1863.

5TH CAVALRY—(1st Ira Harris' Guard)—Part mustered out October, 1864; the rest July 19, 1865.

Armstrong, O. H......Surgeon...135 W. 34th st., New York City. From January, 1865.
Cooper, John R....... " Poughkeepsie, N. Y.......To July, 1862.
Parsons, Wm. W. D..Ass't S.....Fultonville, N. Y...........To June, 1863.
Mead, I. N.............. " Amenia, N. Y ...............From January, 1865.
Woods, Lucius P......Surgeon...Dead.
Webb, E. C............Ass't S.....Homœopathic Hospital, Ward's Island, N. Y. To September, 1863; also 24th Inf.
Goodell, R. H......... " ..................................From May, 1864.

6TH CAVALRY—(2d Ira Harris' Guard)—Consolidated with 15th Cavalry June 17, 1865, and called 2d Provisional Cavalry.

Brundage, Amos H...Ass't S.....Newark, N. J...............To June, 1865.
Curran, Richard..... " Rochester, N. Y...........To 9th Cavalry September, 1864.
Clark, Augustus P...Surgeon...693 Main st., Cambridge, Mass. From May, 1863; also 2d Provisional Cav.
Peters, Joseph A...... " 222 E. 122d st., New York City. Missing January, 1863; also 21st Inf.
*McKay, Lawrence.. " Rochester, N. Y............To Sept., 1862. Dead.
Sanger, Simon C......Ass't S.....Ansonia, Conn..............Dismissed August, 1864.

7TH CAVALRY—(Dodge's Cavalry)—This regiment was consolidated with the 3d Cavalry July 21, 1865, and the force designated 4th Provisional Cavalry.

Wright, F. M............Surgeon...Dead...................................From September, 1864.
Griffin, Bradney......Ass't S.....Dead.
Brown, Wm. R....... " Philadelphia, Pa............From April, 1865.
Bennett, Geo. C......Surgeon...Dead...................................To September, 1864.

7TH CAVALRY—(2d Black Horse Company)—Mustered out March 31, 1862.

Sheldon, Andrew F..Ass't S.....Pultneyville, N. Y ........From November, 1861.
Hubbell, Chas. L......Surgeon...35 1st street, Troy, New York. From October, 1861.

8TH CAVALRY—(Rochester Cavalry)—Mustered out June 27, 1865.

Chapman, James......Surgeon...Medina, N. Y ..................To February, 1862.
Fergerson, N. D...... " Carthage, N. Y..............To December, 1864.
Fuller, Winfield S ....Ass't S.....Fairport, N. Y...............To November, 1862.
Thurston, E. H........ " 584 Wabash avenue, Chicago, Ill. From April, 1865. H. R.
Vosburg, Hiram D... " Lyons, Wayne Co. N. Y..To January, 1864. Dead.
Sickler, Peter E ......Surgeon...Dead.
Adams, Oscar H......Ass't S.....Dead.
Cole, Eli K.............. " Dead...................................To December, 1863.

* Lewis McKay in A. G. R.

NEW YORK—Continued.

9TH CAVALRY—(U. S Lancers, Westfield Cavalry)—The 4th New York Cavalry was consolidated with this regiment February 27, 1865, [March 29, 1865]—Mustered out June 27, 1865.

| | | | |
|---|---|---|---|
| Curran, Richard | Surgeon | Rochester, N. Y. | From September, 1864; also 6th Cav. |
| Spencer, John | " | Westfield, N. Y. | To July, 1862. H. R. for 1861 and 1862. Died December, 1881. |
| Streeter, Buel G. | " | *Warren, Pa. | To 4th Cavalry May, 1863. |
| Bennett, Geo. C. | Ass't S. | Dead. | To May, 1862. |
| Comer, A. T. C. | " | 28 William street, New York City. | From April, 1863. |

10TH CAVALRY—(Porter Guard)—Consolidated with 24th Cavalry June 17, 1865, and called 1st Provisional Cavalry.

| | | | |
|---|---|---|---|
| Bliss, Lyman W. | Ass't S. | Saginaw City, Mich. | To October, 1863. |
| Clark, H. K. | Surgeon | Geneva, N. Y. | From November, 1863. |
| Catlin, C. A. | Ass't S. | Redwood, N. Y. | From March, 1865; also 1st Provisional Cav. |
| Pease, Roger W. | Surgeon | Syracuse, N. Y. | To Surg. U. S. V. October, 1863. |
| Lanning. Oliver | Ass't S. | Dead. | |
| Sickler, Peter E. | " | Dead. | |
| Whedon, G. D. | " | 40 S. Clinton st., Syracuse, N. Y. | To November, 1862. |

11TH CAVALRY—(Scott's Guard)—In service August 31, 1865.

| | | | |
|---|---|---|---|
| Campbell, Alex. W. | Ass't S. | Clyde, Kan. | To June, 1865. Dead. |
| Gray. Charles | Surgeon | Dead. | |
| Ridder, Walter | " | Dead. | |
| Fisher, Chas. L. | Ass't S. | Boston, Mass. | To March, 1863. |

12TH CAVALRY—(3d Ira Harris' Guard)—Mustered out July 19, 1865.

| | | | |
|---|---|---|---|
| Cooper, J. R. | Surgeon | Poughkeepsie, N. Y. | To January, 1863. |
| Nold, John B. | Ass't S. | Boonville, N. Y. | To June, 1865. |
| McDonald, Geo. E. | Surgeon | Schenectady, N. Y. | From July, 1864. |
| Mundy, E. C. | " | Fort Richmond, N. Y. | To May, 1864. |

13TH CAVALRY—(Seymour's Light Cavalry and Tompkins' Cavalry)—Consolidated with 16th Cavalry June 23, 1865, and called 3d Provisional Cavalry.

| | | | |
|---|---|---|---|
| Burdick, James T. | Ass't S. | 458 Gates ave., Brooklyn. N. Y. | From July, 1864. |
| Terry, Chas. H. | " | 540 Washington street, Brooklyn. N. Y. | From Jan., 1865; also 3d Prov. Cavalry. |
| Taylor, B. R. | Surgeon | Nokomis, Ill. | From March, 1864. |
| Woodward, G. F. | " | Dead. | To February, 1864. |
| Eddy, Wm. | Ass't S. | | To May, 1864. |

14TH CAVALRY—(Metropolitan Cavalry and Pierrepont Rifles)—Consolidated with 18th Cavalry June 12, 1865.

| | | | |
|---|---|---|---|
| Lester, Elias | Ass't S. | Seneca. Falls, N. Y. | To August, 1863. |
| Skilton, Julius A. | Surgeon | City of Mexico, Mex. | From December, 1862. |
| Downs, Henry L. | Ass't S. | Dead. | From April, 1863; also 18th Cavalry. |

* Letters returned uncalled for.

## NEW YORK—Continued.

15TH CAVALRY—(Johnson's Cavalry)—Consolidated with 6th Cavalry June 17, 1865, and called 2d Provisional Cavalry.

| | | | |
|---|---|---|---|
| Halsted, Milton A | Ass't S | Jacksonville, Ill | From June, 1864; also 2d Provisional Cavalry. |
| Skiff, Geo. V | Surgeon | 171 W. 45th street, N. Y. city. | From June, 1863; also 12th Inf. |
| Wall, John C | Ass't S | Dead. | |

16TH CAVALRY—(Sprague Light Cavalry)—Consolidated with 13th Cavalry June 23, 1865, and called 3d Provisional Cavalry.

| | | | |
|---|---|---|---|
| Vondersmith, S. P | Ass't S | 420 E. 118th st., N. Y. city. | From October, 1863. |
| Drake, N. S | " | Dead | Dismissed May, 1864. |
| Horniston, J. M | Surgeon | Dead. | |

17TH CAVALRY—(See 1st Veteran Cavalry.)

18TH CAVALRY—(Corning Light Cavalry)—In service August 31, 1865.

| | | | |
|---|---|---|---|
| Gail, Wm. H | Ass't S | Willink, or East Aurora, N. Y. | To February, 1865. |
| Walker, A. C | Surgeon | Greenfield, Mass | To June, 1865; also 133d Inf. |
| Murphy, Robt. P | " | Dead. | |
| Rockwell, Wm | " | Dead. | |
| Downs, H. L | Ass't S | Dead | From April, 1863; also 14th Cavalry. |

19TH CAVALRY—(1st Dragoons and 130th Volunteers)—Mustered out June 30, 1865.

| | | | |
|---|---|---|---|
| Rae, Robert | Ass't S | Portageville, N. Y | From May, 1864. H. R. Also 6th Heavy Artillery. |
| Kneeland, B. T | Surgeon | Nunda, N. Y | From Sept., 1862. H. R. |
| Purchase, J. B | Ass't S | Scottsburgh, N. Y | To February, 1864. |
| Fowler, D. C | " | Oswego, N. Y | From May, 1863. |
| Patterson, J. C | " | So. Livonia, N. Y | To November, 1862. |
| Saunders, Jas. B | " | Detroit, Mich | To January, 1863. |

20TH CAVALRY—(McClellan Cavalry)—Mustered out July 31, 1865.

| | | | |
|---|---|---|---|
| Carter, Norris M | Ass't S | Poughkeepsie, N. Y | To 100th Inf. March, 1865. |
| Hickey, Daniel C | " | Kingston, Canada | From March, 1864. |
| * Madell, Wm. A | Surgeon | Archbild, Pa | From July, 1863. |

21ST CAVALRY—(Griswold's Light Cavalry)—In service August 31, 1865.

| | | | |
|---|---|---|---|
| Huested, Alfred B | Ass't S | Albany, N. Y | From March, 1864. |
| † McLean, Leroy | Surgeon | Troy, N. Y | To October, 1863; also 2d Inf. |
| Draper, Edwin H | Ass't S | Wolcott, N. Y | From March, 1865. |
| Welch, Abraham | " | Maysville, Colo | To 1st Cav. Jan., 1865. Dead. |
| Catlin, Benj. S | Surgeon | Dead | From Oct., 1863; also 2d Infantry. |

* Charges fee $10.
† Did not accompany the 21st Cavalry to the field.

## NEW YORK—Continued.

### 22D CAVALRY—Mustered out August 21, 1865.

Losey, Jesse B.........Ass't S.....Conesus Centre, N. Y.....To July, 1864; re-com. January, 1865.
McShane, Patrick..... " 743 Myrtle ave., Brooklyn, N. Y. To December, 1864.
Van Slyck, D. B......Surgeon...Brookline, Mass.............From November, 1863.
Lee, D. M................Ass't S.....Oxford, N. Y...............From May, 1865.

### 23D CAVALRY—(Mixes' Cavalry Battalion)—Consolidated with 12th Cavalry April 16, 1865.

### 24TH CAVALRY—(Called 1st Provisional Cavalry)—Consolidated with 10th Cavalry June 17, 1865.

George, Chas. L ......Surgeon...Auburn, N. Y...............From September, 1864.
Wilkins, W. E.........Ass't S.....Saratogo Springs, N. Y...To October, 1864.
Buck, Robert.......... " ...............................To June, 1865.
Doolittle, L. L.........Surgeon...Central City, Neb.........To July, 1864.

### 25TH CAVALRY—(Sickles' Cavalry)—Mustered out June 27, 1865.

Dufloo, Armand ......Ass't S.....55 W. 24th st., N. Y. city..To March, 1865; also 70th Inf.
Jones, James D........Surgeon...Died December, 1879.
Sumner, Geo............Ass't S...............................From April, 1864.

### 26TH CAVALRY—(1st Frontier Cavalry)—Mustered out from June 29 to July 7, 1865.

Thompson, Geo. F...Surgeon...Belchertown, Mass.........From April, 1865.

### 2D HEAVY ARTILLERY—(Morgan Artillery)—Mustered out September 29, 1865.

Davis, M. J.............Ass't S.....Lewis, Iowa.................From Jan., 1864; also 4th Heavy Artillery.
How, James C.........Surgeon...Haverhill, Mass..............From December, 1863.
Paine, O. Sprague....Ass't S.....48 E. 31st st., N. Y. city..To 188th Inf. Nov., 1866.
Armstrong, H. A......Surgeon...Winchester, Va...............To November, 1863.
Wiser, Wm. H.........Ass't S.....Dead.............................To January, 1863.
Jackson, Edgar....... " Oyster Bay, L. I., N. Y. (Old.) To March, 1864.
Thoma, Geo. H........ " Eureka, Nev.................From January, 1865.

### 4TH HEAVY ARTILLERY—Mustered out September 26, 1865.

Davis, M. J.............Ass't S.....Lewis, Iowa.................To Oct., 1863; also 2d Heavy Artillery.
Hill, Clayton L......... " Buffalo, N. Y...............From April, 1865.
Kelsey, Charles T..... " Mecklenburgh, N. Y......From September, 1865.
Tompkins, H. C.......Surgeon...Knowlesville, N. Y........From November, 1863.
Williams, F. B.........Ass't S.....Ashland City, Tenn........To July, 1863.
Berky, R. B.............Surgeon...Dead.............................To September, 1862.
Bayles, Geo............. " Orange, N. J..................To March 1863.
Mudie, A. F............Ass't S.....557 Graham st., Brooklyn, N. Y. To July, 1863; also 3d L. Art.
Hendrickson, W. N.. " Wichita, Kan.................To September, 1864.
Lawrence, C. P........ " Victoria, Canada, (old.) To February, 1865.

NEW YORK—Continued.

5TH HEAVY ARTILLERY—Mustered out July 19, 1865.

| Name | Rank | Address | Service |
|---|---|---|---|
| Bowers, Alfred | Ass't S. | 486 Humboldt st., Brooklyn, E. D., N. Y. | From April, 1863. |
| Elliott, Samuel R. | Surgeon | 32 Waverly Place, N. Y. city. | From January, 1865. |
| Hendee, H. S. | Ass't S. | Carthage, N. Y. | To 153d Inf. July, 1864. |
| Smith, J. T. | " | Canandaigua, N. Y. | To May, 1864. |
| Newman, Geo. W. | " | Brooklyn, E. D., N. Y. | From March, 1865. |
| Dilts, George S. | Surgeon | Dead. | |
| Blauvelt, Jas. F. | Ass't S. | 159 Van Buren st., Brooklyn, N. Y. | To September, 1862; also 1st Art. |

6TH HEAVY ARTILLERY—(Anthony Wayne Guard, 135th Infantry—Mustered out August 24, 1865.

| Name | Rank | Address | Service |
|---|---|---|---|
| Wilcox, T. E. | Ass't S. | Care A. G. U. S. A. | To May, 1865. |
| Bendel, Herman | " | Albany, N. Y. | To January, 1865. |
| *Bennett, J. A. | " | 4 Irving Place, N. Y. city. | From April, 1864. |
| Porter, Charles H. | Surgeon | 55 Eagle st., Albany, N. Y. | From Feb., 1863. |
| Rae, Robert | Ass't S. | Portageville, N. Y. | To Jan., 1863; also 19th Cav. |
| Linson, John J. | " | Tarrytown, N. Y. | To February, 1864. |
| Day, E. | " | Grand Tower, Ill. | From December, 1864. |
| Bogart, R. D. | " | Nanuet, N. Y. | To December, 1862. |
| Wood, J. G. | Surgeon | Croton Falls, N. Y. | To January, 1863. |

7TH HEAVY ARTILLERY—Mustered out August 1, 1865.

| Name | Rank | Address | Service |
|---|---|---|---|
| Arnold, J. Newton | Ass't S. | Clyde, N. Y. | To June, 1865. |
| Newcomb. G. H. | Surgeon | Albany, N. Y. | To May, 1865. H. R. G. |
| Pomfret, J. E. | " | Dead | |
| Blaisdell, Wm. | Ass't S. | Dead. | To October, 1862. |
| Snelling, Josiah | " | Peoria, Ill. | From April, 1865. |

8TH HEAVY ARTILLERY—(129th Infantry)—Companies G, H, I, and K transferred to 4th Heavy Artillery June 4, 1865; companies L and M to 10th Inf.; the rest mustered out June 5, 1865.

| Name | Rank | Address | Service |
|---|---|---|---|
| Casey, Francis C. | Ass't S. | Auburn, N. Y. | From May, 1864. |
| Hill, H. C. | " | Lockport, N. Y. | To December, 1862. |
| Leet, James M. | Surgeon | 321 Locust st., St. Louis, Mo. | To October, 1863. |
| Churchill, Alonzo | " | Dead. | |
| Place, Simon G. | Ass't S. | Dead. | |
| Hayes, R. S. | " | | To June, 1863. |
| Freeman, John W. | " | 80 Hansom Place, Brooklyn, N. Y. | To February, 1864. |
| Wiser, W. W. | " | Dead. | To May, 1864. |
| Pegg, Chas. H. | " | Utica, N. Y., (old.) | To November, 1864. |

9TH HEAVY ARTILLERY—Transferred to 2d Artillery June 27, 1865.

| Name | Rank | Address | Service |
|---|---|---|---|
| Brandt, John W. | Ass't S. | Pultneyville, N. Y. | To December, 1864. |
| Chamberlin, D. S. | Surgeon | Lyons, N. Y. | From February, 1865. |
| Dewitt, Byron | Ass't S. | Oswego, N. Y. | From August, 1863. |
| Sabin, Samuel A. | Surgeon | Dead. | |
| Schulte, Otto | Ass't S. | | From April, 1865. |

* In claim No. 331,694 Dr. Bennett says he was not in the army.

NEW YORK—Continued.

10TH HEAVY ARTILLERY—This Regiment, formerly known as the 1st. 2d and 4th Battalions Black River Artillery, was mustered out June 23, 1865, and recruits were transferred to the 6th Heavy Artillery June 27, 1865.

| | | | |
|---|---|---|---|
| Goodall, Addison W. | Ass't S. | 554 Main st., Hartford, Conn. | To June, 1865. |
| *Pope, Benj. F. | " | Care A. G. U. S. A. | From July, 1864. |
| †Trowbridge, W. R. | Surgeon | Waterloo, N. Y. | Not in A. G. R. |
| Copeland, Oliver S. | " | Dead. | |
| Hobbs, Benj. | Ass't S. | Dead. | To March, 1864. |

11TH HEAVY ARTILLERY—Only four companies were organized, which were transferred to the 4th Heavy Artillery.

12TH HEAVY ARTILLERY—Failed to complete.

13TH HEAVY ARTILLERY—Consolidated with 6th Heavy Artillery June 27, 1865.

| | | | |
|---|---|---|---|
| Bennett, Jas. A. | Ass't S. | Prattsburgh, N. Y. | From April, 1863; also 6th H. Artillery. |
| Steele, Aaron J. | Surgeon | 2825 Washington ave., St. Louis, Mo. | From November, 1863. |
| Fontain, Jos. A. | Ass't S. | | From October, 1863. |

14TH HEAVY ARTILLERY—Mustered out June 26, 1865. Hospital records on file at S. G. O.

| | | | |
|---|---|---|---|
| Mullen, Isaac V. | Surgeon | Alexander, N. Y. | From May, 1863. H. R. |
| Morse, Sherman | Ass't S. | Ridgefield, Ill. | To May, 1865. |
| Phillips, Luther | " | Springfield, Pa. (old) | From February, 1864. |

15TH HEAVY ARTILLERY (Companies A, B, C and D were Senge's 3d Battalion German Heavy Artillery)—Mustered out August 22, 1865.

| | | | |
|---|---|---|---|
| Balser, Wm. | Ass't S. | 218 E. 13th street, New York city. | To July, 1863; also 29th and 62d Inf. |
| Patzke, Julius H. | " | Care A. G. U. S. A. | From Jan., 1864. Now Ass't S., U. S. A. |
| Ideler, Hermann | Surgeon | Dead. | |
| Kipp, Chas. J. | Ass't S. | 534 Broad st., Newark, N. J. | To April, 1862. |
| Deane, Chas. T. | " | San Francisco, Cal. | To June, 1863. |
| Greiss, Rudolph | " | | Dismissed Feb., 1865. |

16TH HEAVY ARTILLERY—Mustered out August 21, 1865.

| | | | |
|---|---|---|---|
| Barnum, D. Albert | Ass't S. | Cassville, N. Y. | From March, 1865. |
| Dodge, John L. | Surgeon | Groton, Conn. | From July, 1863. |
| Frame, Solomon V. | Ass't S. | Clayton, N. Y. | From March, 1864. |
| Owen, Edward W. | " | 541 Grand street, Brooklyn, N. Y. | Dismissed Nov., 1864. |

1ST ARTILLERY (Marine)—Disbanded March, 1863.

| | | | |
|---|---|---|---|
| Avery, Amos G. | Ass't S. | Batavia, N. Y. | Missing since Aug., 1862. |
| McLellan, F. | Surgeon | Dead. | |
| Blauvelt, James F. | Ass't S. | 159 Van Buren street, Brooklyn, N. Y. | To October, 1862; also 5th H. Art. |

* Hope, in A. G. R.
† Examined the men at enlistment; kept a record.

## NEW YORK—Continued.

1ST LIGHT ARTILLERY—Mustered out from June 16 to 28, 1865. (Morgan's Light Artillery and Busteed's Chicago Battery formed part of this regiment. Battery M was called Cothran's Battery.)

| | | | |
|---|---|---|---|
| Davis, M. J | Ass't S | Lewis, Iowa | To Dec., 1862; also 2d and 4th H. Art. |
| Pardee, Daniel | Surgeon | Fulton, N. Y | Not in A. G. R. |
| Everts, Franklin | “ | Dead | To October, 1862. |
| Williams, A. A. C | Ass't S | Dead | To April, 1862. |
| McDonell, Edward | “ | Dead | To June, 1862. |

2D ARTILLERY was Heavy Artillery.

3D LIGHT ARTILLERY (19th Infantry)—Mustered out from June 23 to July 29, 1865.

| | | | |
|---|---|---|---|
| Benjamin, Frank W | Ass't S | Mellenville, N. Y | From September, 1864. |
| Dimon, Theodore | Surgeon | Auburn, N. Y | To June, 1863. |
| Knight, Wm. W | “ | Sharon, Conn | To May, 1864. |
| Manly, Bradford S | Ass't S | Potsdam, N. Y | To 1st U. S. C. C. Dec., 1863. |
| Wilson, Alfred D | “ | Dead. | |
| Mudie, Archibald F | “ | 557 Graham ave., Brooklyn, N. Y. | To May, 1865; also 15th Eng. and 4th H. Art. |
| Howard, Benj | | In Europe | To Ass't Surg., U. S. A., August, 1861. |

1ST ENGINEERS (Serrell's Engineers)—H. R. on file at S. G. O.; also at A. G. O.; none prior to 1863.—Mustered out June 30, 1865.

| | | | |
|---|---|---|---|
| Dalrymple, Aaron P | Surgeon | 337 W. 33d street, New York city. | To March, 1862. |
| Garry, James M | “ | Drummondville, Province of Ontario. | From November, 1864. |
| Mudge, Charles | “ | Phelps, N. Y | To October, 1864. |
| Fry, Chas. B | Ass't S | Mattoon, Ill | To June, 1865. |

15TH ENGINEERS (2 years, Sappers and Miners)—Mustered out June 25, 1863.

| | | | |
|---|---|---|---|
| Gibbs, Theron Z | Ass't S | Fort Ann, N. Y. | |
| McNair, James | Surgeon | Dead. | |
| Mudie, Archibald F | Ass't S | 557 Graham ave., Brooklyn, N. Y. | To Jan., 1862; also 3d L. Art. and 4th H. Art. |
| Cochrane, Adam H | “ | San Jose, Cal. | From August, 1862. |

15TH ENGINEERS—Mustered out July 2, 1865.

| | | | |
|---|---|---|---|
| Groat, Cornelius A | Ass't S | Cato, N. Y | From January, 1865. |
| Sualm, Wm. F | “ | 90 La Fayette avenue, Brooklyn, N. Y. | From January, 1865. |
| Gibbs, Theron Z | Surgeon | Fort Ann, N. Y | From August, 1863. |
| Gleason, James H | Ass't S | Syracuse, N. Y | To December, 1864 |

50TH ENGINEERS—(Stuart's Engineers)—Mustered out June 13, 1865. Many men of this regiment were treated in hospital of the 15th Engineers.

| | | | |
|---|---|---|---|
| Baum, A. Clark | Ass't S | Four Mile, N. Y | To January, 1865. |
| Hewitt, Chas. N | Surgeon | Red Wing, Minn | A. W. M. H. R. U. S. Ex. S. |
| Reynolds, R. M | Ass't S | Motor, Kan | From February, 1865. H. R. |
| Potter, Hazzard A | Surgeon | Dead. | |
| Beers, Louis V | Ass't S | | From March, 1863. |
| Hillary, Michael | “ | Saint Stephen's Green, Dublin, Ireland. | To February, 1863. |

NEW YORK—Continued.

1ST INFANTRY—(National Guard)—Mustered out May 25, 1863.

Van Steenburg, W...Ass't S.....Cohoes, N. Y................To 55th Infantry October, 1862.
Howe. John...............Surgeon...Dead.
Carrier, Jos.............Ass't S.......................................To April, 1863.
Benedict, Abel C......     "     .......................................To April, 1863.
Hicks, J. L..............Surgeon...Flushing, N. Y.. ...........To November, 1861.

2D INFANTRY—(1st Troy Regiment)—Mustered out May 26, 1863.

Bontecou, Reed B....Surgeon...Troy, N. Y....................To Surgeon U. S. A. September, 1861. Ex. S.
*McLean, LeRoy....     "     Troy, N. Y....................From January, 1863; also 21st Cav.
Whiton, Henry B.....Ass't S.....Troy, N. Y....................To 60th Inf. Sept., 1863.
Catlin, Benj. S........     "     Dead..........................From August, 1862; also 21st Cavalry.
Camp, Nathan H......     "     Troy, N. Y....................From March, 1863.

3D INFANTRY—(1st Albany Regiment)—Mustered out May 21, 1863, and August 28, 1865.

Johnson, Leonard M..Surgeon...Greene, N. Y.................To August, 1864.
Sullivan, John H......Ass't S.....Haverstraw, N. Y.........Dismissed July, 1865.
Hoff, Alexander H...Surgeon...Dead..............................To September, 1861.
Palmer, John M......     "     Dead.
McDermott, Wm. J..     "     .......................................To 66th Infantry October, 1861.
Van Rensler, J. J.....     "     New Brighton, N. Y......To September, 1862.
Stearns, Chas. W......     "     .......................................To May, 1863.

4TH INFANTRY—(1st Scott Life Guards)—Mustered out May 25, 1863.

Douglass, Geo. C......Ass't S.....Salt Lake City, Utah......From December, 1862.
Lovejoy, Geo. W......Surgeon...646 Palace street, Montreal, Canada. A. W. M.
Welch, Abraham......Ass't S.....Maysville, Colo..............From June, 1862; also 21st Cav. Dead.
Wainright, D. W......Surgeon.......................................To June, 1862.

5TH INFANTRY—(1st Duryea's Zouaves)—Part mustered out May 14, 1863; the rest transferred to 146th Infantry.

Gilbert, Rufus H......Surgeon...New York City..............To Surg. U. S. A. August, 1861.
Freeman, John N.....Ass't S.....80 Hanson Place, Brooklyn, N. Y. From September, 1862.
May, Henry C.........Surgeon...Corning, N. Y................To August, 1862.
Grimes, F. S............Ass't S.......................................From August, 1862.
Doolittle, Frank W...Surgeon.......................................From August, 1862; also 5th Veterans.
Martin, B. Ellis........Ass't S.......................................To February, 1862.
Van Ingen, Jas L.....Surgeon.......................................Dismissed February, '62.

5TH INFANTRY—(Veteran Volunteers)—Mustered out August 21, 1865.

Robinson, John A.....Ass't S.....269 Herkimer st., Brooklyn, N. Y. From October, 1864.
Smith, Orsamus.......Surgeon.......................................From April, 1864.
Doolittle, Frank W...     "     .......................................Missing August 31, 1863.

---

*Adjutant-General's report says McLane, Henry.

## NEW YORK—Continued.

### 6TH INFANTRY—(Wilson's Zouaves)—Mustered out June 25, 1863.

| Name | Rank | Address | Remarks |
|---|---|---|---|
| Pease, Philo C | Surgeon | | From May, 1861. |
| Lynch, Edward | Ass't S. | | From May, 1861. |
| Paterson, Franklin | " | | From December, 1862. |

### 7TH INFANTRY—(2 years)—Steuben Rifles—Mustered out May 8, 1863.

| Name | Rank | Address | Remarks |
|---|---|---|---|
| Gray, Charles | Surgeon | Dead. | |
| Moeller, Edward | Ass't S. | Dead. | |
| Staehly, B. F. | " | | To September, 1862. |
| Jacekh, Gottlieb | " | | To October, 1861. |
| Eisenlord, A. M. T. | Surgeon | | To October, 1862. |
| Nagel, Christopher | Ass't S. | | Dismissed January, 1863. |

### 7TH INFANTRY—Mustered out August 4, 1865.

| Name | Rank | Address | Remarks |
|---|---|---|---|
| Reuss, Peter J | Surgeon | 129 Thompson st,, New York City. | From September, 1864; also 52d Infantry. |
| Buck, Julius | Ass't S. | | From March, 1865. |
| Rodenroth, Albert | " | | Dismissed July 24, 1865. |

### 8TH INFANTRY—(1st German Rifles)—Mustered out April 23, 1863.

| Name | Rank | Address | Remarks |
|---|---|---|---|
| Legler, Theo. H | Ass't S. | | Dismissed Aug., 27, 1862. |
| Frohlich, Mertz | Surgeon | Dead. | |
| Tissot, Max | Ass't S. | Dead. | |
| Welker, Rudolph | Surgeon | | To July, 1861. |
| Krauter, John L | Ass't S. | 742 Flushing avenue, Brooklyn, N. Y. | From October, 1862. |

### 9TH INFANTRY—(1st Hawkins Zouaves)—Mustered out May 20, 1863.

| Name | Rank | Address | Remarks |
|---|---|---|---|
| Humphreys, Geo. H. | Surgeon | 18 W. 10th street, New York city. | From May, 1861. |
| Harding, Wm. L. | Ass't S. | 191 Hudson street, New York city. | A. W. M. |
| White, John P. P. | " | 31 W. 21st street, New York city. | To 10th Inf. May, 1862. |

### 10TH INFANTRY—(National Zouaves)—Mustered out June 30, 1865.

The sick of this regiment were treated in post hospital, Fortress Monroe, in 1861–'62. Report of regimental surgeon on file at Surgeon-General's Office. This regiment had a company J, which was an Engineer corps, commanded by Sergeant William H. Johnson.

| Name | Rank | Address | Remarks |
|---|---|---|---|
| White, John P. P. | Surgeon | 31 W. 21st street, New York city. | Also 9th Inf. |
| Craig, Robert O | " | | From March, 1865; also 148th Inf. |
| Baker, Chas. H | Ass't S. | Jamaica, N. Y. | From January, 1865. |
| Gesner, Brower | Surgeon | | To February, 1865; also 38th Inf. |
| Hunt, John W | " | | To May, 1862. |
| Van Duser, A. E | Ass't S. | Poughkeepsie, N. Y. | To May, 1863. |
| Smith, Orasmus | " | | To May, 1863. |
| Doolittle, Frank W | " | | To 5th Inf. August, 1862. |

### 11TH INFANTRY—(1st Fire Zouaves)—Mustered out June 2, 1862.

| Name | Rank | Address | Remarks |
|---|---|---|---|
| Mitchell, Henry A | Ass't S. | San Francisco, Cal. | To July, 1861. |
| Gray, Chas | Surgeon | Dead. | |
| Forshee, John M | Ass't S. | | A. W. M. |

## NEW YORK—Continued.

12TH INFANTRY—(Independence Guard, Onondaga Regiment)—Part mustered out May 17, 1863; the rest consolidated with 5th Veterans June 2, 1864.

| Name | Rank | Address | Service |
|---|---|---|---|
| Eddy, John L | Ass't S | Olean, N. Y | To May, 1863. |
| Pease, Roger W | Surgeon | Syracuse, N. Y | To August, 1861. |
| Skiff, George V | Ass't S | 24 W. 10th street, New York city. | To May, 1863; also 15th Cav. |
| Hill, Chas. E | A. Ass't S. | Syracuse or McGraw-ville, N. Y. | Private Co. I; also Ass't S. 13th and 188th Inf. |
| Hubbell, Chas. L | Surgeon | Troy, N. Y | To August, 1862. |
| Murphy, Chas. C | " | East Bloomfield, N. Y | To May, 1863. |
| Shipman, A. B | " | | To May, 1862; also 17th Inf. |
| Todd, Geo. B | Ass't S | | To October, 1862. |

13TH INFANTRY—(Rochester Regiment)—Part mustered out May 13, 1863, the rest transferred to 140th Infantry.

| Name | Rank | Address | Service |
|---|---|---|---|
| Avery, Geo. W | Ass't S | Norwich, N. Y | To October, 1862; also 94th Inf. |
| Little, David | Surgeon | Rochester, N. Y | From May, 1861. |
| Mullen, Isaac V | Ass't S | Alexander, N. Y | From August, 1862. |
| Hill, Chas. E | " | Syracuse or McGraw-ville, N. Y. | From November, 1862; also 188th Inf. |

14TH INFANTRY—(1st Oneida Regiment)—Mustered out May 24, 1863.

| Name | Rank | Address | Service |
|---|---|---|---|
| West, Joseph E | Surgeon | Utica, N. Y | To 28th Inf. November, 1862. |
| Churchill, Alonzo | " | Dead. | |
| Shufelt, Philip W | Ass't S | | From August, 1862. |
| Ingraham, Sam'l | " | Palmyra, N. Y | From January, 1863. |

15TH INFANTRY—(See 15th Engineers.)

16TH INFANTRY—(1st Northern New York Regiment)—Mustered out May 22, 1863.

| Name | Rank | Address | Service |
|---|---|---|---|
| Pardee, Chas. L | Ass't S | 172 W. 35th street, New York city. | From September, 1862. |
| Moore, John E | " | Dead. | |
| Crandall, Wm. B | Surgeon | | From May, 1861. |
| Murphy, C. C | Ass't S | | To January, 1863. |

17TH INFANTRY—(2 years)—(Westchester Chasseurs)—Mustered out June 2, 1863, except Company G, transferred to 12th Infantry.

| Name | Rank | Address | Service |
|---|---|---|---|
| Goff, I. Newton | Ass't S | Cazenovia, N. Y | From August, 1862. |
| Weed, Hiland A | " | Jordan, N. Y | To 25th Inf. December, 1861. |
| Shipman, A. B | " | | To 12th Inf. September, 1861. |
| Tice, Lewis | " | | A. W. M. |
| Stewart, James C | Surgeon | Dead. | |

17TH INFANTRY—(Union Sharpshooters, part)—Mustered out July 13, 1865.

| Name | Rank | Address | Service |
|---|---|---|---|
| Stuart, James G | Surgeon | Syracuse, N. Y | To January, 1865. |
| Watson, James L | " | 9 Elm Place, Brooklyn, N. Y. | From March, 1865. |
| Breckaw, Marcus F. | Ass't S | Dead. | |
| Davis, Geo. W | " | Dead. | |

### 18TH INFANTRY—(New York State Rifles)—Mustered out May 28, 1863.

| Name | Rank | Address | Remarks |
|---|---|---|---|
| Bartholf, John H | Ass't S | Care A. G. U. S. A | From October, 1862; now Ass't Surgeon U. S. A. |
| Edmerston, Alex. A. | " | Dead. | |
| Mattimore, Frank I. | " | | From August, 1862. |
| Rice, Nathan P | Surgeon | Custom House, New York city, N. Y. | A. W. M. |

### 19TH INFANTRY—(See 3d Light Artillery.)

### 20TH INFANTRY—(United Turner Rifles)—Mustered out June 1, 1863.

| Name | Rank | Address | Remarks |
|---|---|---|---|
| Steinart, Geo | Ass't S | 207 E. 123d st, N. Y. city. | From August, 1862. |
| Oliver, Alfred S. | " | | To February, 1863. |
| Hausen, Julius | Surgeon | | A. W. M. |
| Heiland, Chas | Ass't S | | Dismissed Oct., 1862. |

### 21ST INFANTRY—(1st Buffalo Regiment, 74th Militia, N. G.)—Mustered out May 18, 1863.

| Name | Rank | Address | Remarks |
|---|---|---|---|
| French, Seth | Surgeon | Sanford, Fla | From Aug., 1863; also 35th Inf. |
| Johnson, T. M | Ass't S | 10 S. Division st., Buffalo, N. Y. | From December, 1862. |
| Peters, Joseph A | " | 222 E. 122d st., N. Y. city. | To 6th Cavalry Oct., 1862. |
| Gibbs, Orestes C | Surgeon | Frewsburgh, N. Y | To January, 1863. |
| Fry, Chas. B | Ass't S | Mattoon, Ill | From April, 1862. |

### 22D INFANTRY—(2d Northern N. Y. Regiment, 2d Troy Regiment)—Mustered out June 19, 1863.

| Name | Rank | Address | Remarks |
|---|---|---|---|
| Holden, Austin W | Ass't S | Glens Falls, N. Y. | Was Captain of Company F until Aug. 24, 1862. H. R. |
| Hutchinson, W. F | Surgeon | Providence, R I | Dismissed Nov., 1862. |
| Bissell, Elias L | " | Buffalo Plains, N. Y | From November, 1862. |
| Goodyear, Miles | Ass't S | | To January, 1863. |

### 23D INFANTRY—(Southern Tier Regiment)—Mustered out May 23, 1863

| Name | Rank | Address | Remarks |
|---|---|---|---|
| Madill, Wm. A | Surgeon | Archbald, Pa | From Aug., 1862. H. R. Charges fee. |
| Churchill, S | " | | To June, 1862. |
| Stilwell, Thos. A | Ass't S | | From September, 1862. |
| Taylor, Wm | " | | From October, 1862. |

### 24TH INFANTRY—(1st Oswego Regiment)—Mustered out May 29, 1863.

| Name | Rank | Address | Remarks |
|---|---|---|---|
| Murdock, Jas. B | Surgeon | Pittsburgh, Pa | From May, 1861. |
| Plumb, S. Hiram | Ass't S | Red Creek, N. Y | To November, 1862. |
| Reynolds, L | " | Oswego, N. Y | To 63d Inf. Jan., 1862. |
| Hall, John D | " | | From August, 1862. |
| Webb, E. Cook | " | Homœopathic Hospital, Ward's Island, N. Y. | From Jan., 1863; also 5th Cav. |

## NEW YORK—Continued.

### 25TH INFANTRY—(Kerrigan Union Rangers)—Mustered out July 10, 1863.

| Name | Rank | Address | Service |
|---|---|---|---|
| Weed, Hiland A | Surgeon | Jordan, N. Y | From Dec., 1861; also 17th Inf. |
| Tallmadge, W. A | Ass't S | Bradford, N. Y | To November, 1862. |
| Welch, Isaac L | " | | To April, 1863. |
| Murphy, Dan'l H | " | | To April, 1862. |
| O'Leary, C. B. | " | | To October, 1861. |
| Fisk, Samuel N | Surgeon | 89 5th street, Brooklyn, N. Y. | To December, 1861. |
| Phillip, Luther | Ass't S | | From December, 1862. |
| O'Neil, Jas. C | " | | Dismissed Sept., 1862. |

### 26TH INFANTRY—(2d Oneida Regiment)—Mustered out May 28, 1863.

| Name | Rank | Address | Service |
|---|---|---|---|
| Steele, Aaron J | Ass't S | 2825 Washington ave, St. Louis Mo. | To 38th Inf. Nov., 1862. |
| Coventry, W. B | Surgeon | | From May, 1861. |
| Searl, I. H | Ass't S | Onondaga, N. Y | From September, 1862. |

### 27TH INFANTRY—Mustered out May 31, 1863.

| Name | Rank | Address | Service |
|---|---|---|---|
| Barnes, Norman S | Surgeon | 712 Carroll avenue, Chicago, Ill | From May, 1861. |
| Morse, Barnett W | Ass't S | Elmira, N. Y | To July, 1862. |
| Steuart, Wm. H | " | | From August, 1862. |

### 28TH INFANTRY—(Niagara Rifles)—Mustered out June 2, 1863.

| Name | Rank | Address | Service |
|---|---|---|---|
| Cushing, Thos | Ass't S | Brooklyn, N. Y | To March, 1862. |
| Helmer, A. M | Surgeon | Waukesha, Wis | To November, 1862. |
| Paine, R. T., Jr | Ass't S | Lockport, N. Y | From December, 1861. |
| West, Joseph E | Surgeon | Utica, N. Y | From Nov. 1862; also 14th Inf. |
| Regan, M. F | Ass't S | Dead. | |

### 29TH INFANTRY—(1st Astor—German Regiment)—Part mustered out June 20, 1863; the rest transferred to 68th Infantry.

| Name | Rank | Address | Service |
|---|---|---|---|
| Balser, Wm | Surgeon | 218 E. 13th street, N. Y. city. | From Jan., 1863; also 15th H. Art. and 62d Inf. |
| Herman, August | Ass't S | 241 E. 49th street, N. Y. city. | To October, 1862. |
| Thormain, Robt | Surgeon | | From Jan., 1863; also 58th Inf. |
| Neuhaus, Chas | " | | To November, 1862. |
| Osborn, Chas. H | Ass't S | 320 W. 35th st., N. Y. city, N. Y. | To January, 1862. |

### 30TH INFANTRY—(2d Astor Regiment)—Part mustered out June 18, 1863; the rest transferred to the 76th Infantry.

| Name | Rank | Address | Service |
|---|---|---|---|
| Chapin, F. L. R | Surgeon | Glens Falls, N. Y | From June, 1861. |
| Deering, Roger M | Ass't S | Dead | |
| Hawks, H. T. | " | 45 E. 30th street, N. Y. city. | From August, 1862. |
| Prentice, Fowler | " | | To 73d Inf. March, 1862. |
| Skilton, Julius | " | | To 87th Inf. Jan., 1862. |

## NEW YORK—Continued.

### 31ST INFANTRY—(Montezuma Battalion)—Mustered out June 4, 1863.

Damainville, L. A....Surgeon...245 W. 52d st., N. Y. city..From November, 1862.
Hamilton, Frank H... " 34 W. 32d st., N. Y. city..To September, 1861; also Lt. 16th Inf.
Stewart, Jos. D........Ass't S.....Fort Miller, N. Y..........To January, 1663.
Pray, O. M............. " ........................................From February, 1863.
*Rippey, John N...... " Lancaster, Ohio.............From January, 1863.

### 32D INFANTRY—(1st California Regiment)—Mustered out July 9, 1863.

Scoon, James H........Ass't S.....Amsterdam, N. Y..........From August, 1862.
Little, W. R..............Surgeon...Dead.
Totten, Gilbert T.....Ass't S...........................................A. W. M.

### 33D INFANTRY—(Ontario Regiment: Company G was called Richmond Guards; Company C, Waterloo Light Guards)—Mustered out June 2, 1863.

Curran, Richard......Ass't S....Rochester, N. Y............From August, 1862.
Dickerson, DeE.......Surgeon...Kansas City, Mo...........A. W. M.
Mulford, S. S........... " 47 W. 31st st, N. Y. city..To November, 1862.
McLachlen, D..........Ass't S..................................................From December, 1862.
Spencer, T. Rush.... Surgeon.................................................To August, 1861.

### 34TH INFANTRY—(Herkimer Regiment)—Mustered out June 30, 1863.

Manley, B. S............Surgeon...Potsdam, N. Y.............From May, 1863.
Knight, Jos. H.........H. Stew...Burgh Hill, Ohio............Mustered out with regiment.
Walter, E. S.............Ass't S.....Dead. To November, 1862.
Sherman, S. N.........Surgeon...Dead.
Miller, J. Hovey.......Ass't S..................................................From December, 1862.

### 35TH INFANTRY—(Jefferson County Regiment)—Mustered out June 5, 1863.

Carpenter, J. B........Ass't S....Gouverneur, N. Y.........To January, 1863.
French, Seth............ " Sanford, Fla.................To 21st Inf. Feb., 1863.
Van Slyck, DeW. C..Surgeon...Cincinnati, Ohio............From June, 1861.
Goodrich, Benj. F.....Ass't S..................................................From May, 1863.

### 36TH INFANTRY—(Washington Volunteers)—Mustered out July 15, 1863.

Hall, Wm. H............Ass't S.....Saratoga Springs, N. Y...A. W. M.
Utter, Albert........... " ........................................To January, 1863.
Dalton, Edward B...Surgeon..................................................To April, 1863.
Mosely, N. R........... " ........................................To Brig. Surg. Oct., 1861.
Radzinsky, L. D......Ass't S.....Mc Keesport, Pa............To December, 1861; also 104th U. S. C. T.

### 37TH INFANTRY—(Irish Rifles)—Mustered out June 22, 1863.

†O'Meagher, Wm......Surgeon...140 E. 117th st., N. Y. city. From October, 1862.
‡Moore, Abraham......................289 Camp st., New Orleans, La.
Schermerhorn, W. B..Ass't S.....Middleville, N. Y..........From September, 1862.
McNulty, John.........Surgeon...344 W. 21st st., N. Y. city, N. Y. To Brig. Surg. Oct., 1861.

---

*Ripper in A. G. R.
†Has list of casualties at Malvern Hill, July 1, 1862.
‡Says he was made Assistant Surgeon after battle of Fair Oaks. Not in A. G. R. as Assistant Surgeon or A. G. of N. Y.

## NEW YORK—Continued.

38TH INFANTRY—(Second Scott Life Guards)—Part mustered out June 22, 1863, the rest transferred to 40th Infantry. The 55th Infantry were consolidated with this regiment December 23, 1862.

| Name | Rank | Address | Service |
|---|---|---|---|
| Devendorf, C. A | Ass't S | Amsterdam, N. Y. or 358 Woodward st., Detroit, Mich. | To June, 1863; also 48th Inf. |
| Robinson, John A | " | 1218 Fulton st., Brooklyn, N. Y. | From September, 1862. |
| Steele, Aaron J | Surgeon | 2825 Washington st., St. Louis, Mo. | From November, 1862; also 26th Inf. |
| Berry, Abraham J | " | Dead. | |
| Gesner, Brower | Ass't S | | To November, 1862; also 10th Inf. |

39TH INFANTRY—(Garibaldi Guards)—Mustered out July 1, 1865.

| Name | Rank | Address | Service |
|---|---|---|---|
| Goodwin, W. W | Ass't S | Brownsville, N. Y. | To April, 1865. |
| Hoyt, Chas. S | Surgeon | Canandaigua, N. Y | From May, 1864; also 126th Inf. |
| Steiger, Emil | Ass't S | Prairie du Chien, Wis | To February, 1864. |
| Wolf, Frederick | Surgeon | St. Louis, Mo | To April, 1864. Dead. |
| Day, Ebenezer | Ass't S | Grand Tower, Ill | To 78th Inf. Sept., 1863. |
| Zander, Leopold | Surgeon | | To December, 1861. |
| Ribbeck, Rudolph | Ass't S | | To May, 1863. |

40TH INFANTRY—(Constitution Guards, Mozart Regiment)—Mustered out July, 1864, and June 27, 1865.

| Name | Rank | Address | Service |
|---|---|---|---|
| Loy, Sam'l N | H. Stew | Aberdeen, Ohio. | |
| Dexter, James E | Surgeon | 453 C st., N.W., Washing-ing, D. C. | To August, 1863. |
| Porter, Chas. H | Ass't S | Albany, N. Y | To February, 1863. |
| Rogers, Obadiah | " | Brockport, N. Y | To January, 1863. |
| Thompson, J. H | Surgeon | 36 E. 30th st., N. Y. city, N. Y. | To August, 1861. |
| Evans, Owen J | " | | From July, 1864. |
| Tobin, Walter | Ass't S | 919 DeKalb ave., Brooklyn, N. Y. | From May, 1863. |
| Campbell, A | Surgeon | | To June, 1864; also 148th Inf. |

41ST INFANTRY—(De Kalb Regiment)—In service August 31, 1865.

| Name | Rank | Address | Service |
|---|---|---|---|
| Shaw, Amos | Ass't S | Jacobstown, N. J | From December, 1862. |
| Brilliantowski, S | Surgeon | Dead. | |
| Sattler, Cornelius | " | Dead. | |
| Thomain, Robert | Ass't S | | To October, 1862. |

42D INFANTRY—(Jackson Guards, Tammany Regiment)—Part mustered out July 13, 1864; the rest transferred to 82d Infantry. H. R. on file at S. G. O.; also at A. G. O.

| Name | Rank | Address | Service |
|---|---|---|---|
| Burr, Wm. J | Surgeon | Newark Valley, N. Y | From May, 1863; also 59th Inf |
| Dinnin, Hugh | H. Stew | 3 Rector st., N. Y. City. | |
| Fossard, Geo. H | Ass't S | Port Jervis, N. Y | To March, 1863; also 56th and 146th Inf. |
| Sawyer, P. R. H | " | Bedford, N. Y | From July, 1863. |
| Osborne, John D | Surgeon | | To April, 1863. |
| Parker, Geo. B | Ass't S | 51 W. 9th st., New York City, N. Y. | To Ass't S. U. S. V. August, 1863. |

## NEW YORK—Continued.

### 43D INFANTRY—(Albany and Yates Rifles)—Mustered out June 27, 1865.

| | | | |
|---|---|---|---|
| Case, Meigs | Surgeon | 17 5th st. S E., Washington, D. C. | To March, 1864. |
| Carpenter, Henry H. | " | Lawrenceville, N. Y. | From March, 1865; also 106th Inf. |
| Norwood, D | H. Stew. | Esperance, N. Y. | M. D. G |
| Smith, Andrew H. | Ass't S. | 22 E. 42d st, or 110 E. 38th st., N. Y. City. | To 94th Inf May, 1862. |
| Eting, Van Vechten | " | Tremont, N. Y. City | To Sept., 1864 Ex. S. |
| Vaughan, C. H. | Surgeon | Des Moines, Iowa | To March, 1865; also 96th Inf. |
| Black, James W. | Ass't S. | Bath, N. Y. | To December, 1862. |
| Thomson, James H. | Surgeon | | To December, 1861. |
| Uglow, James | Ass't S. | Dead. | To 26th U. S. C. T. January, 1864. |

### 44TH INFANTRY—(Ellsworth Avengers, People's Ellsworth Regiment)—Part mustered out October 11, 1864; the rest transferred to 140th and 146th Infantry.

| | | | |
|---|---|---|---|
| Bissell, Elias L. | Ass't S. | Buffalo Plains, N. Y. | To November, 1862. |
| Frothingham, Wm. | Surgeon | St. Nicholas avenue and 157th st., N. Y. City. | Dismissed November, '62. |
| Spencer, D. Carlton | Ass't S. | Augusta, Wis. | From October, 1862. |
| Townsand, M. W. | Surgeon | Bergen, N. Y. | From December, 1862; also 47th Inf. |
| Fearn, Herbert | Ass't S. | Dead. | |

### 45TH INFANTRY—(5th German Rifles)—Transferred to 58th Infantry June 30, 1865.

| | | | |
|---|---|---|---|
| Philler, Hugo | Ass't S. | Waukesha, Wis. | A. W. M. |
| Weise, F. | H. Stew. | Nashville, Tenn. | |
| Feldsbauch, Philip | Ass't S. | | To November, 1862. |
| Rebay, Geo. | " | | A. W. M. |
| Ideler Herman | Surgeon | Dead. | |
| Schoeckel, J. V. F. | " | | From June, 1863, to June, 1865; also 118th Inf. |

### 46TH INFANTRY—(Fremont Rifle Regiment)—Mustered out July 28, 1865.

| | | | |
|---|---|---|---|
| Haak, John W. | Ass't S. | Meadville, Pa. | To January, 1864. |
| Hoevet, Henry | Surgeon | San José, Cal. | To December, 1863. |
| Porteous, Jas. G. | " | Luzerne, N. Y. | From November, 1864; also 118th Inf. |
| Ohnesong, Gustav | Ass't S | | To April, 1865. |

### 47TH INFANTRY—(Imperial Zouaves (part) and Washington Grays)—Mustered out August 30, 1865.

| | | | |
|---|---|---|---|
| Baker, Clarence M. | Ass't S. | 41 Washington Square, S., N. Y. City. | From January, 1864. |
| Smith, Wm. A. | Surgeon | 276 Broad st., Newark, N. J. | From January, 1864 |
| Townsand, M. W. | " | Bergen, N. Y. | To January, 1862; also 44th Infantry. |
| Young, Wm. S. | Ass't S. | Johnstown, N. Y. | To June, 1865. |
| White, Whitman V. | " | 1321 4th ave., N. Y. City. | To December, 1861. |
| Tanner, Wm. H. | Surgeon | Wassaic, N. Y. | To January, 1863. |
| Sickler, Peter E. | " | Dead. | |

## NEW YORK—Continued.

### 48TH INFANTRY—(Continental Guards)—Mustered out September 1, 1865.

| Name | Rank | Address | Remarks |
|---|---|---|---|
| Devendorf, Chas. A. | Surgeon | Amsterdam, N.Y., or 358 Woodward st., Detroit, Mich. | From October, 1864; also 38th and 55th Inf. |
| Humphreys, P. H. | Ass't S. | San Francisco, Cal | To 58th Inf. August, '63. |
| Mulford, Joseph L. | Surgeon | New Brunswick, N. J. | To September, 1864; now U. S. A. |
| Throop, J. Mott | Ass't S. | Lebanon, N. Y. | From May, 1864. |
| Sickler, Peter E. | " | Dead. | |

### 49TH INFANTRY—(2d Buffalo Regiment; Company C was Palmer's Fremont Rifles)—Mustered out June 27, 1865.

| Name | Rank | Address | Remarks |
|---|---|---|---|
| Pickett, John H. | Ass't S. | Elizabeth, N. J. | To October, 1864. |
| Jenkins, John | Surgeon | Shelby, N. Y. | From November, 1864. |
| Hall, James A. | " | Dead. | |
| Potter, Wm. W. | Ass't S. | Dead. | |

### 50TH INFANTRY—(See 50th Engineers, page ——.)

### 51ST INFANTRY—(Shepard's Rifles; two companies were Scott Rifles and two companies were Union Rifles)—Mustered out July 25, 1865.

| Name | Rank | Address | Remarks |
|---|---|---|---|
| Buck, Ephraim W. | Surgeon | Bergen, N. J. | To May, 1862. |
| Bliss, Lyman W. | " | Saginaw City, Mich. | From October, 1863. |
| Dodge, John L. | " | Groton, Conn. | To October, 1862. |
| Leonard, W. H. | " | Worcester, N. Y. | To August, 1863. |
| Vanderhoof, F. D. | Ass't S. | Phelps, N. Y. | To June, 1865. |
| Bird, Francis W. | " | 305 Degrow street, New York City, N. Y. | To October, 1864. |
| Tomey, Chas. W. | " | | To November, 1861. |

### 52D INFANTRY—(German Rangers or Sigel Rifles)—Mustered out July 1, 1865.

| Name | Rank | Address | Remarks |
|---|---|---|---|
| Rappold, Julius C. | Surgeon | 750 Flushing ave., Brooklyn, N. Y. | To November, 1863. |
| Reuss, Peter J. | Ass't S. | 129 Thompson st., New York city. | To December, 1862; also 7th Inf. |
| Frolick, Moritz | Surgeon | Dead. | |
| Bingel, G. A. | Ass't S. | 96 Ten Eyck st., Brooklyn, N. Y. | To March, 1864. |
| Jacobi, Gustavus | " | | To September, 1863. |
| Stieberling, Geo. C. | Surgeon | 45 St. Marks Place, New York city. | To July, 1862 |
| Kaier, Jos. C. | " | | From June, 1865. |
| Althaus, Chas. | Ass't S. | | From March, 1865. |
| Weiler, Ernst | Surgeon | | Dismissed March, 1865. |

### 53D INFANTRY—(De Epineuil Zouaves)—Mustered out March 21, 1862.

| Name | Rank | Address | Remarks |
|---|---|---|---|
| Ewen, Clarence | Ass't S. | Care A. G. U. S. A. | To September, 1862. Not in A. G. R. |
| Phillips, Henry J. | Surgeon | Care A. G. U. S. A. | From October, 1861. Died in 1879. |
| Vanderkeift, B. A. | Ass't S. | Dead. | |
| Dubrieul, Jules | " | | To December, 1861. |

NEW YORK—Continued.

54TH INFANTRY—(Schwarze Jaegers)—In service August 31, 1865.

| Name | Rank | Address | Service |
|---|---|---|---|
| Hagen, Chas. W | Surgeon | 154 Springfield avenue, Newark, N. J. | To October, 1864. |
| Pfifer, Nicholas | Ass't S | 32 Stanton street, New York city. | From October, 1864 |
| Root, Henry | Surgeon | Whitehall, N. Y. | To 58th Inf. Jan , 1863. Mustered out August 1, 1866. |
| Krause, Louis | Ass't S | | To March, 1864 |
| Bott, Frederick | " | La Fargeville, N. Y | To September, 1864. |

55TH INFANTRY—(Lafayette Guard)—Consolidated with the 38th Infantry December 23, 1862.

| Name | Rank | Address | Service |
|---|---|---|---|
| Artand, Theodore | Ass't S | Barrancas, Fla | To September, 1862. |
| Cleveland, Warner | " | Fort Edward, N. Y | From October, 1862, to December, 1862. |
| Devendorf, Chas. A. | " | Amsterdam, N. Y., or 358 Woodward street, Detroit, Mich. | From December, 1862; also 38th and 48th Inf. |
| Van Steenberg, W | Surgeon | Cohoes, N. Y | A. W. M.; also 1st Inf. |
| Petard, Felix | " | | To September, 1862. |

56TH INFANTRY—(Tenth Legion)—In service August 31, 1865.

| Name | Rank | Address | Service |
|---|---|---|---|
| Bradner, Ira S | Ass't S | Middletown, N. Y | From May, 1863. |
| Fossard, Geo. H | Surgeon | Port Jervis, N. Y | To July, 1865; also 42d and 146th Inf. |
| Hardenburg, D. S | Ass't S | Jersey City, N. J | To April, 1865. |
| Turner, A. S | " | 1505 N. Broad st., Philadelphia, Pa | To 103d Inf. November, 1863. |
| Van Etten, Solomon | Surgeon | Port Jervis, N. Y | To September, 1864. |
| Carroll, O. A | Ass't S | Port Jervis, N. Y | Died May, 1879. |

57TH INFANTRY—(National Guard Rifles)—Transferred to 61st Infantry December 2, 1864.

| Name | Rank | Address | Service |
|---|---|---|---|
| McKinn, Robert V | Surgeon | New York city | To December, 1862. |
| Potter, Wm. W | " | Dead. | |
| Winn, T. B | Ass't S | | From July, 1864; also 61st Inf. |
| Neeley, Nelson | " | | To June, 1864. |
| Corry, Robert | " | | To September, 1863. |
| Leach, Geo | Surgeon | | To January, 1862. |
| Dean, Henry C | Ass't S | | To 140th Inf April, 1863. |

58TH INFANTRY—(Polish Legion)—In service August 31, 1865.

| Name | Rank | Address | Service |
|---|---|---|---|
| Humphreys, P. H | Surgeon | San Francisco, Cal | From October, 1863; also 48th Inf. |
| Stein, Chas | Ass't S | 5 Delancey Place, New York city. | From May, 1862. |
| Mücke, Francis | Surgeon | 242 E. 119th street, New York city. | Dismissed Nov., 1862. |
| Haerl, Francis | Ass't S | | To March, 1864. |
| Hessel, Ferdinand | Surgeon | | To April, 1862 |
| Thorman, Robert | " | | To January, 1863; also 29th Inf. |
| Root, Henry | " | Whitehall, N. Y | To October, 1863; also 54th Inf. Mustered out August 1, 1866. |

## NEW YORK—Continued.

59TH INFANTRY—(U. S. Vanguard, Union Guard)—Mustered out June 30, 1865.

| | | | |
|---|---|---|---|
| Burr, Wm. J | Ass't S | Newark Valley, N. Y | To 42d Infantry May, 1863. |
| Darbey, Wm. J | " | 1055 3d ave., New York city. | From February, 1864; also 82d Inf |
| Plumb, S. Hiram | Surgeon | Red Creek, N. Y | Died August, 1880. |
| Uhlein, S P | Ass't S | Kilbourn city, Wis | To April, 1862. |
| Hughes, Jas. W | " | | To 152d Infantry April, 1865. |
| Duane, Henry C | " | | To July, 1863. |
| Myers, John T | Surgeon | Dead | To June, 1864. |
| Colgan, Jos. P | " | 329 Jay street, Brooklyn, N. Y. | To June, 1863. |
| Dougherty, Geo | Ass't S | | Dismissed August, 1863. |

60TH INFANTRY—(Ogdensburgh Regiment and 1st St. Lawrence Regiment)—Mustered out July 17, 1865.

| | | | |
|---|---|---|---|
| Chambers, Wm. B | Ass't S | Edmeston, N. Y | To March, 1863. |
| Gale, James S | Surgeon | Orwell, Vt | To January, 1863. |
| Whiton, Henry B | " | Troy, N. Y | To October, 1864; also 2d Inf. |
| Masses, Smith H | " | | From January, 1865. |
| Burbeck, Chas. H | Ass't S | 22 2d st., Troy, N. Y., or Brunswick, N. Y. | To 102d Inf. November, 1864. |
| Comfort, John E | " | Morrisania, N. Y | From January, 1865. |

61ST INFANTRY (Clinton Guard)—Mustered out July 14, 1865. H. R. on file at A. G. O. prior to April, 1863. H. R. on file at S. G. O; none prior to April, 1863.

| | | | |
|---|---|---|---|
| Tompkins, H. C | Ass't S | Knowlesville, N. Y | To February, 1863. |
| Vogel, Henry C | " | 799 De Kalb avenue, Brooklyn, N. Y. | From January, 1864; also chaplain. |
| Wallace, Theodore C | Surgeon | Cambridge, N. Y | To March, 1864; also 93d Inf |
| Wells, Samuel R | " | Waterloo, N. Y | To July, 1862. |
| Winn, T. B | Ass't S | | From July, 1864; also 57th Inf. |
| Fee, Samuel H | " | | To December, 1862. |
| Merrill, Andrew | " | | To March, 1862. |
| Snow, Asa B | Surgeon | | To February, 1862. |
| Rowland, M. C | " | | From April, 1864. |

62D INFANTRY—(Anderson's Zouaves)—Mustered out August 30, 1865.

| | | | |
|---|---|---|---|
| Balser, Wm | Ass't S | 218 E. 13th st., N. Y. city. | To 29th Inf., Dec., 1862; also 15th Heavy Artillery. |
| Simpson, Geo. B. F | Surgeon | 861 Broad st., Newark, N. J. | To December, 1863. |
| Reagles, James | Ass't S | | From April, 1864. |
| Grimes, Francis S | Surgeon | | To June, 1864. |
| Biblack, Wm. W | Ass't S | | To April, 1863. |
| Bamber, Alex | " | | To April, 1863. |

## NEW YORK—Continued.

63D INFANTRY (Independent Irish Regiment, 3d Regiment Irish Brigade, and Kings County Regiment)—Mustered out June 30, 1865.

| | | | |
|---|---|---|---|
| Elliott, Samuel R | Ass't S | 32 Waverly Place, N. Y. city. | To December, 1862. |
| Reynolds, Lawrence | Surgeon | Oswego, N. Y | From Feb., 1862; also 24th Inf. |
| Smart, Chas | Ass't S | Care of A. G., U. S. A | To Ass't Surg., U. S. A., March, 1864. |
| Gilligan, Michael F | " | 178 Sacket st., Brooklyn, N. Y. | To February, 1862. |
| Hall, Henry D | " | Glen Cove, N. Y | To February, 1863. |
| Ruggles, A. D | " | 230 W. 38th street, New York city. | To July, 1862. |
| Purcell, Jas. J | " | 51 Henry street, New York city. | To June, 1863. |
| Shannahan, D. R | Surgeon | | To February, 1862. |
| Hilliard, Edw. D | Ass't S | | From July, 1864. |

64TH INFANTRY (Cattaraugus Regiment and 64th Militia, N. G.)—Mustered out July 14, 1865. H. R. on file at A. G. O. prior to March 20, 1864. H. R. on file at S. G. O.; none after March 20, 1864.

| | | | |
|---|---|---|---|
| Barr, Geo. W | Surgeon | Titusville, Pa | Dismissed Feb., 1863. |
| Kelsey, Chas. T | " | Mecklenburgh, N. Y | From January, 1865. |
| Kelsey, Dana E | " | | To December, 1864. |
| Russell, John | Ass't S | | From January, 1865. |

65TH INFANTRY—(1st U. S. Chasseurs)—Mustered out July 17, 1865.

| | | | |
|---|---|---|---|
| Grey, John W | Surgeon | Avon Springs, N. Y | To April, 1865; also 98th Inf |
| Kimball, Jas. P | Ass't S | Care of A. G., U. S. A | From January, 1865; also 121st Inf. Now Ass't Surg., U. S. A. |
| McDonald, Wm. O | " | 117 W. 44th street, New York city. | To 27th Connecticut Inf., January, 1863 |
| Stoddart, E. V | " | Rochester, N. Y | To September, 1864. |
| Rogers, John H | " | | Dismissed June, 1863. |
| Lambert, J. Leavitt | " | | From January, 1865. |
| Petheridge, John P | Surgeon | Dead. | |

66TH INFANTRY (Governor's Guard, 6th Militia)—Mustered out August 30, 1865.

| | | | |
|---|---|---|---|
| Wood, Chas. S | Surgeon | 171 W. 47th st., New York city. | To Surg. U. S. V., Sept., 1863. |
| Reno, Griffin | Ass't S | | To October, 1863. |
| McDermott, W. J | Surgeon | | To July, 1865; also 3d Inf. |
| Hewitt, Jas D | Ass't S | | To March, 1862. |
| Van Devere, Albert | Surgeon | Albany, N. Y | From July, 1864. |
| Douglass, Andrew | Ass't S | | From September, 1864. |

67TH INFANTRY (1st Long Island)—Part mustered out July 4, 1864; the rest transferred to 65th Infantry.

| | | | |
|---|---|---|---|
| Adams, Geo. F | Surgeon | St. Louis, Mo | From May, 1862. |
| Staats, Chas. P | Ass't S | Albany, N. Y | From January, 1863. |
| Bassett, Geo. D | " | | To December, 1862. |
| Baker, Lewis F | " | | To August, 1863. |

## NEW YORK—Continued.

### 68TH INFANTRY (Cameron Rifles)—In service August 31, 1865.

| Name | Rank | Address | Remarks |
|---|---|---|---|
| Denicke, Frederick | Ass't S. | 539 California st., San Francisco, Cal. | From July, 1865. |
| Schultz, Louis | Surgeon | 237 E. 34th st., N. Y. city | To March, 1865. |
| Reissberg, H. W | " | Dead. | |
| Laubli, Jacob | Ass't S. | | To November, 1863. |

### 69TH INFANTRY (1st Regiment Irish Brigade)—Mustered out June 30, 1865.

| Name | Rank | Address | Remarks |
|---|---|---|---|
| Meagher, Wm. O | Surgeon | 140 E. 117th street, N.Y. city. | From Jan , 1864. H. R. |
| Reed, James A | Ass't S. | 272 6th ave., N. Y. city | Dismissed March. 1863. |
| Smith, J. Pascal | Surgeon | | To January, 1863. |
| Crosby, A. H | Ass't S. | Lowville, N. Y | To March, 1865. |
| Purcell, Jas. J | " | | From June, 1865. |

### 70TH INFANTRY—(1st Excelsior)—Part mustered out July 1, 1864; the rest transferred to 86th Infantry.

| Name | Rank | Address | Remarks |
|---|---|---|---|
| Ash, James | Surgeon | 1824 Van Pelt st., Philadelphia Pa. | A. W. M. Also 71st Inf. |
| Brown, Harvey E | " | Care A. G. U. S. A. | To Dec., 1862. Now Ass't Surg. U. S. A. |
| Bennett, G. H | Ass't S. | Simco, N. Y | To March, 1863. |
| Dufloo, Armand | " | 55 W. 24th street, N. Y. city. | From June 1863; also 25th Cav. and Lieut. 53d Inf. |
| Tingley, Wm. H | Surgeon | | To August, 1861. |
| Moore, M. Price | Ass't S. | | To May, 1863. |

### 71ST INFANTRY—(2d Excelsior, Jackson's Light Infantry)—Part mustered out June 30, 1864; the rest transferred to 120th Infantry.

| Name | Rank | Address | Remarks |
|---|---|---|---|
| Ash, James | Ass't S. | 1824 Van Pelt st., Philadelphia, Pa. | To 70th Inf. May, 1863. |
| Younglove, John | " | Elizabeth, N. J | From November, 1862. |
| McAllister, Geo. | " | Dead. | |
| McGovan, John J | Surgeon | Dead. | |
| Perkins, E. T | " | | From May, 1863; also 72d Inf. |

### 72D INFANTRY—(3d Excelsior)—Part mustered out ———, 1864; the rest transferred to 120th Infantry.

| Name | Rank | Address | Remarks |
|---|---|---|---|
| Leighton, N. W. | Ass't S. | 143 Taylor st., Brooklyn, N. Y. | To October, 1862. |
| Townsend, Geo. D | " | Boston, Mass. | Missing since Oct., 1863. |
| Simpson, F. W | " | | Dismissed May, 1864. |
| Perkins, E. T | " | | To 71st Inf. May, 1863. |
| Irwine, Chas. K | Surgeon | Dead. | |

### 73D INFANTRY—(4th Excelsior and 2d Fire Zouaves)—Mustered out June 29, 1865.

| Name | Rank | Address | Remarks |
|---|---|---|---|
| Adams, Oliver B | Ass't S. | Warsaw, N. Y | Missing since April, 1863. |
| Searl, I. N | Surgeon | Onondaga, N. Y | From June, 1865. |
| Ackley, G. J | Ass't S. | | From April, 1865. |
| Boswick, H. P | Surgeon | | To February, 1862. |
| Ridgway. Frank | Ass't S. | | To 74th Inf. July. 1863. |
| Prentice, Fowler | Surgeon | | To May, 1865; also 30th Inf. |

## NEW YORK—Continued.

**74TH INFANTRY**—(5th Excelsior)—Part mustered out June 26, 1864; the rest transferred to 40th Infantry.

Calhoun, Jas. T.......Surgeon...Dead.
Ridgeway, Frank..... " ........................From July, 1863; also 73d Inf.
Stewart, Jos. D........Ass't S.....Fort Miller, N. Y .........From June, 1863.
Kauffman, John F... " ........................To November, 1862.
Lodge, Chas.............Surgeon........................To May, 1863.
Masson, Louis .........Ass't S........................To June, 1862.

**75TH INFANTRY**—(Auburn Regiment)—Mustered out August 31, 1865. This regiment served as Mounted Infantry from November, 1863, to May 31, 1864.

Benedict, M. D ........Surgeon...Syracuse, N. Y..............To November, 1864.
Root, Wm. W......... " Mason, Mich........ .........From August, 1865.
Treadway, F. S.......Ass't S.....Dead........................To November, 1864.
Powers, Cyrus......... " Died March, 1880.
Blaisdell, Westley.... " Dead........................To July, 1863.

**76TH INFANTRY**—(Cortland County Regiment)—Part mustered out December, 1864; the rest transferred to 147th Infantry.

Barnes, Nelson R.....Ass't S.....Cincinnatus, N. Y.........To 184th Inf. Nov., 1864.
Fisbee, C. M............ " Brushland, N. Y............To March, 1863.
Hamilton, C. A........ " Savannah, N. Y............From May, 1863; transferred to 147th Inf. Jan., 1865; also 91st Inf.
Lakeman, Wm. H..... " Rochester, N. Y............Dismissed Nov., 1862.
Nelson, Judson C.....Surgeon...Truxton, N. Y.............To July, 1862.
Metcalf, Geo. W...... " Dead.

**77TH INFANTRY**—(Saratoga and Bemis Heights Regiment)—Mustered out June 27, 1865.

Perry, John L.........Surgeon...Saratoga Springs, N. Y...To January, 1862.
Stevens, Geo. T....... " 33 W. 33d street, N. Y. city. To Dec., 1864. H. R.
Thompson, J. G....... " Angola, N. Y................From December, 1864.
Fay, John W............Ass't S.....Detroit, Mich................To December, 1862.
De Long, Wm. A...... " 285 S 2d st., Brooklyn, N. Y. To December, 1864.
Campbell, A.............Surgeon........................To February, 1863.

**78TH INFANTRY**—(Cameron Highlanders)—Consolidated with the 102d Infantry June 29, 1864.

Fuller, Winfield S....Surgeon...Fairport, N. Y................From July, 1863, to June 1864.
Sheldon, A. F..........Ass't S.....Pultneyville, N. Y.........To October, 1862.
Day, Ebenezer......... " Grand Tower, Ill...........From July, 1863, to June, 1864; also 39th Inf.
Gray, Eldred P........Surgeon........................To September, 1864.
Day, Henry L .........Ass't S.....Arcade, N. Y...............To December, 1862.

**79TH INFANTRY**—(79th Militia, National Guard, Highlanders)—Mustered out July 14, 1865.

Heffron, Henry G..—H. Stew...Chicago, Ill..................Also Capt. Co. B and Lt. Col.
Fitch, Andrew T......Surgeon...Dead.
McDonald, J. E....... " Dead.
Norval, James......... " Dead.
Melville, Andrew......Ass't S........................To April, 1863.
McLetchie, A.......... " ........................To April, 1862.
Mead, Richard I...... " ........................To May, 1864.
McKay, David ......... " Dallas, Texas................To May, 1864; also 29th U. S. C. T.

NEW YORK—Continued.

80TH INFANTRY—(20th Militia and Ulster Guard)—In service August 31, 1865.

| Name | Rank | Residence | Service |
|---|---|---|---|
| Gates, Howard E | Ass't S | Ellenville, N. Y., or Litchfield, Conn. | To 189th Inf., Nov., 1864. |
| Loughran, R | Surgeon | Kingston, N. Y | From October, 1861. |
| Taylor, Wm | Ass't S | Canastota, N. Y | From July, 1863. |
| Tuthill, Robert K | " | Poughkeepsie, N. Y | To 145th Inf. April, 1863. |
| Humphrey, C. L | " | Spring Valley, N. Y | To June, 1865. |

81ST INFANTRY—(2d Oswego Regiment)—Mustered out August 31, 1865.

| Name | Rank | Residence | Service |
|---|---|---|---|
| Buck, Ephraim W | Ass't S | Bergen, N. J | To A. S. U. S. V. July, 1864. |
| Miller, J. N | Surgeon | Highland, N. Y | From March, 1865; also 120th Inf. |
| Macfarlane, C | Ass't S | Oswego, N. Y | To 115th Inf. Sept., 1863. |
| Oliver, John N | " | Essex, N. Y | From January, 1865. |
| Rice, Wm. H | Surgeon | Phœnix, N. Y | Died January, 1881. |
| Earl, Geo. W | Ass't S | Tully, N. Y | To March, 1863. |

82D INFANTRY (2d Militia)—Mustered out June 25, 1864; veterans and recruits transferred to the 59th Inf.

| Name | Rank | Residence | Service |
|---|---|---|---|
| Darbey, Wm. J | Ass't S | 1055 3d ave., N. Y. city | From Feb., 1864; also 59th Inf. |
| Ferguson, Jas. F | " | 5 Waverly Place, N. Y. city | To December, 1862. |
| Plumb S. H | Surgeon | Red Creek, N. Y | Died August, 1881. |
| Powell, Alfred | " | Dead. | |
| Lewis, Morgan L | Ass't S | | To October, 1863. |
| Fitch, Wm. R | " | | To October, 1863. |
| Lewis, Wm. C | Surgeon | | To July, 1862 |
| McCullough, J. R | Ass't S | | Dismissed Feb., 1864. |

83D INFANTRY—(9th Militia)—Mustered out August, 1864; veterans and recruits transferred to the 97th Inf.

| Name | Rank | Residence | Service |
|---|---|---|---|
| McFarland, S. F | Ass't S | Oxford, N. Y | To Oct., 1862; not in A. G. R. |
| Nordguist, C. J | Surgeon | Tuckahoe, N. Y | A. W. M. H. R. |
| Pinkney, Howard | Ass't S | 24 E. 41st st., N. Y. city | To December 1862. |
| Bigelow, J. R | Surgeon | Washington, D. C | To June, 1861. Not in A. G. R. |
| Ketcham, Abram | Ass't S | | To June, 1864. |

84TH INFANTRY—(Brooklyn Chasseurs and 14th Militia)—Mustered out June 2, 1864; veterans and recruits transferred to the 5th Veteran Infantry.

| Name | Rank | Residence | Service |
|---|---|---|---|
| Farley, Jas. M | Surgeon | 90 Pulaski st., Brooklyn, N. Y. | To June, 1863. |
| Fisher, John H | H. Stew | 90 Pulaski st., Brooklyn, N. Y. | |
| House, Alfred | Ass't S | Sycamore, Ill | To August, 1863. |
| Horniston, Jos. M | Surgeon | Dead. | |
| Larabee, David | " | Dead | |
| Swalm, Wm. F | Ass't S | 90 LaFayette ave., Brooklyn, N. Y. | To November, 1862. |
| Farley, Henry L | " | | To June, 1863. |
| Joslin, C. C | " | Johnstown, N. Y | To January, 1864. |
| Dewey, David B | " | | To April, 1863. |

## NEW YORK—Continued.

### 85TH INFANTRY—Mustered out June 27, 1865.

Helme, Thos..........Surgeon...Guilderland, N. Y..........From April, 1865; also 148th Inf.
Smith, Wm. M.......... " Angelica or Stapleton, N. Y. To June, 1863.
Lewis, John D..........Ass't S....Dead.
Palmer, John M....... " Dead.

### 86TH INFANTRY—(Steuben Rangers)—Mustered out June 27, 1865.

Bendoll, Herman......Surgeon...Albany, N. Y................To May, 1865.
Darrall, Clinton B...Ass't S....Morgan City, La............A. W. M.
Jemison, John S......Surgeon...Hornellsville, N. Y.........To Nov., 1864. H. R.
Wylie, Farand.........Ass't S.....Bath, N. Y.......................To Surg. 155th Inf. Oct., 1863.
Larabee, David........ " Dead.

### 87TH INFANTRY—(Brooklyn Rifles, 13th Militia)—Consolidated with the 40th Volunteers September 6, 1862.

Cleveland, Warren...Surgeon...Fort Edwards, N. Y......To January, 1862.
Knight, Wm............Ass't S..........................................From December, 1861.
Skilton, Julius A......Surgeon..........................................A. W. M. Also 30th Inf.

### 88TH INFANTRY—(5th Irish Brigade)—Mustered out June 30, 1865.

Reynolds, Frank......Surgeon...Care A. G. U. S. A.........To Aug., 1863; also 2d U. S. Vet. Inf. Retired.
Stillman, John T..... " Brookfield, N. Y............From Jan., 1865; also 147th Inf.
Powell, Richard...... " Died May, 1872.

### 89TH INFANTRY—(Dickinson Guard)—Mustered out August 3, 1865.

Allen, James............Ass't S.....Richford, N. Y...............To November, 1864.
Smith, Wm. A......... " 276 Broad st., Newark, N. J. To 103d Inf. Dec., 1862.
Squire, Truman H....Surgeon...Elmira, N. Y..................To May, 1865.
Shaw, M. E.............Ass't S..........................................To October, 1863.

### 90TH INFANTRY—(McClellan Rifles)—In service August 31, 1865.

Chapman, James......Ass't S.....Medina, N. Y..................To April, 1862.
Stub, Arnold............Surgeon...136 Dean st., Brooklyn, N. Y. From January, 1865.
Patterson, J. F.........Ass't S..........................................From April, 1865.
Hoffman, E. S.........Surgeon...Died in 1876.
Kinnie, Wm.............Ass't S.....Dead.
Kleine, Lewis.......... " ...........................................Dismissed March 15, 1865.

### 91ST INFANTRY—(Columbia County Regiment and McClellan Chasseurs)—Mustered out July 3, 1865.

Hamilton, Chas. A...Ass't S.....Savannah, N. Y............From May, 1863; also 142 Inf.
Hill, C. Judson....... " Utica, N. Y.....................To November, 1864.
Morris, Robert........Surgeon...Ogdensburgh, N. Y.......From December, 1861.
Myers, John T........Ass't S.....Dead.
Clunie, Wm............ " ...........................................To March, 1865.

## NEW YORK—Continued.

92D INFANTRY—(Excelsior Rifle Battalion, Potsdam Regiment, and 2d St. Lawrence Regiment)—Mustered out January 7, 1865.

Crukshank, W. H....Ass't S.....Lisbon Centre, N. Y......To September, 1862.
Thompson, Thomas.. " Mesilla, New Mexico......From June, 1864.
Edmerston, Alex. A..Surgeon...Dead.
Hewett, Henry....... " Dead.
Mansfield, Wm. Q....Ass't S.....Dead.
Clarke, Caleb ......... " ..............................To June, 1863.

93D INFANTRY—(Morgan's Rifles)—Mustered out June 29, 1865.

Bailey, Lorenzo W...Ass't S.....Mill Port, N. Y............From April, 1865.
Smith, Strabridge.....Surgeon...South America...............Probably dead.
Wallace, Theo. C......Ass't S.....Cambridge, N. Y..........To 61st Infantry March, 1863.
Crampton, Henry E.. " 221 2d avenue, New York City. To February, 1863.
Loomis, Alden......... " ..............................To February, 1863.
Wilcox, Francis M... " ..............................To May, 1864.

94TH INFANTRY—(Sackett's Harbor Regiment and Bell Jefferson Rifles)—H. R. on file at A. G. O. prior to 1864. H. R. on file at S. G. O.; none prior to 1864—Mustered out July 18, 1865.

Avery, George W.....Surgeon.. Norwich, N. Y..............To September, 1864; also 13th Inf.
*Chamberlain, D. C.. " Norwood, Mich.............To March, 1865.
Smith, Andrew H..... " 110 E. 38th street, New York City. To February, 1862; also 43d Infantry.
Derby, Edmund G...Ass't S.....Orange City, Fla...........To September, 1864.
Seymour, E. G......... " Hermon, N. Y...............To January, 1863.
De Wolfe, Dan'l O...H. Stew...Sackett's Harbor, N. Y.
Brown, John T........Ass't S.....Kerney, Junction, Nebr..To Assistant Surg. U. S. V. July, 1864.
Goodale, Charles......Surgeon...Dead.

95TH INFANTRY—(Warren Rifles)—Mustered out July 16, 1865.

Ramsay, Geo. M......Surgeon...Clokey, Pa....................From December, 1862.
Sloat, Spencer S...... " Haverstraw, N. Y..........To October, 1862.
Hadden, James........ " 202 W. 11th street, New York City. To August, 1862.
Sargent, Thos. B......Ass't S.......................................From February, 1864.
Sibley, James W...... " ..............................To September, 1862.

96TH INFANTRY—(Macomb Regiment, Plattsburg Regiment)—In service August 31, 1865.

Brady, Robert W......Surgeon...Honesdale, Pa................From July, 1865.
Hines, Marshall........Ass't S.....North Potsdam, N. Y.....To January, 1865.
Davignon, F. J........Surgeon.. Alleged dead.
Vaughan, C. H.........Ass't S.....Des Moines, Iowa..........To 43d Inf. May, 1864.
Muller, J. Henry......A. A. S....Dansville, N. Y.

97TH INFANTRY—(Boonville Regiment and Conkling Rifles)—Mustered out July 18, 1865.

Chambers Wm. B...Surgeon...Edmeston, N. Y.............To February, 1865.
Ferguson, Nelson D.. " Carthage, N. Y.............To March, 1862.
Hough, Franklin B... " Lowville, N. Y...............To March, 1863.
Isham, Nelson.........Ass't S.....Little Falls, N. Y.........To November, 1863.
Little, George S.......Surgeon...171 Carlton ave., Brooklyn, N. Y. From May, 1865.
Hurd, Willard O......Ass't S.....Gilsum, N. H..................To June, 1865.
Marvin, Lewis J......Surgeon.......................................To July, 1862.
Cornish, Aaron.......Ass't S.........................................Dismissed September,'62.

* David A., in A. G. R.

## NEW YORK—Continued.

98TH INFANTRY—Mustered out August 31, 1865.

Benton, James D......Surgeon...Syracuse, N. Y..............From March, 1865; also 111th Inf.
Balsh, Galusha B......Ass't S.....Yonkers, N. Y........ ......To August, 1862; also 2d Vet Cav.
Crary, Charles W..... " Lake City, Minn.............To June, 1863: also Capt.
Gray, John W......... " Avon Springs, N. Y.......To 65th Infantry November, 1864.
Howland, Hiram...... " Plattekill, N. Y.............To June, 1865.
Van Rensaeller, J J..Surgeon...New Brighton, N. Y.......To February, 1865.
Davids, Wm. G....... " Dansville, N. Y............To September, 1862.

99TH INFANTRY—(Naval Brigade and Union Coast Guard)—Mustered out July 15, 1865.

Ensign, Samuel.......Ass't S.....Arborville, Nebr..........To May, 1863.
Wilson, James.........Surgeon.........................................To July, 1864.
Chambers, James A..Ass't S...........................................From February, 1865.
Whiteford, Alfred H.. " Died in 1873.
Johnson, Chas. M..... " Watertown, N. Y..........To July, 1864.

*100TH INFANTRY—(2d Regiment Eagle Brigade)—Mustered out August 28, 1865.

Carter, Norris M......Surgeon...Poughkeepsie, N. Y.......From March, 1865; also 20th Cav.
Kittenger, Martin S.. " Lockport, N. Y.............To January, 1865.
Murray, Wm. D.......Ass't S.....Tonawanda, N. Y.........To July, 1864.
Tryon, A. W.......... " Lockport, N. Y.............To September, 1863.
Schofield, Edwin...... " ..........................................From July, 1864.

101ST INFANTRY (1st Regiment Union Brigade)—Consolidated with the 37th Infantry December 24, 1862.

Van Slyke, D. B......Surgeon...Brookline, Mass.............From December, 1862.
Streeter, Mifflin H....Ass't S....Granville, N. Y.............From August, 1862.
Fellows, Milton A.... " ..........................................From March, 1862.
Cunnyngham, T......Surgeon..........................................Dismissed October, 1862.

102D INFANTRY (12th Militia, Van Buren Light Infantry)—Mustered out July 21, 1865.

Bogardus, J. C.........Ass't S.....Rosendale, N. Y............To December, 1862.
Goodrich, Chas. S....Surgeon...414 W. 22d st., N. Y. city..To May, 1862.
Burbeck, Chas. H..... " Brunswick, N. Y., or 22 2d st., Troy, N. Y. From Nov., 1864; also 60th Inf.
Failing, E. P..........Ass't S...........................................From December, 1864.
Lord, C. H...............Surgeon.........................................To October, 1864.
Applegate, Lewis.....Ass't S...........................................To U. S. V. Sept., 1864.
Vanderkieft, B. A.....Surgeon.........................................To March, 1863.

103D INFANTRY (Seward Infantry, Union Grenadiers—part)—In service August 31, 1865.

Steinach, Adelrich...Surgeon...122 Allen st., N. Y. city..To April, 1865. H. R.
Smith, Wm. A........ " 276 Broad st., Newark, N. J. To Oct., 1863; also 89th Inf.
Turner, Albert S...... " 1505 Broad st., Phila., Pa. To Jan., 1865; also 56th Inf.
Kraenter, John L.....Ass't S.....Germany.......................To May, 1862.
Hedler, Franz L......Surgeon...New York city........ ......To August, 1862.
Tissot, Max..............Ass't S....Dead.
Baalon, Herman...... " ..........................................To April, 1865.
Ebner, Chas. W.......Surgeon.........................................To August, 1862.
Schoeckel, J. V. F...Ass't S...........................................To 45th Inf., June, 1863.

* Andrew B. Morey, late Ord. Sergt. Co. C. has a diary containing valuable information. P. O. address, 758 John Street, Elmira, N. Y.

## NEW YORK—Continued.

### 104TH INFANTRY (Wadsworth Guard)—Mustered out July 17, 1865.

| | | | |
|---|---|---|---|
| Chase, Enos G | Surgeon | Boulder, Col | To Dec., 1864. Dead. |
| Landon, Douglas S | Ass't S | Soldiers and Sailors' Home, Bath, N. Y. | To November, 1862. |
| Richmond, Chas. H. | Surgeon | Livonia, N. Y | From December, 1864. |
| Rugg, Geo. S | Ass't S | Elizabeth, N. J | To June, 1865. |
| Pendergast, Patrick | " | | From June, 1863. |
| Ladue, Edmund K | " | | From February, 1864. |
| Himrod, D. G. | " | | To May, 1863. |

### 105TH INFANTRY—Consolidated with the 94th Infantry March, 1863.

| | | | |
|---|---|---|---|
| Chamberlain, D. A | Surgeon | Norwood, Mich | From Nov., 1863; also 94th Inf. |
| Casey, James W | Ass't S | Rochester, N. Y | From November, 1862. |
| Brown, John T | " | Kerney Junction, Neb | From September, 1862; also 94th Inf. |

### 106TH INFANTRY—Mustered out June 22, 1865.

| | | | |
|---|---|---|---|
| Carpenter, Henry H. | Ass't S | Lawrenceville, N. Y | To 43d Infantry March, 1865. |
| Freeman, John N | Surgeon | 80 Hanson st., Brooklyn, N. Y. | From February, 1864. |
| Skinner, Calvin S | " | Malone, N. Y | To December, 1863. |
| Freeman, Julius A | Ass't S | | From February, 1865. |

### 107TH INFANTRY—Part mustered out June 5, 1865; the rest transferred to the 60th Infantry.

| | | | |
|---|---|---|---|
| Flood, John M | Ass't S | Elmira, N. Y | To September, 1863. |
| Flood, Patrick H | Surgeon | Elmira, N. Y | From July, 1862. |
| Hewett, James D | Ass't S | Woodbourne, N. Y | Dismissed May, 1863. |

### 108TH INFANTRY—Mustered out May 28, 1865.

| | | | |
|---|---|---|---|
| Ely, Wm. S | Ass't S | Rochester, N. Y | To U. S. V. Sept., 1863. |
| Wafer, Francis M | Surgeon | Kingston, Canada | From July, 1864. |
| Whitbeck, John F | " | Rochester, N. Y | To January, 1863. |
| Arner, Thos | Ass't S | | To January, 1863. |
| Munson, Owen | Surgeon | Dead. | |
| Stevenson, Robert | Ass't S | | From December, 1864. |

### 109TH INFANTRY—Mustered out June 4, 1865.

| | | | |
|---|---|---|---|
| French, S. H | Ass't S | Amsterdam, N. Y | To June, 1864. |
| Johnson, Wm. E | Surgeon | Waverly, N. Y | From February, 1864. |
| White, Asa J | Ass't S | Newfield, N. Y | From September, 1864. |
| Churchill, Seymour | Surgeon | | To January, 1864. |
| Hunt, Sanford B | " | Newark, N. J | To March, 1863. |

### 110TH INFANTRY—Mustered out August 28, 1865.

| | | | |
|---|---|---|---|
| Bates, N. W | Ass't S | Central Square or Hastings, N. Y. | From February, 1865. |
| Rice, Alfred | Surgeon | Hannibal, N. Y | From August, 1864. |
| Green, Tobias J | Ass't S | Parish, N. Y | To November, 1862. |
| Huntington, Elia A. | " | | To June, 1863. |
| Livingston, Allen C. | Surgeon | | To January, 1864. |

## NEW YORK—Continued.

111TH INFANTRY—Mustered out June 3, 1865; recruits transferred to 4th Heavy Artillery.

Benton, Jas. D.........Ass't S.....Syracuse, N. Y.............To 98th Inf. March, 1865.
Hopkins, D. S......... " Dead.
Vasburgh, Wm........Surgeon...Dead.
Frisbie, Chas. M.......Ass't S.....Friendship, N. Y............From April, 1863.

112TH INFANTRY—(Chatauqua Regiment)—Mustered out June 13, 1865.

Boyd, Edson...........Ass't S.....Harmony, N. Y............To November, 1863.
Mead, Chas............... " Dead.
Thomas, Jeffrey R... " ...................................To December, 1862.

113TH INFANTRY—(See 7th Heavy Artillery.)

114TH INFANTRY—Mustered out June 8, 1865.

Beecher, Harris H.....Ass't S.....Norwich, N. Y..............From Sept., 1862. H. R.
Crary, Chas. W........ " Lake City, Minn............To October, 1864.
Wagoner, Levi P......Surgeon...Dead.
Beardsley, H. G.......Ass't S.........................................To February, 1863.

115TH INFANTRY—Mustered out July 17, 1865.

Macfarlane, C..........Surgeon...Oswego, N. Y...............From Sept., 1863; also 81st Inf.
Peters, Samuel.........Ass't S....Cohoes, N. Y..................To January, 1863.
Sutton, Richard E....Surgeon...Rome, N. Y.....................To June, 1863.
Watson, Jas. L........Ass't S.....9 Elm Place, Brooklyn, N. Y. To March, 1865.
Rector, Pierson....... " ...................................To 127th Inf. Feb., 1864.
Perry, John L., Jr... " ...................................To August, 1863.
Ingerson, H. H....... " ...................................To October, 1863.

116TH INFANTRY—Mustered out June 8, 1865.

Howe, Carey W.......Ass't S....Cowlesville, N. Y..........To January, 1863.
Hutchins, C. B.........Surgeon...843 Mission street, San Francisco Cal. From May, 1864.
Lynde, Uri C...........Ass't S.....Buffalo, N. Y................To October, 1863.
Shaw, M. E............ " Ripley, N. Y.................To May, 1864

117TH INFANTRY—Mustered out June 8, 1865.

Carpenter, H. W......Surgeon...Oneida, N. Y.................To Nov., 1864. U. S. Ex. S.
Day, Warren E........Ass't S.....Bradshaw, Arizona........From June, 1863.
Loomis, Edward......Surgeon...Oneida, N. Y.................To April, 1863. U. S. Ex. S.
Mowris, James A...... " La Fayette, N. Y..........From January, 1865.
Ingraham Samuel.....Ass't S....Palmyra, N. Y...............To October, 1862.

118TH INFANTRY—(Adirondack Regiment)—Mustered out June 13, 1865.

Porteous, Jas. G......Ass't S.....Luzerne, N. Y...............To 46th Inf. Nov., 1864.
Wilson, Melvin W.... " Dutch Flat, Cal...........To October, 1864.
Moores, John H.......Surgeon..........................................To April, 1864.
Preston, John C......Ass't S...........................................From January, 1865.
Mansfield, Wm. Q...Surgeon...Dead.

## NEW YORK—Continued.

### 119TH INFANTRY—Mustered out June 7, 1865.

Fulda, Albin............Ass't S....502 E. 14th st., N. Y. city. Dismissed June, 1863.
Kennedy, L. W........Surgeon...Dead.
Brueninghausen, C... " 108 Waverly Place, N. Y. city. To February, 1863.
Utterhart, Carl........Ass't S..........................................To 9th U. S. C. T. Nov., 1864.
Ayme, Henry..........Surgeon...Dead.
Hewett, Jas. D ........ " 125 W. 13th st., N. Y. city. Dismissed June, 1863.

### 120TH INFANTRY—Mustered out June 3, 1865.

Miller, John N.........Ass't S.....Highland, N. Y..............To 81st Inf. March, 1865.
Van Hovenburg, J.O.Surgeon...Westfield (Staten Island,) N. Y. To December, 1862.
Van Steenburg, W... " Cohoes, N. Y................Dead.
Hogan, Ed. K.........Ass't S.....294 Madison ave., N. Y. city. To August, 1864.

### 121ST INFANTRY—Mustered out June 25, 1865.

Hotaling, I. W.........Ass't S.....Somerset, N. Y..............To August, 1863.
Kimball, Jas. P........ " Care A. G. U. S. A........Also 65th Inf. Now Ass't Surg. U. S. A.
Slocom, John O.......Surgeon...Camillus, N. Y..............From July, 1863; also 122d Inf.
Valentine. S. B.......Ass't S.....Dead.
Walker, E. J.......... " Dead.
Bassett, Wm............Surgeon Binghamton, N. Y.........To September, 1862.
Holt, Daniel M.........Ass't S....Dead.

### 122D INFANTRY—Mustered out June 23, 1865.

Knapp, Edwin A.....Surgeon...Jamesville, N. Y ............From May, 1864. H. R.
Slocum, John O.......Ass't S.....Camillus, N. Y..............To Surg. 121st Inf. July, 1863.
Tefft, Nathan R......Surgeon...Onondaga, N. Y............To April, 1864.
Sanders, Jas. Jr.......Ass't S.........................................From October, 1864.

### 123D INFANTRY—Mustered out June 8, 1865.

Corning, Leonard.....H. Stew...Fort Ann, N. Y.
*Chapman, Jas........Surgeon...Medina, N. Y................From May, 1863.
Moneypenny, J........ " Cambridge, N. Y..........To March, 1863.
Connelly, R. S. .......Ass't S....Dead.
Kennedy, L ............ " Dead.

### 124TH INFANTRY—(American Guard and Orange Blossoms)—Mustered out June 3, 1865. H. R. on file at S. G. O.; not on file prior to August 15, 1863.

Montfort, R. V. K...Surgeon...Newburgh, N. Y ...........From March, 1865.
Thompson, John H... " Goshen, N. Y................Dismissed Nov., 1864.
Marshall, Edward....Ass't S.........................................Dismissed August, 1863.
Fox, Edward C........ " ......................................From April, 1865.

* Not with regiment after December 27, 1863. On Staff 1st Brigade, 2d Division, 12th Army Corps.

NEW YORK—Continued.

125TH INFANTRY—Mustered out June 5, 1865; recruits transferred to 4th Heavy Artillery. Some of the H. R. were lost at Spottsylvania. H. R. on file at S. G. O.; none prior to January 1, 1864.

| | | | |
|---|---|---|---|
| Aiken, Washington | Ass't S | Troy, N. Y | From August, 1862. |
| Cooper, W. S | Surgeon | Troy, N. Y | From August. 1862. |
| Owen, Geo. H | Ass't S | | To March, 1865. |
| Allen, Chas. S | " | Greenborough, N. Y | To December, 1862. |
| Benedict, Abijah G | " | | To November, 1862. |

126TH INFANTRY—Mustered out June 3, 1865. H. R. on file at A. G. O. and S. G. O; none prior to December 10, 1862, in S. G. O.

| | | | |
|---|---|---|---|
| Hoyt, Charles S | Surgeon | Canandaigua. N. Y | To 39th Inf May, 1864. |
| Peltier. Pierre D | Ass't S | Hartford, Conn | To November, 1863. |
| Pasco, Ferdinand M | " | Red Creek, N. Y | From November, 1864. |
| Hammond, F. M | Surgeon | Penn Yan, N. Y | A. W. M. |

127TH INFANTRY—(National Volunteers)—Mustered out June 30, 1865.

| | | | |
|---|---|---|---|
| Cutter, Geo. R | Surgeon | Corner 2d ave. and 13th st., New York city. | From September, 1862. |
| Dayton, Chas. B | Ass't S | East Hampton, N. Y | From December, 1862. |
| Rowland. Elbert | " | Olney, Ill | To March, 1864. |
| Rector, Pierson | " | | To December, 1864; also 115th Inf. |
| Hageman, Thos. G | H. Stew | Bridgeport, Conn. | |

128TH INFANTRY—Mustered out July 12, 1865. H R on file at S. G. O.; also in A. G. O., covering 1864.

| | | | |
|---|---|---|---|
| Andrus, Chas. H | Ass't S | Metuchen, N. J | To 176th Inf. Aug, 1864. |
| Crawe, J. Mortimer | Surgeon | Watertown, N. Y | From February, 1865; also 157th Inf. |
| Deming, Willard F | Ass't S | 6 Charles street. New York city. | To June, 1864. |
| Past, Wm. H. B | " | | From October. 1864. |
| Cole, Palmer C | Surgeon | 254 W. 42d street, New York city. | To September, 1864. |
| Cole, Henry B | Ass't S | | To May, 1863. |

129TH INFANTRY—(See 8th Heavy Artillery.)

130TH INFANTRY—(See 19th Cavalry.)

131ST INFANTRY—(1st Metropolitan Guards)—Mustered out July 26, 1865.

| | | | |
|---|---|---|---|
| Newton. Homer G | Ass't S | Sherburne, N. Y | From February, 1864. |
| Bates, Henry G | " | | To September, 1863. |
| Squires, Wm. W | " | | To November, 1863 |
| Buel, Wm. P | Surgeon | | From September, 1862. |

132D INFANTRY—(2d Regiment Empire Brigade)—Mustered out June 29, 1865.

| | | | |
|---|---|---|---|
| Mansfield, John R | Ass't S | Wakefield, Mass | To February, 1863. |
| Rice, Pitkin B | Surgeon | Dead. | |
| Groninger, Lewis C | Ass't S | | To June, 1863. |
| Dusenberry, H. L | " | | To August, 1863. |
| Cutland, Wm. F. G | " | | To April, 1863. |

## NEW YORK—Continued.

133D INFANTRY—(2d Metropolitan Guards)—Mustered out June 6, 1865.

Watts, Robert, Jr.....Surgeon...49 W. 36th street, New York city. From September, 1862.
Walker, A. C..........Ass't S.....Greenfield, Mass..........To 18th Cav. Oct., 1864.
Hasbrouck, S. E ..... " Marlborough, N. Y.........From Dec., 1862. Dead.

134TH INFANTRY—Consolidated with 102d Infantry June 1, 1865. Officers mustered out.

Cutter, J. L............Ass't S.....Bolivar, N. Y..................To January, 1864.
Douglass, Geo. C......Surgeon...Salt Lake, Utah............From April, 1865; also 1st Cav.
Fanning, Nelson...... " Catskill, N. Y...............To May, 1863; old and feeble.
Hoag, Wm. H..........Ass't S.... Manhassett, L. I., N. Y..To November, 1864.
Murphy, Peter M...... " Albany, N. Y...............A. W. M.
Joseph, Alexander... " ..................................To March, 1864.
Cartwright, S. S...... " Roxbury, N. Y.............To December, 1862.

135TH INFANTRY—(See 6th Heavy Artillery.)

136TH INFANTRY—Mustered out June 13, 1865.

Amsden, Edwin ......Surgeon...Allegan, Mich...............From December, 1864.
Hovey, Bleeker L..... " 35 N. Fitzhugh street, Rochester, N. Y. To October, 1864.
Warner, Chas. F......Ass't S.....Mankato, Minn.............To July, 1864.
Smith, John R......... " ..........................................To July, 1864.

137TH INFANTRY—Consolidated with the 102d Infantry June 1, 1865. Officers mustered out.

Farrington, John M..Surgeon...Trumansburgh, N. Y......To August, 1863. H. R.
Hutchinson, Edwin.. " Utica, N. Y.................. From September, 1863; also 3d Md. Inf.
*Hand, Stephen M...Ass't S....Norwich, N. Y..............Dismissed March, 1863.
Hubbard, Truman....H. Stew...Owego, N. Y.
Redfield, Geo. S......Ass't S.....Equinunk, Pa ..............From January, 1865; also Capt. Co. L.

138TH INFANTRY—(See 9th Heavy Artillery.)

139TH INFANTRY—Mustered out June 19, 1865.

Burt, Asahel, Jr .....Surgeon...Wakefield, Kan .............From January, 1864.
Brady, Robert W .....Ass't S.....Honesdale, Pa...............From January, 1864.
Thompson, J. Harry..Surgeon...Rome, Italy ...................To December, 1863.
Watson, Jas. L.........Ass't S.....9 Elm Place, Brooklyn, N. Y. To November, 1863.

140TH INFANTRY (Monroe County Regiment)—Mustered out June 3, 1865.

Lord, Mathias L ......Ass't S.....Rochester, N. Y ............From February, 1863.
Menzie, Geo. Leroy .. " Verona, N. Y.................From March, 1863.
Moon, Jos. F...........H. Stew...Scottsville, N. Y.
Paine, O. Sprague....Ass't S.....48 E. 31st st., New York City. Dismissed January, 1863.
Slayton, Wm C ..... " Spencertown, N. Y........To December, 1862.
Dean, Henry C........Surgeon...................................From April, 1863; also 57th Inf.

*Sherman M. Hand, in A. G. R.

## NEW YORK—Continued.

### 141ST INFANTRY—Mustered out June 8, 1865.

| | | | |
|---|---|---|---|
| Babcock, Moses T | Ass't S | Hammondsport, N. Y | From September, 1862. |
| Beakes, Geo. M | Surgeon | Bloomingburgh, N. Y | From October, 1863. |
| Greemman, O. G | Ass't S | Horseheads, N. Y | From September, 1862. |
| Robinson, Jos. W | Surgeon | Hornellsville, N. Y | To June, 1863. |
| Sawyer, Harris C | H. Stew | Hornellsville, N. Y. | |

### 142D INFANTRY—Mustered out June 7, 1865.

| | | | |
|---|---|---|---|
| Boland, Herman A | Ass't S | Lawrenceville, N. Y | To January, 1863. |
| Ellsworth, Chas. E | H Stew | Hammond, N. Y. | |
| McFalls, David | Surgeon | Park City, Utah Ter | From Sept., 1862. H. R. |
| Powell, Hans | Ass't S | Dead | |
| Rice, Westley T | " | Dead. | |

### 143D INFANTRY (Sullivan Regiment)—Mustered out July 20, 1865.

| | | | |
|---|---|---|---|
| Craft, Herman | Ass't S | Stone Ridge, N Y | To April, 1864. |
| *Matthews, David | Surgeon | 206 West 15th st., New York City. | From September, 1862. |
| Carroll, O. A | " | Died May, 1879. | |
| Edsall, Henry M | " | Dead. | |
| Stuart, Wm. H | Ass't S | Norwich, N. Y | From June, 1864. |

### 144TH INFANTRY—Mustered out June 25, 1865.

| | | | |
|---|---|---|---|
| Bundy, Oliver T | Ass't S | Deposit, N. Y | A. W. M. |
| Leal, John R | Surgeon | Paterson, N. J | A. W. M. |
| Bryce, Wm. M | Ass't S | Dead. | |

1

### 45TH INFANTRY (Stanton Legion)—Disbanded December 9, 1863; members transferred to the 107th, 123d and 150th Infantry.

| | | | |
|---|---|---|---|
| Tuthill, Robert K | Surgeon | Poughkeepsie, N. Y | From April, 1863; also 80th Inf. |
| Rockwell, Wm | " | Dead. | |
| May, Henry A | Ass't S | | From September, 1862. |
| Le Duc, Edmund K | " | | From January, 1863. |
| O'Leary, C. B | " | Albany, N. Y | To January, 1863. |

### 146TH INFANTRY (Halleck's Infantry and 5th Oneida Regiment)—Mustered out July 16, 1865.

| | | | |
|---|---|---|---|
| Fossard, Geo. H | Ass't S | Port Jervis, N. Y | To 56th Inf. Nov., 1864; also 42d Inf. |
| Flandreau, Thos. M | Surgeon | Rome, N. Y | A. W. M. |
| Fenwick, Robert | Ass't S | Junction, N. J | From June, 1863. |
| Thomas, P. Henry | H. Stew | Utica N. Y. | |
| Sommers, Albert M | Ass't S | Deansville, N. Y | To December, 1862. |
| Bass, E. C | " | Cazenovia, N. Y | To August, 1863. |
| Morris, Wm. H. H | " | Utica, N Y | From February, 1865. |
| Bradish, Jas. S | " | | Dismissed May, 1863. |

### 147TH INFANTRY—Mustered out June 7, 1865; recruits transferred to 91st Infantry.

| | | | |
|---|---|---|---|
| Coe. Algernon S | Surgeon | Oswego, N. Y | From September, 1862. |
| Hamilton, Chas. A | Ass't S | Savannah, N. Y | From May, 1863; also 76th and 91st Inf. |
| Stillman, J. T | " | Brookfield, N. Y | To 88th Inf. Jan., 1865. |
| †Greene, S. W | " | Wellsville, N. Y | From February, 1865. |
| Place, Simon G | " | Dead. | |

* H. R. from March 9 to April 5, 1865.
† Formerly private Co. D, 15th New York.

## NEW YORK—Continued.

### 148TH INFANTRY—Mustered out June 22, 1865.

| | | | |
|---|---|---|---|
| Carpenter, Calvin H. | Surgeon | Geneva, N. Y. | From August, 1863. |
| Helme, Thos. | Ass't S. | Guilderland, N. Y. | To 85th Inf. April, 1865. |
| Simmons, E. W. | Surgeon | Canandaigua, N. Y. | To February, 1863. |
| Seelye, F. B. | Ass't S. | Rushville, N. Y. | To March, 1863 |
| Bellows, Jas. W. | Surgeon | | To August, 1863. |
| Craig, Robert O. | Ass't S. | | To 10th Inf., March, 1865. |
| Campbell, Augustus. | " | | To 40th Inf., Aug., 1863. |

### 149TH INFANTRY—Mustered out June 12, 1865.

| | | | |
|---|---|---|---|
| Kendall, Jas. V. | Surgeon | Baldwinsville, N. Y. | From August, 1862. |
| Nims, Horace | Ass't S. | Manlius, N. Y. | To March, 1863. |
| Adams, Henry F. | " | Dead. 2d Oct 1862 | |
| Phillips, Albert W. | " | | 24th Nov. 1863 To November, 1863 |

### 150TH INFANTRY—Mustered out June 8, 1865; recruits transferred to 60th Inf.

| | | | |
|---|---|---|---|
| Campbell, C. M. | Surgeon | Poughkeepsie, N. Y. | A. W. M. |
| Pierce, Henry | Ass't S. | Pawling, N. Y. | To April, 1864. |
| Hamill, Alex. | " | Baldwinsville, N. Y. | From March, 1865. |
| Cook, S. G. | " | | To October, 1864. |

### 151ST INFANTRY—(Independent Rifles)—Mustered out June 20, 1865.

| | | | |
|---|---|---|---|
| Cotes, John R. | Surgeon | Batavia, N. Y. | From May, 1863. |
| Leonard, A. M. | " | Lockport, N. Y. | To April, 1863. |
| Onderdonk, D. W. | Ass't S. | Ridgeway Corners, N. Y. | To April, 1863. |
| Steiner, George | " | | To July, 1863. |

### 152D INFANTRY—Mustered out July 13, 1865.

| | | | |
|---|---|---|---|
| Ingham, Silas A. | Surgeon | Little Falls, N. Y. | To September, 1864 |
| Corbin, E. Lyon | Ass't S. | 2d Auditor's Office, Washington, D. C. | From April, 1864. |
| Hughes, J. W. | Surgeon | | From April, 1865; also 59th Inf. |
| Ward, S. W. | Ass't S. | | To March, 1864. |
| Comstock, L. S. | Surgeon | | To Jan., 1865; also 155th Inf. |
| Miller, Adam | Ass't S. | Jordanville, N. Y. | To October, 1863. |
| Blood, N. M. | " | | To January, 1863. |

### 153D INFANTRY—Mustered out October 2, 1865.

| | | | |
|---|---|---|---|
| Alexander, J. H. | Ass't S. | Hermon, N. Y. | To August, 1863. |
| Hendee, H. S. | Surgeon | Carthage, N. Y. | To Feb., 1864; also 5th H. Art. |
| Snow, N. L. | " | Albany, N. Y. | From March, 1864. |
| Sweeney, James | Ass't S. | 192 N. 6th st., Brooklyn, N. Y. | From June, 1864. |

### 154TH INFANTRY—Mustered out June 11, 1865.

| | | | |
|---|---|---|---|
| Bosley, George H. | Ass't S. | 231 W. 49th st., N. Y. city. | From January, 1865. |
| Day, Dwight W. | Surgeon | Eau Claire, Wis. | From January, 1865. |
| Rugg, Corydon C. | Ass't S. | Jamestown, N. Y. | To October, 1864. |
| *Van Aernam, H. | Surgeon | Franklinville, N. Y. | To November, 1864. |

*M. C. and ex-Commissioner of Pensions.

## NEW YORK—Continued.

### 155TH INFANTRY—(Part of Corcoran's Irish Legion)—Mustered out July 15, 1865.

Wylie, Farand ......... Surgeon... Bath, N. Y. ........................ To Dec., 1864; also 86th Inf.
Louisberry, S. S. ....... " ........................................ From Jan., 1865; also 170th Inf.
Harris, Newton C.... Ass't S..... Schuylersville, N. Y. ....... From Jan., 1865.
Nolan, Patrick......... Surgeon........................................ To September, 1863.
Comstock, L. C........ Ass't S........................................ To 152d Inf. Nov., 1864.

### 156TH INFANTRY—(Mountain Legion)—In service August 31, 1865.

Smith, George C...... Surgeon... Rondout, N. Y. ............... From April, 1864.
Webster, Wm. S...... Ass't S..... Liberty, N. Y. ................. To April, 1864.
Laurie, C. M. M. ...... " ........................................ To September, 1864.
Percy, Edward R..... Surgeon........................................ To January, 1864.

### 157TH INFANTRY—Mustered out July 10, 1865.

Beebe, Frank D....... Ass't S..... Hamilton, N. Y. ...... ...... To November, 1863.
Crawe, J. M............ " Watertown, N. Y. .......... To 128th Inf. Feb., 1865.
Holcombe, B. R. ....... " Whitehall, N. Y ............. From February, 1865.
Hendrick, H. C........ Surgeon... McGranville, N. Y. ......... From August, 1862.

### 158TH INFANTRY—(1st Empire Brigade)—Mustered out June 30, 1865.

Murphy, C. H.......... Surgeon... Dead.
De Landre, G........... " Care of Dr. J. Robinson, 150 Grand st., N.Y. city. From December, 1862.
Towner, W. D......... Ass't S........................................ To September, 1863.
Stitler, Isaac W........ " ........................................ To November 1864
McGrath, Edward.... " ........................................ To April, 1863.

### 159TH INFANTRY—In service August 31, 1865.

Briggs, Caleb C........ Surgeon... Union Springs, Ala......... From October, 1862.
Provost, Wm. Y...... " Greenpoint, L. I., N. Y.. To July, 1865.
Robertson, C........... " Albany, N. Y. .................. To November, 1863.

### 160TH INFANTRY—In service August 31, 1865.

Fordyce, B. A ........ Ass't S..... Union Springs, N. Y...... To January, 1865.
Armstrong, D. H ..... " Died in 1880.
Powers, Cyrus......... Surgeon... Died March, 1880.
Fitzimmons, P......... " ........................................ From April, 1865.
Reynolds, G. W....... Ass't S..... Morley, N. Y. .................. To May, 1863.

### 161ST INFANTRY—In service August 31, 1865.

Beard, George M...... H. Stew... Millport, N. Y.
Darling, Louis ......... Surgeon... Lawrenceville, Pa ......... To April, 1864.
Dolson, Joseph S...... Ass't S..... Bath, N. Y. ..................... To July, 1863.
Murray, Wm. D........ Surgeon... Tonawanda, N. Y. .......... A. W. M.
Stoddard, P. K......... Ass't S.... Prattsburgh, N. Y ........ From September, 1863.
Pierce, Charles M..... " ........................................ To October, 1863.

### 162D INFANTRY—(3d Metropolitan Guards)—In service August 31, 1865.

Eager, Wm. B., Jr... Surgeon... Middletown, N. Y. ......... To February, 1864.
VanDeWarker, E. E.. " Syracuse, N. Y. ....... ..... From August, 1864. H. R.
Adams, James L..... Ass't S..... Phelps, N. Y. .................. To February, 1864.
Hozier, Wm. H........ Surgeon........................................ To April, 1864.
Mecham, Wm. G...... Ass't S........................................ To May, 1865.
Brown, David M...... " ........................................ To December, 1862.

## NEW YORK—Continued.

163D INFANTRY—(3d Regiment Empire Brigade)—Consolidated with the 73d Infantry January 20, 1863.

Dufloo, Armand.......Ass't S.....55 W. 24th street, New York City. From September, 1862; also 25th Cav. 70th Inf. and Lt. 53d Inf.
Marmon, Paul D......Surgeon.......................................A. W. M.

164TH INFANTRY—(Part of, Irish Legion; Phœnix Regiment)—Mustered out July 15, 1865.

Hasbruck, Jos. L......Surgeon...242 S. 3d st, Brooklyn, N. Y. From November, 1864.
Regan, Matthew F... " Dead.
Wall, John C..........Ass't S.....Dead.

165TH INFANTRY—(2d Duryee's Zouaves)—Mustered out September 1, 1865.

Ferguson, James F...Surgeon...5 Waverly Place, New York City. To March, 1864.
Hubbard, Geo. C...... " Hornellsville, N. Y.......From September, 1864.

166TH AND 167TH INFANTRY—Failed to complete.

168TH INFANTRY—(19th Militia)—Mustered out October 31, 1863.

Root, E. B...............Ass't S.....Painesville, Ohio............From April, 1863.
Leighton, Jacob M...Surgeon...Dead.

169TH INFANTRY—Mustered out July 19, 1865.

Knowlson, John......Surgeon...Poultney, Vt................From October, 1862.
Murphy, Peter M.....Ass't S.....Albany, N. Y......... .....To February, 1864.
Reynolds, P. L. F.... " Albany, N. Y..............To December, 1863.
Parker, John T........ " Alleged dead................From January, 1865.
Meadville, Austin..... " ...................................To January, 1865.
Smith, Clark............ " ...................................To August, 1863.
Skinner, Jos. T........ " ...................................To February, 1863.

170TH INFANTRY—(Part of Irish Legion)—Mustered out July 15, 1865.

Olmstead, Sam'l H..Surgeon...192 Union st., Brooklyn, N. Y. From December, 1864.
Douglas, Frederick... " Dead.
Heath, Allen S......... " 945 Lexington avenue, N. Y. City. To January, 1864.
Lounsberry, Seth S..Ass't S....................................... To 155th Inf. Jan., 1865.
O'Flaherty, John..... " Hartford, Conn.............From January, 1865.

171ST AND 172D INFANTRY—Failed to complete.

173D INFANTRY—(4th Metropolitan Guards, 4th National Guards)—Mustered out October 18, 1865.

Leighton, N. W.......Surgeon...143 Taylor street, Brooklyn, N. Y. To September, 1864.
Mather, W. H.........Ass't S.....Suffield or Hartford, Conn. To March, 1864.
Sweeny, John.......... " Bloomington, Ill........... From January, 1865.
* Baldwin, Nelson A..Surgeon...168 Franklin ave., Brooklyn, N. Y. From January, 1865.

* Assistant Surgeon from November, 1862.

## NEW YORK—Continued.

174TH INFANTRY—(5th National Guards)—Consolidated with 162d Infantry February 9, 1864.

Hazier, Wm. H........Surgeon........................................From June, 1863.
Kent, Prentiss J......Ass't S........................................From December, 1862.
Guernsey, Desault....Surgeon........................................To May, 1863.

175TH INFANTRY—Mustered out November 27, 1865.

Becket, Thomas.......Ass't S.....Albany, N. Y....................To June, 1863.
Fearn, Herbert.......Surgeon...196 Clermont st., Brooklyn, N. Y. From November, 1863.
Bausch, Charles.......Ass't S........................................To October, 1863.
McClintock, E......... " ........................................To July, 1864
O'Leary, C. B........ Surgeon...Albany, N. Y....................To September, 1863.

176TH INFANTRY—(Ironsides)—In service August 31, 1865.

Andrus, Charles H...Surgeon...Metuchen, N. J.............From August, 1864; also 128th Inf.
Throop, J. Mott.......Ass't S.....Lebanon, N. Y.............To November, 1863.
Steele, Albert F.......Surgeon........................................Dismissed October, 1864.
Willetts, Andrew J... " ........................................To November, 1863.

177TH INFANTRY—Mustered out September 10, 1863.

Boulware, Jeptha R..Ass't S.....Albany, N. Y.................From November, 1862.
Craig, William H......Surgeon...Albany, N. Y.................From October, 1862.
Young, Oscar H.......Ass't S........................................From November, 1862.

178TH INFANTRY—In service August 31, 1865.

Cooper, Henry C......Surgeon...81 John st., New York city. From May, 1865.
Weiss, Conrad.........Ass't S.....Mount Vernon, N. Y.....Dismissed August, 1864.
Tanner, Wm. A.......Surgeon........................................To November, 1864.

179TH INFANTRY—Mustered out June 8, 1865.

Bailey, Wm. C........ Ass't S.....Adams Centre, N. Y......To 186th Inf. Oct., 1864.
Robinson, Jos. W.....Surgeon...Hornellsville, N. Y........From May, 1864.
Rose, P. E..............Ass't S.....Anoka, Minn..................From November, 1864.

180TH AND 181ST INFANTRY—Failed to complete.

182D INFANTRY—(69th N. G. A.)—Mustered out July 15, 1865.

Dwyer, John............Surgeon...224 E. 112th st., New York city. To August, 1863.
Ewen, Clarence ......Ass't S.....Care A. G. U. S. A.........To October, 1863; now Ass't Surg. U. S. A.
Crowley, Patrick..... " New York city..............From November, 1864.
Nealis, Wm. T.........Surgeon...Dead...................................From October, 1864.
Spencer, John A...... " Dublin, Ireland...............To September, 1864.

183D INFANTRY—Failed to complete.

184TH INFANTRY—Mustered out June 29, 1865.

Barnes, Nelson R.....Surgeon...Cincinnatus, N. Y.........From Nov., 1864. H. R. Also 76th Infantry.
Kinne, Theo. Y........Ass't S ...Paterson, N. J................From November, 1864.

## NEW YORK—Continued.

### 185TH INFANTRY—Mustered out May 29, 1865.

| | | | |
|---|---|---|---|
| Bradford, Wm. M | Ass't S | Marathon, N. Y | From Oct., 1864. U. M. |
| Crary, Chas. W | Surgeon | Lake City, Minn | From October, 1864. |
| Newcomb, G. L | Ass't S | 337 E. 18th street, New York city. | From October, 1864. |

### 186TH INFANTRY—Mustered out June 2, 1865.

| | | | |
|---|---|---|---|
| Bailey, Wm. C | Surgeon | Adams Centre, N. Y | From Oct., 1864; also 179th Infantry. |
| Coleman, Jas. C | Ass't S | Goshen, N. Y | From March, 1865. |
| Carlisle, Eber S | " | Omar, N. Y | To February, 1865. |
| Shaw, Jas. N | " | | To February, 1865. |

### 187TH INFANTRY—Mustered out July 1, 1865.

| | | | |
|---|---|---|---|
| Sonnick, Peter L | Surgeon | Buffalo, N. Y | From September, 1864. |
| Wachter, E. Wm | Ass't S | | From January, 1865. |

### 188TH INFANTRY—Mustered out July 1, 1865.

| | | | |
|---|---|---|---|
| Hill, Chas. E | Ass't S | McGrawville, N. Y | From May, 1865. |
| Paine, O. Sprague | Surgeon | 47 W. 31st street, New York city. | From Nov., 1864; also 2d H. Artillery. |
| Spencer, G. O | Ass't S | Cleveland, Ohio | To December, 1864. |

### 189TH INFANTRY—Mustered out May 30, 1865.

| | | | |
|---|---|---|---|
| Horton, J. G | Surgeon | Whitesville, N. Y | Not in A. G. R. U. S. Ex. S. |
| Gates, Howard E | " | Litchfield, Conn | From Nov., 1864; also 80th Inf. |
| Lanning, Henry | Ass't S | Oakis, Japan | From January, 1865. |
| Grasse, Sidney G | " | Dead. | |

### 190TH INFANTRY—Mustered out May 3, 1865.

| | | | |
|---|---|---|---|
| Denick, Frederick | Surgeon | San Francisco, Cal | From March, 1865. |

### 191ST INFANTRY—Mustered out May 3, 1865.

### 192D INFANTRY—Mustered out August 28, 1865.

| | | | |
|---|---|---|---|
| Haskins, Henry R | Surgeon | Albany, N. Y | From February, 1865. |

### 193D INFANTRY—In service August 31, 1865.

| | | | |
|---|---|---|---|
| Tankie, A. H | Ass't S | In Utica Insane Asylum, New York. | From March, 1865. |
| Armstrong, D. H | Surgeon | Died in 1880. | |
| Phinney, Lorenzo | Ass't S | Watkins, N. Y | From April, 1865. |

### ENFANS PERDUS—Was consolidated with the 47th and 48th Infantry January 30, 1864.

| | | | |
|---|---|---|---|
| Harrison, Benj | Surgeon | | A. W. M. |
| Vandrey, Etinne | Ass't S | | To November, 1863. |
| Costello, Ernest | " | | Missing since April, 1862. |
| Conilly, Guent | " | | Missing since April, 1862. |

Hospital records of Park Barracks, New York city, are with Adjutant General of New York.

## NORTH CAROLINA.

### 1st Infantry—Mustered out June 27, 1865.

| | | | |
|---|---|---|---|
| Maynard, D. A | Ass't S. | | From May, 1865. |
| Sulter, Julius C | Surgeon | | From December, 1864. |
| Menninger, H. J | Ass't S. | 97 Strand street, cor. of Jay, Brooklyn, N. Y. | To 2d Inf. Feb., 1864. |

### 2d Infantry—Consolidated with the 1st Infantry February 27, 1865.

| | | | |
|---|---|---|---|
| Menninger, H. J | Surgeon | 97 Strand street, cor. of Jay, Brooklyn, N. Y. | To Feb., 1865; also 1st Inf. |

### 2d Infantry—(Mounted Infantry)—Mustered out August 16, 1865.

| | | | |
|---|---|---|---|
| Sams, Anson B | Con't S. | Marion Springs, N. C | Not in A. G. R. U. M. |
| Barritt, J. J | Ass't S. | | To June, 1864. |

### 3d Infantry—(Mounted Infantry)—Mustered out August 8, 1865.

| | | | |
|---|---|---|---|
| Doake, Sam'l S. | Ass't S. | Camp Creek, Tenn | From March, 1865. |
| Roberts, Marion | " | Flat Creek, N. C | From March, 1865. |
| Perry, Jas. A | H. Stew. | Knoxville, Tenn | M. D. |

## OHIO.

### 1st Cavalry—Mustered out September 13 and 26, 1865.

| | | | |
|---|---|---|---|
| Wirth, Rudolph | Surgeon | Columbus, Ohio | To May, 1862; also 9th Inf. |
| Cannan, John | " | London, Ohio | Dead. |
| Cowan, Wilson V. | " | Hardin, Ohio | To Oct., 1864; also 34th Inf. |
| McDill, John B | Ass't S. | | To Feb., 1863; also 63d Inf. |

### 2d Cavalry—Mustered out from September 11 to October 12, 1865.

| | | | |
|---|---|---|---|
| Cook, Mathias | Ass't S. | Utica, N. Y. | From May, 1865. |
| Smith, Joseph T | Surgeon | Collinwood, Ohio | To March, 1865. |
| Noble, Havilah B. | Ass't S. | 17 Warren st., Baltimore, Md. | To March, 1865; also 4th Cav. and 196th Inf. |
| Brisbine, N. B | Surgeon | | From July, 1865; also 123d Infantry. |
| Taylor, Alfred | " | | To April, 1863. |
| McReynolds, W. H. | " | | To June, 1865. |

### 3d Cavalry—Mustered out August 5, 1865.

| | | | |
|---|---|---|---|
| Boyd, Wm. B. | Surgeon | Monmouth, Ill | From Dec., 1864. H. R. |
| Cuykindall, M. C. | " | Bucyrus, Ohio | To Nov., 1864. U. S. Ex. S. |
| Selby, Stephen F | Ass't S. | Williamson, N. Y. or Solon, Ohio. | To November, 1863. |
| Bickett, Wm. W. | " | Washington, Ohio. | From April, 1864. |
| Moore, David K. | " | | To December, 1862. |

### 4th Cavalry—Mustered out July 5, 1865.

| | | | |
|---|---|---|---|
| Field, Orestes G. | Surgeon | Midway, Ohio | From Nov., 1864; also 5th Inf. |
| James, Lucian A. | " | 7th and Mound sts, Cincinnati, Ohio. | To September, 1864. |
| Weist, Jacob R. | Ass't S. | Richmond, Ind | To Surg. 1st U. S. C. T. Sept., 1863. U. S. Ex. S. |
| Noble, Havilah B. | " | 17 Warren st., Baltimore, Md | To Dec., 1862; also 2d Cav. and 196th Inf. |
| McMillen, Thos. | " | | To July, 1862. |
| Biggs, Cyrus F. H. | " | | From November, 1864. |

OHIO—Continued.

5TH CAVALRY—Mustered out October 30, 1865.

| Name | Rank | Residence | Service |
|---|---|---|---|
| Rannells, D. V. | Ass't S. | McArthur, Ohio | To May, 1865 |
| Sprague, George | " | | To November, 1864. |
| Thornton, Chas. | Surgeon | | To September, 1864. |
| McMillan, Wm | " | Lexington, Ohio | From October, 1865. |
| Shohoney, A. J. | Ass't S. | | From February, 1865. |

6TH CAVALRY—Mustered out August 7, 1865.

| Name | Rank | Residence | Service |
|---|---|---|---|
| Knowlton, A. P. | Ass't S. | Olmstead Falls, Ohio | To December, 1863. |
| Rezner, Wm. B. | Surgeon | Cleveland, Ohio | To Nov., 1864; also 11th Cav. |
| Marr, James C | Ass't S. | Niles, Ohio | To Sept, 1862; also 173d Inf. |
| Rockwell, A. D. | Surgeon | | From December, 1864. |
| Kibele, Cuno | Ass't S. | | From April, 1865. |

7TH CAVALRY—Mustered out July 4, 1865.

| Name | Rank | Residence | Service |
|---|---|---|---|
| Train, Isaac | Surgeon | Pomeroy, Ohio | From Oct., 1862. Dead. |
| Krapt, John | Ass't S. | Caldwell or Bremen, O. | From January, 1865; also 160th Inf. |
| Barrett, Perry G. | " | Hood's River, Oregon | To Surg. 31st U. S. C. T. October, 1864. |

8TH CAVALRY—(Formerly 44th Infantry)—Mustered out July 30, 1865.

| Name | Rank | Residence | Service |
|---|---|---|---|
| Davis, B. F. | Ass't S. | Tontogany, Ohio | Form March, 1863. |
| Rodgers, John H. | " | Springfield, Ohio | To Surg. 104th Inf. Feb., 1863. |
| Steele, Henry K | Surgeon | Denver, Col | To October, 1864. |
| Luce, Douglas | Ass't S. | Bonta, Cal. | To January, 1864. |
| Bowland, Milton J. | Surgeon | | From Oct., 1864; also 71st Inf. |
| Hazeltine, Lewis H. | Ass't S. | | From May, 1865. |

9TH CAVALRY—Mustered out July 20, 1865.

| Name | Rank | Residence | Service |
|---|---|---|---|
| Finch, Cyrus M. | Surgeon | Portsmouth, Ohio | From December, 1863. |
| Pinney, Charles H | Ass't S. | Council Bluffs, Iowa | From April, 1864. |
| McMillen, Wm | " | Massillon, Ohio | A. W. M |
| Thorpe, Jas C. | " | | Dismissed April, 1864. |

10TH CAVALRY—Mustered out July 24, 1865.

| Name | Rank | Residence | Service |
|---|---|---|---|
| Gardner, Jas F. | Ass't S. | West Brookfield, Ohio | To January, 1865. |
| Hawes, Michael | Surgeon | Claysville, Ohio | A. W. M. |
| Valentine, M. | Ass't S. | Etna, Ohio | To Oct., 1863; also 182d Inf. |
| Hall, Wm. G. | " | | To September, 1863. |

11TH CAVALRY—Mustered out July 14, 1866.

| Name | Rank | Residence | Service |
|---|---|---|---|
| Underhill, Geo. C. | Surgeon | La Grange, Ohio | To April, 1865. |
| Rezner, Wm. B. | " | Cleveland, Ohio | Transferred to 6th Cav. June, 1863 |
| Marr, J. C. | Ass't S. | | To September, 1862. |
| Finfrock, John H. | " | | To April, 1865. |
| Zeigler, Albert F. | " | | To April, 1865. |

12TH CAVALRY—Mustered out November 14, 1865.

| Name | Rank | Residence | Service |
|---|---|---|---|
| Brooke, Geo. W | Surgeon | Ellsworth, Ohio | To August, 1865. |
| Hunt, Abram H. | Ass't S. | Wooster, Ohio | To U S Navy March, 1865. |
| Russell, A. J. | " | Hannibal, Mo. | 1863–'64–'65. Not in A. G. R. |
| Pease, Geo. W. | Surgeon | 713 W. Jackson street, Chicago, Ill. | From October, 1865; also 197th Infantry. |
| Hughes, Wallace K. | " | | From September, 1865. |

OHIO—Continued.

13TH CAVALRY—Mustered out August 10, 1865.

| | | | |
|---|---|---|---|
| Richardson, N. S. | Surgeon | Macon, Mo | From November, 1864; also 118th Infantry. |
| Downey, Robt. C. | Ass't S. | Sarahsville, Ohio | To April, 1865. |
| Wilson, Wm. J. | " | Berlin Township, Mahoning County, Ohio. | From May, 1865. |

1ST HEAVY ARTILLERY—Mustered out July 25, 1865.

| | | | |
|---|---|---|---|
| Beard, Henry C. | Surgeon | Lucasville, Ohio | From January, 1865. |
| Firestone, John L. | " | Salem, Ohio | From September, 1862. |
| Hard, Elbridge G. | Ass't S. | Medina, Ohio | To August, 1864. |
| Lafferty, Nelson B. | " | Cherry Fork, Ohio | To January, 1865 |
| Albright, Strickland. | " | Abilene, Kans | To August, 1863; also 2d Heavy Artillery. |
| Carey, Geo. A. E. | " | 213 Plum street, Cincinnati, Ohio. | From February, 1865. |

2D HEAVY ARTILLERY—Mustered out August 23, 1865.

| | | | |
|---|---|---|---|
| Albright, Strickland. | Surgeon | Abilene, Kans | From August, 1863; also 1st Heavy Artillery. |
| Kendig, Eli V. | Ass't S. | Hayesville, Ohio | From September, 1864. |
| Morgan, John. | " | Cadiz, Ohio | From Nov., 1864: also 32d and 172d Inf. |
| Dwyer, Rufus A. | " | New Petersburgh, Ohio. | To September, 1864, also 175th Infantry. |
| Powers, Frank E. | " | | To Surg. 180th Infantry, October, 1864. |

1ST LIGHT ARTILLERY—Mustered out from June 15 to July 31, 1865.

| | | | |
|---|---|---|---|
| Stanton, Byron | Ass't S. | 610 Freeman street, Cincinnati, Ohio. | To December, 1862; also 114th and 120th Inf. |
| Ames, Chas. E | " | | To December, 1865; also 14th and 60th Infantry. |
| Swartzwelder, A. C. | Surgeon | Waco, Tex | To December, 1862. |

9TH INDEPENDENT BATTERY—Mustered out July 25, 1865.

| | | | |
|---|---|---|---|
| Johnston, Wm. W. | Ass't S. | Eureka Springs, Ark | Not in A. G. R. Had charge in 1862; also 85th Ind. |

1ST INFANTRY—Part mustered out September 24, 1864; veterans and recruits transferred to 18th Veterans October 31, 1864

| | | | |
|---|---|---|---|
| *Fletcher, Robert | Surgeon | Office Surgeon General U. S. A. | A. A. Surg. U. S. A. |
| Barr, Jacob C. | " | Springfield, Ohio | From March, 1864. |
| Brockett, And. J. | Ass't S. | Bristolville, Ohio | From May, 1864. |
| Wilson, Albert | " | Sidney, Ohio | To Surg. 113th Infantry, September, 1863. |

2D INFANTRY—Part mustered out October 10, 1864; veterans and recruits transferred to 18th Veterans October 31, 1864.

| | | | |
|---|---|---|---|
| Miller, Benj. F | Surgeon | 70 W. 8th st., Cincinnati, Ohio. | From March, 1862. |
| Wade, Daniel E. | " | 86 Everett st., Cincinnati, Ohio. | To January, 1862. |
| Carmichael, Wm. A. | Ass't S. | | A. W. M. |
| Shannon, Thos. J. | " | Dead | To Surg. 116th Infantry, August, 1863. |

* In charge of General Hospital No. 7, Nashville, to November, 1863.

OHIO—Continued.

3D INFANTRY—Mustered out June 21, 1864.

| Name | Rank | Residence | Remarks |
|---|---|---|---|
| Peck, Wm. L. | Surgeon | Indianapolis, Ind. | A. W. M. Also 114th Inf. |
| Seys, Henry H | Ass't S. | Springfield, Ohio | Missing since May, 1862; also 15th Infantry. |
| Clason, T. C | " | | To August, 1863. |
| Race, Wesley H. | " | Mansfield, Ohio | From October, 1863. |

4TH INFANTRY—Part mustered out June 21, 1864; veterans and recruits consolidated with those of 8th Infantry to form 4th Battalion Ohio Infantry.

| Name | Rank | Residence | Remarks |
|---|---|---|---|
| Laird, John B. | Ass't S. | Millsborough, Pa. | To July, 1863. |
| Morrison, Francis W. | Surgeon | Delaware, Ohio | From November, 1863. |
| Cantwell, Jacob Y. | Ass't S. | Decatur, Ala | To August, 1861; also 82d Infantry. |
| Gray, Barzilla | " | | Tr'fd to 4th Batt'n May, 1864. |
| Longwell, Albert | " | | To November, 1862. |
| McAbee, Harry M. | Surgeon | | To September, 1863. |

4TH BATTALION—Mustered out July 12, 1865.

| Name | Rank | Residence | Remarks |
|---|---|---|---|
| Gray, Barzilla | Ass't S. | | From May, 1864; also 4th Infantry. |

5TH INFANTRY—Mustered out July 26, 1865.

| Name | Rank | Residence | Remarks |
|---|---|---|---|
| Tibbals, Wm. F. | Ass't S. | Cincinnati, Ohio | To Sept., 1864. Dead. |
| Jenner, Alexander E. | Surgeon | Dayton, Ohio | From September, 1864. |
| Bellows, Curtis J. | Ass't S. | Fayette, Mich | To Sept., 1862; also 7th Infantry. |
| Field, O. G | " | Midway, Ohio | To Oct., 1863; also 4th Cavalry. |
| Junkin, Jas. D | " | | From April, 1865. |
| Ball, Alfred | Surgeon | Zanesville, Ohio | To June, 1864. |
| Greenleaf, Chas. | Ass't S. | | Missing since June, 1861. |

6TH INFANTRY—Mustered out June 23, 1864.

| Name | Rank | Residence | Remarks |
|---|---|---|---|
| Bedell, Israel | Ass't S. | Mt. Vernon, Ohio | From September, 1863. |
| Loving, Starling | Surgeon | Columbus, Ohio | To October, 1861. |
| Stephens, A. H. | " | National Military Home, Montgomery Co., Ohio. | A. W. M. |
| Ames, Fisher W. | Ass't S. | 137 Plum street, Cincinnati, Ohio. | To June, 1863; also 14th U. S. C. T. |
| Fountain, W. W. | " | | To August, 1863; also 88th Inf. |

7TH INFANTRY—Mustered out June, 1864; veterans and recruits transferred to the 5th Infantry.

| Name | Rank | Residence | Remarks |
|---|---|---|---|
| Bellows, Curtis J. | Surgeon | Fayette, Mich. | From December, 1862; also 5th Inf. |
| Denig, Chas. E | Ass't S. | Columbus, Ohio | To September, 1862. |
| Ferguson, John C. | " | | From May, 1863. |
| Williams, David | " | Alexandria, Ohio | From August, 1863; also 56th Inf. |
| Cushing, Henry K. | Surgeon | 12 Euclid avenue, Cleveland, Ohio. | To September, 1861. |
| Salter, Francis | " | Dead | To November, 1862. |
| Hitchcock, Eliezer | Ass't S. | Williamsfield, Ohio | To June, 1863. |

OHIO—Continued.

8TH INFANTRY—Mustered out July 13, 1864; veterans and recruits consolidated with those of 4th Infantry to form 4th Battalion.

| Name | Rank | Address | Service |
|---|---|---|---|
| Brenton, Jos. L. | Surgeon | Beloit, Wis, or North Georgetown, Ohio. | From March, 1863. |
| Pollock, Jas. S. | Ass't S. | Belle Centre, Ohio | From August, 1863. |
| McEbright, Thos. P. | Surgeon | Akron, Ohio | To January, 1863. |
| Culver, Benj. F. | Ass't S. | Vincent, Ohio | To February, 1863; also 148th Inf. |
| Tuttle, Freeman A. | " | Geneva, Ohio | To March, 1864. |
| Sexton, Samuel | " | 9th ave. and 36th street, New York city. | To October, 1862. |
| Tappan, Benj. | Surgeon | | To March, 1862. |

9TH INFANTRY—Mustered out June 7, 1864.

| Name | Rank | Address | Service |
|---|---|---|---|
| Beers, Adam M. | Ass't S. | New Comerstown, Ohio | From August, 1863; also 92d Inf. |
| Wirth, Rudolph | " | Columbus, Ohio | To September, 1861; also Surg. 1st Cavalry. |
| Soellheim, Conrad | Surgeon | Cincinnati, Ohio | From May, 1863. |
| Boyle, Chas. E. | " | | To April, 1863. |

10TH INFANTRY—Mustered out June 3, 1864.

| Name | Rank | Address | Service |
|---|---|---|---|
| Muscroft, Chas. S. | Surgeon | 333 John street, Cincinnati, Ohio. | To June, 1863. |
| Shaw, Homer C. | " | Homer, Ill. | From July, 1863. |
| Van Deman, Jos. H. | Ass't S. | Chattanooga, Tenn | To May, 1864. |
| Powers, Francis E. | " | | To May, 1863. |

11TH INFANTRY—Mustered out June 11, 1865.

| Name | Rank | Address | Service |
|---|---|---|---|
| Gill, Henry Z. | Ass't S. | Jerseyville, Ill. | To Surg. 95th Inf. July, 1862. |
| McCurdy, John | Surgeon | Youngstown, Ohio | To April, 1864; also 23d Inf. U S. Ex. S. |
| Gabriel, Jonas F. | " | Piqua, Ohio | To September, 1862. |
| Hudson, Samuel | Surgeon | Medina, Ohio | To October, 1862. |
| McNutt, Alex C. | " | Caledonia, Ohio | To February, 1863. |
| Sidwell, N. Henry | " | | To June, 1864. |

12TH INFANTRY—Mustered out June 11, 1864; veterans and recruits transferred to the 23d Infantry.

| Name | Rank | Address | Service |
|---|---|---|---|
| Buck, Silas T. | Ass't S. | Wellsville, Mo. | From May, 1863. |
| Reidnour, W. T. | Surgeon | Toledo, Ohio | To December, 1862. |
| **Graham, N. F.* | " | U. S. Pension Office | From February, 1863. |
| Carpenter, John E. | H. Stew. | U. S. Pension Office | M. D. |
| Kay, Horace P. | Ass't S. | Died September, 1881 | A. W. M.; also 18th Veterans. |
| Webb, Jas. D. | " | Dead | To December, 1862. |
| Holmes, Wm. W. | Surgeon | Dead. | |
| Swaine, Chas. H. | Ass't S. | | To September, 1861. |

13TH INFANTRY—Part mustered out June 26, 1864; the rest December 5, 1865.

| Name | Rank | Address | Service |
|---|---|---|---|
| Jones, Allen | Surgeon | Kinsman, Ohio | To June, 1864. |
| Thrift, Rob't W. | Ass't S. | Lima, Ohio | To Surg. 49th Inf. Aug., 1861. |
| Seeds, Silas M. | " | | From May, 1865. |
| Turney, Sam'l D. | Surgeon | Circleville, Ohio | To Surgeon U. S. Vols. March, 1863. |
| Chase, Elmore Y. | Ass't S. | | To September, 1862. |
| Smith, Jeremiah W. | " | Wellington, Ohio | To April, 1863. |
| McCready, Jas. | " | Monroe, Ohio | To June, 1864. |
| Moore, John K. | " | | To June, 1864. |

* Assistant Medical Referee, U. S. Pension Office.

OHIO—Continued.

14TH INFANTRY—Mustered out July 11, 1865.

Coons, Israel A........Surgeon...Spring Hill, Kan...........Three months' service; also 38th Inf.
Daniels, Waldo C..... " 754 Michigan ave, Chicago, Ill. To November, 1862.
Eaton, Chas. M.......Ass't S....Ithaca, Mich....................To March, 1863.
Nash, E. King........Surgeon...Montrose, Ohio..............From March, 1865.
Sloat, Geo. E.......... " U. S. Pension Office.......To Nov., 1864. H. R.
Ames, Chas. E........Ass't S.................................To 60th Inf. May, 1864; also 1st Light Artillery.

15TH INFANTRY—Mustered out November 21, 1865.

Clark, Wm. M.........Surgeon...Caldwell, Ohio..............From November 1864.
Kelley, Wm. J.........Ass't S.....Toledo, Ohio..................To September, 1864.
Young, J. B........... " Patterson Ohio................From April, 1865.
Seys, Henry H.......Surgeon...Springfield, Ohio...........To Aug., 1864; [also 3d Inf.
Welsh, David..........Ass't S.................................To Surg. 33d Inf April, 1863.
Ferris, Orrin...........Surgeon...Upper Sandusky, Ohio...To March, 1862; also 123d Inf.
Hall, D. S.............. " ..................................To July, 1862.
Liggett, Geo. T........Ass't S.................................To July, 1862.

16TH INFANTRY—Mustered out October 31, 1864.

Brashear, B. B.........Surgeon...Akron, Ohio...................From December, 1861.
Chas. Byron S..........Ass't S......Akron, Ohio...................Also 53d U. S. C. T. Dead.
Vandervoort, J. W... " Harveysburgh, Ohio.......From August, 1864.
Pomeroy. Orange..... " Charden, Ohio..............To March, 1864.
Ellsberry, I. N.,........ " ..................................Dismissed Sept., 1863.

17TH INFANTRY—Mustered out July 16, 1865.

Benedict, D. D.........Surgeon...Norwalk, Ohio...............From July, 1865.
Kyle, John G........... " Xenia, Ohio....................Three months' service. Dead.
Schenck, W. L......... " Osage City, Kans............To December, 1862.
Sinnett. E................Ass't S.....Granville, Ohio...............To January, 1862.
Herrick, Henry........Surgeon.................................To December, 1864.
Fowler, J. E............ " ..................................To May, 1865.

18TH INFANTRY—Mustered out November 9, 1864; veterans and recruits consolidated with those of 35th Infantry to form 18th Veteran Infantry.

French, Chas. H......Ass't S.....McArthur, Ohio.............From Feb., 1863.
Johnson, W. P.........Surgeon...Cor. Broad & Arch sts, Philadelphia, Pa. From September, 1861.
Mills, Wm. W..........Ass't S.....Gallipolis, Ohio..............To February, 1864

18TH VETERAN INFANTRY—Mustered out October 9, 1865.

Baxter, Sam'l A......Ass't S.....Lima. Ohio....................From June. 1865.
Kay, Horace P.........Surgeon...Died Sept., 1881............From April, 1865; also 12th Inf.
Newell, Arthur C.....Ass't S.................................From May, 1865.

19TH INFANTRY—Mustered out October 24, 1865.

Failor. Benj. M........Surgeon...Newton, Iowa...............To April. 1865. Ex. S.
McNeilley. Rob't......Ass't S.................................To August, 1862.
Hurxthal, F. T.......Surgeon.................................To March. 1863.
Sowers, Adam H......Ass't S.....Canal Fulton, Ohio.........From April. 1865.

OHIO—Continued.

20TH INFANTRY—Mustered out July 15, 1865.

Guthrie, James W....Ass't S.....Aberdeen, Ohio..............A. W. M.
Hill, Edward L........Surgeon...Oxford, Ohio..................To October, 1864.
Fricker, Henry P...... " Ashtabula, Ohio ............From October, 1864.

21ST INFANTRY—Mustered out July 25, 1865.

Eames, Wm, M........Surgeon...Ashtabula, Ohio.............To October, 1862; also 157th Inf. U.S. Ex. S.
Young, Daniel S...... " 248 W. 7th st., Cincinnati, Ohio. From December, 1862.
Payne, William C....Ass't S..............................................To August, 1863.
Gray, Richard, Jr..... " ...................................................To June, 1865.

22D INFANTRY—Mustered out August 28, 1865.

Brown, Aaron M......Ass't S.....Cincinnati, Ohio ............To November. 1864.
Bell, John B...........Surgeon.............................................To February, 1862.*
Gilmore, Wm. H......Ass't S.....Fair Haven, Ohio ..........To May, 1863.
Foote, Henry E.......Surgeon.............................................To November, 1864.

23D INFANTRY—Mustered out July 26, 1865.

Barrett, Jos. E.........Ass't S....Wooster, Ohio................To Surg. 194th Infantry March, 1865.
McCurdy, John........ " Youngstown, Ohio.........To Surg. 11th Inf. Nov., 1862.
Webb, Jos. T...........Surgeon...Fremont, Ohio...............From July, 1861. Dead.
King, Elmore Y ......Ass't S...............................................From April, 1865.
McClure, Jas.......... " Albany, Ohio.................A. W. M.

24TH INFANTRY—Mustered out June 17 to 24, 1864.

Cooke, Jabez M........Surgeon...Adams, Ind.....................From June, 1863.
Weeks, Geo. R......... " Little Rock, Ark............To Surg. U. S.Vols. Feb., 1863; also 25th Inf.
Smith, Henry Y ......Ass't S...............................................To June, 1863.
Howland, Eran M.... " ...................................................From September, 1863.

25TH INFANTRY—Mustered out June 18, 1866.*

Hendrix, H. W.........Ass't S....Lexington, C. H., S. C....On duty from Sept., 1865, to March, 1866; not in A. G. R.
Meyers, Louis G.......Surgeon...Cleveland, Ohio.............To July, 1864.
Walton, Wm............ " Clarington or Woodsfield. Ohio. From September, 1864.
Wilson, Eli M..........Ass't S....Falls City, Neb................From September, 1864.
Gregorie, I. McP......Surgeon...McPhersonville. S. C......Not in A. G. R.
Weeks, Geo. R.........Ass't S.....Little Rock, Ark.............To Surg. 24th Inf. July, 1861.
Andrews, L. G......... " ...................................................To May, 1863.

26TH INFANTRY—Mustered out October 21, 1865.

Carr, Jas. G ............Ass't S.....Clark's, Ohio .................From October, 1864.
Stimmell, M. M........Surgeon...Kenton, Ohio..................To May. 1863; also 135th Inf.
Rush, David............ " Celina, Ohio...................To June, 1865.
Sabine, Andrew.......Ass't S.. ..Marysville, Ohio ............To Feb., 1863; also 76th Inf.
Slusser, Lewis ........Surgeon...Canton, Ohio .................From July, 1865; also 69th Inf.
McGavran, Wm. B... " ...................................................To September. 1864.
Richards, Daniel......Ass't S.....New Philadelphia, Ohio..To February, 1863.

---

* Original Co. D detached as 12th Battery Ohio Light Artillery March 17, 1862. New Co. D organized.

OHIO—Continued.

27TH INFANTRY—Mustered out July 11, 1865.

| | | | |
|---|---|---|---|
| Denise, J. C | Surgeon | Omaha, Neb | To November, 1864. |
| Sprague, Jas | Ass't S | London, Ohio | To April, 1864. |
| Young, Isaac | Surgeon | London, Ohio | From November, 1864. |
| Thrall, Wm. R | “ | | To March. 1863 |
| Chapel, John L | Ass't S | | From April, 1865. |

28TH INFANTRY—Part mustered out July 23, 1864; the rest July 6, 1865.

| | | | |
|---|---|---|---|
| Denig, Chas. E | Surgeon | Columbus, Ohio | To July, 1864. |
| Hachenberg, Geo. P | Ass't S | Austin, Tex | To February, 1863. |
| Jenner, Alex. E | “ | Dayton, Ohio | To July, 1864. |
| Saal, Gerhardt | Surgeon | | To January, 1863. |
| Schoenbein, A | Ass't S | | To March, 1863. |

29TH INFANTRY—Mustered out July 13, 1865.

| | | | |
|---|---|---|---|
| Haines, E. P | Surgeon | Elyria, Ohio | Dead. |
| Fifield, Amos K | “ | Conneaut, Ohio | To August, 1864. |
| Miser, Thos B | “ | Martinsburgh, Ohio | From July, 1865. |
| Burrows, S. S | Ass't S | Geneva, Ohio | To Jan., 1863; also 177th Inf |
| Hosack, Cyrus | “ | | To August, 1863; also 183d Inf. |

30TH INFANTRY—Mustered out August 13, 1865.

| | | | |
|---|---|---|---|
| Beverly, P. F | Ass't S | 3d ave., Columbus, Ohio | To April, 1863. |
| Potter, Jos. B | Surgeon | Canal Winchester, Ohio | From November, 1861. |
| Richards, Chas. B | Ass't S | Binghamton, N Y | To October, 1864. |
| Stocker, Solomon | H. Stew | Gnadenhutten, Ohio. | |
| Grier, Henry T | Surgeon | | To Nov., 1861; also 60th Inf. |

31ST INFANTRY—Mustered out July 20, 1865.

| | | | |
|---|---|---|---|
| Chapel, Elias S | Surgeon | East Claridon, Ohio | From January, 1865. |
| Mountz, Jas. L | Ass't S | Morrow, Ohio | To Jan., 1863; also 144th Inf. |
| Arter, Jason R | Surgeon | | To September, 1864. |
| Varney, Royal W | Ass't S | | From April, 1863. |

32D INFANTRY—Mustered out July 20, 1865.*

| | | | |
|---|---|---|---|
| Brundage, A. H | Surgeon | Xenia, Ohio | To September, 1864. |
| Morgan, John | Ass't S | Cadiz, Ohio, or Tower Hill, Ill | To Feb., 1864. also 172d Inf. and 2d H. Art. |
| Sheldon, Silas E | “ | Topeka, Kan | To March, 1863; also 104th Inf. |
| Mowry, John N | Surgeon | Mansfield, Ohio | To January, 1862. |
| Buchannan, Jas. G | “ | | To January, 1863. |
| Grimes, Lewis A | Ass't S | | To July, 1864. |
| Clark, Chambers K | “ | | From June, 1865. |
| Bond, Thos. P | Surgeon | | From October, 1864; also 66th Inf. |

33D INFANTRY—Mustered out July 12, 1865.

| | | | |
|---|---|---|---|
| Mussey, F. B | Surgeon | Portsmouth, Ohio | To October, 1862. |
| Mossenneier, B | Ass't S | 552 Elm street, Cincinnati, Ohio. | To October, 1863. |
| Welsh, David | Surgeon | | To September, 1864; also 15th Inf. |
| Smith, Lionel J | “ | | From Nov., 1864; also 39th Inf. |
| Ropp, Wm. T. | Ass't S | | From January, 1864. |
| Phelps, Alonzo J | “ | | To Brig. Surg. April, 1862. |
| Hair, John H | “ | | To July, 1863. |

* Original Co. F detached as 26th Battery December 22, 1863; new company organized.

OHIO—Continued.

34TH INFANTRY—Consolidated with 36th Infantry February 24, 1865.

| Name | Rank | Residence | Remarks |
|---|---|---|---|
| Ayers, John H | Surgeon | Urbana, Ohio | From August, 1862. |
| Schilling, J. Philip | Ass't S | Louisville, Ohio | From June, 1864; also 88th Inf. |
| Clark, Wm. R. S | Surgeon | Blufton, Ohio | To Aug., 1862; also 86th Inf. (six months). |
| Miller, Chas. A | Ass't S | Court and Baymiller sts., Cincinnati, Ohio. | To September, 1864. |
| Cowan, Wilson V | " | Hardin, Ohio | To Feb., 1864; also 1st Cav. |
| Cantwell, Jas. S | Surgeon | | Missing December, 1861. |

35TH INFANTRY—Mustered out from August 26 to September 28, 1864; veterans and recruits transferred to the 18th Veteran Infantry.

| Name | Rank | Residence | Remarks |
|---|---|---|---|
| Gordon, P. A | Surgeon | Meilan or Mansfield, Ohio. | To November, 186[illegible]. |
| Wright, Chas. O | Ass't S | 76 W. 8th street, Cincinnati, Ohio. | To June, 1864 |
| Morris, Francis D | Surgeon | | A. W. M. |
| Landis, A. H | Ass't S | | A. W. M. |

36TH INFANTRY—Mustered out July 27, 1865.

| Name | Rank | Residence | Remarks |
|---|---|---|---|
| Dickinson, John | Ass't S | 33 Sibley street, or 146 Oranto st., Cleveland, Ohio. | To Surgeon 195th Inf. March, 1865. |
| Holcomb, B. F | " | Jackson C. H., Ohio | From April, 1865. |
| Whitford, Jas. H | Surgeon | Garnett, Kans | To March, 1863. H. R. |
| Barr, Robert N | " | | To February, 1862; also 87th Inf. (3 months). |
| Mackenzie, Colin | Ass't S | | To May, 1863. |
| Welch, Jas. P | " | | To September, 1864. |

37TH INFANTRY—Mustered out August 7, 1865.

| Name | Rank | Residence | Remarks |
|---|---|---|---|
| Arnold, Wm | Surgeon | Brownsville, Neb | To July, 1863; also 74th Inf. |
| Hohly, Fred'k | " | Toledo, Ohio | From May, 1864. |
| Ringler, Eugene | Ass't S | Saginaw, Mich | To Surgeon 106th Inf. March, 1864. |
| Schenck, Julius | Surgeon | 248 Pearl st., Cleveland, Ohio. | To November, 1862. |
| Billhardt, A. W | Ass't S | Upper Sandusky, Ohio | To October, 1864. |
| Gessner, Louis | " | Fremont, Ohio | To January, 1863. |
| Schenck, Conrad | Surgeon | | To June, 1862. |
| Pfeiffer, Nicholas | Ass't S | | To October, 1862. |
| Weidenbach, Aug | Surgeon | | Dismissed March, 1864. |

38TH INFANTRY—Mustered out July 12, 1865.

| Name | Rank | Residence | Remarks |
|---|---|---|---|
| Coons, Israel A | Surgeon | Spring Hill, Kans | To August, 1863. |
| Haller, Jas | " | Burlingame, Kans | To January, 1865. |
| Powell, H. B | " | Arrow Rock, Mo | From February, 1865. |
| Brooks, Theodore D | Ass't S | | To March, 1865. |

39TH INFANTRY—Mustered out July 9, 1865.

| Name | Rank | Residence | Remarks |
|---|---|---|---|
| Foster, Christian | Ass't S | Hamilton, Ohio | To Surgeon 58th Inf. November, 1862. |
| Follette, John A | Surgeon | 31 Milk st., Boston, Mass. | From November, 1862. |
| Smith, Lionel J | Ass't S | | To Surgeon 33d Inf. November, 1864. |
| Nixon, Oliver W | Surgeon | | To May, 1862. |
| McArthur, Thos. W | " | Chillicothe, Mo | To Sept., 1862. Ex. S. |
| Andrews, Wm. J | Ass't S | | From April, 1865. |
| Starr, Pierre S | " | | A. W. M. |

## OHIO—Continued.

**40TH INFANTRY**—Mustered out October, November, and December, 1864; veterans and recruits transferred to 51st Infantry December 10, 1864.

| Name | Rank | Address | Service |
|---|---|---|---|
| Beach, John N | Surgeon | West Jefferson, Ohio | To December, 1864 |
| Isaminger, And. E | Ass't S | Leadville, Col. | To December, 1864. |
| Kalb, Joseph C | " | Henry, Ill | To January, 1863; also 42d Inf. |
| Matchett, Wm. H | " | Greenville, Ohio | To October, 1864; also 186th Inf. |
| McBride, Alex | Surgeon | Berea, Ohio | To April, 1862; also 88th Inf. (3 months). |

**41ST INFANTRY**—Mustered out November 27, 1865.

| Name | Rank | Address | Service |
|---|---|---|---|
| Hart, Albert G | Surgeon | 37 Jennings ave., Cleveland, Ohio | To November, 1864. H. R. |
| Hill, John | " | Senecaville, Ohio | From Dec. 1864; also 75th, 86th and 139th Inf. |
| Cleveland, Thos. G | " | | To May, 1862. |
| Catlin, Wm. C | Ass't S | | To February, 1863; also 86th Inf. (6 months). |
| Bugh, John W | " | | To January, 1864 |
| Cheney, Benj. H | " | | To August, 1864. |
| Tupper, Chas. E | " | Ottawa, Ohio | From November, 1864. |
| Hubbard, John C | Surgeon | | To August, 1862. |

**42D INFANTRY**—Mustered out September 30 to December 2, 1864; veterans and recruits transferred to 96th Infantry.

| Name | Rank | Address | Service |
|---|---|---|---|
| Kalb, Jos. C | Surgeon | Henry, Ill | To August, 1864; also 40th Inf. |
| McFadden, H | Ass't S | Pharisburgh, Ohio | From January, 1864. |
| Pomerene, Joel | Surgeon | Millersburgh, Ohio | To July, 1863. Dead. |
| Harmon, Jos. W | Ass't S | | To November, 1862. |
| Driscol, John W | " | | To July, 1863. |

**43D INFANTRY**—Mustered out July 13, 1865.

| Name | Rank | Address | Service |
|---|---|---|---|
| Capehart, Henry | Surgeon | Bridgeport, Ohio | Not in A. G. R. |
| Morrow, Corridon | Ass't S | Bainbridge, Ohio | To March, 1864. |
| Poe, Chas. E | " | Ravenna, Ohio | From April, 1864. |
| Rose, Francis M | Surgeon | Faribault, Minn | From May, 1862. |
| McDermont, C. C | " | | Missing March, 1862. |
| Bell, Wm. S | Ass't S | U. S. Pension Office | To March, 1864. |
| Anderson, Wesley | " | | From March, 1865. |

**44TH INFANTRY**.—(See 8th Cavalry.)

**45TH INFANTRY**—Mustered out June 12, 1865.

| Name | Rank | Address | Service |
|---|---|---|---|
| Besse, Henry | Ass't S | Delaware, Ohio | To November, 1862; also 145th Inf. |
| Kearney, Thos. H | Surgeon | 209 West 7th street, Cincinnati, Ohio. | From August, 1862. |
| Hill, Robert J | Ass't S | 414 Washington ave., St. Louis, Mo. | From March, 1863, Secretary Board U. S. Ex. S. |
| Sheldon, Julius J | " | Beattie, Kansas | To November, 1864. |

**46TH INFANTRY**—Mustered out July 22, 1865.

| Name | Rank | Address | Service |
|---|---|---|---|
| Halderman, Davis | Surgeon | In Scotland | From February, 1865. |
| McFadden, Thos | " | Westerville, Ohio | To August, 1862. |
| Smedley, D. P | " | | To December, 1864. |
| Hagan, Chas. J | Ass't S | | From March, 1865. |

OHIO—Continued.

47TH INFANTRY—Mustered out August 11, 1865.

| | | | |
|---|---|---|---|
| Barlow, A. C. | Ass't S. | Fort Scott, Kans. | To November, 1862. |
| Huber, Jacob | " | Pana, Ill. | From April, 1863. H. R. |
| Spies, Geo. A. | Surgeon | | To April, 1862; also 106th Inf. |
| Hoeltze, Augustus | Ass't S. | | To January, 1863. |
| Davidson, Andrew | " | | To July, 1863. |
| Bonner, S. P. | Surgeon | 189 W. 7th street, Cincinnati, Ohio. | To December, 1864. |

48TH INFANTRY BATTALION—Mustered out May 9, 1866.

| | | | |
|---|---|---|---|
| Baird, Thos. C. | Ass't S. | | From July, 1863; also 114th Inf. |
| Willis, Plynn A. | Surgeon | | To March, 1862; also 48th and 83d Inf. |

48TH INFANTRY—Consolidated with the 83d Infantry January 17, 1865.

| | | | |
|---|---|---|---|
| Johnson, A. T. | Ass't S. | New Vienna, Ohio | To March, 1863. |
| Wiles, C. H. | " | Six Miles, or Hardinsburgh, Ind. | From April, 1863. |
| Willis, Plynn A. | Surgeon | Belle Point, Ohio | From March, 1863; also 83d Inf. |
| Carey, Milton T. | " | | To March, 1863. |
| Watt, William | Ass't S. | Kenton, Ohio | To January, 1864. |

49TH INFANTRY—Mustered out November 30, 1865.

| | | | |
|---|---|---|---|
| Corey, John M. | H. Stew. | Fremont, Ohio | H. R. |
| Park, Wm. H. | Surgeon | Bois D'Arc, Mo. | From Oct., 1864. H. R. |
| Thrift, Robt. W. | " | Lima, Ohio | To September, 1864. |
| Spencer, Sam'l H. | Ass't S. | Cortland, Ohio | To July, 1865. |
| Lung, Henry B. | " | | To March, 1864. |

50TH INFANTRY—Mustered out July 26, 1865.

| | | | |
|---|---|---|---|
| Keifer, Geo. | Surgeon | Troy, Ohio | To December, 1863. |
| Woods, Jos. T. | " | Toledo, Ohio | From Aug., 1862; also 99th Inf. |
| Sadler, Geo. | Ass't S. | Ravenna, Ohio | From June, 1864; also 99th Inf. |
| Cole, Nehemiah B. | " | | To April, 1865. |
| Crawford, S. K. | Surgeon | | To December, 1864. |

51ST INFANTRY—Mustered out October 3, 1865.

| | | | |
|---|---|---|---|
| Hagan, Martin | Ass't S. | St. Paul, Minn. | To Nov., 1862; also 161st Inf. |
| Woodworth, M. C. | Surgeon | Ellsworth, Wis. | To July, 1864. |
| Wing, E. D. W. C. | " | Fall City, Neb., or Mt. Vernon, Ohio | From July, 1864. |
| Jennings, R. P. | Ass't S. | | From March, 1863. |
| Weagley, L. E. | " | | From May, 1865. |

52D INFANTRY—Mustered out June 3, 1865.

| | | | |
|---|---|---|---|
| Hill, Nathan S. | Surgeon | Neville, Ohio | From Jan., 1865; also 121st Inf. |
| Simpson, S. A. | Ass't S. | | From June 1864. |
| Morse, Joel | Surgeon | | To May, 1863. |
| Duff, Henry M. | " | Calion, Ohio | To September, 1864. |

## OHIO—Continued.

### 53D INFANTRY—Mustered out August 11, 1865.

| Name | Rank | Residence | Service |
|---|---|---|---|
| Cake, Wm. M | Surgeon | Fostoria, or West Independence, Ohio. | To September, 1864. |
| Lair, John | " | Chillicothe, or Dayton, Ohio. | From January, 1865 |
| Bing, James P | Ass't S | Portsmouth, Ohio | To August, 1862. |
| Van Harlingen, R. L. | " | Lebanon, Ohio | To Surg. 70th Inf. Nov., 1863. |
| Hani, Wm. F | " | Middlebury, Ind | From July, 1865; also 175th Inf. |

### 54TH INFANTRY—Part mustered out November, 1864; the rest August 15, 1865.

| Name | Rank | Residence | Service |
|---|---|---|---|
| Brent, C. P | Surgeon | 133 W. 8th street, Cincinnati, Ohio. | To January, 1865. |
| Harper, T. L | Ass't S | 394 Wade street, Cincinnati. Ohio | To August, 1863. |
| Baggs, James | Surgeon | Ontario, Ohio | From March, 1865. |

### 55TH INFANTRY—Mustered out July 11, 1865.

| Name | Rank | Residence | Service |
|---|---|---|---|
| Hebble, Joseph | Surgeon | Springfield, Ohio | From November, 1864. |
| Myers, James C | Ass't S | Attica, Ohio | From April, 1865. |
| Kling, Jay | Surgeon | Monroeville, Ohio | To October, 1864. |
| Spooner, H K | Ass't S | Republic, Ohio | To Surg. 61st Inf. Nov. 1863. |

### 56TH INFANTRY—Mustered out April 25, 1866.

| Name | Rank | Residence | Service |
|---|---|---|---|
| King, Wilson N | Surgeon | Abilene, Kans | To August, 1863. |
| McFarland, P. M | Ass't S | Centralia, Ill | From September, 1865. |
| McGreer, John F | H. Stew | Sholer's Mills, Ohio. | |
| Payne, W. C | Ass't S | | To April, 1862. |
| Williams, David | Surgeon | Alexandria, Ohio | To Nov., 1864; also 7th Inf. |

### 57TH INFANTRY—Mustered out August 14, 1865.

| Name | Rank | Residence | Service |
|---|---|---|---|
| Le Fevre, N. D | Surgeon | Anna Station or Careysville, Ohio. | Not in A. G. R. |
| Woodruff, L | Ass't S | Alton, Ohio | To April, 1862. |
| Knauff, J. H | " | | To April, 1864. |
| Messenger, A. C | Surgeon | | To November, 1864. |
| Millikan, Robert H | " | | From January, 1865. |
| Frazer, Daniel M | Ass't S | | From April, 1865. |

### 58TH INFANTRY—Part mustered out January 14, the rest September 16, 1865.

| Name | Rank | Residence | Service |
|---|---|---|---|
| Forster, Christian | Surgeon | Hamilton, Ohio | To Jan., 1865; also 39th Inf. and 6th Light Artillery April and May, 1862. |
| Ringler, Eugene | Ass't S | Saginaw, Mich | To May, 1862; also 106th Inf. |
| King, W. H | | Abilene, Kan | Not in A. G. R. |
| McElwee, E. A | Ass't S | | To December, 1862. |
| Dayton, Eli | " | | To January, 1865. |
| Schallern, Reiner | Surgeon | | To September, 1862. |

### 59TH INFANTRY—Mustered out from June 28 to July 16, 1865.

| Name | Rank | Residence | Service |
|---|---|---|---|
| Gordon, Sidney C | Ass't S | Georgetown, Ohio | To November, 1864; also 189th Inf. |
| McChesney, A. C | Surgeon | 142 W. 8th street, Cincinnati Ohio. | To November, 1864. |
| Wilbur, Charles T | Ass't S | | To June, 1862; also 95th Inf. |
| Swingley, Frederick | " | | To November, 1862. |
| Barber, N. J | " | | To November, 1864. |

OHIO—Continued.

60TH INFANTRY—(1 year)—Mustered out November 10, 1862.

| Name | Rank | Residence | Remarks |
|---|---|---|---|
| Noble, David | Surgeon | Hillsborough, Ohio | From October, 1861. U. S. Ex. S. |
| Grier, Henry T | Ass't S | | A. W. M.; also 30th Inf. |
| Dwyer, R. A | " | New Petersburgh, Ohio | To May, 1862. |

60TH INFANTRY—Mustered out July 28, 1865.

| Name | Rank | Residence | Remarks |
|---|---|---|---|
| Ames, Charles E | Surgeon | | From June, 1864; also 14th Inf. and 1st Light Artillery. |
| Thompson, James F | Ass't S | | From May, 1865. |
| Evans, John M | " | Clarksburgh, Ohio | From January, 1865. |

61ST INFANTRY—Consolidated with 82d Infantry March 31, 1865.

| Name | Rank | Residence | Remarks |
|---|---|---|---|
| Pearce, Enoch | Surgeon | Steubenville, Ohio | To Surg. U. S. V. Sept., 1863. |
| Spooner, Henry K | " | Republic, Ohio | From November, 1863; also 55th Inf. |
| Culver, Lucius P | Ass't S | Riversville, Ohio | From November, 1863; also 82d Inf. |
| Conlin, J. J | " | | To September, 1863. |

62D INFANTRY—Consolidated with 67th Infantry September 1, 1865.

| Name | Rank | Residence | Remarks |
|---|---|---|---|
| Barlow, Augustus C | Surgeon | Fort Scott, Kan | From March, 1863. |
| Culbertson, H | Con't S | Zanesville, Ohio | H. R. for 1862. |
| Sayler, John H | Ass't S | Groveport, Ohio | From February, 1864; dismissed Sept. 25, 1865. |
| Truman, John | " | 67 Richmond street, Cincinnati, Ohio. | To June, 1863. |
| Wolfley, William I | " | 140 C street N. E., Washington, D. C. | To Surgeon U. S. Vols. June, 1864. |
| Hood, Charles H | Surgeon | | To January, 1863. |
| Haynes, Thomas J | Ass't S | | To September, 1862. |

63D INFANTRY—Mustered out July 8, 1865

| Name | Rank | Residence | Remarks |
|---|---|---|---|
| Monohan, A. B | Surgeon | Jackson C. H., Ohio | Dead. |
| Crane, Isaac L | " | | To January, 1862. |
| Marsh, John O | Ass't S | | To Nov. '62, also 153d Inf. |
| McDill, John B | " | | To May, '65; also 1st Cav. |

64TH INFANTRY—Part mustered out from December 10, 1864, to May 31, 1865. Final muster-out December 3, 1865.

| Name | Rank | Residence | Remarks |
|---|---|---|---|
| Mack, Henry O | Surgeon | Benzonia, Mich | To August, 1862. |
| Miller, Volney G | Ass't S | Lawrence, Kan | To May, 1863. |
| Potter, Amos | " | Paola, Kan | To November, 1863; also 156th Inf. |
| McMahon, A. M | Surgeon | San Jose, Cal | To July, 1864. |
| Anderson, Hugh P | " | | From August, 1864. |
| Quinn, Moses H | Ass't S | | From August, 1864. |

65TH INFANTRY—Mustered out November 30, 1865.

| Name | Rank | Residence | Remarks |
|---|---|---|---|
| Gill, John C | Ass't S | Cleveland, Ohio | To June, 1862; also 114th and 120th Inf. |
| Cruthers, John H | Surgeon | Delaware, Ohio | From March, 1865; also 88th Inf. |
| Todd, John M | " | Highland or New Lisbon, Ohio. | To December, 1864 |
| Patterson, Wm. E | Ass't S | Dungannon, Ohio | To October, 1865. |
| Patterson, Wilson S | " | Hillsborough, Ohio | To May, 1864 |
| Kyle, John G | Surgeon | Xenia, Ohio | To August, 1862; also 17th Inf. Dead |
| McCulley, Wm. A | Ass't S | Independence, Kan | To Surgeon 2d U. S. C. T. November, 1863. |

## OHIO—Continued.

### 66TH INFANTRY—Mustered out July 15, 1865.

| Name | Rank | Residence | Remarks |
|---|---|---|---|
| Brock, Jesse W | Surgeon | Leavenworth, Kan | From Sept, 1862. H. R. |
| Ludlum, B. F. | Ass't S. | Miamiville, Ohio | From March, 1863. |
| Bond, Thos. P | Surgeon | | To September, 1862; also 32d Inf. |

### 67TH INFANTRY—Mustered out December 7, 1865.

| Name | Rank | Residence | Remarks |
|---|---|---|---|
| Combs, Alfred S | Ass't S. | Thurman, Ohio | To May, 1865. |
| Forbes, Samuel F | Surgeon | Toledo, Ohio | To October, 1863. |
| Westfall, Jas | " | Minerva, Ohio | Dead. |
| Coston, Chauncey | Ass't S. | | To March, 1863. |
| Layton, John H. | " | | Dismissed Oct., 1865. |

### 68TH INFANTRY—Mustered out July 10, 1865.

| Name | Rank | Residence | Remarks |
|---|---|---|---|
| Bigham, John G | Surgeon | Millersburgh Ohio | From December, 1864. |
| Harrison, E. B | " | Napoleon, Ohio | To June, 1864. |
| Massie, Wm | Ass't S. | Paris, Ill | To August, 1864. |
| Voorhies, L. B | " | Mount Gilead, Ohio | Not in A. G. R. |
| Chase, S. C. | " | | To October, 1862. |
| Berkley, B. F. | " | | To December, 1862. |

### 69TH INFANTRY—Mustered out July 17, 1865.

| Name | Rank | Residence | Remarks |
|---|---|---|---|
| Janos, H. H. | H. Stew | Hamilton, Ohio. | |
| Stephenson, R | Surgeon | Manchester, Ohio | From May, 1865. |
| Slusser, Lewis | " | Canton, Ohio | To Feb., 1865; also 26th Inf. |
| Haynes, Moses H | Ass't S. | Seven Mile, Ohio | To Sept., 1862; also 167th Inf. |
| Frost, Milton, A | " | Bellevue, Ohio | To February, 1863. |

### 70TH INFANTRY—Mustered out August 14, 1865.

| Name | Rank | Residence | Remarks |
|---|---|---|---|
| Farrell, Thos. J | Ass't S. | Columbus, Ohio | To Dec., 1864. Dead. |
| Jaeger, Fred'k | " | E. Toledo or Elmore, O. | To January, 1864. |
| Van Harlingen, R.I. | Surgeon | Lebanon, Ohio | From Nov., 1863; also 53d Inf. |
| Montgomery, Wm | H. Stew | Manchester, Ohio. | |
| Swain, Chas. H | Surgeon | Toledo, Ohio | To August, 1863. Dead. |

### 71ST INFANTRY—Mustered out November 30, 1865.

| Name | Rank | Residence | Remarks |
|---|---|---|---|
| Hoagland, C. N | Surgeon | New York city | From November, 1863. |
| Crane, Wm. W | Ass't S. | Tippecanoe City, Ohio | To January, 1865. |
| Duncan, A. E | H. Stew | Yellow Springs, Ohio. | |
| Bowland, M. J | Ass't S. | | Missing Aug., 1862; also 8th Cav. |
| Wakefield, S. R | " | | To June, 1865. |

### 72D INFANTRY—Part mustered out December 14, 1864, the rest September 11, 1865.

| Name | Rank | Residence | Remarks |
|---|---|---|---|
| Rice, John B | Surgeon | Fremont, Ohio | To December, 1864. |
| Kaul, Wm. M | Ass't S. | | To June, 1864. |
| Caldwell, Wm | " | | To January, 1865. |
| Goodson, John W | " | Bellevue, Ohio | Dismissed March, 1863. |

### 73D INFANTRY—Part mustered out December 30, 1864, the rest July 20, 1865.

| Name | Rank | Residence | Remarks |
|---|---|---|---|
| Himes, Isaac N | Surgeon | 121 Prospect st., Cleveland, Ohio | To December, 1864. |
| Preston, John C | " | Cleveland, Ohio | From April, 1865. |
| Richeson, Wm | Ass't S. | Canal Dover, Ohio | To June, 1864. |
| Sigafoos, Jas | " | Bradford, Ohio | To October, 1862. |
| Steer, Smith D | " | Burton, Ohio | From April, 1865. |
| Safford, Jonas P | Surgeon | Keokuk, Iowa | Dismissed Dec., 1862. |

OHIO—Continued.

74TH INFANTRY—Mustered out July 10, 1865.

| | | | |
|---|---|---|---|
| Arnold, Wm | Ass't S | Somerset, Ohio | To Nov., 1862; also 37th Inf. |
| Dickson, M. M | Surgeon | Johnson's Corners, Ohio | From January, 1865. |
| Moore, Clarke A | Ass't S | | From June, 1865. |
| Steele, Ebenezer W | " | | To June, 1862. |
| Brelsford, Jas. R | Surgeon | | To November, 1864. |
| Williams, A. L | Ass't S | | Dismissed January, 1864. |

75TH INFANTRY—Mustered out from November 16, 1864, to July 27, 1865.

| | | | |
|---|---|---|---|
| Hart, Samuel | Surgeon | Marietta, Ohio | To May, 1863. |
| Ingram, John | " | Vineland, N. J. | To January, 1865. |
| Owen, Henry W | Ass't S | Huron Co., Ohio | To Nov., 1862; county auditor. |
| Wilson, Chas. L | Surgeon. | Atlanta, Ga | To Oct., 1863; also 141st Inf. |
| Hill, John | Ass't S | Senecaville, Ohio | To May, 1863; also 41st, 86th, and 139th Inf. |
| Wren, Daniel B | " | | To July, 1864. |

76TH INFANTRY—Mustered out July 15, 1865.

| | | | |
|---|---|---|---|
| *HOOD, THOS. B | Ass't S | U. S. Pension Office | To January, 1863. |
| Mendenhall, S. C | " | Frazeysburgh, Ohio | From Feb., 1863; also 78th Inf. |
| Sabine, Andrew | Surgeon | Marysville, Ohio | From Feb., 1863; also 26th Inf. |
| Smith, Geo. E | Ass't S | | To June, 1863. |

77TH INFANTRY—Part mustered out December 10, 1864, to January 3, 1865. Final muster out March 8, 1866.

| | | | |
|---|---|---|---|
| Lund, G. J | H. Stew | Marietta, Ohio. | |
| Wall, Andrew | Surgeon | Cambridge, Ohio | From September, 1864. |
| Warfield, Jas. W | " | Belmont, Ohio | To May, 1864. Dead. |
| Jones, Y. H | Ass't S | Cadiz, Ohio | To December, 1864. |

78TH INFANTRY—Part mustered out January 12, the rest July 11, 1865.

| | | | |
|---|---|---|---|
| Beach, Wm. M | Ass't S | London, Ohio | To Surg. 118th Inf. June, 1864. |
| Mendenhall, S. C | " | Frazeysburgh, Ohio | To April, 1862; also 76th Inf. |
| Peckham, Geo. F | " | Elyria, Ohio | From June, 1864. |
| Webb, Ralph D | " | Logan, Ohio | From April, 1865. |
| Reeves, Jas. S | Surgeon | Niles, or East Tawas, Mich. | From January, 1862. |
| Wortman, J. D | Ass't S | Cadiz, Ohio | To February, 1863. |
| De Forrest, E. C | " | | To November, 1863. |

79TH INFANTRY—Mustered out June 9, 1865.

| | | | |
|---|---|---|---|
| Jones, John E | Ass't S | 1295 E. Front st., Cincinnati, Ohio. | From May, 1863. |
| Langdon, H. H | Surgeon | Columbia, or Akron, Ohio. | From March, 1863. |
| Elstun, W. P | " | | To February, 1863. |
| Swander, Wm. H | Ass't S | | To December, 1863. |

* Medical referee U. S. Pension Office.

## OHIO—Continued.

### 80TH INFANTRY—Mustered out August 13, 1865.

Bombach, G............Ass't S....Ripley, Ohio....................To July, 1863.
Buell, E. P...........Surgeon...New Philadelphia, Ohio..To January, 1865.
Buvinger, C. W........ " 4407 Butler street, Pittsburgh, Pa. From April, 1865.
Tope, Hiram G.........Ass't S.....Lamartine, Ohio............From July, 1865.
Lee, Samuel............ " Coshocton, Ohio............To September, 1862.

### 81ST INFANTRY—Part mustered out September 26, 1864; the rest July 13, 1865.

Jacobs, Wm. C.........Surgeon...Akron, Ohio....................A. W. M.
Whittaker, John......Ass't S.....5th and Vine sts., Cincinnati, Ohio To November, 1864.
Lannue, Wm. H......Surgeon........................................To March, 1862.
McLean, Robt. G..... " ........................................To November, 1862.
Shaffer, Hiram M.....Ass't S........................................To Aug., 1864; also 187th Inf.

### 82D INFANTRY—Mustered out July 24, 1865.

*Cantwell, J. Y ......Surgeon...Decatur, Ala.................To Surg. U. S. Vols. July, 1864.
Culver, Lucius P...... " Riversville, Ohio............From July, 1865; also 31st Inf.
Hedges, Wm. B........Ass't S.....Delaware, Ohio.............From May, 1864; also 86th (6 months) Inf.
Meyers, Chas. W......Surgeon...Clinton, Iowa..................To May, 1865.
Munson, A. W.........Ass't S.....Kenton, Ohio...................To April, 1863, also 188th Inf.
Shaffer, W. B.......... " ........................................To December, 1861.

### 83D INFANTRY—Part mustered out July 24, 1865; veterans and recruits consolidated with those of 114th Infantry to form 48th Battalion.

Cassady, Geo..........Ass't S.....Cleves, Ohio....................To Surg. 182d Inf. April, 1865.
Wilkerson, M .......... " Clinton Co., Ohio..........To August, 1863.
Wiles, Christian H... " Six Mile, or Hardinsburgh, Ind..................... From April, 1863; also 48th Inf.
Willis, Plynn A........Surgeon...Belle Point, Ohio..........From March, 1863; also 48th Inf.
McGrew, John S...... " ........................................To July, 1864.

### 84TH INFANTRY—(3 months)—Mustered out September 20, 1862.

Leonard, B. B.........Surgeon...West Liberty, Ohio.........From June, 1862.
Thompson, J. W......Ass't S.....Died while in 10th Cav. Nov., 1864. From June, 1862.

### 85TH INFANTRY—(3 months)—Mustered out September 23 and 27, 1862.

Brown, L. C.............Surgeon...Painesville, Ohio............From June, 1862.
Darby, John E.........Ass't S.....Cleveland, Ohio .............From June, 1862.

### 86TH INFANTRY—(3 months)—Mustered out September, 25, 1862.

Hill, John ...............Surgeon...Senecaville, Ohio..........From June, 1862; also 41st, 75th, and 139th Inf.
Mowry, John N.......Surgeon...Moorefield, Ohio............From June, 1862.

---

*In charge of Hospital, 11th Army Corps.

## OHIO—Continued.

### 86TH INFANTRY—(6 months)—Mustered out February 10, 1864.

| Name | Rank | Residence | Remarks |
|---|---|---|---|
| Hill, John | Ass't S | Senecaville, Ohio | From Aug., 1863; also 41st, 75th and 139th Inf. |
| Hedges, Wm. B. | " | Delaware, Ohio | From Sept., 1863; also 82d Inf. |
| Smith, Jas. W | Surgeon | Wellington. Ohio | Not in A. G. R. |
| Clark, Wm. R. S | " | Blufton, Ohio | From July, 1863; also 34th Inf. |
| Catlin, Wm. C | Ass't S | | To Sept., 1863; also 41st Inf |

### 87TH INFANTRY—(3 months)—Mustered out from October 1 to 4, 1862.

| Name | Rank | Residence | Remarks |
|---|---|---|---|
| Barr, Robert N | Surgeon | | From June, 1862; also 36th Inf. |
| Miller, Orlando C | Ass't S. | Jackson C. H., Ohio | From May, 1862. |

### 88TH INFANTRY—Mustered out July 3, 1865.

| Name | Rank | Residence | Remarks |
|---|---|---|---|
| Cruthers, John H | Ass't S. | Delaware, Ohio | To April, 1865; also 65th Inf. |
| Schilling, J. Phil | " | Louisville, Ohio | From May, 1865; also 34th Inf. |
| Warner, Henry E | Surgeon | | From March, 1865. |
| Fountain, Wm. W | Ass't S | | From March, 1865; also 6th Inf. |

### 89TH INFANTRY—Mustered out June 7, 1865.

| Name | Rank | Residence | Remarks |
|---|---|---|---|
| Bradley, Harvey | Surgeon | Felicity, Ohio | To June, 1863. |
| Crew, Sam'l B | " | 146 6th st. S. W., Washington, D. C. | From June, 1863. |
| Purdum, Elijah F | Ass't S | | From August, 1863. |
| Spence, Colon | " | | To May, 1863. |

### 90TH INFANTRY—Mustered out June 13, 1865.

| Name | Rank | Residence | Remarks |
|---|---|---|---|
| Carpenter, H. W | Ass't S | Lancaster, Ohio | To May, 1863; also 187th Inf. |
| Tipton, Richard H | Surgeon | Darbyville, Ohio | From August, 1862. |
| O'Hanlon, Chas. P | Ass't S | East Fairfield, Ohio | A. W. M. |
| Wylie, Jefferson L | " | Ripley, Ohio | To November, 1862. |
| Coates, John G | " | | To December, 1863. |

### 91ST INFANTRY—Mustered out June 24, 1865.

| Name | Rank | Residence | Remarks |
|---|---|---|---|
| Carpenter, Geo. H | Surgeon | Athens, Ohio | To May, 1863. |
| Warwick, John B | " | Lucasville, Ohio | From August, 1863. |
| Newton, Wm. S | Ass't S | Gallipolis, Ohio | To Surgeon 193d Inf. March, 1865. |
| Wellous, G. S | " | Barnesville, Ohio | From August, 1863. |
| Alling, David G | " | | From March, 1865. |

### 92D INFANTRY—Mustered out June 10, 1865

| Name | Rank | Residence | Remarks |
|---|---|---|---|
| Beers, Adam H | Ass't S | New Comerstown, Ohio | From September, 1864. |
| Colton, Josiah D | Surgeon | Marietta, Ohio | From August, 1862. |
| Sisson, Nelson B | Ass't S | Porter Village, or Pine Grove, Ohio | To August, 1864. |
| Howel, Thos. D | " | | To April, 1863. |

### 93D INFANTRY—Part mustered out June 8, 1865, the rest transferred to 41st Infantry.

| Name | Rank | Residence | Remarks |
|---|---|---|---|
| Weaver, Jas. M | Surgeon | National Military Home, Montgomery Co, Ohio. | From September, 1864. |
| Brooks, Martin L, jr. | Ass't S | 98 Public Square, Cleveland, Ohio | From April, 1865. |
| Ashman, Geo P | Surgeon | | To August, 1864. |
| Bowers, Ezer D | Ass't S | Columbus, Ohio | To March, 1865. |

## OHIO—Continued.

### 94TH INFANTRY—Mustered out June 5, 1865.

Gibson, W B..........Surgeon...Topeka, Kans. ...............From December, 1863.
Lockett, I. N...........H. Stew...New Madison, Ohio.
Sinnet, Edwin.........Surgeon...Granville, Ohio..............To September, 1863.
Humphreville D.W..Ass't S.....Waterville, Kans............From April, 1864.
Fouts, Louis C......... " ..................................To April, 1863.

### 95TH INFANTRY—Mustered out August 14, 1865.

Gill, Henry Z..........Surgeon...Jerseyville, Ill..............To Surgeon U. S. Volunteers May, 1864.
Wilbur, Chas. T....... " ..................................From July, 1864: also 59th Inf.
Gaines, Wm. M........Ass't S..................................A. W. M.
Hoover, Enoch P...... " ..................................To April, 1864.

### 96TH INFANTRY—Mustered out July 7, 1865.

Henderson, D. W.....Surgeon...Marysville, Ohio............To April, 1863.
Hess, John F........... " Mount Vernon, Ohio......From September, 1863.
Ramage, Geo. W......Ass't S.....Round Grove, Ill............To December, 1864.
Sullivan, Wm J....... " Urbana, Ohio...................To February, 1863.

### 97TH INFANTRY—Part mustered out June 10, 1865, the rest transferred to 26th Infantry.

Gordon, Thos. W......Surgeon...Georgetown, Ohio..........To May, 1864.
Stewart, Thos. A...... " ..................................From August, 1864.
Cadwell, Jos. W.......Ass't S..................................From April, 1863.
Edwards, Jas. T...... " West Carlisle, Ohio........To December, 1862.

### 98TH INFANTRY—Mustered out June 1, 1865.

Sharp. Wm. T .........Ass't S.....Cadiz, Ohio...................To September, 1863.
West, Henry.............Surgeon...St. Clairsville, Ohio........To October, 1863.
Lewis, T. N ...... .....Ass't S..................................To February, 1863.
McCracken, Wm. A..Surgeon..................................From May, 1864.
Simons, Chas. P.......Ass't S....Cambridge, Ohio. ...........From May, 1864.

### 99TH INFANTRY—Consolidated with 50th Infantry December 31, 1864.

Sadler, Geo...............Ass't S.....Ravenna, Ohio..............From June, 1864. H. R. Also 50th Inf.
Woods, J. T ..............Surgeon...Toledo, Ohio..................From Aug., 1862; also 50th Inf.
Clemons, P. H.........Ass't S.....U. S. Pension Office.......To Surgeon, 17th U. S. C. T. Nov., 1863.
Stover, Samuel T..... " ..................................To April, 1864.
Wood, Geo. T.......... " ..................................Dismissed Oct., 1862.

### 100TH INFANTRY—Mustered out June 20, 1865.

Collamore, Geo. A...Surgeon...Toledo, Ohio....................From August, 1862.
Johnson, Robt.........Ass't S....Milford, Mich...................A. W. M.
Brown, Elijah J.......H. Stew...Junction, Ohio.
Thacker, Wm. H......Ass't S..................................To October, 1863.

### 101ST INFANTRY—Mustered out June 12, 1865.

Cook, Thos. M.........Surgeon...Sandusky, Ohio..............From August '62. H R.
Russell, Hiram H.....Ass't S..................................From April, 1865: also 138th Inf.
Zingling, Geo. S...... " ..................................To January, 1863.
Caswell, Walter....... " ..................................To July, 1863.
Lacey, Henry T....... " ..................................To November, 1864.

OHIO—Continued.

102D INFANTRY—Mustered out June 30, 1865.

| Name | Rank | Residence | Remarks |
|---|---|---|---|
| Beach, Wm. | Ass't S. | Madison or London, O. | Not in A. G. R. |
| Mitchell, Geo. | " | Mansfield, Ohio | From August, 1862. |
| Patterson, A. V. | Surgeon | Mansfield, Ohio | From September, 1862. U. S Ex. S. |
| Irwin, Aaron J. | Ass't S. | Dead | To Surg. 2d Tenn. Mt'd Inf., April, 1864. |

103D INFANTRY—Mustered out June 12, 1865.

| Name | Rank | Residence | Remarks |
|---|---|---|---|
| Griswold, L. D. | Surgeon | Elyria, Ohio | To August, 1864. |
| Butler, Geo. O. | Ass't S. | 92 Scoville st., Cleveland, Ohio. | To May, 1863. |
| Casebeer, Jacob B. | " | Auburn, Ind. | From March, 1865. |
| Brinkerhoff, D. H. | Surgeon | Fremont, Ohio | From August, 1864. |
| Stansbury, R. S. | Ass't S. | | To January, 1864; also 155th Inf. |

104TH INFANTRY—Mustered out June 17, 1865.

| Name | Rank | Residence | Remarks |
|---|---|---|---|
| *Boynton, D. T. | Surgeon | Knoxville, Tenn. | To May, 1865. |
| Rodgers, John H. | " | Springfield, Ohio | To December, 1864; also 8th Cav. U. S. Ex. S. |
| Sheldon, Silas E. | Ass't S. | Topeka, Kan. | A. W. M. Also 32d Inf. |
| McKenzie, N. K. | " | Wellsville, Ohio | To January, 1863. |
| Johnson, R. P. | " | Canton, Ohio | To February, 1863. |
| Thomas, K. G. | Surgeon | | To December, 1862. |

105TH INFANTRY—Mustered out June 3, 1865.

| Name | Rank | Residence | Remarks |
|---|---|---|---|
| Fowler, Chas. N. | Surgeon | Youngstown, Ohio | A. W. M. |
| Turnbull, John | Ass't S. | Bellbrook, Ohio | From July, 1863. |
| Taft, Harvey S. | " | Marquette, Mich. | To August, 1863. |
| Paulding, Jos. G. | " | | To April, 1863. |

106TH INFANTRY—Mustered out June 29, 1865.

| Name | Rank | Residence | Remarks |
|---|---|---|---|
| Ringler, Eugene | Surgeon | Saginaw, Mich. | From March, 1864. H. R. Also 58th Inf. |
| Westbrook, A. E. | Ass't S. | Ashley, Ohio | From August, 1863. |
| Spies, Geo. A. | Surgeon | | To February, 1863; also 47th Inf. |
| Schroen, Adolph | " | New Richmond, Ohio. | To January, 1864. |

107TH INFANTRY—Mustered out July 10, 1865.

| Name | Rank | Residence | Remarks |
|---|---|---|---|
| Knaus, John | Surgeon | Care A. G. U. S. A. | From March, 1864. |
| Schill, Franz | Ass't S. | 44 W. 7th st., Cincinnati, Ohio. | From May, 1864. |
| Shopp, Hubert | Surgeon | | To November, 1863; also 108th Inf. |
| Wannenwetsch | Ass't S. | | To February, 1863. |
| Niedermeyer, H. | " | River Road, Cincinnati, Ohio. | To July, 1863; also 27th U. S. C. T. |

108TH INFANTRY—Mustered out June 9 and July 22, 1865.

| Name | Rank | Residence | Remarks |
|---|---|---|---|
| Matzdorff, A. | Ass't S. | Cincinnati, Ohio | Dead. |
| Zipperlen, A. | Surgeon | 23 Webster st., Cincinnati, Ohio. | From August, 1862. |
| Shopp, Hubert | Ass't S. | | To Surgeon 107th Infantry, June, 1863. |
| Mills, Lucius | " | | To April, 1865. |
| Ulrich, Henry | " | Dead | To July, 1864. |
| Hettich, C. F. | " | | Dismissed December, '62. |

* U. S. Pension Agent.

## OHIO—Continued.

109TH INFANTRY—Failed to complete; men transferred to 113th Infantry.

### 110TH INFANTRY—Mustered out June 25, 1865.

McCandliss, R. R.....Surgeon...Emporia, Kan.................From July, 1863.
Park, Wm. H..........Ass't S.....Elyria, Ohio..................From July, 1864.
Ebersole, E. P.........  "  Lewisburgh, Ohio..........From September, 1864.
Pixley, Sumner........Surgeon...Peninsula, Ohio.............To May, 1863.
Owen, Thos. C.........Ass't S....Richmond, Ohio.............To April, 1864.
Pinkerton, Alex. W..  "  ..................................To August, 1864.

### 111TH INFANTRY—Mustered out June 27, 1865.

Chalfant, Caleb M....Ass't S.....326 Pearl st., Cleveland, Ohio. To Surgeon 107th U. S. C. T. September, 1864.
Brewer, Lyman A....Surgeon.....................................From September, 1862.
Mock, John W.........Ass't S......................................From August, 1864.

112TH INFANTRY—Failed to complete.

### 113TH INFANTRY—Mustered out July 6, 1865.

Black, Jas. R..........Surgeon...Newark, Ohio.................To July, 1863.
Wilson, Albert.........  "  ..................................From September, 1863; also 1st Inf.
Bassett, Hiram H.....Ass't S.....Mt. Pleasant, Ohio.........To Surgeon 121st Infantry April, 1865.
Harlow, Alonzo.......  "  ..................................To May, 1863.
Tipton, Thomas C...  "  Williamsport, Ohio.........To June, 1863
Kemp, Geo. W.........  "  Marseilles, Ohio.............To October, 1863.

### 114TH INFANTRY—Mustered out July 31, 1865; veterans and recruits transferred to 48th Battalion.

French, Otis E ........Surgeon...Denver, Col.....................To December, 1864.
Gill, John C ............  "  Cleveland, Ohio.............From June, 1865; also 65th and 120th Inf.
Peck, Wm. L...........Ass't S.....Indianapolis, Ind............To Surg. 3d Inf. Nov., 1862.
Stanton, Byron........Surgeon...610 Freeman st., Cincinnati, Ohio. To May, 1865; also 120th Inf. and 1st L. Art.
Baird, Thos. C... .....Ass't S......................................From July, 1863; also 48th Bat.
Bean, Asa A............  "  ..................................To April, 1863.
Lenardson, H..........  "  ..................................To June, 1863.

### 115TH INFANTRY—Mustered out June 22, 1865.

Brenton, Jos. L........Ass't S.....North Georgetown, Ohio..To Surg. 8th Inf. March, 1863.
Johnson, Henry B....Surgeon...Beloit, Wis.........................To February, 1865.
Jones, Wm. H ........  "  Jeffersonville, Ohio.........From March, 1865.
Reed, John W.........Ass't S.....Barnesville, Ohio............From September, 1864.
Patterson, A. J........  "  ..................................To November, 1863.

### 116TH INFANTRY—Mustered out June 14, 1865.

Brown, Josiah L .....Ass't S....Green Spring, Ohio........To October, 1864.
Smith, T. Curtis ......Surgeon...Aurora, Ind.....................From December, 1864.
Waterman, H. C......Ass't S.....Middleport, Ohio............Not in A. G. R.
Sampsell, Jas. A......  "  Columbiana Co., Ohio.....From January, 1865.
Johnson, Jas............  "  Cheshire, Ohio.................To February, 1863.
Hudson, J. Q. A......  "  ..................................To March, 1863.

117TH INFANTRY—(See 1st Heavy Artillery.)

OHIO—Continued.

118TH INFANTRY—Mustered out June 24, 1865.

| | | | |
|---|---|---|---|
| Beach, Wm. M | Surgeon | London, Ohio | From June, 1863; also 78th Inf. |
| Patterson, J. E | Ass't S | Maple Hill, Ohio | From January, 1865. |
| Phillips, Wm. H | Surgeon | Kenton, Ohio | To May, 1864 |
| Richardson, N. S | Ass't S | Macon, Mo | To Surg. 13th Cav. Nov., 1864. |
| Bodman, H. A | " | | To December, 1862. |
| Schaffer, Wm. B | " | | To February, 1864. |

119TH INFANTRY—Failed to complete its organization. Men transferred to 124th Infantry.

120TH INFANTRY—Consolidated with 114th Infantry November 27, 1864.

| | | | |
|---|---|---|---|
| Hammond, J. W | Surgeon | Wellsville, Ohio | To August, 1863. |
| Stanton, Byron | " | 610 Freeman st, Cincinnati, Ohio. | A. W. M. Also 114th Inf. and 1st L. Art. |
| Stoufer, C. C | Ass't S | West Salem, Ohio | To January, 1864. |
| Gill, John C | " | Cleveland, Ohio | From March, 1864; also 65th and 114th Inf. |
| Taggart, Wm. W | Surgeon | Wooster, Ohio | To November, 1862. |

121ST INFANTRY—Mustered out June 8, 1865.

| | | | |
|---|---|---|---|
| Keyes, B. W | H. Stew | Marysville, Ohio | Belonged to 121st or 122d Vol. |
| Hill, Nathan S | Ass't S | Neville, Ohio | To Surg. 52d Inf. Jan., 1865. |
| Williams, Thos B | Surgeon | Delaware, Ohio | To March, 1865. Dead |
| Bassett, Hiram H | " | Mt. Pleasant, Ohio | From April, 1865; also 113th Inf. |
| Scoville, Selden S | Ass't S | | To May, 1863. |

122D INFANTRY—Mustered out June 26, 1865.

| | | | |
|---|---|---|---|
| Houston, Wm. M | Surgeon | Urbana, Ohio | From Jan., 1863. H. R. |
| Richards, Alva | Ass't S | New Lexington, Ohio | To Surg. 126th Inf. Dec., 1864. |
| Bryant, Wilson G | " | Springfield, Ohio | To Surg. 197th Inf. May, 1865. |
| Reamay, T. A | Surgeon | Zanesville, Ohio | To January, 1863. |
| Keyes, Beverly W | H. Stew | Marysville, Ohio. | |

123D INFANTRY—Mustered out June 12, 1865.

| | | | |
|---|---|---|---|
| Hyatt, Wm. B | Surgeon | Marshallville, Ohio | From December, 1864. |
| Williams, Jas. H | Ass't S | Ada, Ohio | To January, 1864. |
| Brisbine, N. B | " | | From March, 1864; also 2d Cav. |
| Ferris, Orrin | Surgeon | | To November, 1864; also 15th Inf. |

124TH INFANTRY—Mustered out July 9, 1865.

| | | | |
|---|---|---|---|
| Patterson, DeW. C | Surgeon | 919 I st., N.W., Washington, D. C. | From May, 1863. |
| Smith, Jas. W | " | Wellington, Ohio | To Jan., 1863; also 129th Inf. (6 mos.) and 150th (3 mos.) |
| Bidwell, T. S | Ass't S | | From May, 1863. |
| Morse, David A | " | Midway, Ohio | To Aug., 1863; also 162d Inf. |

OHIO—Continued.

125TH INFANTRY—Mustered out September 25, 1865.—Co. A mustered out June 8, and Co. B June 20, 1865.

| | | | |
|---|---|---|---|
| McHenry, Henry | Surgeon | Napoleon, Ohio | To June, 1865. |
| Yates, Porter | Ass't S. | Port Clinton, Ohio | To May, 1863; also 128th Inf. U. S. Ex. S. |
| Buchanan, Jas. G. | " | | To January, 1865; also 32d Inf. |
| Darby, John E. | " | | To S. 42d U. S. C. T. May, 1864; also 85th Inf. (3 months). |
| McKim, Wm. E. | Surgeon | | From March, 1865. |

126TH INFANTRY—Mustered out June 25, 1865.

| | | | |
|---|---|---|---|
| Ely, J. Sykes | Surgeon | Barnesville, Ohio | To June, 1864. U.S. Ex.S. |
| Estep, Wm. | " | Loydsville, Ohio | To February, 1864. |
| Richards, Alva | " | New Lexington, Ohio | From December, 1864; also 122d Inf. |
| Worley, Joshua | Ass't S | | From July, 1864. |
| Weed, Ithamar B. | Surgeon | | To November, 1864. |
| Alcorn, Jas. P | Ass't S | | Dismissed March, 1863. |

127TH INFANTRY—(See 5th U. S. C T.)

128TH INFANTRY—Mustered out July 13, 1865.

| | | | |
|---|---|---|---|
| Woodbridge, T | Surgeon | Fort Peck (via Fort Buford, Dak. Ter.) | From September, 1862. |
| Yates, Porter | Ass't S. | Green Springs or Port Clinton, Ohio. | From January, 1864; also 125th Inf. |
| Tripp, Wm | " | Carroll Co., Ohio | From January, 1864. |

129TH INFANTRY—(6 months)—Mustered out from March 4 to 10, 1864.

| | | | |
|---|---|---|---|
| Smith, Jas W | Ass't S. | Wellington, Ohio | From August, 1863. H. R; also 124th and 150th Inf. |
| Campbell, John | " | Delhi, Ohio | From August, 1863; also 178th Inf. |
| Weber, G C. E | Surgeon | | To November, 1863. |

130TH INFANTRY—(100 days)—Mustered out September 22, 1864.

| | | | |
|---|---|---|---|
| Hathaway, Calvin | Ass't S. | Edgerton, Ohio | From May, 1864. |
| Thorn, Samuel S | Surgeon | Toledo, Ohio | From May, 1864. |

131ST INFANTRY—(100 days)—Mustered out August 25, 1864.

| | | | |
|---|---|---|---|
| Britton, Orson | Surgeon | | From May, 1864. |
| Lathrop, Levi B | Ass't S | | From May, 1864. |

132D INFANTRY—(100 days)—Mustered out September 10, 1864.

| | | | |
|---|---|---|---|
| Sullivan, Wm. J | Surgeon | Urbana, Ohio | From May, 1864. |
| Edward, Richard | Ass't S. | Ridgeway, Ohio | From May, 1864; also 177th Inf. |
| Matson, Albert F. | " | | From May, 1864. |

133D INFANTRY—(100 days)—Mustered out August 20, 1864.

| | | | |
|---|---|---|---|
| Landon, C. P. | Surgeon | Westerville, Ohio | From May, 1864. |
| McConnel, R. N | Ass't S. | Upper Sandusky, Ohio | From May, 1864. |
| Ridenour, David | " | | From May, 1864. |

OHIO—Continued.

134TH INFANTRY—(100 days)—Mustered out August 31, 1864.

Baker, Benj. F.........Ass't S.....St. Paris, Ohio...............From May, 1864.
Spain, Jas. F.........Surgeon.......................................From May, 1864.
Wells, Allen W.......Ass't S.......................................A. W. M.

135TH INFANTRY—(100 days)—Mustered out September 1, 1864.

Stimmell, M. M........Surgeon...Kenton, Ohio.................From May, 1864; also 26th Inf.
Gregory, D. H.........Ass't S.....Newark, Ohio................Dead.
Jones, Wm. Jr......... " ..........................................From May, 1864.

136TH INFANTRY—(100 days)—Mustered out August 31, 1864.

Boylan, Aaron.........Ass't S....Milford Centre, Ohio......From June, 1864.
Reed, William......... " Iberia, Ohio...................From May, 1864; also 176th Inf.
Hewitt, S. M............Surgeon...Winton Place, Ohio.......From July, 1864.

137TH INFANTRY—(100 days)—Mustered out August 19, 1864.

Culbertson, Jas. C...Ass't S.....281 W. 7th street, Cincinnati, Ohio. From July, 1864.
Davis, Wm. B..........Surgeon...310 Elm street, Cincinnati, Ohio. From May, 1864.
Hunt, Charles........ Ass't S.....Wooster, Ohio...............To July, 1864; also 169th Inf.

138TH INFANTRY—(100 days)—Mustered out September 1, 1864.

Wilson, Chas. P......Surgeon.......................................From May, 1864.
Fuller, Amos B........Ass't S.....Loudonville, Ohio..........From June, 1864.
Russell, Hiram H..... " ..........................................From June, 1864; also 101st Inf.

139TH INFANTRY—(100 days)—Mustered out August 26, 1864.

Hill, John...............Surgeon...Senecaville, Ohio...........From May, 1864; also 41st, 75th, and 86th Inf.
McKennon, B. F......Ass't S.....Lewistown, Ohio............From May, 1864.

140TH INFANTRY—(100 days)—Mustered out September 3, 1864.

Rathburn, D. C........Surgeon...Middleport, Ohio...........From May, 1864. G.

141ST INFANTRY—(100 days)—Mustered out September 3, 1864.

Johnston, Jas. ....... Ass't S.....Kyger, Ohio..................From May, 1864.
Wilson, Chas. L......Surgeon...Atlanta, Ga....................From May, 1864; also 75th Inf.

142D INFANTRY—(100 days)—Mustered out September 2, 1864.

King, Wilson N........Surgeon...Abilene, Kan..................From May, 1864.
Stamp, Jacob...........Ass't S.....Mt. Vernon, Ohio..........From May, 1864.

143D INFANTRY—(100 days)—Mustered out September 13, 1864.

Lee, Sam'l H...........Surgeon.......................................From May, 1864.
Chandler, G. M........Ass't S.....Akron, Ohio .................From June, 1864.

144TH INFANTRY—(100 days)—Mustered out August 31, 1864.

Mounts, Jas. L........ Surgeon...Morrow, Ohio................From May, 1864; also 31st Inf.
Baker, Edward F.....Ass't S.....600 N. Wells st., Chicago, Ill. From May, 1864; also 183d Inf.
White, G. M............ " ..........................................From May, 1864.

## OHIO—Continued.

### 145TH INFANTRY—(100 days)—Mustered out August 24, 1864.

Besse, Henry..........Surgeon...Delaware, Ohio..............From May, 1864; also 45th Inf.
Janney, John D.......Ass't S...................................From May, 1864.
Starr, Moses L......... " Shenandoah, Ohio.........From May, 1864.

### 146TH INFANTRY—(100 days)—Mustered out September 7, 1864.

Drake, Isaac L.........Surgeon...Lebanon, Ohio................From May, 1864.
Evans, Otho, Jr ..... Ass't S....Franklin, Ohio................From May, 1864.
Sellers, Amos.......... " Waynesville, Ohio ...... . From May, 1864.

### 147TH INFANTRY—(100 days)—Mustered out August 30, 1864.

Coleman, Horace......Surgeon...Troy, Ohio....................From May, 1864. U. S. Ex. S.
Hershiser, H. K........Ass't S...................................From June, 1864.

### 148TH INFANTRY—(100 days)—Mustered out September 14, 1864.

Beebe, Wm...............Surgeon...Barlow, Ohio. ...............From May, 1864.
Culver, Benj. F........Ass't S.....Vincent, Ohio ................From May, 1864; also 8th Inf.

### 149TH INFANTRY—(100 days)—Mustered out August 30, 1864.

Brown, Wm. A ........Surgeon...933 New York avenue, Washington, D. C. From May, 1864; also 176th Inf.
Miesse, Benj. F........Ass't S.....Chillicothe, Ohio............From May, 1864.

### 150TH INFANTRY—(100 days)—Mustered out August 23, 1864.

Smith, Jas. W .........Surgeon...Wellington, Ohio .........From May, 1864; also 124th and 129th Inf.
Dutton, Chas. F......Ass't S...................................From May, 1864.
Armstrong, J. F...... " 427 Pearl street, Cleveland, Ohio. From May, 1864.

### 151ST INFANTRY—(100 days)—Mustered out August 27, 1864.

Kelch, Jas. R...........Ass't S.....Tarlton, Ohio ..................From May, 1864.
Harper, Wm. H ......Surgeon...Lima, Ohio......................From May, 1864.
Holloway, A. G. .....Ass't S.....Wauseon, Ohio..............From May, 1864.

### 152D INFANTRY—(100 days)—Mustered out September 2, 1864.

Williamson, J. C......Surgeon...Versailles, Ohio..............From May, 1864.
Jobes, John A .........Ass't S ....Palestine, Ohio..............From May, 1864.

### 153D INFANTRY—(100 days)—Mustered out September 9, 1864.

Combs, John S.........Surgeon...Owensville, Ohio............From May, 1864.
Marsh, John O.........Ass't S...................................From May, 1864; also 63d Inf.

### 154TH INFANTRY—(100 days)—Mustered out September 1, 1864.

Watt, George..........Surgeon...Xenia, Ohio.....................From May, 1864.
McClung, Leigh.......Ass't S.....Xenia, Ohio ....................From May, 1864.

### 155TH INFANTRY—(100 days)—Mustered out August 27, 1864.

Stansbury, R. S.......Surgeon...................................From Aug., 1864; also 103d Inf.

OHIO—Continued.

156TH INFANTRY—(100 days)—Mustered out September 1, 1864.

| | | | |
|---|---|---|---|
| Miller, Volney G | Surgeon | Lawrence, Kans | From May, 1864; also 64th Inf. |
| Robinson, Jas. N | Ass't S. | | From May, 1864. |
| Evans, Caleb S | " | Hill Grove, Ohio | From May, 1864. |

157TH INFANTRY—(100 days)—Mustered out September 2, 1864.

| | | | |
|---|---|---|---|
| Eames, Wm. M | Surgeon | Ashtabula, Ohio | From May, 1864; also 21st Inf. |
| Eagle, Thos. B | Ass't S. | | From May, 1864. |
| Fisher, Benj. H | " | | From May, 1864. |

158TH INFANTRY—Failed to complete.

159TH INFANTRY—(100 days)—Mustered out August 22 and 24, 1864.

| | | | |
|---|---|---|---|
| Chambers, Rob't | Surgeon | Chandlersville, Ohio | From May, 1864. |
| Holden, Wm. H | Ass't S. | New Lexington, Ohio | From May, 1864. |

160TH INFANTRY—(100 days)—Mustered out September 7, 1864.

| | | | |
|---|---|---|---|
| Holcomb, C. B | Ass't S. | Bremen, Ohio | From May, 1864; also 192d Inf. |
| Kraps, John | Surgeon | Caldwell, or Bremen, Ohio. | From May, 1864; also 7th Cav. |

161ST INFANTRY—(100 days)—Mustered out September 2, 1864.

| | | | |
|---|---|---|---|
| Thompson, S. R | Ass't S. | Uhrichsville, Ohio | Not in A. G. R. |
| Tucker, Henry C | " | El Paso, Kans | From May, 1864. |
| Hagan, Martin | Surgeon | St. Paul, Minn | From May, 1864; also 51st Inf. |

162D INFANTRY—(100 days)—Mustered out September 4, 1864.

| | | | |
|---|---|---|---|
| Morse, D. A | Surgeon | Midway, Ohio | From May, 1864; also 124th Inf. |
| Whitacre, Thos. H | Ass't S. | Magnolia, Ohio | From May, 1864. |
| Miller, David H | " | | From May, 1864. |

163D INFANTRY—(100 days)—Mustered out September 10, 1864.

| | | | |
|---|---|---|---|
| Carter, Jas. O | Ass't S. | Lincoln, Nebr | From May, 1864. |
| McMillen, D. C | " | Mansfield, Ohio | From May, 1864. |
| Sutherland, Alex | Surgeon | Mansfield, Ohio | From May, 1864. |

164TH INFANTRY—(100 days)—Mustered out August 27, 1864.

| | | | |
|---|---|---|---|
| Hale, Robert W | Surgeon | Fostoria, Ohio | From May, 1864. |
| Schaffner, John F | Ass't S. | Willshire, Ohio | From May, 1864. |
| Yingling, Geo. S | " | Tiffin, Ohio | From May, 1864. |

165TH INFANTRY—(100 days)—Mustered out August 31, 1864.

| | | | |
|---|---|---|---|
| Mallory, Henry | Surgeon | Hamilton, Ohio | From June, 1864. |
| Wolff, Solomon | Ass't S. | Wilmoth, Ohio | From June, 1864. |

166TH INFANTRY—(100 days)—Mustered out September 9, 1864.

| | | | |
|---|---|---|---|
| Carr, Jas. G | Ass't S. or Lt | Clark's, Ohio | Not in A. G. R. as Ass't Surg. |
| Ebright, Thos. M | Surgeon | Akron, Ohio | From May, 1864. |
| Sykes, Wm H | Ass't S. | Plymouth, Ohio | From May, 1864. |
| Newkirk, Henry C | " | | From May, 1864. |

OHIO—Continued.

167TH INFANTRY—(100 days)—Mustered out September 8, 1864.

Haynes, Moses H......Surgeon.........................................From May, 1864; also 69th Inf.

Ferguson, Jas. S......Ass't S.....Camden, Ohio ...............From May, 1864.

168TH INFANTRY—(100 days)—Mustered out September 8, 1864.

Granger, Benj. D......Surgeon...Russell Station, Ohio......From May, 1864; also 175th Inf

Smith, Chas. H.........Ass't S.....Kenton, Ohio.................From June, 1864.

169TH INFANTRY—(160 days)—Mustered out September 4, 1864.

Beauregard, Peter....Surgeon...Fremont, Ohio...............From May, 1864.
McCarty, Oliver C....Ass't S.....Polk, Ohio.....................From July, 1864; also 181st Inf.

Hunt, Charles ......... " Wooster, Ohio ..............From July, 1864.

170TH INFANTRY—(100 days)—Mustered out September 10, 1864.

Crawford, Jas. B......Surgeon...Uhrichsville, Ohio..........From May, 1864.

171ST INFANTRY—(100 days)—Mustered out August 20, 1864.

Applegate, F. C.......Surgeon...Windham, Ohio..............From May, 1864.
Miner, Albert G.......Ass't S.....Niles, Ohio.....................From May, 1864.
Pitman, Benj. F....... " Cincinnati, Ohio..............From May, 1864.

172D INFANTRY—(100 days)—Mustered out September 3, 1864.

Morgan, John..........Surgeon...Cadiz, Ohio.....................From June, 1864; also 2d H. Art. and 32d Inf.

Wyman, George ......Ass't S.....Topeka, Kas....................From June, 1864; also 173d Inf.

Mosher, E. B........... " ........................................ From June, 1864.

173D INFANTRY—(1 year)—Mustered out June 26, 1865.

Marr, Jas. C...........Surgeon...Niles Ohio.........................From September, 1864; also 6th Cav.

Morris, Joseph.........Ass't S....Columbus Grove, Ohio...From September, 1864.
Wyman, George...... " Topeka, Kan....................From October, 1864; also 172d Inf.

174TH INFANTRY—(1 year)—Mustered out June 28, 1865.

Morrison, F. W........Surgeon...Delaware, Ohio...............From September, 1864.
Starr, Mitchell.........Ass't S....Shenandoah ...................From Sept., 1864. H. R.
Monroe, Chas. E...... " ........................................From April, 1865.

175TH INFANTRY—(1 year)—Mustered out June 27, 1865.

Dwyer, Rufus A......Surgeon...New Petersburgh, Ohio..From October, 1864; also 2d Heavy Artillery.

Granger, Benj. D.....Ass't S.....Russell Station, Ohio......A. W. M. Also 168th Infantry.

Hani, Wm. F.......... " Middleburgh, Ind..........To May, 1865; also 53d Inf

176TH INFANTRY—Mustered out June 14, 1865.

Brown, Wm. A........Surgeon...933 New York avenue, Washington, D. C. From September, 1864; also 149th Inf.

Fiser, Chas. M.........Ass't S.....Fort Wayne. Ind., or Liberty, Ohio. From January, 1865.

Reed, Wm............... " Iberia, Ohio.....................From January, 1865; also 136th Inf.

## OHIO—Continued.

### 177TH INFANTRY—(1 year)—Mustered out June 24, 1865.

| Name | Rank | Residence | Service |
|---|---|---|---|
| Burrows, S. S. | Surgeon | Geneva, Ohio | From October, 1864; also 29th Inf. |
| Edwards, Richard | Ass't S. | Ridgeway, Ohio | From October, 1864. H. R. Also 132d Inf. |
| Leslie, A. J. | H. Stew. | Cleveland, Ohio. | |
| Rogers, Harvey N. | Ass't S. | | From April, 1865. |
| Bivins, W. A. | " | New Hope, Ohio | To November, 1864. |

### 178TH INFANTRY—(1 year)—Mustered out June 29, 1865.

| Name | Rank | Residence | Service |
|---|---|---|---|
| Booth, Edwin. | Ass't S. | Crestline, Ohio | From September, 1864. Dead. |
| Campbell, John | Surgeon | Uniontown, Ohio | From September, 1864; also 129th Inf. |
| Taylor, Robert | Ass't S. | | From September, 1864. |

### 179TH INFANTRY—(1 year)—Mustered out June 17, 1865.

| Name | Rank | Residence | Service |
|---|---|---|---|
| Willson, Wm. H. | Surgeon | Greenfield, Ohio | From September, 1864. |
| Logue, M. H. | Ass't S. | | From September, 1864. |
| La Force, H. C. | " | | From April, 1865. |
| Inman, F. W. | " | | To February, 1865. |

### 180TH INFANTRY—(1 year)—Mustered out July 12, 1865.

| Name | Rank | Residence | Service |
|---|---|---|---|
| Case, Calvin D. | Ass't S. | Hoge, Kan | To January, 1865. |
| Powers, Frank E. | Surgeon | | From October, 1864; also 2d H. A. |
| Bolard, Jas. N. | Ass't S. | | From October, 1864. |

### 181ST INFANTRY—(1 year)—Mustered out July 14, 1865.

| Name | Rank | Residence | Service |
|---|---|---|---|
| Wolff, S. B. | Surgeon | | From October, 1864. |
| Force, Alfred | Ass't S. | | From October, 1864. |
| McCarty, Oliver C. | " | Polk, Ohio | From October, 1864; also 169th Inf. |

### 182D INFANTRY—(1 year)—Mustered out July 7, 1865.

| Name | Rank | Residence | Service |
|---|---|---|---|
| Cassady, George | Surgeon | Cleves, Ohio | From April, 1865; also 83d Infantry. |
| Iler, Abraham H. | Ass't S. | Blue Balls, Ohio | From October, 1864. |
| Thompson, Thos. J. | " | Erie, Mich | From April, 1865. |
| Valentine, Milton | Surgeon | Etna, Ohio | To March, 1865; also 10th Cav. |
| Willett, Peter | Ass't S. | | To March, 1865. |

### 183D INFANTRY—(1 year)—Mustered out July 17, 1865.

| Name | Rank | Residence | Service |
|---|---|---|---|
| Baker, Edward F. | Ass't S. | 600 N. Wells street, Chicago, Ill. | From November, 1864; also 144th Inf. |
| Plunkett, F. C. | " | Lowell, Mass | From November, 1864. |
| Hosack, Cyrus | Surgeon | | From November, 1864; also 29th Inf. |

### 184TH INFANTRY—(1 year)—Mustered out September 20, 1865.

| Name | Rank | Residence | Service |
|---|---|---|---|
| Shaw, Henry H. | Ass't S. | Mt. Gilead, Ohio | From February, 1865. U. S. Ex. S. |
| Meyer, Louis G. | Surgeon | | From February, 1865. |
| Richardson, R. A. | Ass't S. | Anna, Ohio | From February, 1865. |
| Price, Emmett W. | " | Randolph, Ohio | To June, 1865. |

OHIO—Continued.

185TH INFANTRY—(1 year)—Mustered out September 26, 1865.

Bowers, E. Dillon....Surgeon...Columbus, Ohio............From March, 1865.
Bodle, Foster..........Ass't S..........................From February, 1865.
Welsh, Jas. H.......... " ..........................From June, 1865.

186TH INFANTRY—(1 year)—Mustered out September 18, 1865.

Matchett, Wm. H.....Surgeon...Greenville, Ohio............From March, 1865; also 40th Inf.
Hargreaves, Wm......Ass't S..........................From March, 1865.
Coleman, Thos. M.... " ..........................From March, 1865.

187TH INFANTRY—Mustered out January 20, 1866.

Carpenter, H. W......Ass't S.....Lancaster, Ohio............From July, 1865; also 90th Inf.
Patterson, Theo. H...Surgeon...12 Centre ave., Chicago, Ill. From July, 1865.
Shaffer, Wm. B........Ass't S..........................From May, 1865.
Shaffer, Hiram M.....Surgeon..........................To June, 1865; also 81st Inf.

188TH INFANTRY—(1 year)—Mustered out September 21, 1865.

Munson, A. W .........Surgeon...Kenton, Ohio...............From March, 1865; also 82d Inf.
Landon, Hannibal ...Ass't S.....Remington, Ind.............From March, 1865.
Wheaton, John M.... " Columbus, Ohio.............From March, 1865.

189TH INFANTRY—Mustered out September 28, 1865.

Gordon, Sidney C.....Surgeon...Georgetown, Ohio ..........From March, 1865; also 59th Inf.
Otwell, Curtis ..........Ass't S.....Greenville, Ohio ............From March, 1865.
Otwell, L. S. B......... " ..........................From March, 1865.

190TH INFANTRY—Failed to complete its organization.

191ST INFANTRY—(1 year)—Mustered out August 27, 1865.

Willis, George .........Ass't S.....Brooklyn, Ill ...............From March, 1865.
Warfield, J. W.........Surgeon..........................From March, 1865.
McKinnon, B. F......Ass't S.....Lewistown, Ohio...........From March, 1865.

192D INFANTRY—(1 year)—Mustered out September 1, 1865.

Parker, Wm. S.........Surgeon...Piqua, Ohio.................From March, 1865.
Holcomb, C. B.........Ass't S.....Bremen, Ohio...............From March, 1865; also 160th Inf.
Martin, H. B............ " Tiffin, Ohio..................From March, 1865.

193D INFANTRY—(1 year)—Mustered out August 4, 1865.

Newton, Wm. S ......Surgeon...Gallipolis, Ohio.............From March, 1865; also 91st Inf.
Brown, Ambrose......Ass't S.....Grand Ledge, Mich........From March, 1865.
Waste, J. P ............ " ..........................From March, 1865.

194TH INFANTRY—(1 year)—Mustered out October 24, 1865.

Barrett, Jos. E.........Surgeon...Wooster, Ohio................To July, 1865; also 23d Inf.
Livers, Thos. J ........ " ..........................From July, 1865.
Franks, Jacob T.......Ass't S..........................To April, 1865.
Graham, Benj. F...... " Minneapolis, Minn .........To October, 1865.

## OHIO—Continued.

### 195TH INFANTRY—(1 year)—Mustered out December 18, 1865.

| Name | Rank | Address | Service |
|---|---|---|---|
| Dickinson, John | Surgeon | 146 Oranto st., Cleveland, Ohio. | From March, 1865; also 36th Inf. |
| Elson, David B | Ass't S. | | From March, 1865. |
| Strain, Hugh S | " | | From March, 1865. |

### 196TH INFANTRY—(1 year)—Mustered out September 11, 1865.

| Name | Rank | Address | Service |
|---|---|---|---|
| Noble, Havilah B | Surgeon | 17 Warren st., Baltimore, Md. | From March, 1865; also 2d and 4th Cav. |
| Shields, Chas. J | Ass't S. | | From March, 1865. |
| Driscoll, J. W | " | | From March, 1865. |

### 197TH INFANTRY—(1 year)—Mustered out July 31, 1865.

| Name | Rank | Address | Service |
|---|---|---|---|
| Pease, Geo. W | Ass't S. | 713 W. Jackson st., Chicago, Ill. | From April, 1865; also 12th Cav. |
| Bryant, Wilson G | Surgeon | | From April, 1865; also 122d Inf. |
| Lawrence, Amos | Ass't S. | | From April, 1865. |

### 198TH INFANTRY—Mustered out May 8, 1865.

## OREGON.

### 1ST CAVALRY—Mustered out from May 26 to November 20, 1866.

| Name | Rank | Address | Service |
|---|---|---|---|
| Watkins, Wm. H | Surgeon | Portland, Oregon | To December, 1864. |
| Steele, A. H | " | Olympia, Wash. T | Not in A. G. R. |
| Carpenter, Horace | Ass't S. | | To 1st Inf. March, 1865. |
| Holton, David H | " | | To March, 1863. |
| Stower, Edward | Surgeon | | To July, 1866. |

### 1ST INFANTRY—Mustered out from October 31, 1865, to July 19, 1867.

| Name | Rank | Address | Service |
|---|---|---|---|
| Carpenter, Horace | Surgeon | Salem, Oregon | To Dec, 1865; also 1st Cav. |
| Whittemore, Sam'l | Ass't S. | | To February, 1866. |

## PENNSYLVANIA.

### 1ST CAVALRY—Consolidated with 6th and 17th Cavalry to form the 2d Provisional Cavalry June 17, 1865.

| Name | Rank | Address | Service |
|---|---|---|---|
| Hotchkin, G. B | Ass't S. | Morrisdale, Pa | To September, 1864. |
| Tuft, R. H | " | Elkton, Md | From July, 1863; also 2d Provisional Cavalry. |
| Kelly, Hiram N | " | Nicholson. Pa | To June, 1863. |
| Calver, Geo. W. H | " | Florence, N. J | To August, 1862; also 147th Inf. |
| Stanton, David | Surgeon | | To Surg. U. S. V. Nov., 1862. |
| Atkinson, Lewis E | Ass't S. | | To September, 1864. |

### 1ST PROVISIONAL CAVALRY—Mustered out July 13, 1865.

| Name | Rank | Address | Service |
|---|---|---|---|
| Grumbine, Wm | Ass't S. | Annville, Pa | A. W. M.; also 20th Cav. |
| Donnelly, Edward | Surgeon | 139 Grant street, Pittsburgh, Pa. | From November, 1864; also 2d Cav. and 2d and 5th Reserves. |
| Nissley, S. R | Ass't S. | | From April, 1865; also 2d Cav. |

PENNSYLVANIA—Continued.

2D CAVALRY—(59th Volunteers)—Consolidated with 20th Cavalry to form 1st Provisional Cavalry June 17, 1865.

| Name | Rank | Address | Remarks |
|---|---|---|---|
| Weidman, W. M | Surgeon | 214 S. 5th street, Reading, Pa. | To October, 1864; also 11th Cav. |
| Haesler, C. H | " | Pottsville, Pa | Not in A. G R; also 20th Cav. |
| Davidson, F. B | Ass't S | Fleetville, Pa | To 45th Inf June, 1865. |
| Donnelly, Edward | Surgeon | 139 Grant street, Pittsburgh, Pa. | From November, 1864; also 1st Prov. Cav. and 2d and 5th Reserves. |
| Walter, P. S. P | Ass't S | Nazareth, Pa | To December, 1863. |
| Taggart, Wm. H | Surgeon | 1931 Spruce street, Philadelphia, Pa. | To September, 1862. |
| Nissley, S. R | Ass't S | | From April, 1865; also 1st Provisional Cav. |
| Strawn, Jas. J | " | | To July, 1864. |

2D PROVISIONAL CAVALRY—Mustered out August 7, 1865.

| Name | Rank | Address | Remarks |
|---|---|---|---|
| Tuft, R. H | Ass't S | Elkton, Md | From July, 1863; also 1st Cav. |
| Swift, Daniel D | Surgeon | 724 South 21st street, Philadelphia, Pa. | A. W. M.; also 6th Cav. and 126th Inf. |
| Yocum, Jos. J | Ass't S | Ashland, Pa | From April, 1865; also 6th Cav. |

3D CAVALRY—(Also called Young's Kentucky Light Cavalry)—Transferred to 5th Cavalry May 8, 1865.

| Name | Rank | Address | Remarks |
|---|---|---|---|
| Sherwood, T. H | Ass't S | Cor. Butler and Broad sts., Philadelphia, Pa. | To 27th Inf. April, 1863. |
| Tate, T H | " | Gettysburg, Pa | To August, 1864. |
| Wester, O. J | Surgeon | Germantown, Pa | Not in A. G. R. |
| Stewart, J. L | " | Erie, Pa | To March, 1862. |
| Ridgely, Thos. H | Ass't S | | To December, 1861. |
| Durant, H. J | " | | From March, 1863; also 5th Cav. |
| Hezless, Wm. B | Surgeon | | To August, 1864. |

3D PROVISIONAL CAVALRY—Mustered out October 31, 1865.

| Name | Rank | Address | Remarks |
|---|---|---|---|
| Lynch, N. R | Ass't S | 1201 Jefferson street, Philadelphia, Pa. | From March, 1864; also 22d Cav. and 176th Inf. |
| Finley, S. M | " | Harrisburgh, Pa | From April, 1864; also 22d Cav. |
| Williams, S. C | Surgeon | | From December, 1864; also 18th Cav. |

4TH CAVALRY—(64th Volunteers)—Mustered out July 1, 1865.

| Name | Rank | Address | Remarks |
|---|---|---|---|
| Bushley, F. A | Ass't S | Greencastle, Pa | To November, 1863. |
| McCoy, J. A | Surgeon | Osage Agency, Ind. Ter. | From April, 1865. |
| Skeels, Jas S | " | Albion, Pa | From March, 1865. |
| Price, W. B | " | New Berlin, Ill | From February, 1865. |
| Junkin, John M | " | Easton, Pa | To February, 1865; also 56th Inf. |
| Marsh, N. F | " | | To November, 1862; also 5th Inf. |
| King, S. Charles | Ass't S | | To November, 1862; also 5th Cav. |
| Morrison, James M | " | | To 48th Inf. November, 1862. |
| Lyons, John C | Surgeon | | To 56th Inf. January, 1863. |
| Wager, Peter | Ass't S | | To 5th Cav. March, 1863; also 177th Inf. |

## PENNSYLVANIA—Continued.

5TH CAVALRY—(Cameron Dragoons and 65th Volunteers)—Mustered out August 7, 1865.

| Name | Rank | Address | Service |
|---|---|---|---|
| Hughes, John W | Ass't S | Blairsville, Pa | From December, 1864. |
| Todd, W. C | Surgeon | Manayunk, Pa | To August, 1864; also 66th Inf. |
| Yarrow, Thos. J | Ass't S | 1315 Girard ave., Philadelphia, Pa. | To March, 1862. |
| King, S. Chas | " | | To 4th Cav. April, 1862. |
| Bryant, James | Surgeon | | To November, 1861. |
| Jaquith, F. S | " | | To February, 1862. |
| Yarrow, Henry C | Ass't S | | To February, 1862. |
| Wager, Peter | " | | To February, 1863; also 4th Cav. and 177th Inf. |
| Durant, H. J | " | | From March, 1863; also 3d Cav. |
| Heany, Patrick | Surgeon | | To November, 1864; also 66th Inf. |
| Wagoner, John F | Ass't S | | To February, 1862. |
| Curtis, Henry R | " | | To May, 1865. |
| Parker, Clifford J | " | | Dismissed Sept., 1863. |
| Sallman, Earnest | " | | Dismissed March, 1865. |

6TH CAVALRY—(70th Volunteers and Rush's Lancers)—Consolidated with the 1st and 17th Cavalry to form 2d Provisional Cavalry June 17, 1865.

| Name | Rank | Address | Service |
|---|---|---|---|
| Ellis, C. M | Ass't S | Elkton, Md | To January, 1863. |
| Moss, Wm | Surgeon | Chestnut Hill, Pa | To October, 1862. |
| Morrison, T. S | Ass't S | Coatesville, Pa | To June, 1863. |
| Engler, Geo. S | " | Bethlehem Pa | To June, 1864. |
| Swift, Daniel D | Surgeon | 724 South 21st st., Philadelphia, Pa. | A. W. M. Also 2d Prov. Cav. and 126th Inf |
| Henderson, Wm. B | Ass't S | | From March to June, 1865. |
| Yocum, Jos. J | " | | From April, 1865; also 2d Provisional Cavalry. |
| Wyeth, A. R | Surgeon | | To October, 1861. |
| Prieson, A | Ass't S | Lock Haven, Pa | To October, 1862. |

7TH CAVALRY—(80th Volunteers)—Mustered out August 23, 1865.

| Name | Rank | Address | Service |
|---|---|---|---|
| Hezlep, Wm. B | Surgeon | Allegheny or Bakerstown, Pa. | From June, 1865; also 6th Heavy Artillery. |
| Speer, A. M | " | 212 Penn st., Pittsburgh, Pa. | To June, 1863. |
| Jung, Theo. J | Ass't S | | From May, 1863; also 124th Inf. |
| Brety, Geo. B | " | | From July, 1865. |
| Shirner, R. S | Surgeon | | From March, 1863. |
| Harris, Geo. T | Ass't S | | To September, 1864. |

8TH CAVALRY—(89th Volunteers)—Consolidated with 16th Cavalry July 24, 1865.

| Name | Rank | Address | Service |
|---|---|---|---|
| Chritzman, H. G | Ass't S | Welch Run, Pa | To October, 1864; also 57th Inf. |
| Everhart, I. F | Surgeon | Scranton, Pa | From Feb., 1865; also 16th Cav. |
| Mitchell, S. B. W | " | 132 Arch st., Philadelphia, Pa. | Dead. |
| Wells, J. R | Ass't S | 5142 Lancaster avenue, Philadelphia, Pa. | To March, 1863. |
| Lightner, Sam'l B | " | | From Feb. to July, 1865. |

PENNSYLVANIA—Continued.

9TH CAVALRY—(92d Volunteers and Lochiel Cavalry)—Mustered out July 18, 1865.

| Name | Rank | Residence | Service |
|---|---|---|---|
| Robins, O. M. | Surgeon | Shamokin, Pa. | To August. 1864. |
| Rice, Wm. | Ass't S. | Rome, Pa. | From April, 1865. |
| Sutton, R. S. | " | Pittsburgh, Pa. | To January, 1864. |
| Walker, S. C. | Surgeon | Fountaindale, Pa. | From Aug., 1864. H. R. |
| Jenkins. J. M. | Ass't S. | | To November, 1862. |
| Moore, Jas. | " | | To May, 1865. |

10TH CAVALRY—Failed to complete.

11TH CAVALRY—(108th Volunteers and Harland's Iowa Cavalry)—Mustered out August 13th, 1865.

| Name | Rank | Residence | Service |
|---|---|---|---|
| Harlan, G. C. | Surgeon | 1806 Chestnut st., Philadelphia, Pa. | To September, 1864. |
| Nagle, H. M. | " | Reading, Pa. | From December, 1864. |
| Weidman, W. M. | Ass't S. | 214 S. 5th st., Reading, Pa. | To January, 1862; also 2d Cav. |
| Nebinger, A. R. | " | 1018 S. 2d st., Phila., Pa. | From July, 1864; also 158th Inf. |
| Applegate, J. W. | " | | To August, 1862. |
| Donor, Wm. J. | " | | To February, 1864. |

12TH CAVALRY—(113th Volunteers)—Mustered out July 20, 1865.

| Name | Rank | Residence | Service |
|---|---|---|---|
| Schoales, J. D. | Surgeon | 1428 N. 11th st., Philadelphia, Pa. | From April, 1862. |
| Allen, J. C. | Ass't S. | 2418 Market st., Phila., Pa. (Removed.) | From February, 1863. |
| Lashell, T. B. | " | Meadville, Pa. | To December, 1862. |
| Cruice, Rob't B. | " | 731 N. 17th st., Phila., Pa. | To July, 1862. |
| Foster, O. D. | " | | From May, 1865. |
| Bowes, M. F. | " | | To 209th Inf. Sept., 1864; also 51st Inf. |

13TH CAVALRY—(117th Volunteers)—Mustered out July 14, 1865.

| Name | Rank | Residence | Service |
|---|---|---|---|
| Moore, C. W. | Ass't S. | Sterling, Nebr. | To September, 1864. |
| Osborn, Wm. F. | Surgeon | Burlington, Kas. | From Jan., 1865; also 11th Inf. |
| Nyce, N. J. | Ass't S. | | From April, 1865. |
| Stanton, J. C. | " | | To May, 1865. |
| Lummiss, Geo. B. | Surgeon | | To Nov., 1864; also 71st Inf. |

14TH CAVALRY—(Stanton Cavalry and 159th Volunteers)—Mustered out August 24, 1865.

| Name | Rank | Residence | Service |
|---|---|---|---|
| McCabe, J. W. | Ass't S. | Vanceport, or Pittsburgh, Pa. | To December, 1864. |
| Wynne, Wm. B. | Surgeon | Parker's Landing, Pa. | To Feb., 1865; also 53d Inf. |
| Seiler, John P. | Ass't S. | | From March, 1865. |
| Worthington, C. W. | Surgeon | | To July, 1865. |

15TH CAVALRY—(160th Volunteers)—Mustered out June 21, 1865, except Company A, mustered out July 18, 1865.

| Name | Rank | Residence | Service |
|---|---|---|---|
| Alexander, J. W. | Surgeon | Morganza, Md., or Canonsburgh, Pa. | From October, 1862; also 85th Inf. |
| Mish, Geo. F. | Ass't S. | Middletown, Pa. | From October, 1862 |
| Say, Eli J. | " | | From April, 1863. |

## PENNSYLVANIA—Continued.

### 16TH CAVALRY—(161st Volunteers)—Mustered out August 11, 1865.

| Name | Rank | Residence | Service |
|---|---|---|---|
| Carey, Ezrah | Ass't S. | Prosperity, Pa | To October, 1863. |
| Coxe, Thos. C | " | Chatham, Pa | From April, 1865. |
| Everhart, I. F. | Surgeon | Scranton, Pa | From February, 1865; also 8th Cav. |
| Ellershaw, Wm | Ass't S. | 959 N. 3d st., Phila., Pa | From March, 1865. |
| Le Moyne, Francis | Surgeon | 157 4th st., Pittsburgh, Pa | To July, 1865; also 9th Inf. |
| Herman, A. F. | Ass't S. | | To March, 1865. |
| Cominger, W. H | Surgeon | | To December, 1863. |

### 17TH CAVALRY—(162d Volunteers)—Consolidated with 1st and 6th Cavalry to form 2d Provisional Cavalry June 17, 1865.

| Name | Rank | Residence | Service |
|---|---|---|---|
| DeWitt, J. Wilson | Ass't S. | St. George, Del | From April, 1863, to June, 1865. |
| Walborne, Isaac | Surgeon | Myerstown, Pa | To September, 1863; also 83d Inf. |
| Moore, James B. | Ass't S. | Philadelphia, Pa | To July, 1863. |
| Pomeroy, Geo. B. | Surgeon | | A. W. M. Also 110th Infantry. |
| Gardner, T. S. | " | | To April, 1864; also 62d Inf. |

### 18TH CAVALRY—(163d Volunteers)—Consolidated with 22d Cavalry to form 3d Provisional Cavalry June 24, 1865.

| Name | Rank | Residence | Service |
|---|---|---|---|
| Marks, John J | Surgeon | Lewistown, Pa | From December, 1863; also 205th Inf. |
| McCurdy, J. R | Ass't S. | Clinton or Florence, Pa | From January, 1865. |
| Sharp, W. W | Surgeon | Amity, Pa | From October, 1864; also 140th Inf |
| Williams, Samuel C. | " | | From December, 1864; also 3d Prov. Cav. |
| Withers, Geo. W | Ass't S. | | To March, 1864. |

### 19TH CAVALRY—(180th Volunteers)—In service August 31, 1865.

| Name | Rank | Residence | Service |
|---|---|---|---|
| Reed, A. G. | Surgeon | 815 N. 10th street, Philadelphia, Pa. | To August, 1864; also Lieut 134th Vols. |
| Albright, Francis G. | " | Lancaster, Pa | To March, 1865; also 79th Inf. |
| Noyes, Laman A | Ass't S. | St. Paul Island, Alaska | From October, 1863. |

### 20TH CAVALRY—(181st Volunteers)—Consolidated with 2d Cavalry to form 1st Provisional Cavalry June 17, 1865.

| Name | Rank | Residence | Service |
|---|---|---|---|
| Grumbine, Wm | Ass't S. | Annville, Pa | A. W. M. Also 1st Prov. Cav. |
| Gray, Samuel G. | " | Washington Boro', Pa | To February, 1865. |
| Haesler, C. H. | " | Pottsville Pa | Not in A. G. R. Also 2d Cav. |
| Walls, Aug. G | Surgeon | Clinton, Pa | A. W. M. |

### 21ST CAVALRY—(182d Volunteers)—Mustered out July 8, 1865

| Name | Rank | Residence | Service |
|---|---|---|---|
| Kitchen, Elias C | Ass't S. | Brumfieldville or Oil City, Pa. | To January, 1865; also 155th Inf. |
| Kohler, Fred S. | " | Reedsville, Pa | From March, 1865. |
| King, W. Howard | Surgeon | Greencastle, Pa | From August, 1863; also 149th Inf. |
| Rewalt, L. L. | Ass't S. | Wrightsville, Pa | From February, 1865. |

PENNSYLVANIA—Continued.

22D CAVALRY—(185th Volunteers)—Consolidated with 18th Cavalry to form 3d Provisional Cavalry June 24, 1865.

Phelps, W. C..........Surgeon...2048 Vine st. or 327 N. 18th st., Philadelphia. From April, 1864; also 11th Inf

Lynch, N. R..........Ass't S.....1201 Jefferson st., Philadelphia, Pa. From March, 1864; also 3d Prov. Cav. and 176th Inf.

Finley, S. M.......... " Harrisburgh, Pa..........From April, 1864; also 3d Prov. Cav.

2D HEAVY ARTILLERY—(112th Volunteers)—In service August 31, 1865.

Bartine, David H......Surgeon...Merchantsville or Princeton, N. J. From August, 1864; also 112th Inf.

Dewitt, A. T..........Ass't S.....Riverside, Pa. ...............From November, 1863.

Graham, John......... " 326 5th st, Philadelphia, Pa. From July, 1865.

Griswold, Elisha...... " Sharon, Pa..................To July, 1864.

Wevill, R. H........... " ..................................To December, 1861.

Rossenberger, S....... " 1722 N. 7th street, Philadelphia, Pa. To March, 1863.

Kirk, Lewis R......... " Rising Sun, Md............To November, 1863; also 26th and 131st Inf.

Lowe, Jas. A.......... " Dead ..........................To June, 1865.

Linton, Jas. D......... " ..................................To June, 1862.

3D HEAVY ARTILLERY—(152d Volunteers)—Cos. A and B mustered out July 11, 1865, and Co. H July 25, 1865; the rest in service August 31, 1865.

Bancroft, F. J....... Surgeon...Denver, Colo................A. W. M. Also 76th Inf. U. S Ex. S.

Kern, Francis J.......Ass't S.....Shenandoah, Pa...........To 188th Infantry April, 1864.

Vandersloot, F. W... " Nittany, Pa.....................From November, 1863.

Brownfield B. T...... " Smithfield, Pa ................Dismissed October, 1863.

Ruttger, C.............. " ..................................Dismissed July, 1865.

5TH HEAVY ARTILLERY—(204th Volunteers)—Mustered out June 30, 1865.

Greenlee, David R...Ass't S.....Meadville, Pa..................From September, 1864.

McCann, Jas........... " 229 Pa ave., Pittsburgh, Pa. From September, 1864.

Barber, John..........Surgeon...Sharon, Pa......................From September, 1864; also 1st Res.

6TH HEAVY ARTILLERY—(212th Volunteers)—Mustered out June 12, 1865.

Taylor, Wm............Ass't S.....Towanda, Pa....................From September, 1864.

Hezlep, W. B..........Surgeon...Bakerstown, or Allegheny, Pa. From October, 1864; also 7th Cavalry.

Rea, James L..........Ass't S.........................................From September, 1864.

1ST LIGHT ARTILLERY.

Shippen, Edward.....Surgeon...1205 Walnut st., Philadelphia, Pa. To U. S. Vols. Sept., 1862.

Reily, Jas. R ..........Ass't S.........................................127th Inf. Sept., 1862; also 179th Inf.

Price, M. F.............Surgeon.........................................To September, 1863.

1ST RESERVES INFANTRY—(30th Volunteers)—Mustered out June 11, 1864.

Read, L. W..............Surgeon...Norristown, Pa..............To June, 1863.

Chapin, Sam'l F......Ass't S.....Wattsburgh, or Erie, Pa. To 139th Inf. Sept., 1862.

Barber, John...........Surgeon...Sharon, Pa..................From Feb., 1864; also 5th Heavy Artillery.

Chilson, S. L..........Ass't S.........................................From Aug., 1862; also 74th and 190th Inf.

Brennemen, E......... " ..................................To December, 1861.

## PENNSYLVANIA—Continued.

2D RESERVES INFANTRY—(31st Volunteers)—Mustered out June 16, 1864.

| Name | Rank | Address | Remarks |
|---|---|---|---|
| Coleman, A G | Ass't S | Limerick Station, Pa | A. W. M. |
| Basehore, D. W | " | West Fairview. Pa | To November, 1862. |
| Donnelly, E | Surgeon | 139 Grant street, Pittsburgh, Pa. | From April, 1862; also 1st Prov. Cav. and 2d Cav 5th Res |
| Reed, Thos. B | " | 1427 Walnut st, Philadelphia, Pa. | To Surgeon U. S Vols. April, 1862. |
| Lodge, John W | Ass't S | Cor. Lancaster and Marion avenues, Philadelphia, Pa. | To October, 1861. |
| Malone, John | " | | To Nov., 1862; also 71st Inf. |

3D RESERVES INFANTRY—(32d Volunteers)—Mustered out June 17, 1864.

| Name | Rank | Address | Remarks |
|---|---|---|---|
| Collins, Jas | Surgeon | Philadelphia, Pa | To April, 1864. U. S. Ex. S. |
| Rice, Geo. I | Ass't S | Lamoille, Ill | To January, 1863. |
| Welch, Stanton A | " | Asbury. N. J | From January, 1863. |
| Burchfield, J. P | " | Penn ave., Pittsburgh, Pa. | From May, 1863. |
| Pancoast, Geo. L | " | | To Surg. U. S. V. Oct., 1861. |
| Colston, H. S | " | | To 81st Inf. Sept., 1862. |
| Orr, Samuel S | " | | To March, 1863. |

4TH RESERVES INFANTRY—(33d Volunteers)—Mustered out June 17, 1864.

| Name | Rank | Address | Remarks |
|---|---|---|---|
| Davis, Wm. H | Surgeon | Horsehead, N. Y | From Dec., 1862; also 5th Res. |
| Patze, Adolphus | " | Franklin House, Washington, D. C. | To November, 1862. |
| Dickerson, W. T. W | Ass't S | Media, Pa | To July, 1862. |
| Ritter, Fred. D | " | Athens, Pa | To August, 1862. |
| Brinton, Wm. B | " | West Chester, Pa | To May, 1864; also 184th Inf. |
| Griesener, J. B | " | | To February, 1863. |
| Bulkeley, J. E | " | Wilkesbarre, Pa | From November, 1862. |

5TH RESERVES INFANTRY—(34th Volunteers)—Mustered out June 13, 1864.

| Name | Rank | Address | Remarks |
|---|---|---|---|
| Carpenter, J. T | Surgeon | Pottsville, Pa | To U. S. Vols Sept., 1861. |
| Witman, Harry T | Ass't S | Indianapolis, Ind., or Reading, Pa | From Sept., 1863; also 195th Inf |
| Davis, Wm. H | " | Horseheads, N. Y | To 4th Reserves Dec., 1862. |
| Donnelly, Edward | " | 139 Grand street, Pittsburgh, Pa. | To 2d Res. April, 1862; also 1st Prov. and 2d Cav. |
| Lane, Sam'l G | Surgeon | Chambersburgh, Pa | To March, 1864. |
| Grim, Henry A | " | Allentown, Pa | From April, 1864; also 12th Res. and 190th Inf. |
| Marsh, N. F | Ass't S | | To 4th Cav. Oct., 1861. |
| Groff, J. M | " | | To July, 1863. |
| Johnson, C. O | " | | To September, 1863. |

6TH RESERVES INFANTRY—(35th Volunteers)—Mustered out June 11, 1864.

| Name | Rank | Address | Remarks |
|---|---|---|---|
| Corson, J. K | Ass't S | Care A. G. U. S. A | From March, 1863. Ass't S. U. S. A. |
| Bower, Charles | Surgeon | | From July, 1861. |
| Bishop, J. L | Ass't S | | To 7th Reserves Feb., 1863. |
| Jones, Z. Ring | " | | To 63d Inf. August, 1862; also 195th Inf. |
| Atkinson, N. J | " | | Dismissed March, 1863. |

## PENNSYLVANIA—Continued.

### 7TH RESERVES INFANTRY—(36th Volunteers)—Mustered out June 16, 1864.

| Name | Rank | Residence | Remarks |
|---|---|---|---|
| Green, Alfred W | Surgeon | Meadville, Pa | To Jan., 1863; also 186th Inf. |
| Hornet, Volney | Ass't S | Camptown, Pa | From September, 1862. |
| Ross, Robt. W | " | Shepherdstown, Pa | Dismissed April, 1863. |
| Jones Thos. | " | Dead | To 8th Res. Sept., 1862. |
| Bishop, J. L | Surgeon | | From Feb., 1863; also 6th Res. |

### 8TH RESERVES INFANTRY—(37th Volunteers)—Mustered out May 24, 1864.

| Name | Rank | Residence | Remarks |
|---|---|---|---|
| Allman, F. O | Ass't S | Charleston, S. C | To July, 1862; also 9th Res. |
| Rugh, J. W | " | New Alexandria, Pa | To May, 1863. |
| McCormick, E C | " | | From June, 1863. |
| Hayne, T | " | | Dissmissed October, 1862. |
| Kline, G. H | " | | Dismissed March, 1863. |
| Litchtenthaller, H. A. | Surgeon | | To March, 1862. |

### 9TH RESERVES INFANTRY—(38th Volunteers)—Mustered out May 12, 1864.

| Name | Rank | Residence | Remarks |
|---|---|---|---|
| Phillips, J. A | Surgeon | 57 Grant st., Pittsburgh, Pa. | From June, 1861. |
| LeMoyne, Francis | Ass't S | 157 4th st., Pittsburgh, Pa. | To 16th Cav. Jan., 1864. |
| Allman, F. O | " | Charleston, S. C. | Dismissed Jan., 1863; also 8th Reserves. |
| Akley, Benj. F | " | | From February, 1864. |
| Martin, Henry F | " | | To 123d Inf. Aug., 1862. |
| Sigmond, A. M | " | Shinnerville, Pa | To November, 1863 |

### 10TH RESERVES INFANTRY—(39th Volunteers)—Mustered out June 11, 1864.

| Name | Rank | Residence | Remarks |
|---|---|---|---|
| McKinney, David | Ass't S | New Brighton, Pa | To 134th Inf. Sept., 1862. |
| Rohrer, Benj | Surgeon | 478 Germantown ave., Philadelphia Pa. | Dead. |
| Patton, J. R | H. Stew | Huntingdon, Pa. | |
| Barr, Benj | Ass't S | 643 North 13th st, Philadelphia, Pa. | From July, 1862; charges fee $25. |
| Buckley, Wm. C | " | | To August, 1863. |

### 11TH RESERVES INFANTRY—(40th Volunteers)—Mustered out June 13, 1864.

| Name | Rank | Residence | Remarks |
|---|---|---|---|
| Kurtz, Samuel L | Ass't S | Reading, Pa | To 55th Inf. June, 1862. |
| Marbourg, J. L | " | Bedford, Pa | To November, 1862. U. S. Ex. S. |
| Lyons, Wm | Surgeon | 1312 N. Front st. Phila., Pa. | To 191st Inf. June, 1864. |
| Ballentine, D W | Ass't S | | To February, 1862. |
| DeBenneville, J. S | Surgeon | 1716 Pine st., Phila., Pa. | To November, 1863. |
| Cole, Ashton J | Ass't S | Mansfield, Pa | From January, 1864. |

### 11TH INFANTRY—Mustered out July 1, 1865.

| Name | Rank | Residence | Remarks |
|---|---|---|---|
| Anawalt, J. W | Ass't S | Greensburgh, Pa | To 132d Inf. Oct., 1862. H. R. |
| Beechlee, H. B | Surgeon | Harrisburg[illegible] | Not [illegible] G. R. |
| Osborn, Wm. F | Ass't S | Burlingto[illegible] | To 13th Cav. Feb., 1865. |
| Rankin, John M | " | Richla[illegible] | From January, 1865. |
| Morris, Thos G | " | Liverpoo[illegible] | To November, 1862 |
| Phelps, Wm. C | " | 2048 Vine st. [illegible] 27 N. 18th st., Phila. Pa. | To April, 1864; also 22d Cav. |
| Jackson, R M. S | Surgeon | | To April, 1863. |
| Fortney, Chas. D | Ass't S | | To March, 1865. |

## PENNSYLVANIA—Continued.

### 12th Reserves Infantry—(41st Volunteers)—Mustered out June 11, 1864.

| Name | Rank | Address | Remarks |
|---|---|---|---|
| Taylor, William | Ass't S. | Towanda, Pa | To December, 1862. |
| Beaver, Daniel R | " | Conshohocken, Pa | From April, 1864. |
| Grim, Henry A | " | Allentown, Pa | To 5th Reserves April, 1864; also 198th Inf. |
| Clark, Isaac | Surgeon | | From May, 1863. |
| Thorne, Wm. H | Ass't S. | Lebanon, Pa | To U. S. V. April, 1862. |
| Crawford, J. B | " | | To September, 1862. |
| Shearer, James M | " | Dillsburgh, Pa | To August, 1863. |

### 13th Reserves Infantry—(42d Volunteers and 1st Rifles)—Mustered out June 11, 1864.

| Name | Rank | Address | Remarks |
|---|---|---|---|
| Comfort, J. J | Surgeon | Blackwoodtown or Atlantic City, N. J. | To 190th Inf. May, 1864; also 121st Inf. |
| Freeman, S. D | " | Southport, Pa | To Surg. U. S. V. Oct., 1862. |
| Humphrey, Wm. F | Ass't S. | Osceola, Pa | To 149th Inf Sept, 1862. |
| Crouch, Daniel O | " | Connellsville, Pa | To June, 1863. |
| Jones, Wm. B | " | 8th & Tasker sts., Phila., Pa. | To November, 1862. |
| Warner, J. E | " | | Dismissed Aug., 1863. |
| Butler, Lafayette | " | | To 190th Inf. May, 1864; also 125th Inf. |

From the 14th to the 22d Infantry, inclusive, were three-months' Regiments.

### 23d Infantry—Mustered out September 8, 1864; recruits and veterans transferred to the 82d Infantry.

| Name | Rank | Address | Remarks |
|---|---|---|---|
| Gross, S. W | Surgeon | 1112 Walnut st. Phila., Pa. | Not in A. G. R. |
| Roller, Wm. C | " | Hollidaysburgh, Pa | A. W. M. |
| Clarke, Anson T | Ass't S. | Worth, Pa | From May, 1863. |
| Campbell, C. F. H | Surgeon | | To Surg. U. S. V. Nov., 1864. |
| McGrath, John | " | | To Jan., 1862; also 78th Inf. |
| Fundenburg, G. B | " | | To March, 1862. |
| Yeomans, Geo | Ass't S. | Ashland, Pa | To March, 1865. |
| Tusting, Robert | " | | Dismissed August, 1863. |

The 24th and 25th Infantry were three-months' Regiments.

### 26th Infantry—Mustered out June 18, 1864; veterans and recruits transferred to the 99th Infantry.

| Name | Rank | Address | Remarks |
|---|---|---|---|
| Craig, William | Ass't S. | 1711 Cherry st Phila., Pa. | From April, 1863. |
| Mintzer, John W | Surgeon | 1036 Race st., Phila., Pa. | To Surg. U. S. V. June, 1863. |
| Gross, H. S | Ass't S. | 616 S. 9th st., Phila., Pa. | To October, 1863. |
| Alexander, J. W | " | Cannonsburgh, Pa | To June, 1862. |
| Kirk, Lewis R | Surgeon | Rising Sun, Md | From Nov., 1863; also 131st Inf. and 2d H. Art. |
| Shultz, Solomon S | " | | To June, 1863; also 75th Inf. |
| Cohen, Jules B | Ass't S. | | To June, 1862. |
| Magnin, Jules A. F | " | | To December, 1862. |
| Hopkins, Samuel | " | | To February, 1862. |
| Newcomer, David | " | | To July, 1862. |

PENNSYLVANIA—Continued.

27TH INFANTRY—Mustered out June 11. 1864; veterans and recruits transferred to the 109th Infantry, except Co. F to Co. C, 73d Infantry.

| | | | |
|---|---|---|---|
| Heller, Henry | Surgeon | 428 N. Fifth st., Philadelphia, Pa. | To September, 1861. |
| Sherwood, Thos. H | " | Cor. Beaver st. and Germantown ave., Philadelphia, Pa. | From May, 1863; also 3d Cav. |
| Ginkinger, W. H. H | Ass't S | 969 N. 6th st., Phila., Pa | From August, 1862. |
| Heller, Max | Surgeon | | To April, 1863. |
| Gominger, Wm. H | " | | To October, 1862. |
| Heckel, Edw'd P | Ass't S | Vincent, Pa | From March, 1863. |

28TH INFANTRY—Mustered out July 18, 1865.

| | | | |
|---|---|---|---|
| Goodman, H. E | Surgeon. | 1427 Chestnut st., Philadelphia, Pa. | To U. S. V. May, 1864. President Bd. Ex. S. |
| Kemble, Jos | H. Stew | Philadelphia, Pa | M. D. |
| Smith, Wm. F | Ass't S | Airville, Pa | To 73d Inf. Dec., 1864 |
| Altman, Wm | Surgeon | Punxsutawney, Pa | From May, 1864. |
| Logan, Samuel | Ass't S | Greensburgh, Pa | To October, 1862. |
| Dorland, Wm. M | " | 4034 Locust st. Phila., Pa | To November, 1862. |
| Light, A. H | " | Lebanon, Pa | From May, 1864. |
| Mullen, John H | " | Phœnixville, Pa | To April, 1863. |

29TH INFANTRY—Mustered out July 11, 1865.

| | | | |
|---|---|---|---|
| Bender, Jacob S | Ass't S | Carlisle, Pa | From May, 1863 |
| Jackson, Geo. W | " | | To 53d Inf. March, 1863. |
| Dowling, James P | " | | To Ass't S. U. S. V. Nov., 1864. |
| Duffee, John H | Surgeon | | To November, 1861. |
| Wolfe, Joseph A | " | | From December, 1861. |

From the 30TH to the 40TH INFANTRY, inclusive, were three-months' Regiments.

45TH INFANTRY—Mustered out July 17, 1865.

| | | | |
|---|---|---|---|
| Davidson, Francis B | Surgeon | Fleetville, Pa | From June, 1865; also 2d Cav. |
| Christ, Theo. S | " | Chester, Pa | To October, 1864. |
| Maxwell, John K | Ass't S | Worthington, Pa | To August, 1864. |
| Weistling, Rob't R | " | Huntingdon, Pa | To February, 1863 |
| Yundt, Winfield S | " | Lancaster, Pa | To May, 1865. |
| Potter, Geo. L | Surgeon | Bellefonte, Pa | To July, 1862. Dead |
| Styer, Charles | Ass't S | | To Jan., 1863; also 99th Inf. |
| Iddings, C. E | " | | To June, 1865. |

46TH INFANTRY—Mustered out July 16, 1865.

| | | | |
|---|---|---|---|
| Tracy, Geo. P | Surgeon | Burlington, Pa | From May, 1865; also 90th Inf. |
| Burke, Geo. W | Ass't S | New Castle, Pa | From Jan., 1863. Died 1874. |
| McDonough, James | " | California, Pa | From Jan. 1863. Dead. |
| Quick, Lavington | Surgeon | | To U. S. V. from Dec., 1861. |
| Coover, J. B | Ass't S | Killed Sept., 1864. | To 6th Cav. Jan., 1863. |
| Holmes, Daniel | Surgeon | | To March, 1862. |
| Rodgers, Wm. C | " | | To May, 1863. |

## PENNSYLVANIA—Continued.

### 47TH INFANTRY—In service August 31, 1865.

| Name | Rank | Residence | Service |
|---|---|---|---|
| Bailey, Elijah W | Surgeon | Pennington, N. J | To September, 1864. |
| Sturdevant, S. B | “ | Wilkes Barre, or Providence, Pa. | From March, 1865; also 84th and 139th Inf. |
| Scheetz, J. H | Ass't S. | Pottstown, Pa | To September, 1864. |
| Weiland, Christian F. | “ | Hilton Head, S. C | From December, 1864. |
| Shindel, John Y | “ | Middleburgh, Pa | From February, 1865. |
| Adler, Lewis H | “ | 1301 Arch st, Phila., Pa. | To September, 1862. |
| Reiber, Wm. F | “ | Berrien Springs, Mich | To January, 1865. |

### 48TH INFANTRY—Mustered out July 17, 1865.

| Name | Rank | Residence | Service |
|---|---|---|---|
| Blackwood, W. R. D. | Surgeon | 246 N. 20th st, Phila., Pa. | From April, 1863; also 149th Inf. |
| Culver, J. B | Ass't S. | Towanda, Kans | From January, 1864. |
| Aschom, John P | Surgeon | Renova, Pa | To Feb., 1862; also 54th and 116th Inf. |
| Morrison, James M | Ass't S. | | Dismissed August, 1863; also 4th Cav. |
| Smyser, Eugene M | “ | | From April, 1864. |
| Reber, Charles F | Surgeon | | To February, 1863. |
| Bushong, Israel | Ass't S. | New Holland, Pa | To September, 1862. |
| Maloney, A. J | “ | | To December, 1862. |
| Husten, John M | “ | | To June, 1863. |

### 49TH INFANTRY—Mustered out July 15, 1865.

| Name | Rank | Residence | Service |
|---|---|---|---|
| Spratt, G. R | Surgeon | Coatesville, Pa | From April, 1864. |
| Gobrecht, W. H | “ | Cincinnati, Ohio | To Jan., 1863. Dead. |
| Knox, S. B. P | “ | Santa Barbara, Cal | To July, 1865. |
| Sample, S. R | Ass't S. | Intercourse, Pa | To December, 1862. |
| Sides, Benj. F | “ | Lancaster, Pa | To January, 1863. |
| Wilson, C. H | Surgeon | Berwick, Pa | To October, 1864. |
| Huber, John F | Ass't S. | | To 131st Inf. Oct., 1862. |

### 50TH INFANTRY—Mustered out July 30, 1865.

| Name | Rank | Residence | Service |
|---|---|---|---|
| Book, Wm. P | Ass't S. | Bradford, Pa | To September, 1864. |
| McKibbin, D. J | Surgeon | Ashland, Pa | To Surg. U. S. V. Feb., 1862. |
| Vickers, Jos. P | Ass't S. | Cincinnati, Ohio | To July, 1864. |
| Wilson, Frank P | “ | East Toledo, Ohio | From March, 1865. |
| Siemens, C. J | Surgeon | | To March, 1864; also 76th Inf. |
| Kollock, John M | “ | | To June, 1865; also 118th Inf. |

### 51ST INFANTRY—Mustered out July 27, 1865.

| Name | Rank | Residence | Service |
|---|---|---|---|
| Hosack, J. P | Surgeon | Mercer, Pa | To July, 1863; also 101st Inf. |
| Shurlock, Wm. C | “ | Darlington or Harrisburgh, Pa, or Fargo, Dak. Ter | To June, 1865; also 100th Inf. |
| Cress, James | Ass't S. | Woodberry, Md | From February, 1865. |
| Livergood, John | Surgeon | Lancaster, Pa | To December, 1861. |
| Reinholdt, John B | Ass't S. | New Castle, Pa | To June, 1865. |
| Noble, James D | “ | | To August, 1862. |
| Bowes, Manning F | Surgeon | | From June 1865; also 12th Cav. & 209th Inf. |
| Duffell, Chas. L | Ass't S. | | To November, 1864. |

## PENNSYLVANIA—Continued.

### 52D INFANTRY—Mustered out July 12, 1865

| Name | Rank | Address | Service |
|---|---|---|---|
| Flowers, John | Surgeon | Kent County, Del | From April, 1865. U. M. |
| Kauffman, J. H. | Ass't S. | Annville, Pa | From June, 1864. |
| McCandless, J. G. | " | 18 Centre ave., Pittsburgh, Pa. | To August, 1862. |
| Sargent, Rufus | " | 1609 Mt. Vernon street, Philadelphia, Pa. | To May, 1864. |
| Crawford, John B. | Surgeon | Wilkes Barre, Pa | To May, 1864 |
| Dana, Chas. H. | Ass't S. | Tunkhannock, Pa | To October, 1863. |
| Woods, Wm. S. | Surgeon | | To May 1863. |

### 53D INFANTRY—Mustered out June 30, 1865.

| Name | Rank | Address | Service |
|---|---|---|---|
| Burchfield, J. P. | Ass't S. | Clearfield, Pa | To 83d Inf. April, 1862. |
| Spayd, Charles W. | Surgeon | Wilkes Barre, Pa | From August, 1864. |
| Wynne, Wm. B. | Ass't S. | Parker's Landing, Pa | To October, 1862; also 14th Cav. |
| McKinnon, M. I. | Surgeon | York, Pa | To January, 1863. |
| Gatchell, Jacob C. | Ass't S. | Martinsville, Pa | From October, 1864. |
| Ironberger, J. H. | Surgeon | | To January, 1862. |
| Jackson, Geo. W. | " | | To Aug., 1864; also 29th Inf. |

### 54TH INFANTRY—Mustered out July 15, 1865.

| Name | Rank | Address | Service |
|---|---|---|---|
| Allen, John M. | Surgeon | Chester, Pa | To October, 1864. |
| Aschom, John P. | " | Renova, Pa | To May, 1865; also 48th and 116th Inf. |
| Fruit, John C. | Ass't S. | Jerseytown, Pa | To May, 1864. |
| Lewis, George R. | " | Indiana, Pa | To 61st Inf. Oct., 1863. Ex. S. |
| Hall, Wm. E. | " | Renovo, Pa | From May, 1864. |
| Matthews, A. W. | " | | To 128th Inf. Nov., 1862. |

### 55TH INFANTRY—Mustered out August 30, 1865.

| Name | Rank | Address | Service |
|---|---|---|---|
| Brandt, J. B. | Surgeon | Llewellyn, Pa | From Sept., 1864. Also 110th & 175th Inf. I. |
| Christy, H. C. | Ass't S. | 225 Segar st., Cleveland or Toledo, Ohio. | To 58th Inf. Oct., 1863. |
| Merritt, David | Surgeon | 2032 Bainbridge street, Philadelphia, Pa. | To August, 1864. |
| Ramsey, J. S. | Ass't S. | 719 S. 16th st., Philadelphia, Pa. | To 130th Inf. Oct., 1862. |
| Johnson, Ovid M. | " | | To August, 1864 |
| Lauer, Charles F. | " | | To September, 1864. |
| Noetling, John | " | | To June, 1865. |
| Boyer, Sam'l S. | " | | From February, 1865. |

### 56TH INFANTRY—Mustered out July 1, 1865.

| Name | Rank | Address | Service |
|---|---|---|---|
| Pennsyl, Philip H. | Ass't S. | Alleghany Co., Md | From October, 1864. |
| McCleary, J. P. | Surgeon | Milton, Pa | To September, 1862. |
| Junkin, John M. | " | Easton, Pa | To 4th Cav. Jan., 1863. |
| Shoemaker, J. T. | " | 31st st. and Gray's Ferry Road, Phila., Pa. | From March, 1865; also 88th Inf. |
| Lyons, John C. | " | | To Dec., 1864; also 4th Cav. |
| Nebinger, W. P. | Ass't S. | Lewisberry, Pa | To October, 1864. |
| Stitzell, Geo | " | | To August, 1863 |
| Culver, W. Wesley | " | | To February, 1863. |
| Nebaker, John G. | " | | To September, 1862. |
| Wilson, James P. | Surgeon | Dead | To April, 1862. |

PENNSYLVANIA—Continued.

57TH INFANTRY—Mustered out June 29, 1865.

| Name | Rank | Address | Service |
|---|---|---|---|
| Jack, Wm | Ass't S | Jacksonville, Pa | From June, 1864; also 84th Inf. |
| Chritzman, H. G | Surgeon | Welch Run, Pa | From November, 1864: also 8th Cav. |
| Lyman, J. W | " | Towanda, Pa | To Lieut Col. 203d Inf., Sept., 1864. |
| Kennedy, David D | Ass't S | Oxford, Pa | To Surg. 133d Inf., February. 1863. |
| Leet, Fred. H | " | Greenville, Pa | To September. 1863. |
| Downs, Thos. A | " | 4032 Market street, Philadelphia, Pa. | To March, 1864. |
| Cassell, J. K | " | | From September, 1864. |
| Miller, J. Elliott | " | Butler near Penn street, Pittsburgh, Pa. | To December, 1862. |
| Fisher, A. W | " | | To August, 1862. |

58TH INFANTRY—In service August 31, 1865.

| Name | Rank | Address | Service |
|---|---|---|---|
| Christy, H. C | Surgeon | Toledo, or 225 Segar st., Cleveland. Ohio. | From October, 1863; also 55th Inf. |
| Nichols, P. J | Ass't S | Londonderry, Pa | To 97th Inf. March, 1865. |
| Wright, A. W | Surgeon | Chester, Pa | To September, 1863. |
| Cummins, L. C | Ass't S | | To September, 1862; also 125th Inf. |
| Campbell, Wm. H | " | | To July, 1863. |

The 59TH and 60TH INFANTRY were three-months' organizations.

61ST INFANTRY—Mustered out June 28, 1865.

| Name | Rank | Address | Service |
|---|---|---|---|
| Lewis, G. R | Surgeon | Indiana, Pa | From October, 1863; also 54th Inf. U. S. Ex S. |
| Tindle, R. M | " | 129 Penna ave., Pittsburgh, Pa | To August, 1863. |
| Herr, Ambrose J | Ass't S | Lancaster. Pa | To 68th Inf., Sept., 1862. |
| Kinlin, Wm. W | " | Waddam's Grove, Ill | From December, 1864. |
| Freeland, J. B | " | | To January, 1863. |
| Riddle, John W | " | | To September, 1864 |
| McFadden, James A | " | | To September, 1864. |

62D INFANTRY—Mustered out July 13, 1865; veterans and recruits transferred to 155th Infantry.

| Name | Rank | Address | Service |
|---|---|---|---|
| Kerr, James | Surgeon | 1611 Carson st., Pittsburgh, Pa. | From July, 1861. |
| Wilson, Jos. F | Ass't S | 826 Arch st., Phila., Pa | To April. 1864. |
| Gardner, T. S | " | | To October, 1863; also Surg. 17th Cav. |
| Webb, Joseph P | " | | To September, 1862. |
| Martin, Wallace D | " | Harrisburgh, Pa | To October, 1863. |
| Zeigler, P. M | " | | From November. 1863. |

63D INFANTRY—Mustered out September 9, 1864; veterans and recruits transferred to the 99th Infantry, and subsequently to the 105th Infantry.

| Name | Rank | Address | Service |
|---|---|---|---|
| McFadden, James | Ass't S | 404 Fairmount avenue, Philadelphia, Pa | To June, 1862. |
| McMorris, N. C | " | Duncannon, Pa | From August, 1863. |
| Farrell, Gerald D. O | " | 716 E. Cumberland st., Philadelphia, Pa. | From April, 1863; also 215th Infantry. |
| Rodgers, James K | Surgeon | Dead | To July, 1862 |
| Jones, Z Ring | " | | From Jan., 1863; also 6th Reserves and 195th Inf. |
| Worthington, W. H | " | Dead | To 99th Inf., Feb., 1862. |
| Crawford, John T | " | | To Surg. U. S. V. October, 1861. |

## PENNSYLVANIA—Continued.

For 64TH INFANTRY see 4th Cavalry; for 65TH INFANTRY see 5th Cavalry.

### 66TH INFANTRY—Consolidated with 73d and 99th Infantry March, 1862.

| | | | |
|---|---|---|---|
| Todd, W. C. | Surgeon | Manayunk, Pa | Transferred to 5th Cav. March, 1862. |
| Heaney, Patrick | Ass't S | | A. W. M. Also 5th Cav. |

### 67TH INFANTRY—Mustered out July 17, 1865.

| | | | |
|---|---|---|---|
| Barr, Robert | Surgeon | Indiana, Pa | To November, 1864. |
| Thornton, Thos. C | " | Lewisburgh, Pa | From April, 1865; also 138th Inf. |
| Pettinos, James W | Ass't S | 1918 Christian st., Philadelphia, Pa. | To June, 1863. |
| Corson, Thos F | " | | To May, 1865. |

### 68TH INFANTRY—In service August 31, 1865.

| | | | |
|---|---|---|---|
| Herr, Ambrose J | Surgeon | Lancaster, Pa | From September, 1863; also 61st Inf. |
| Shaw, James | Ass't S | 1721 Wallace st., Philadelphia, Pa. | From December, 1864. |
| Wilson, John C | " | Conemaugh, Pa | To October, 1864; also 206th Inf. |
| Curran, Thos M | " | | To December, 1862. |
| McIlvain, John E | " | | To September, 1863. |

### 69TH INFANTRY—Mustered out July 1, 1865.

| | | | |
|---|---|---|---|
| Wadsworth, H. A | Ass't S | 1753 Frankford Road, Philadelphia, Pa. | Dismissed January, 1863. |
| Burmeister, Fred. F | Surgeon | 1942 Frankford avenue, Philadelphia, Pa. | From December, 1862; also 73d Inf. |
| Mc Niell, B. A | Ass't S | | To August, 1864. |
| Bombaugh, Chas. C | Surgeon | | To September, 1862. |
| Corson, Elwood M | Ass't S | | To September, 1863. |
| Smith, Chas. J | " | | From October, 1864. |

### 70TH INFANTRY—(See 6th Cavalry.)

### 71ST INFANTRY—(Also called Baker's 1st California Infantry)—Mustered out July 2, 1864.

| | | | |
|---|---|---|---|
| Robison, G. R. B | Ass't S | Sharpsburgh, Pa | From May, 1863. |
| Dwinelle, Justin | " | | To 106th Inf. Sept., 1861. |
| Linton, Herman B | " | 548 N. 10th st., Phila., Pa. | To 175th Inf. Nov., 1862. |
| Lummis, G. B. | " | | To 13th Cav. Sept., 1862. |
| Marshall, C. P | " | | To April, 1864. |
| Baker, Alfred C | Surgeon | | To August, 1862. |
| Munger, S B | Ass't S | | To November, 1861. |
| Aiken, John | Surgeon | | From April, 1863. |
| Malone, John | " | | Dismissed Feb, 1863; also 2d Res. |

### 72D INFANTRY—Mustered out August 24, 1864.

| | | | |
|---|---|---|---|
| Houston, I. W | Ass't S | Collamer, Pa | To October, 1862. |
| Rizer, Martin | Surgeon | Philadelphia, Pa | From August, 1861. |
| Burr, Richard | " | 1644 N. 8th st., Phila., Pa. | To February, 1862. |
| Jones, A. Stokes | Ass't S | Ottsville, Pa | From Aug, 1862; also 200th Inf. |
| Hayes, Joshua R | Surgeon | 1360 Richmond street Phila., Pa. | To Aug, 1862; also 187th Inf. |

## PENNSYLVANIA—Continued.

### 73D INFANTRY—Mustered out July 14, 1865.

| Name | Rank | Address | Remarks |
|---|---|---|---|
| Armstrong, J. A | Ass't S | Camden, N. J | To 75th Inf. Oct., 1862. Ex. S. |
| Gunkle, Wm | Surgeon | Philadelphia, Pa | To Nov., 1864. Dead. |
| Smith, Wm. F | " | Airville, Pa | From Dec., 1864; also 28th Inf |
| Trexler, J. S | Ass't S | Kutztown, Pa | To January, 1865. |
| Wilson, John H | " | Bethlehem, Pa | To March, 1864. |
| Rex, George | Surgeon | 2118 Pine st., Philadelphia, Pa | To Sept., 1861. A. G. reports missing |
| Burmeister, F. F | Ass't S | 1942 Frankford avenue, Philadelphia, Pa. | To 69th Inf. Dec., 1862. |
| Blake, I. A. D | " | 2514 N. 10th st., Phila., Pa. | From February, 1865. |

### 74TH INFANTRY—Mustered out August 29, 1865.

| Name | Rank | Address | Remarks |
|---|---|---|---|
| Cadwell, Dan'l G | Ass't S | Care A. G. U. S A | To October, 1863. |
| Stockton, G. B | " | North East, Pa | From May, 1865. |
| Pillichody, F. | Surgeon | Buchanan, Pa | To February, 1864. |
| Saylor, O. L | Ass't S | Schuylkill Haven, Pa | To January, 1863. |
| Swartzlander, F | " | Doylestown, Pa | To October, 1864. |
| Chilson, S. L | Surgeon | | From June, 1865; also 1st Res. and 190th Inf. |
| Giseman, Geo. S | Ass't S | | To October, 1862 |
| Siddall, Hugh W | Surgeon | | To Oct., 1864; also 85th Inf. |
| Gueuste, F | Ass't S | | Dismissed Dec., 1861. |

### 75TH INFANTRY—Mustered out September 1, 1865.

| Name | Rank | Address | Remarks |
|---|---|---|---|
| Armstrong, J. A | Surgeon | Camden, N J | To Sept., 1864; also 73d Inf Ex. S. |
| Koerper, E. A | " | Fort McKinney, Wash. Ter., care A. G. U. S. A. | From October, 1864. |
| Mish, P. B | Ass't S | Lebanon, Pa | From December, 1864 |
| Shultz, S. S | " | | To 26th Inf. June, 1863. |
| Barry, Wm. A | " | | To Jan., 1864; tr'f. to 98th Inf. |
| Long, M. S | " | Mertztown, Pa | To January, 1863. |
| Nicholas, John T | " | | To March, 1863. |
| Beekin, Charles. | Surgeon | 244 N. 5th st., Phila., Pa. | To October, 1862. |

### 76TH INFANTRY—Mustered out July 18, 1865.

| Name | Rank | Address | Remarks |
|---|---|---|---|
| Backhus, C. W | Surgeon | Three Rivers, Mich | A. W. M. Also 99th and 203d Inf. |
| * Bancroft, F. J | Ass't S | Denver, Colo | To 3d Heavy Art. Sept., 1862. |
| Leit, Nathan Y | Surgeon | Scranton, Pa | To June, 1865. |
| Lefever, Isaac | Ass't S | Harrisburgh, Pa | From October, 1864. |
| Scholl, E. R | Surgeon | Reading, Pa | To Feb., 1863. U. S. Ex. S. |
| Withers, M. A | " | Pittston, Pa | To July, 1864. |
| Siemens, C. J | Ass't S | | To 50th Inf. March, 1862. |
| Keeley, Edwin | " | | To May, 1863. |
| Schlosser, A | " | | To September, 1864. |

### 77TH INFANTRY.—In service August 31, 1865.

| Name | Rank | Address | Remarks |
|---|---|---|---|
| Downey, J. B | Ass't S | Carrigo Springs, Tex | To 78th Inf. Aug., 1863. |
| McCandless, J. N | Surgeon | Prescott, Ariz | From February, 1864. |
| Adair, James T | Ass't S | | From March, 1864 |
| Maurer, Jocob S | " | | To November, 1862. |
| Potter, Thos. B | " | Phillipsburgh, Pa | To April, 1862 |
| Irish, Franklin | Surgeon | | To February, 1864. |

* Was at hospital, Harrisburgh, Pa., four years, and Fortress Monroe, Va., three years.

## PENNSYLVANIA—Continued.

### 78TH INFANTRY—Mustered out September 21, 1865.

Downey, J B.........Surgeon...Carrigo Springs, Tex......To April, 1864; also 77th Inf.
Kosack, Wm. T.. ..... " Oakland, Pa..................Not on A. G. R
Bailey, Wm. D......... " Dillsburgh, Pa................To November, 1864.
Morris, F. B...... .....Ass't S.....2013 Germantown ave, Philadelphia, Pa. To July, 1865.
Miller, Victor D ...... " Mason and Dixon, Pa.....To March, 1863.
Walton, John T.......Surgeon...Buffalo, N. Y.................From June, 1865; also 103d Inf Dead.
McCollough, W. P...Ass't S..........................................To November, 1864.
Bollinger, O. B........ " Saegers own, Pa............To June. 1865.
Ross, Elijah A......... " ..........................................To January, 1863.
McGrath, John.........Surgeon..........................................To June, 1863; also 23d Inf.
Marks, John I ......... " Lewistown, Pa...............To Aug., 1862; also 205th Inf.

### 79TH INFANTRY—Mustered out September 11, 1865.

Albright, F. G..........Ass't S.....Lancaster, Pa...............To Nov., 1864; also 9th Cav.
Wright, W. M..........Surgeon...Geneva, N. Y..................To December, 1864.
White, W. H...... .... " Bloomfield, N. J............From January. 1865.
Phillips, Thomas H...Ass't S ..........................................From Jan., 1865; also 175th Inf.

### 80TH INFANTRY—(See 7th Cavalry)

### 81ST INFANTRY—Mustered out June 29, 1865.

Norris, John C.........Surgeon...1307 Girard ave., Phila...From October. 1864.
Graham, Samuel......Ass't S.....Butler. Pa.......................From Dec., 1864; also 174th Inf.
Houston, John.........Surgeon...Marietta, Pa.....................To September, 1864.
Gardiner. Wm. A..... " ..........................................To August, 1862.
Kimball, J. P.......... Ass't S..........................................To January, 1862.
Colston, H. S..........Surgeon..........................................To Dec., 1862; also 3d Inf.
Beshler, J. B...........Ass't S..........................................Dismissed March, 1863; also 88th Inf.

### 82D INFANTRY—Mustered out July 13, 1865

Richardson, J. R......Surgeon...610 S. 4th st., Phila., Pa..To January, 1865.
Clarke, D. D............ " Philadelphia, Pa............To November, 1862.
Foote, Richard ........Ass't S ....Carbondale, Pa..............To January, 1864.
Thomas, Joseph.......Surgeon...Quakertown, Pa ...........From July, 1865; also 118th Inf.
Emanuel, Louis M... " ..........................................To September, 1864.
Miller, James..........Ass't S..........................................From Jan., 1865; also 115th Inf.
Brous, Henry K....... " ..........................................From February, 1865.

### 83D INFANTRY—Mustered out June 28, 1865.

Allen, E. P.............Surgeon...Athens, Pa.......................To March, 1863; also 141st Inf
Burchfield, J. P.......Ass't S.....Clearfield, Pa.................From April, 1863; also 53d Inf.
Faulkner, Wm.........Surgeon...Erie, Pa...........................To October, 1862.
Stockton, T. C. M.....Ass't S....Cross Creek Village, Pa..From May, 1864.
Stewart. W. S......... " 17th & Filbert sts., Philadelphia, Pa. To Sept., 1864; also 123d Inf
Walborne Isaac....... " Meyerstown, Pa.............To January, 1863; also 17th Cav.
Wotring, Jonathan... " Newark, Ohio ................To May, 1863.
Thompson, Michael.. " ..........................................To May, 1863.
Belknap, D. E......... " ..........................................To June, 1862.

PENNSYLVANIA—Continued.

84TH INFANTRY—Consolidated with 57th Infantry January 13, 1865.

| Name | Rank | Residence | Service |
|---|---|---|---|
| Hoop, G. F. | " | Idaho Springs, Colo., or Phillipsburgh, Pa. | To September, 1863. |
| Jack, Wm | Ass't S. | Jacksonville, Pa | From June, 1864; also 57th Inf. |
| Norman, J. P. | " | Monongahela City, Pa. | To July, 1864. |
| Sturdevant, Sam'l B. | Surgeon | Wilkes Barre, or Providence, Pa. | From Aug, 1864; also 47th and 139th Inf. |
| McClure, James D. | Ass't S. | Baxter Springs, Kans. | To 147th Inf. May, 1863. |
| Redlick, Chas. A. W. | " | Sharpsburgh, Pa | To 136th Inf. Sept., 1862. |
| Thompson, G. W. | " | Mapleton, Pa. | To August, 1862. |
| Waggoner, John S. | Surgeon | | To April, 1864. |

85TH INFANTRY—Mustered out November 22, 1864, veterans and recruits transferred to 188th Infantry.

| Name | Rank | Residence | Service |
|---|---|---|---|
| Alexander, J. W. | Surgeon | Morganza, Md., or Cannonsburgh, Pa. | To Oct., 1863; also 15th Cav. |
| Kurtz, Sam'l L. | " | Reading, Pa | From June, 1862; also 11th Res. |
| Levis, J. C. | Ass't S. | Bridgewater, Pa | To June, 1862. |
| Laidley, J. B. | Surgeon | Carmichael, Pa. | To May, 1862. |
| Sandt, Samuel | Ass't S. | Easton, Pa | From August, 1862. |
| Siddall, Hugh W. | " | | To Surg. 74th Inf. April, 1864. |

86TH INFANTRY—Failed to complete.

87TH INFANTRY—Mustered out June 29, 1865.

| Name | Rank | Residence | Service |
|---|---|---|---|
| Helwig, T. A. | Surgeon | Minersville, Pa | From February, 1865. H. R. Also 128th Inf. |
| McKinney, D. F. | " | Frederick, Md | To October, 1864. |
| Steadman, Horace C. | Ass't S. | Mifflinburgh, Pa | To January, 1864. |
| Campbell, Bernard J. | " | | From March, 1865. |
| Hoover, Nicholas M. | " | North Hope, Pa | From April, 1865. |
| McCurdy, Francis F. | Surgeon | | Dismissed February, 1864. |

88TH INFANTRY—Mustered out June 30, 1865.

| Name | Rank | Residence | Service |
|---|---|---|---|
| Seltzer, John H. | Surgeon | 227 S. 5th st Phila., Pa. | To July, 1862. |
| Hayes, Jos. H. | Ass't S. | Lock Haven, Pa | To 90th Inf. Jan, 1864. |
| McAlear, M. B. | " | N. E. cor. Front and Dauphin sts., Phila., Pa. | From April, 1865; also 104th Inf. |
| Rawlings, J. W. | Surgeon | | From Feb., 1863; also 118th Inf. |
| Mitchell, Geo. H. | Ass't S. | | To August, 1862. |
| Beshler, J. B. | " | | To June, 1862; also 81st Inf. |
| Shoemaker, Jos. T. | " | 31st st. and Gray's Ferry Road, Phila., Pa. | To 56th Inf. March, 1865. |

89TH INFANTRY—(See 8th Cavalry.)

90TH INFANTRY—Consolidated with 11th Infantry November 26, 1864.

| Name | Rank | Residence | Service |
|---|---|---|---|
| Hayes, J. H | Surgeon | Lock Haven, Pa | From Jan., 1864; also 88th Inf. |
| Tracy, Geo. P | Ass't S. | Burlington, Pa | To July, 1863; also 46th Inf. |
| Griffiths, David S. | " | Bedford, Pa | From March, 1863. |
| Stille, A. Owen | " | Dead | To 23d Inf. March, 1862. |
| Shreeve, J. R. | Surgeon | | To December, 1863. |
| Duncan, Thos. F. | Ass't S. | | To September, 1862. |
| Kemp, Joshua S. | " | Littlestown, Pa. | To November, 1862. |

## PENNSYLVANIA—Continued.

### 91st Infantry—Mustered out July 10, 1865.

Keir, Wm. G............Surgeon...28 N. 38th st., Phila., Pa. From April, 1864; also 135th Inf.
Houghton, C. W .....Ass't S.....1528 N. 17th st., Phila., Pa To Sept., 1862; also 124th and 214th Inf.
Hewitt J. M............ " ........................................From June, 1865.
Young, John .......... " ........................................Dismissed May, 1863; also 183d Inf.
Thomas, T. C.. ........ " ........................................Dismissed May, 1863.
Oldmixon, Geo. S..... " ........................................To March, 1865.
Knight, Isaac D........Surgeon........................................To April, 1864.

### 92d Infantry—(See 9th Cavalry.)

### 93d Infantry—Mustered out June 27, 1865.

Bennett, A. D.........Ass't S.....New Washington, Pa......From December, 1864.
Mays, G. W.............. " Philadelphia, Pa..........To February, 1863.
Simmington, R. S....Surgeon...Danville, Pa...............To August, 1862.
Umberger, E. R...... " Lebanon, Pa...............From Oct., 1863. Dead.
Dickson, John M......Ass't S.....Care A. G. U. S. A.........To October, 1864; also 213th Inf.
Worthington, W. H..Surgeon...Dead.........................Dismissed August, 1863.

### 94th Infantry—Failed to complete.

### 95th Infantry—Mustered out July 17, 1865.

McGlaughlin, C. C...Surgeon...Cor. 5th and Pine sts., Philadelphia, Pa. From December, 1864.
Litz, Jefferson.........Ass't S....Kylertown, Pa...............From March 1865.
Kelly, E B. P.........Surgeon...Perth Amboy, N. J.......To November, 1864.
Laney, T. M.........Ass't S........................................To July 1864; also 206th Inf.

### 96th Infantry—Mustered out October 21, 1864; veterans and recruits transferred to 95th Infantry.

Bland, D. W............Surgeon...Pottsville, Pa.............From Sept., 1861. H. R.
Light, Sam'l B.........Ass't S........................................From October, 1863.
Nugent, W .............. " ........................................To September, 1862.
Egle, Wm ................ " ........................................To March, 1863.
Shamms, J. R.......... " ........................................To August, 1863.

### 97th Infantry—Mustered out August 28, 1865.

Everhart, J. R.........Surgeon...West Chester, Pa............To November, 1864.
Morrison, W. C........Ass't S.....Cochranville, Pa............To January, 1865.
Nichols, P. J...........Surgeon...Londonderry, Pa...........From March, 1865; also 58th Infantry.
Miller, Geo. W.........Ass't S.....Lampeter, Pa...............To April, 1864.

### 98th Infantry—Mustered out June 29, 1865.

Boisnor, J M...........Surgeon...1308 N. 6th street, Philadelphia, Pa. To April, 1863. Dead.
Oliver, G. P...........Ass't S.....936 N. 5th street, Philadelphia, Pa. To 111th Infantry January, 1863.
Goerhig, Wm........... " Williamsport, Pa...........To June, 1865.
Hughes, Isaac..........Surgeon........................................To September, 1863; also 102d Inf.
Buckmann, E D...... " ........................................To November, 1863.
Barry, Wm. A......... " ........................................A. W. M. Also 75th Inf.

## PENNSYLVANIA—Continued.

### 99TH INFANTRY—Mustered out July 1, 1865.

| | | | |
|---|---|---|---|
| Backhus, C. W. | Ass't S. | Three Rivers, Mich. | To October, 1864; also 76th and 203d Inf. |
| Butcher, B. F. | " | 771 S. 10th st., Phila, Pa. | To January, 1863. |
| Dickerson, M. T. W. | Surgeon | Media, Pa | To January, 1863. |
| Hoffman, J. M. | Ass't S. | 420 Franklin st., Reading, Pa. | To 155th Infantry September, 1862. |
| Updegrove, Silas | Surgeon | 804 Marshall st., Philadelphia, Pa | To November, 1864; also 157th Inf. |
| Lotz, Geo. | Ass't S. | | To June, 1863. |
| Rodgers, Jas. K. | Surgeon | | To 63d Inf. Feb., 1862. |
| Worthington, W. H. | " | Dead | To May, 1862; also 63d Inf. |
| Gallagher, J. H. | Ass't S. | | To June, 1865. |
| Styer, Charles | Surgeon | | Dismissed March, 1863; also 45th Inf. |
| Boyer, David P. | " | | From December, 1864. |

### 100TH INFANTRY—Mustered out July 24, 1865.

| | | | |
|---|---|---|---|
| Card, James C. | Ass't S. | Philadelphia, Pa | To June, 1864 Dead. |
| Durant, H. B. | " | Claryville, Pa. | To March, 1865. |
| Ludington, Horace | Surgeon | 317 Elm st., Cincinnati, Ohio or 2008 Burt st., Omaha, Neb | To September, 1864. |
| Mass, Abraham | " | Neosho, Pa. | From October, 1864. |
| Shurlock, Wm. C. | Ass't S. | Harrisburgh or Darlington, Pa. or Fargo, Dak. Ter. | To 51st Inf Dec., 1863. |
| Rossiter, J. P. | " | | To 129th Inf Sept., 1862. |
| Gross, F. H. | Surgeon | S. 11th, cor. Walnut st., Phila., Pa. | To Surg. U. S. V. Oct., 1861. |

### 101ST INFANTRY—Mustered out July 25, 1865.

| | | | |
|---|---|---|---|
| McPherson, Wm. | Ass't S. | 349 Wharton st., Phila., Pa. | From August, 1863; also 137th Inf. |
| Rush, D. G. | Surgeon | 51 W. Washington st., Chicago, Ill. | To May, 1865. |
| Frick, A. P. | Ass't S. | Fort Steel or Fort Laramie, Wyoming Ter. | To 103d Inf. Nov., 1862. |
| Hosack, J. P. | Surgeon | Mercer, Pa | To 51st Inf. Feb., 1862. |
| Bretz, Geo. Z. | Ass't S. | | From August, 1862. |

### 102D INFANTRY—Mustered out June 2, 1865.

| | | | |
|---|---|---|---|
| McCormick, S. C. | Ass't S. | Duluth, Minn. | A. G. R. M[illegible], August, 1862; also 202d Inf. |
| Morrison, M. P. | Surgeon | Monongahela City, Pa | From September, 1863. |
| Crawford, C. C. V. A. | Ass't S. | Village Green, Pa | To November, 1864. |
| Pennepacker, J. J. | " | | From May, 1865 |
| Fleming, Wm. J. | Surgeon | 2207 Callowhill street, Phila., Pa. | Dismissed August, 1862. |
| Roberts, J. H. | Ass't S. | 138 Cassen street, Pittsburgh, Pa. | To June, 1865. |
| Hughes, Isaac | " | | To 98th Inf. May, 1863. |

### 103D INFANTRY—Mustered out August 25, 1865.

| | | | |
|---|---|---|---|
| Frick, A. P. | Surgeon | Fort Steel, or Fort Laramie, Wyo. Ter. | To Jan., 1865; also 101st Inf. |
| Stavely, Wm. R. | " | Lahoska, Pa. | To November, 1862. |
| Marshall, D. M. | Ass't S. | Brady, Pa | To 167th Inf. Jan., 1863. |
| Walton, John T. | " | Buffalo, N. Y. | To 78th Inf. May, 1865. Dead. |
| Jacobs, Theodore | " | | To June, 1862; also 187th Inf. |
| Meredith, J. Q. A. | Surgeon | | From July, 1862. |

## PENNSYLVANIA—Continued.

### 104TH INFANTRY—Mustered out August 25, 1865.

| | | | |
|---|---|---|---|
| McAlear, M. B | Ass't S | N.E. cor. Front & Dauphin sts., Phila., Pa. | To June, 1864; also 88th Inf. |
| Peek, Wm. A | Surgeon | Waymart, Pa | To July, 1862. |
| Robinson, W. T | " | 1920 Mt. Vernon street, Phila., Pa. | A. W. M. |
| Hendrie, W. Scott | Ass't S | Holmesburg, Pa | To November, 1862. |
| Cadwallader, D. W | " | | To 169th Inf Jan., 1863. |
| Brush, Platt E | Surgeon | | From April, 1863. |

### 105TH INFANTRY—Mustered out July 11, 1865.

| | | | |
|---|---|---|---|
| Heichhold, Alex. P | Surgeon | Special A. P. O. Dep't, Brookville. Pa. | To September, 1862. |
| Smith, Wm. F | Ass't S | Airville, Pa | To October 1862. |
| Ewing. Geo. E | " | | To 115th Inf. April, 1863. |
| Vaughn. Aaron C | " | | To September. 1864. |
| Taylor, Jos | " | 1538 Wallace st., Phila., Pa. | From June, 1865. |
| Wenger, Adam | Surgeon | | From June, 1865. |

### 106TH INFANTRY—Part mustered out September 10, 1864; the remainder June 30, 1865.

| | | | |
|---|---|---|---|
| Leidy, Philip | Ass't S | 526 Marshall st., Phila., Pa. | To Sept., 1862; also 119th Inf. |
| Gates, E. D | " | Fairvew, Pa | From September, 1862. |
| Alexander, Hugh | " | | To October, 1862. |
| Dwinelle, Justin | Surgeon | | To Sept., 1864; also 71st Inf. |
| McLean, H. D | Ass't S | 1531 Pine st., Phila., Pa | To December, 1863. |

### 107TH INFANTRY—Mustered out July 13, 1865.

| | | | |
|---|---|---|---|
| Dana, R. S | Surgeon | Morrisville, Pa | From May, 1865. |
| Hutchinson, J. F | " | Harrisburgh, Pa | To March, 1865. |
| Reichard, P. L | Ass't S | Allentown, Pa | From April, 1865. |
| Worrall, H. G | " | | To 173d Inf. Nov., 1862. |
| Westcott, E. R | " | | To April 1863. |
| Sherdown, A. M | " | | To December, 1863. |
| Frow, John G | Surgeon | | To August, 1862. |

### 108TH INFANTRY—(See 11th Cavalry.)

### 109TH INFANTRY—Consolidated with 111th Infantry March 31, 1865.

| | | | |
|---|---|---|---|
| Matlock, W. H | Ass't S | Downingtown, Pa | To May, 1862. |
| Dunn, J. L | Surgeon | Titusville, Pa | From March, 1862. H. R. Also 111th Inf. |
| Brubaker, D. M | Ass't S | Mifflin, Pa | To January, 1865. |
| Hassenplug, J. H | " | 511 N. 10th st., Phila., Pa. | To October, 1863. |

### 110TH INFANTRY—Mustered out June 28, 1865.

| | | | |
|---|---|---|---|
| Palm, P. R | Ass't S | Allentown, Pa | To 137th Inf. Dec., 1862. |
| Hays, David S | Surgeon | Hollidaysburg, Pa. | To June, 1865. |
| Church, Wm | Ass't S | Meadville, Pa | To Surg. 141st Inf. Sept., 1862. Dead |
| Wilson, Chas. H | " | Berwick, Pa | To Surg. 49th [illegible] [illegible]ch, 1863. |
| Brandt, J. B | " | Llewellyn, Pa | To Surg. 55th I[illegible] [illegible]pt., 1864; also 175th Inf. J. |
| Pomeroy, Geo. B | " | | To Surg. 17th Cav., May, 1864. |
| McCormick, Jas. F | " | | From October, 1864. |

## PENNSYLVANIA—Continued.

### 111TH INFANTRY—Mustered out July 19, 1865.

| | | | |
|---|---|---|---|
| Dunn, J. L. | Surgeon | Titusville, Pa. | To April, 1865; also 109th Inf. |
| Ake, Joseph H | Ass't S. | Williamsburg, Pa. | To April. 1865. |
| Stickland, D. H. | Surgeon | Erie, Pa | From May, 1865. |
| Oliver, Geo. P. | " | 936 N. 5th st., Phila., Pa. | To July, 1864; also 98th Inf. |
| Stokes, James. | Ass't S. | Upper Dublin, Pa. | To January, 1863. |
| Bradfield, Geo. M. | " | Blain, Pa. | From June, 1865. |
| Conrad, H. F. | " | | To 174th Inf. February, 1863. |
| Stewart, W. B | Surgeon | | To November, 1862. |

### 112TH INFANTRY—(See 2d Heavy Artillery.)

### 113TH INFANTRY—(See 12th Cavalry.)

### 114TH INFANTRY—Mustered out May 29, 1865

| | | | |
|---|---|---|---|
| Bartine, D. H. | Ass't S. | Princeton or Merchantville, N. J. | To 2d H. Art. August, 1864. |
| Cummins, J. M. | Surgeon | Industry or Ligonier, Pa. | From July, 1862. |
| Hawk, James A | Ass't S. | | From March, 1863. |
| Kelly, Thos. J | " | | To 142d Infantry February, 1863. |

### 115TH INFANTRY—Consolidated with 110th June 22, 1864.

| | | | |
|---|---|---|---|
| Bartram, T. L | Ass't S | 1613 Richmond street, Philadelphia, Pa. | A. W. M. |
| Blakeslee, W. R | Surgeon | Coatesville, Pa. | Dismissed March, 1863. |
| Miller, James | Ass't S. | | From April, 1863; also 82d Infantry. |
| Ewing, Geo. E | Surgeon | | From April, 1863; also 105th Infantry. |
| McCullough, J. A. | Ass't S. | | To December, 1862. |

### 116TH INFANTRY—Cos. A to E mustered out June 3, 1865, the rest July 14, 1865.

| | | | |
|---|---|---|---|
| Hartman, Wm. B. | Surgeon | St. Mary's, Pa | To June, 1865. |
| Aschom, John P | " | Renovo, Pa. | To March, 1863; also 54th and 48th Inf. |
| Cunningham, D. S. | Ass't S. | | To October, 1864. |
| Rawlings, John W. | " | | To Jan., 1863; also 88th Inf. |
| Boyle, Philip A. | " | 1452 N. 2d st., Phila., Pa. | To February, 1863. |

### 117TH INFANTRY—(See 13th Cavalry.)

### 118TH INFANTRY—Mustered out June 1, 1865; recruits transferred to 91st Regiment.

| | | | |
|---|---|---|---|
| Thomas, Jos. | Surgeon | Quakertown, Pa. | From August, 1862; also 82d Inf. |
| Crouse, J. L | Ass't S. | | From September, 1864. |
| Rowland, N. L | " | | To December. 1863. |
| Kollock, J. M. | " | | To 50th Inf. Sept., 1864. |

### 119TH INFANTRY—Mustered out June 19, 1865.

| | | | |
|---|---|---|---|
| Leidy, Philip. | Surgeon | 526 Marshall st., Philadelphia, Pa. | From September, 1862; also 106th Inf. |
| Mitchell, Geo. W. | Ass't S. | Andersonburgh, Pa. | From February, 1863. |
| Newman, Thos. | " | | From December, 1862. |
| Byington, W. C. | " | | To 183d Infantry March, 1864. |

## PENNSYLVANIA—Continued.

### 120TH INFANTRY—Failed to complete.

### 121ST INFANTRY—Mustered out June 2, 1865.

| | | | |
|---|---|---|---|
| Davis, F. F. | Ass't S. | S. Oil City, Pa. | From September, 1863; also 168th Inf. |
| Comfort, J. J. | " | Atlantic City or Blackwoodtown, N. J. | To 13th Reserves Dec., 1862; also 190th Inf. |
| Kerr, P. M. | " | Holt, Pa. | To January, 1863. |
| Hottenstein, H. P. | Surgeon | Selin's Grove, Pa. | To October, 1862. |
| Cady, Chas. E. | Ass't S. | Corner 6th and York sts., Phila., Pa. | To September, 1862; also 138th Inf. |
| Wilson, Alex. | " | | Dismissed August, 1863. |
| Ramsay, J. A. | Surgeon | | From November, 1862. |

### 122D INFANTRY—(9 months)—Mustered out May 15 and 16, 1863.

| | | | |
|---|---|---|---|
| Burg, Washington | Ass't S. | Brickersville, Pa. | From September, 1863; also 207th Inf. |
| Hogendobler, I. C. | " | | From September, 1862; also 143d Inf. |
| Lane, Wm. C. | Surgeon | | From September, 1862. |

### 123D INFANTRY—(9 months)—Mustered out May 13, 1863.

| | | | |
|---|---|---|---|
| Stewart, Samuel S. | Ass't S. | Stewart's Station, or Cavettsville, Pa. | From September, 1862. |
| Stewart, Wm. S. | " | 17th and Filbert sts., Philadelphia, Pa. | From March, 1863; also 83d Inf. |
| Angle, J. S. | " | Sunbury, Pa. | To January, 1863 |
| Martin, Henry F. | Surgeon | | From Sept., 1862; also 9th Reserves. |

### 124TH INFANTRY—(9 months)—Mustered out May 16, 1863.

| | | | |
|---|---|---|---|
| Houghton, C. W. | Surgeon | 1528 N. 17th st., Philadelphia, Pa. | From Sept., 1862; also 91st and 214th Inf. |
| Martin, J. R. | Ass't S. | Stewartstown, Pa. | From August, 1862. |
| Harshberger, A. | " | Milroy, Pa. | To 166th Inf. Dec., 1862; also 149th inf |
| Jung, Theo. J. | " | | From Jan., 1863; also 7th Cav. |

### 125TH INFANTRY—(9 months)—Mustered out May 18, 1863.

| | | | |
|---|---|---|---|
| Cummins, Lewis C. | Surgeon | | From Sept., 1863; also 58th Inf. |
| Davis, Augustus | Ass't S. | | From December, 1862. |
| Butler, Lafayette | " | | From Feb., 1863; also 13th Res. and 190th Inf. |
| Freay, John | " | | To October, 1862. |
| Davidson, Francis B. | " | | To November, 1862. |

### 126TH INFANTRY—(9 months)—Mustered out May 20, 1863.

| | | | |
|---|---|---|---|
| Nugent, Wash'n G. | Surgeon | Pittston, Pa. | From October, 1862. |
| Swift, Daniel D. | Ass't S. | 724 S. 21st st., Phila., Pa. | From Aug., 1862; also 2d Prov. and 6th Cav. |
| Grube, Frank | " | | From August, 1862. |

### 127TH INFANTRY—(9 months)—Mustered out May 29, 1863.

| | | | |
|---|---|---|---|
| Vastine, J. H. | Ass't S. | Danville, Pa. | From August, 1862. |
| Horner, E. H. | Surgeon | Turbotville, Pa. | From March, 1863. |
| Reily, James R. | " | | To 179th Inf. Jan., 1863; also 1st Lt. Art. |

PENNSYLVANIA—Continued.

128TH INFANTRY—(9 months)—Mustered out May 19, 1863.

Helwig, T. A..........Ass't S.....Minersville, Pa..............From August, 1862; also 87th Inf.
Potteiger, J. B........ " Hamburgh, Pa...............To January, 1863.
Kauffman, J. H....... " Minersville, Pa..............A. W. M. Also 52d and 151st Inf.
Mathews, A. W.......Surgeon....................................From Nov., 1862; also 54th Inf.

129TH INFANTRY—(9 months)—Mustered out May 18, 1863.

Rossiter, J. B..........Surgeon....................................From Sept., 1862; also 100th Inf.
Schittler, Otto .........Ass't S.....................................From August, 1862.
Long, J. G.............. " ....................................Dismissed Nov., 1862.

130TH INFANTRY—(9 months)—Mustered out May 21, 1863.

Ramsey, John S.......Surgeon...1930 Pine st, or 719 S. 16th st., Phila., Pa. From Oct., 1862; also 55th Inf.
Longenecker, J. H...Ass't S.....................................From September, 1862.
Winter, Peter.......... " ....................................A. W. M.
Haupt, Fred. S........ " Sunbury, Pa................. To February, 1863.

131ST INFANTRY—(9 months)—Mustered out May 23, 1863.

Huber, J. F............Surgeon....................................From Oct., 1863; also 49th Inf.
Kirk, Lewis R.........Ass't S.....Rising Sun, Md.............From Aug., 1862; also 26th Inf. and 2d H. Art.
Evans, David J....... " ....................................From August, 1862.

132D INFANTRY—(9 months)—Mustered out May 24, 1863.

Anawalt, J. W.........Surgeon...Greensburgh, Pa............A. W. M. H. R. Also 11th Inf.
Wagonseller, B. F ...Ass't S.. Selin's Grove, Pa ..........Missing Aug., 1862; also 139th and 201st Inf.
Hoover, G. W.......... " Lewistown, Pa................From Sept., 1862. Dead.
Thompson, G. K...... " Wellsboro, Pa...............From August, 1862.
Oberholtzer, Levi.....Surgeon...................................To Jan., 1863; also 139th and 147th Inf.

133D INFANTRY—(9 months)—Mustered out May 21 to 26, 1863.

Stathem, Thos. E.....Ass't S.....Greenwich, N. J............From August, 1862.
Kennedy, D. D........Surgeon...Oxford, Pa....................From Feb., 1863; also 57th Inf.
Thompson, Wm........Ass't S....Centre Moreland, Pa......From December, 1862.
Keyes, John W........ " ....................................Dismissed January, 1863.

134TH INFANTRY—(9 months)—Mustered out May 26, 1863.

McKinney, David .....Surgeon...New Brighton, Pa.........From Aug., 1862; also 10th Inf.
Cobb, J. W.............Ass't S....Binghamton, N. Y.........From August, 1862.
McCormick, Sam'l.... " ....................................From September, 1863.

135TH INFANTRY—(9 months)—Mustered out May 24, 1863.

Hottenstein, C. D.....Surgeon...3522 Market st., Philadelphia, Pa. From August, 1862.
Keir, Wm. G...........Ass't S.....28 N. 38th st., Phila., Pa..From Aug., 1862; also 91st Inf.
Marr, Wm. H.......... " ....................................From September, 1862.

## PENNSYLVANIA—Continued.

### 136TH INFANTRY—(9 months)—Mustered out May 29, 1863.

| Name | Rank | Residence | Remarks |
|---|---|---|---|
| Eston, Elisha C | Ass't S | 1639 N. 11th st., Phila., Pa. | To December, 1862. |
| Young, P. B | " | Crestline, Ohio | From January, 1863. |
| Redlick, C. A. W | Surgeon | Sharpsburgh, Pa | To Sept., 1862; also 84th Inf. |
| Funderburg, W. F | Ass't S | | To 176th Inf. Dec., 1862. |

### 137TH INFANTRY—(9 months)—Mustered out June 1, 1863.

| Name | Rank | Residence | Remarks |
|---|---|---|---|
| Palm, P. R | Surgeon | Allentown, Pa | From Dec., 1862; also 110th Inf. |
| McPherson, Wm | Ass't S | 349 Wharton st., Phila., Pa. | From Sept., 1862; also 101st Inf. |
| Whitney, M. G | " | Kingston, Pa | To April, 1863. |

### 138TH INFANTRY—Mustered out June 23, 1865.

| Name | Rank | Residence | Remarks |
|---|---|---|---|
| Cady, Chas. E | Surgeon | Cor. 6th and York sts., Phila. | From Jan., 1864; also 121st Inf. |
| Thornton, T. C | Ass't S | Lewisburgh, Pa | To Surg. 67th Inf. April, 1865. |
| Tomlinson, T. P | " | | From May, 1865. |
| Herrington, C. P | Surgeon | | To December, 1863. |

### 139TH INFANTRY—Mustered out June 21, 1865.

| Name | Rank | Residence | Remarks |
|---|---|---|---|
| Chapin, S. F | Surgeon | Wattsburgh or Erie, Pa | From September, 1862, to June, 1865. H. R. Also 1st Inf. |
| Wagonseller, B. F | Ass't S | Selin's Grove, Pa | To 158th Inf. Feb., 1863; also 132d and 201st Inf. |
| Sturdevant, S. B | " | Wilkes Barre or Providence, Pa. | To 84th Inf. July, 1864; also 47th Inf. |
| Oberholtzer, Levi | " | | To 132d Inf. Dec., 1862; also 147th Inf. |
| Patton, J. R | " | Clarksville, Pa | From April, 1863. |

### 140TH INFANTRY—Mustered out May 31, 1865.

| Name | Rank | Residence | Remarks |
|---|---|---|---|
| Sharp, W. W | Ass't S | Amity, Pa | To 18th Cav. Jan., 1864. |
| Wishart, J. W | Surgeon | 30, 6th ave., Pittsburgh, Pa. | From Oct., 1862; U. S. Ex. S. |
| Hill, Benj. F | Ass't S | Candor, Pa | From Nov., 1862. |

### 141ST INFANTRY—Mustered out May 28, 1865.

| Name | Rank | Residence | Remarks |
|---|---|---|---|
| Allen, E. P | Ass't S | Athens, Pa | To 83d Inf. Dec., 1862. |
| Beyerle, W. G | " | Bernville, Pa | From December, 1864. |
| Church, Wm. | Surgeon | Meadville, Pa | To September, 1864. Died March, 1879 |
| Denison, F. C | " | Mehoopany, Pa | From December, 1864 |

### 142D INFANTRY—Mustered out May 29, 1865.

| Name | Rank | Residence | Remarks |
|---|---|---|---|
| Asay, Lambert J | Ass't S | Visalia, Cal | To 208th Inf. Sept., 1864. |
| Humphrey, C. E | " | Bethlehem, Pa | To 143d Inf. March, 1865. |
| Halsey, R. C | " | | Dismissed March, 1863. |
| Kelly, Thos. J | Surgeon | | From Feb., 1863; also 114th Inf. |
| Barr, A. M | Ass't S | | From April, 1865. |

## PENNSYLVANIA—Continued.

### 143D INFANTRY—Mustered out June 12, 1865.

| | | | |
|---|---|---|---|
| Brobst, Edward | Ass't S | Leesport, Pa | From December, 1864. |
| Humphrey, C. E | Surgeon | Bethlehem, Pa | From April, 1865; also 142d Inf. |
| Hogendobler, I. C | Ass't S | | To U. S. V. Sept., 1864; also 122d Inf. |
| Reamer, F. C | Surgeon | | To February, 1865. |
| Scott, David L | Ass't S | | To April, 1864. |
| Fulton, James | " | New London, Pa | To April, 1864; also 139th Inf. |

### 144TH INFANTRY—Failed to complete.

### 145TH INFANTRY—Mustered out May 31, 1865.

| | | | |
|---|---|---|---|
| Potter, Geo. L | Surgeon | Bellefonte, Pa | A. W. M. Dead. |
| Whildin, J. S | Ass't S | Philadelphia, Pa | To 208th Inf. Feb., 1865. |
| Taylor, I. N | " | Girard, Pa | From March, 1865. |
| Pilgrim, S. V | " | 108 Columbia st., N. Y. city. | To Sept., 1862; also 81st U. S. C. T. |
| Richards, D. W | " | Applebachsville, Pa | To November, 1864. |

### 146TH INFANTRY—Failed to complete.

### 147TH INFANTRY—Mustered out July 6 and 15, 1865.

| | | | |
|---|---|---|---|
| Calver, G. W. H | Ass't S | Florence, N. J | A. W. M. Also 1st Cav. |
| Longshore, W. R | Surgeon | Hazleton, Pa | From December, 1863. |
| McClure, J. D | " | Baxter Springs, Kans | To Nov., 1863; also 84th Inf. |
| Obenholtzer, L | " | | Dismissed March, 1863; also 132d and 139th Inf. |

### 148TH INFANTRY—Mustered out June 1, 1865.

| | | | |
|---|---|---|---|
| Allen, John W | Ass't S | Altoona, Pa | From May, 1864. |
| Hamilton, A. T | " | Lewistown, Pa | From February, 1863. |
| Fisher, C. P. W | " | Boalsburgh, Pa | To June, 1863. |
| Davis, U. Q | Surgeon | Milton, Pa | From December, 1862. |

### 149TH INFANTRY—Mustered out June 24, 1865.

| | | | |
|---|---|---|---|
| Humphrey, Wm. F | Surgeon | Osceola, Pa | To January, 1865; also 13th Inf. |
| * Harshberger, A | " | Milroy, Pa | From Feb., 1865; also 124th and 166th Inf. |
| Hunter, W. G | Ass't S | Bucksville, Pa | To 211th Inf. September, 1864. |
| Blackwood, W. R. D | " | 246 N. 20th street, Philadelphia, Pa. | To 48th Inf. April, 1863. |
| King, W. Howard | " | Greencastle, Pa | To Surgeon 21st Cavalry July, 1863 |
| Riggs, D. W | " | Alleghany, Pa | To February, 1865. |
| Graham, John | " | 326 S. 15th street, Philadelphia, Pa. | To April, 1865. |

### 150TH INFANTRY—Mustered out June 23, 1865.

| | | | |
|---|---|---|---|
| Morris, J. L | Ass't S | Amboy, Ohio | From January, 1864. |
| O'Hara, Michael | Surgeon | 31 S. 16th street, Philadelphia, Pa. | To April, 1863. |
| Strauss, Henry | " | | From December, 1863 |
| Fulton, James | Ass't S | | To 143d Inf. November, 1862. |
| Henderson, Mathew | " | | To June, 1863. |
| Quinan, P. A | Surgeon | | Dismissed November, '63. |

* Has sick reports from November 13, 1864, to June 24, 1865.

## PENNSYLVANIA—Continued.

### 151ST INFANTRY—(9 months)—Mustered out July 27, 1863.

Blakeslee, Amos C...Surgeon...Nicholson or Glenwood, Pa. From March, 1863.
Kauffman, Jonas H...Ass't S....Annville or Minersville, Pa. From June, 1863; also 52d and 128th Inf.
Underwood, W. J..... " ..................................From November, 1862.

### 152D INFANTRY—(See 3d Heavy Artillery.)

### 153D INFANTRY—(9 months)—Mustered out July 24, 1863.

Stout, Abraham.......Ass't S.....Bethlehem, Pa...............From October, 1862.
Kohler, J. P............ " Bethlehem, Pa...................From October, 1862.
Neff, Henry H.........Surgeon.......................................From October, 1862.

### 154TH INFANTRY—(9 months)—Mustered from September 29 to October 21, 1863. (No Surgeons in A. G. R.)

### 155TH INFANTRY—Mustered out June 2, 1865.

Wilson, W. S.......... Ass't S.....Jersey City, N. J.............To 210th Inf. September, 1864.
Hoffman, J. M.........Surgeon...420 Franklin st., Reading, Pa. Dismissed March, 1863; also 99th Inf.
Kitchen, E. C.......... " Brumfieldville, or Oil City, Pa. From January, 1865; also 21st Cav.
Reed, J. A. E.......... " Lancaster, Pa................To January, 1865.
Tewksbury, A. D.....Ass't S.....Ashley, Pa.....................From July, 1864.
Thompson, C. K...... " Wellsboro', Pa...............From March, 1865.

### 156TH INFANTRY—Failed to complete and was consolidated with 157th.

### 157TH INFANTRY—Transferred to the 191st Infantry March 21, 1865.

Updegrove, Silas......Ass't S.....804 Marshall st., Philadelphia, Pa. To February, 1863; also 99th Inf.

### 158TH INFANTRY—(9 months)—Mustered out August 12, 1863.

Wagonseller, B F....Surgeon...Selin's Grove, Pa...........From February, 1863; also 132d, 139th & 201st Inf.
Leet, Nathan Y.......Ass't S.....Scranton, Pa..................From November, 1862.
Nebinger, A. R...... " ........................................From December, 1862; also 11th Cav.

### 159TH, 160TH, 161ST, 162D, and 163D INFANTRY—(See 14th, 15th, 16th, 17th, and 18th Cavalry.)

### 164TH INFANTRY—Failed to complete.

### 165TH INFANTRY—(9 months)—Mustered out July 28, 1863.

Heckel, F. W..........Surgeon...Vincent, Pa.......................From December, 1862.
Nealy, Shaw F.........Ass't S...............................................From October, 1862.
Wilson, R. A.......... " .........................................From May, 1863.

### 166TH INFANTRY—(9 months)—Mustered out July 28, 1863.

Harshberger, A.. .....Surgeon...Milroy, Pa.........................From December, 1862; also 124th & 149th Inf.
Swartz, Joseph........Ass't S.....Duncannon, Pa...............To June, 1863.
Whitman, A. H....... " .........................................From February, 1863.

## PENNSYLVANIA—Continued.

### 167TH INFANTRY—(9 months)—Mustered out August 12, 1863.

Marshall, D. M.........Surgeon...Brady. Pa.....................A. W. M. Also 103d Inf.
Stearly, J. B...........Ass't S.....Reading, Pa ..................To March, 1863.
Batdorf, D. T........... " ......................................From May, 1863; also 199th Inf.
Henderson, Wm. A.. " ......................................To April, 1863.

### 168TH INFANTRY—(9 months)—Mustered out July 25, 1863.

Christy, R. W.........Surgeon...Hollidaysburgh, Pa........A. W. M. Dead.
Davis, F. F.. ...........Ass't S.....Oil City, Pa...................From October, 1862; also 121st Inf.
Rea, Alexander M... " West Middletown, Pa.....From June, 1863.

### 169TH INFANTRY—(9 months)—Mustered out July 26 and 27, 1863.

Batchelor, W. C......H. Stew...Girard, Pa.
Rhoades, T. J. B......Ass't S....Boyerstown, Pa...........From December, 1862. G.
Rhoads, Reuben B... " Reading, Pa..................From Dec., 1862; also 104th Inf.
Cadwallader, D. W..Surgeon........................................From January, 1863; also 104th Inf.

### 170TH INFANTRY—Failed to complete.

### 171ST INFANTRY—(9 months)—Mustered out August 8, 1863.

Deming, H. D.........H. Stew...Wellsboro', Pa.
Lashells, Theo. B....Surgeon...Meadville, Pa................From December, 1862; also 12th Cav.
Hull, W. B..............Ass't S.....Williamsport, Pa...........From November, 1862.
Culver, Z. D.......... " ......................................From May, 1863.
Pollock, Thos. C...... " ......................................Dismissed Dec., 30, 1862.

### 172D INFANTRY—(9 months)—Mustered out July 31 and August 1, 1863.

Cole, C. H...............Surgeon...Sheshequin, Pa..............From December, 1862
Miller, Jacob M.......Ass't S..........................................From October, 1862.

### 173D INFANTRY—(9 months)—Mustered out August 18, 1863.

Long, Hiram...........Ass't S ...Sunbury, Pa ................From November, 1862; also 205th Inf.
Worrall, H. G.........Surgeon...Dead.......................................From November, 1862.
Barstow, D. H.........Ass't S..........................................From November, 1862.

### 174TH INFANTRY—(9 months)—Mustered out August 7, 1863.

Graham, Samuel......Ass't S.....Butler, Pa.......................From January, 1863; also 81st Inf.
Rankin, A. H.......... " Sandusky, Ohio...............To January, 1863.
Kitchen, F. A......... " Toledo, Ohio.................Missing since June 30, 1863.
Conrad, H. F.. ........Surgeon........................................From February, 1863; also 111th Inf.

### 175TH INFANTRY—(9 months)—Mustered out from August 7, 1863.

Evans, John F.........Ass't S.....Pottstown, Pa................From November, 1862.
Brandt, J. B............Surgeon...Llewellyn, Pa................From February, 1863; also 55th Inf. I.
Phillips, Thos. H.....Ass't S..........................................From June, 1863: also 79th Inf
Linton, H. B...........Surgeon........................................To January, 1863; also 71st Inf.

PENNSYLVANIA—Continued.

176TH INFANTRY—(9 months)—Mustered out from August 17 to 19, 1863.

| | | | |
|---|---|---|---|
| Lynch, N. R. | Ass't S. | 1201 Jefferson street, Philadelphia, Pa. | From November, 1863. H. R.; also 3d Prov. and 22d Cav. |
| Fundurberg, W. F. | Surgeon | | From December, 1862; also 136th Inf. |

177TH INFANTRY—(9 months)—Mustered out August 4 to 7, 1863.

| | | | |
|---|---|---|---|
| Mitchell, G. V. | Surgeon | Kishacoquillas, Pa | To February, 1863. |
| Jack, Wm | Ass't S. | Jacksonville, Pa | From November, 1862; also 57th and 84th Inf. |
| Flowers, John | " | | From January, 1863; also 52d Inf. |
| Wager, Peter | Surgeon | | From February, 1863; also 4th and 5th Cav. |

178TH INFANTRY—(9 months)—Mustered out August, 1863.

| | | | |
|---|---|---|---|
| Swayze, Geo. H. B. | Ass't S. | 256 Columbia st., or 1828 Colorado ave., Philadelphia, Pa. | From November, 1862. |
| Mays, Geo | Surgeon | 1939 Ridge ave., Philadelphia, Pa. | From May, 1863. |
| Peck, Wilbur F. | Ass't S. | Waymart, Pa | From November, 1862. |

179TH INFANTRY—(9 months)—Mustered out from July 21 to 27, 1863.

| | | | |
|---|---|---|---|
| Reily, Jas. R. | Surgeon | | From September, 1862; also 1st Light Artillery and 127th Inf. |
| Frick, Wm. S. | Ass't S. | 821 8th street, Philadelphia, Pa. | From December, 1862. |

180TH, 181ST, and 182D INFANTRY—(See 19th, 20th, and 21st Cavalry.)

183D INFANTRY—Mustered out July 13, 1865.

| | | | |
|---|---|---|---|
| Moody, Horace M. | Ass't S. | East Smithfield, Pa | From April, 1864. |
| Young, John | " | | From April, 1865; also 91st Inf. |
| Byington, Wm. C. | Surgeon | | From March, 1864; also 119th Inf. |
| Richey, Jas. A. | Ass't S. | | To October, 1864. |

184TH INFANTRY—Mustered out July 14, 1865.

| | | | |
|---|---|---|---|
| Brinton, Wm. B. | Surgeon | West Chester, Pa | From July, 1864; also 4th Reserves. |
| Morris, T. G. | Ass't S. | Liverpool, Pa. | To August, 1864. U. S. Ex. S. |
| Marshall, Robt. C. | " | Newport, Pa | From April, 1864. |

185TH INFANTRY—(See 22d Cavalry.)

186TH INFANTRY—Mustered out August 15, 1865.

| | | | |
|---|---|---|---|
| Green, Alfred W. | Surgeon | Meadville, Pa | From April, 1864; also 7th Reserves. |
| Pfeiffer, Geo. S. F. | Ass't S. | | From March, 1864. |
| Gale, Eli H. | " | | From May, 1864. |

PENNSYLVANIA—Continued.

187TH INFANTRY—Mustered out August 3, 1865.

Mahon, James T......Ass't S.....Newton Hamilton, Pa.....From January, 1865.
Webb, W. W.......... " Wellsborough, Pa.........To September, 1864.
Fruit, John C..........Surgeon...Jerseytown, Pa..............From July, 1864; also 54th Inf.
Jacobs, Theo..........Ass't S.............................................From October, 1864; also 103d Inf
Hayes, J. R. .......... " .............................................To Sept., 1864; also 72d Inf.

188TH INFANTRY—In service August 31, 1865.

Atkinson, Louise E...Surgeon...Mifflintown, Pa.............From October, 1864.
Leighton, W. H........Ass't S.....Lowell, Mass ................From April, 1864.
Kern, Francis J........Surgeon...Shenandoah, Pa ............To July, 1864; also 3d Heavy Artillery.

189TH INFANTRY—Failed to complete.

190TH INFANTRY—Mustered out June 28, 1865.

Comfort, J. J..........Surgeon...Atlantic City, N. J.........From Dec., 1862; also 13th Inf.
Chambers, J J.........Ass't S.............................................To July, 1864.
Butler, Lafayette..... " ............................................. To June, 1864; also 13th Res. and 125th, Inf.
Chilson, S. L .......... " .............................................To June, 1865; also 1st Res. and 74th Inf.

191ST INFANTRY—Mustered out June 28, 1865.

Lyons, Wm.............Surgeon...1312 N. Front st., Phila., Pa A. W. M. Also 11th Reserves.
Beaver, D. R.. ........Ass't S.....Conshohocken, Pa .........From July, 1864.
Wylie, Arthur.......... " .............................................From August, 1864.

192D INFANTRY—Mustered out August 24, 1865.

Coleman, A. G........Surgeon...Limerick, Pa.................From March, 1865; also 2d Reserves.
Umbstaetter, E. S....Ass't S.....107 Ross st., Pittsburgh, Pa. From May, 1865.
Main, Geo. T.......... " .............................................From April, 1865.

193D and 194TH INFANTRY—100 days' organizations.

195TH INFANTRY—In service August 31, 1865.

Whitman, H. T........Ass't S.....Indianapolis, Ind. or Reading, Pa. From March, 1863; also 5th Reserves
Jones, Z. Ring.........Surgeon...........................................From March, 1865; also 6th and 63d Inf.

196TH and 197TH INFANTRY—100 days' organizations.

198TH INFANTRY—Mustered out June 4, 1865.

Thompson, Wm.......Ass't S.....Centre Moreland, Pa......From September, 1864.
Becker, A. D........... " Bethlehem, Pa................From January, 1865
Grim, H. A...............Surgeon ..Allentown, Pa................A. W. M Also 5th and 12th Reserves.

199TH INFANTRY—Part mustered out June 28, 1865, the rest transferred to 188th Infantry.

Barr, Benj................Surgeon...643 N. 13th st., Phila., Pa. From Oct., 1864; also 10th Res. Charges fee.
Batdorf, Dan'l T.... .Ass't S............................................. From Oct., 1864; also 167th Inf.
McGinness, J. S....... " .............................................From January, 1865.

## PENNSYLVANIA—Continued.

### 200TH INFANTRY—(1 year)—Mustered out May 30, 1865.

Boyer, Alonzo H .....Ass't S.....Philadelphia, Pa............From December, 1864.
Snyder, P. C........... " Ellendale, Pa.................From September, 1864.
Jones, A. Stokes....Surgeon...Lebanon, N. J................From Sept., 1864; also 72d Inf.

### 201ST INFANTRY—(1 year)—Mustered out June 21, 1865.

Litchfield, A. F........Ass't S.....North Newberg, Mich ...From February, 1865.
Wagenseller, B. F....Surgeon...Selin's Grove, Pa...........From Sept., 1864; also 132d, 139th, and 158th Inf.
Henderson, James...Ass't S.... Hummelstown, Pa.........Dismissed Dec., 1864.
McCreary, John H... " ..........................................From September, 1864.

### 202D INFANTRY—(1 year)—Mustered out August 3, 1865.

McCormick, S. C......Surgeon...Duluth, Minn.................From Sept., 1864; also 102d Inf.
Becker, A. D...........H. Stew...Bethlehem, Pa...............Also Ass't S. 198th Inf.
Campbell, William...Ass't S..........................................From September, 1864.
Culver, W. W.......... " ..........................................From October, 1864.

### 203D INFANTRY—(1 year)—Mustered out June 22, 1865.

Backhus, C. W.........Surgeon.. Three Rivers, Mich.........Missing since May, 1865; also 76th and 99th Inf.
Steckel, E. F...........Ass't S....Emaus, Pa.....................From September, 1864.
Hunter, H. D.......... " ..........................................Dismissed April, 1865.

### 204TH INFANTRY—(See 5th Heavy Artillery.)

### 205TH INFANTRY—(1 year)—Mustered out June 2, 1865.

Long, Hiram............Surgeon...Sunbury, Pa..................From March, 1865. H.R. Also 173d Inf.
Marks, John I.......... " Lewistown, Pa ..............To March, 1865; also 18th Cav. and 78th Inf.
Seem, A. A...............Ass't S.....Ackermantown, Pa........From April, 1865.
Noel, Agideous........ " Square Corner, Pa.........From September, 1864.

### 206TH INFANTRY—(1 year)—Mustered out June 26, 1865.

Alter, David............Ass't S....Freeport, Pa..................From September, 1864.
Wilson, John C......... " Conemaugh, Pa.............From Sept., 1864; also 68th Inf.
Laney, Thos. M.. .....Surgeon..........................................A. W. M. Also 95th Inf.

### 207TH INFANTRY—(1 year)—Mustered out May 31, 1865.

Burg, Washington....Surgeon...Brickerville, Pa..............From Sept., 1864; also 122d Inf.
Lindley, Henry S......Ass't S..........................................From September, 1864.
Linn, A. E .............. " ..........................................From September, 1864.

### 208TH INFANTRY—(1 year)—Mustered out June 1, 1865.

Asay, J. Lambert.....Surgeon...Visalia, Cal......................To Dec., 1864; also 142d Inf.
Kaempfer, S. O........Ass't S.....Selin's Grove, Pa ..........From September, 1864.
Whildin, J. Stiles.....Surgeon...Philadelphia, Pa............From Feb., 1865; also 145th Inf.
Wyeth, A. R...........Ass't S..........................................To March, 1865; also 6th Cav.
Snivelly, Whitmer ... " 73 6th ave., Pittsburgh, Pa. From March, 1865.

PENNSYLVANIA—Continued.

209TH INFANTRY—(1 year)—Mustered out May 31, 1865.

Barday, Jos. D.........Ass't S.....Langmont, Colo., or Brownsville, Pa. From September, 1864.
Vankirk, T. R......... " McKeesport, Pa ............From September, 1864.
Bowes, M. F............Surgeon.......................................From Oct., 1864; also 12th Cav.

210TH INFANTRY—(1 year)—Mustered out May 31, 1865.

Bard, C. L ..............Ass't S....121 Clay st., San Francisco, Cal. From September, 1864.
Raub, Jacob F......... " Mt. Bethel, Pa............. From September, 1864.
Wilson, Stockton W..Surgeon...Jersey City, N. J...........From Oct., 1864: also 155th Inf.

211TH INFANTRY—(1 year)—Mustered out June 2, 1865.

Hunter, W. G.........Surgeon...Bucksville, Pa................From Sept., 1864; also 149th Inf.
Steckel, A. P.......... Ass't S.......................................From September, 1864.
Smith, J. Henderson. " ........................................A. W. M.

212TH INFANTRY—(See 6th Heavy Artillery.)

213TH INFANTRY—(1 year)—In service August 31, 1865.

Dickson, John M......Surgeon...Care Adjutant General U. S. A. From March, 1863; also 93d Inf.
Jefferies, D. W.........Ass't S....Chester, Pa.....................A. W. M.
Weirick, W. H ......... " ........................................From April, 1865.

214TH INFANTRY—(1 year)—In service August 31, 1865.

Houghton, C. W......Surgeon...1528 N. 17th st., Philadelphia, Pa A. W. M. Also 91st and 124th Inf.
De Long, D. R.........Ass't S....Stone Church, Pa..........A. W. M.
Eldridge, C. R......... " ........................................A. W. M.

215TH INFANTRY—(1 year)—Mustered out July 31, 1865.

Farrell, G. D. O.......Ass't S.....716 E. Cumberland st., Philadelphia, Pa. A. W. M. Also 63d Inf.
Bair, John A........... " ........................................A. W. M.
Hawks, Jas. A ........Surgeon.......................................From April, 1865.

## RHODE ISLAND.

*1ST CAVALRY—Mustered out August 3, 1865.

Newell, Timothy......Surgeon...Providence, R. I...........To May, 1862. H. R.
Greeley, Jas. B ........ " Nashua, N. H ...............To August, 1862
Mann, A. A.............Ass't S.....Central Falls, R. I.........To November, 1864.
Utter, Albert.......... " Plainfield, N. J...............A. W. M. Jan., 1863, to Aug., 1865.
Wilbor, Wm. H........Surgeon...Dead...................................To January, 1865.

2D CAVALRY—Officers mustered out July 12, 1863; men transferred to 1st Louisiana Cavalry August 24, 1863.

King, Howard W......Surgeon...Providence, R. I...........Not in A. G. R.
Stanton, N. B.........Ass't S.......................................A. W. M.

---

* Four companies—I, K, L, and M—permanently detached to serve as New Hampshire Cavalry January, 7, 1864.

## RHODE ISLAND—Continued.

### 3D CAVALRY—In service August 31, 1865.

| Name | Rank | Residence | Remarks |
|---|---|---|---|
| Budlong, John B | Surgeon | Centredale, R. I | A. W. M. |
| Monroe, Geo. A | Ass't S | | To April, 1865. |
| Swan, Lyman L | " | Providence, R. I | From April, 1865. |
| Taylor, Frank L | " | | To May, 1864. |

### 1ST and 2D HEAVY ARTILLERY were Infantry.

### 3D HEAVY ARTILLERY—Mustered out from June 9 to August 27, 1865.

| Name | Rank | Residence | Remarks |
|---|---|---|---|
| Peckham, Fenner H. | Surgeon | Bristol, R. I | To March, 1862; also 2d Lieut. 12th Inf. |
| Kenyon, Job | Ass't S | River Point, R. I. | Jo January, 1863. |
| Lamson, Horace S | " | Providence. R. I | To August, 1864 |
| Grosvenor, Jos. W | " | Lockport, N. Y | To April, 1865; also 11th Inf. |
| Burton, Geo. S | Surgeon | Coventry, or Anthony, R. I. | To June, 1865. |
| Stickney, Horatio G. | " | Dead. | |

### 4TH HEAVY ARTILLERY was Infantry.

### 5TH HEAVY ARTILLERY—Part mustered out December, 1864; the rest June 26, 1865.

| Name | Rank | Residence | Remarks |
|---|---|---|---|
| Green, Jerome B | Surgeon | Providence, R. I | From January, 1865. |
| Warren, Ephraim L. | " | Medford, Mass | To November, 1863. |
| Potter, Albert | " | Chepachet, R. I | To December, 1864. |

### 1ST LIGHT ARTILLERY—Part mustered out August 27, 1864; the rest from June 12 to July 17, 1865.

| Name | Rank | Residence | Remarks |
|---|---|---|---|
| Thurston, Wm. T | Surgeon | Providence, R. I | To April, 1863. |
| Merrill, John H | " | Westerly, R. I | To March, 1864. |
| Bradford, Francis S. | Ass't S | | To July, 1862. |

### 1ST INFANTRY—(3 months.)

### 2D INFANTRY—Part mustered out July 17, 1864; the rest July 13, 1865.

| Name | Rank | Residence | Remarks |
|---|---|---|---|
| Carr, Geo. W | Surgeon | Providence, R. I | To June, 1864. U. S. Ex. S. |
| Harris, James | Ass't S | Japan | Missing since Oct., 1861; also 7th Inf. |
| Bolles, Lucius S | " | | To September, 1863. |
| Smith, Wm. F | Surgeon | | From March, 1865. |
| Wheaton, Francis L. | " | Providence, R. I | Dismissed Sept., 1862. |
| Jones, Morris E | Ass't S | | To April, 1863. |

### 3D INFANTRY—(See 3d Heavy Artillery.)

### 4TH INFANTRY—Part mustered out October 15, 1864; the rest transferred to 7th Infantry.

| Name | Rank | Residence | Remarks |
|---|---|---|---|
| Dedrick, Albert C | Ass't S | Centreville, R. I | A. W. M. |
| Millar, Robert | " | Providence, R. I | To August, 1864. H. R. U. S. Ex. S. |
| Rivers, Henry W | Surgeon | Dead. | |
| Smalley, Geo. L | Ass't S | | To September, 1862. |

### 5TH INFANTRY—(See 5th Heavy Artillery.)

### 6TH INFANTRY—Failed to complete.

## RHODE ISLAND—Continued.

### 7TH INFANTRY—Mustered out July 13, 1865.

Harris, James..........Surgeon...Japan..............................To June, 1865; also 2d Inf.
Sprague, Albert G...Ass't S....Warwick or Providence, R. I. To June, 1865.
Langworth, Geo. A..A. H. S.....Hope Valley, R. I.
Peckham, S. F......... " Providence, R. I.
Corey, Chas. G........Ass't S.....Dead.
Gaylord, Wm. A ..... " Pawtucket, R. I.............To January, 1863.

### 8TH INFANTRY—Failed to complete.

### 9TH INFANTRY—(3 months)—Mustered out September 2, 1862.

King, Henry............Surgeon...Providence, R. I............From May, 1862; also 12th Inf.

### 10TH INFANTRY—(3 months)—Mustered out September 1, 1862.

Wilcox, Geo. D........Surgeon...Providence, R. I............Not in A. G. R.

### 11TH INFANTRY—Mustered out July 13, 1863.

Perry, Thos. W........Surgeon...3 Aborn st., Providence, R. I. From Oct., 1862. H. R.
Grosvenor, Jos. W...Ass't S.....Lockport, N. Y.............From October, 1862; also 3d H. A.
Taft, Geo. H........... " Charlton, Mass..............From October, 1862.

### 12TH MILITIA—(9 months)—Mustered out July 29, 1863.

Carpenter, Beoni......Surgeon...Pawtucket, R. I............From Oct., 1862. Dead.
King, Henry.............Ass't S.....Providence, R. I............To May, 1863; also 9th Inf., 3 months.
Fletcher, Sam'l M..... " Alleged dead.
Hutchinson, P. H..... " Dead.............................To April, 1863.

## TENNESSEE.

### 1ST CAVALRY—(4th Infantry)—Mustered out April and June, 1865.

Green, Wm. F.........Surgeon...Clarksville, Tenn...........To May, 1865; also 2d Mich. Cav.
Reed, John L...........Ass't S....Giddings, Tex................To June, 1865.
Logan, Pleasant W...Surgeon...Stanford, Ky..................To December, 1862; also 19th Ky. Inf.
Jones, John T......... " Nashville, Tenn...........To June, 1863. Dead.
Jones, James H........Ass't S.....West Point, Ky..............To June, 1863; also 12th Cav.
Rankin, Wm. T....... " Dead...............................To February, 1865.

### 2D CAVALRY—Mustered out July 6, 1865.

Carrick, Anthony L..Surgeon...154 Broadway, Cincinnati, Ohio. From December, 1862.
Jerolds, Marcus F.....Ass't S.....Clear Creek, Tenn.........From August, 1862.
Mays, John W......... " Dead...............................From June, 1863.

### 3D CAVALRY—Mustered out August 3, 1865

Lyle, J. Nat............H. Stew...Dandridge, Tenn............Dead.
McCoy, Henry C .....Ass't S.....Algona, Iowa..................To May, 1865
Sowers, John A.......Surgeon........................................From May, 1863.
Campbell, Jas. M.....Ass't S.....Elizabeth, Tenn............To June, 1864.

## TENNESSEE—Continued.

4TH CAVALRY—Mustered out July 12, 1865. H. R. on file at A. G. O. Specific call necessary.

| Name | Rank | Residence | Remarks |
|---|---|---|---|
| Hale, E. B | Ass't S | Talbott, Tenn | From July, 1863. |
| Padget, B. W | H. Stew | Ooltewah, Tenn. | |
| Matlock, R. H | Ass't S | | From June, 1864. |
| Brown, John G | Surgeon | | From August, 1863. |

5TH CAVALRY—(1st Middle Tennessee Cavalry)—Mustered out August 14, 1865.

| Name | Rank | Residence | Remarks |
|---|---|---|---|
| Hickman, T. G | Surgeon | Vandalia, Ill | To January, 1863. |
| Bill, Curtis H | " | | From November, 1864. |
| Meconnekin, W H | Ass't S | | To August, 1864. |
| Moffett, Wm. H | " | | From June, 1864. |
| Everrett, John | H. Stew | Smallman, Tenn. | |

6TH CAVALRY—(6th West Tennessee Cavalry)—Mustered out July 26, 1865.

| Name | Rank | Residence | Remarks |
|---|---|---|---|
| Purdy, Job | Ass't S | Purdy, Tenn | Not in A. G. R. |
| Williams, Thos | Surgeon | Jacksonville, Fla | Dismissed May, 1865. |
| Tidwell, J. F | H. Stew | Attila, Ill. | |
| Tanner, L O | Ass't S | | From March, 1865. |
| Cashon, P. A | " | Cashon, Tenn | From April, 1865. |
| Marvin, Jos. E | " | | To July, 1864. |
| Bell, Job | " | Purdy, Tenn | To March, 1865. |
| Huddleston, John | H. Stew | Crab Orchard, Ill. | |

7TH CAVALRY—Mustered out October 26, 1863, and August 9, 1865.

| Name | Rank | Residence | Remarks |
|---|---|---|---|
| Arbuckle, E | Ass't S | Henry Station, Tenn | A. W. M. H. R. |

8TH CAVALRY—Mustered out September 11, 1865.

| Name | Rank | Residence | Remarks |
|---|---|---|---|
| Brady, Jas. W | Surgeon | Shawnee, Ohio | A. W. M. |
| Finn, E A | Ass't S | Pawnee City, Neb | From Sept., 1863. Dead. |
| Depew, Elbert S | H. Stew | Slaughter, Tenn. | |
| Estes, Joseph | " | Jonesboro', Tenn. | |
| Wheeler, C | Ass't S | Jonesboro', Tenn | From May, 1864. President Examining Board. |
| Smith, Wm | " | Chuck Valley, Tenn | To January, 1864. |

9TH CAVALRY—Mustered out September 11, 1865.

| Name | Rank | Residence | Remarks |
|---|---|---|---|
| Duncan, [illegible]. E | Ass't S | Yellow Springs, Ohio | From February, 1864. |
| Hunt, Wm | Surgeon | Cleveland, Tenn | To March, 1865. Died Feb., 1882. |
| Mathes, Wm. T | H. Stew | Strawberry Plains, Tenn. | |
| Divine, John W | Ass't S | Tazewell, Tenn | A. W. M. Also 11th Cav. |
| Brandon, G. R | Surgeon | Knoxville, Tenn | From May, 1863; also 11th Cav. Dead. |

10TH CAVALRY—Mustered out August 1, 1865.

| Name | Rank | Residence | Remarks |
|---|---|---|---|
| Freeman, Brook B | Ass't S | Westville, Ind | From May, 1864. |
| Leonard, John R | " | Jalapa, Tenn | To February, 1865. |
| Spencer, Wm | Surgeon | Monticello, Ind | From April, 1864; also 73d Ind. Inf. Ex. S. |
| Saines, Jas. G | Ass't S | | To April, 1864. |

11TH CAVALRY—Consolidated with 9th Cavalry January 9, 1865.

| Name | Rank | Residence | Remarks |
|---|---|---|---|
| Divine, John W | Ass't S | Tazewell, Tenn | A. W. M. Also 9th Cav. |
| Brandon, G. A | Surgeon | Knoxville, Tenn | From May, 1863; also 9th Cav. Dead. |

## TENNESSEE—Continued.

12TH CAVALRY—Mustered out October 7, 1865.

| | | | |
|---|---|---|---|
| Mitchell, J. B. | Surgeon | South Pueblo, Colo. | To Feb., 1865; also 5th Kentucky Cav. |
| Price, Curtis E | " | Care A. G. U. S. A | From March, 1865. Now Ass't Surg. U. S. A. |
| Jones, Jas. H | Ass't S. | West Point, Ky | To May, 1865; also 1st Cav. |

13TH CAVALRY—Mustered out September 5, 1865.

| | | | |
|---|---|---|---|
| Cameron, Jas. M | Ass't S. | Elizabethon, Tenn | To July, 1865. |
| Crosswhite, A. L | H. Stew | Stump Knob, Tenn. | |
| Blackburn, L. P | Ass't S. | Key Station, Tenn | To July, 1865. |
| Matlack, Wm H | Surgeon | | From September, 1864. |
| Hobbs, Jas. H | " | | To August, 1864. |

14TH CAVALRY—Only one company was organized, which was transferred to 6th Cavalry.

BRADFORD'S BATTALION—The members that were not captured or killed at Fort Pillow were formed into one company and transferred to the 14th Cavalry as Company A, subsequently to the 6th Cavalry as Company E.

1ST LIGHT ARTILLERY—Mustered out from July 20 to August 3, 1865.

| | | | |
|---|---|---|---|
| Mitchell, R. P | Surgeon | Rogersville, Tenn | From October, 1863. |
| Brown, Owen M | Ass't S. | War Gap, Tenn | A. W. M. |

1ST INFANTRY—Mustered out September 17, 1864, and August 8, 1865.

| | | | |
|---|---|---|---|
| Davidson, B. F. | Ass't S. | Mouth of Wolf, Tenn | To November, 1864. |
| Rodgers, Wm A | " | Graveston, Tenn | To 3d Inf April, 1862. |
| Norwood, E. M | " | Lexington, Ky | To Surg. 4th Inf. June, 1864. |
| Stanford, R. L | Surgeon | | To Surgeon U. S. Vols. November, 1861. |
| McMillan, Carr W | " | | To September, 1864. |

1ST MOUNTED INFANTRY—Mustered out from December 13, 1864, to July 22, 1865.

| | | | |
|---|---|---|---|
| Clements, C. C | Ass't S. | Springfield, Mo | From April 1864; also 4th Mounted Inf. Ex. S |
| Shayer, Chas. C | Surgeon | Leavenworth, Kan | From April 1864, also 8th Mounted Infantry. |

2D INFANTRY—Mustered out August 3, 1865.

| | | | |
|---|---|---|---|
| Shrady, John | Surgeon | 1974 Madison ave., New York city. | To October, 1864. |
| Leber, F. C | Ass't S. | | To October, 1862. |
| Neat, Andrew | Surgeon | New Albany, Ind. | To October, 1862. |
| White, J. P | Ass't S. | | To October, 1864. |
| Larey, J. A. J | " | | To October, 1864. |

2D MOUNTED INFANTRY—Mustered out from October 14, 1864, to June 27, 1865.

| | | | |
|---|---|---|---|
| Ellis, Jonathan | Ass't S. | Birmingham, Ky | To January, 1865. |
| *Hogle, Lorenzo D | " | Nashville, Tenn | From March, 1864. |
| Fouts, Louis C | Surgeon | | From June, 1864. |

3D INFANTRY—Mustered out February 23, 1865.

| | | | |
|---|---|---|---|
| Rodgers, Wm. A | Surgeon | Graveston, Tenn | To July, 1864; also 1st Inf |
| Haughey, Thos | " | | From September, 1864. |
| Blankenship, Jno. P. | Ass't S. | Maryville, Tenn | To April, 1863. |

*Was Acting Assistant Surgeon at General Hospital No. 11, Nashville, Tenn., in 1863-'4.

## TENNESSEE—Continued.

### 4TH INFANTRY—Mustered out August 2, 1865.

Sweeney, Robt. E...Lt. Co. D..Eureka Springs, Ark., or Chanute, Kan.............From January, 1864. Said to have been detailed as Surgeon.
Norwood, Edw. M...Surgeon...Lexington, Ky..............From June, 1864; also 1st Inf.
*Farquharson, R. J.. " Des Moines, Iowa..........To March, 1864.
Tadlock, Alex. B.....Ass't S.....Knoxville, Tenn............To Dec., 1863. Ex. S.
Kelly, J. M..............A. A. S.....Nortonville, Kan...........April, 1864.
Hale, E. B.............. " Talbott, Tenn...............April, 1865.
Cavener, Wm.........Ass't S..............................................To June, 1865.
Locke, Matt. T....... " ..............................................Dismissed April, 1864.
Lusk, L. H. P.........H. Stew.. Johnson City, Tenn.

### 4TH MOUNTED INFANTRY—Mustered out June 1 and August 25, 1865.

Clements, C. C.........Surgeon...Springfield, Mo.............From March, 1865; also 1st Mounted Infantry. Ex. S.
Knight, Sampson.....Ass't S.....Dead.

### 5TH INFANTRY—Mustered out from March 29 to June 30, 1865.

McMillon, Geo. W...Surgeon...Osage Mission, Kan........To April, 1864.
Everett, John C......Ass't S.....Liberty, Tenn................To July, 1864.
Lea, Albert T..........Surgeon..............................................From June, 1864.

### 5TH MOUNTED INFANTRY—Mustered out from July 12 to 17, 18 5.

Remage, Geo. W......Surgeon...Paulding, Ohio .............To February, 1865.
Smith, Geo. C.........Ass't S.....Ridgway, Ill..................To May, 1865; also 2d Lieut. 14th Illinois Cav.
Parkinson, John A...Surgeon...Riceville, Tenn .............From February, 1865.

### 6TH INFANTRY—Mustered out from April 27 to May 17, 1865.

Maupin, Ayres.........Surgeon...Well Springs, Tenn........From April, 1862.
Mills, John.............Ass't S..............................................From August, 1863.
Walker, Richard...... " ..............................................To June, 1863.

### 6TH MOUNTED INFANTRY—Mustered out June 30, 1865.

Lyle, Jas. Nat.........Ass't S.....Dandridge, Tenn...........Dead.

### 7TH INFANTRY—Officers mustered out; men transferred to other regiments July 31, 1863.

### 7TH MOUNTED INFANTRY—Mustered out July 27, 1865.

Collins, Enoch..........Ass't S.....Rhea Springs, Tenn.......Died April, 1881.

### 8TH INFANTRY—Mustered out June 30, 1865.

Sparks, Joseph.........Surgeon...Ucando Hotel, Nicholasville, Ky. A. W. M.
Snodgrass, Jesse......Ass't S..............................................A. W. M.
Hunt, Wm...............Surgeon..............................................To August, 1863.
Wood, Joseph ....... Ass't S....Boonshill, Tenn ...........To November, 1864.

### 8TH MOUNTED INFANTRY—Mustered out August 17, 1865.

Shayer, Chas. C......Surgeon...Leavenworth, Kan.........From April, 1865; also 1st Mounted Infantry.

### 9TH INFANTRY—Consolidated with the 1st West Tennessee Cavalry and known as the 6th Cavalry.

*Secretary State Board of Health.

TENNESSEE—Continued.

10TH INFANTRY—Mustered out May 25 and June 10 and 23, 1865.

| | | | |
|---|---|---|---|
| Knaffi, Rudolph | Surgeon | Knoxville, Tenn | A. W. M. Dead. |
| Knaffii, Louis | Ass't S. | | From October, 1863. |
| Murphy, Andrew J. | " | | From April, 1864. |
| Kelly, Alanson W. | " | Leadville, Col., or Chicago, Ill. | To 59th Illinois March, 1863. |
| O'Reilly, John J. | " | Louisville, Ky | To March, 1864. |

TEXAS.

1ST CAVALRY—Mustered out November, 4, 1865.

| | | | |
|---|---|---|---|
| Short, Wesley | Surgeon | Gilmer, Tex | To August, 1864; also 26th Indiana Inf. |
| Farmer, John C. | Ass't S. | | To December, 1863. |
| Southworth, M. A. | Surgeon | | From November, 1863; also 2d Cav. |

2D CAVALRY—Consolidated with 1st Cavalry September 10, 1864.

| | | | |
|---|---|---|---|
| Southworth, M. A. | Surgeon | | From November, 1863; also 1st Cav. |

VERMONT.

The Adjutant General of Vermont states, under date of August 11, 1881: "There is a carefully prepared statement of the casualties * * * (2d Vermont Brigade) at Gettysburgh, Pa."

1ST CAVALRY—Mustered out August 9, 1865.

| | | | |
|---|---|---|---|
| Clark, Almon | Surgeon | Sheboygan, Wis | From April, 1865. H. R. Also 10th Inf. U. S. Ex. S |
| Edson, P. O'm | Ass't S. | 109 Warren st., Roxbury, Mass. | To April. 1864; also 16th and 17th Inf. |
| Hall, Elmer J. | " | Morrisville, Vt | To Sept., 1864. U. S. Ex. S |
| Nims, Edward B. | " | Northampton, Mass. | From May, 1864. U. M. |
| Holdredge, F. H. | H. Stew. | Irasburgh, Vt. | |
| Brush, Geo | " | Brockville, Canada. | |
| Gale, Geo. S | Surgeon | Dead. | |

1ST HEAVY ARTILLERY—(11th Volunteers.) Mustered out August 25, 1865.

| | | | |
|---|---|---|---|
| Kidder, C. W. B | Surgeon | Vergennes, Vt | To September, 1863. |
| Porter, Edward O. | Ass't S. | Cornwall, Vt | To January, 1865. |
| *Harrington, J. L. | Surgeon | Halifax, Vt. | From March. 1865. |
| Park, C. B., Jr | Ass't S. | Grand Junction, Iowa | To June, 1865. H. R. Also 16th Inf. |
| Bourne, Chas. W. | " | Boston, N. Y. | To June, 1865 |
| Meigs, John J. | " | Elko, Nev | To Surg., 3d Inf. Nov., 6, 1864. |

* H. R. from July, 1864, to last of August, 1865.

## VERMONT—Continued.

### 2D BATTERY LIGHT ARTILLERY.

List of surgeons with battery, as reported by Surgeon General U. S. A. May 23, 1882.

| | | | |
|---|---|---|---|
| Kimball, G | Surgeon | Lowell, Mass | Dec., 1861, and March, 1862. |
| Thompson, A. J | Ass't S. | Salem, Mass | September, 1862. Dead. |
| Whitmore, C. W | A. A. S | Gardiner, Me | December, 1862. |
| Smith, G. C. | Ass't S. | Rondout, N. Y | May and June, 1863. |
| Ward, E. F. | " | 200 W. 38th st., N. Y. city. | July and August, 1863. |
| Huntington, R. M. | " | Boone, Iowa | Sept. to Dec , 1863. |
| Reynolds, Albert | " | Independence, Iowa | November, 1863. |
| Palmer, D. E. | A. A. S | Tuftonboro, N. H. | Jan. to April, 1864. |
| Fish, John | Surgeon | Auburn, Ohio | April and May, 1864. |
| Coad, M | Ass't S | Williamstown, Mich. | June to Nov., 1864. |
| Berthell, J. P. | A. A. S. | 112 Brown st., Phila., Pa. | January to May, 1865. |
| Herrick, L. C. | Ass't S. | Woodstock, Ohio | June and July, 1865. |
| Brownell, W. R. | Surgeon | Dead | June, 1862. |
| Gihon, John H | Ass't S. | Dead | September, 1862. |
| Smith, R. K | Surgeon | Dead | January, 1863. |
| Dean, C. A | Ass't S. | | April, 1863. |
| Brown, Henry W | Surgeon | Dead | April and Nov., 1864, to Jan., 1865. |

### 3D BATTERY—(See List of Surgeons.)

### 3D BATTERY LIGHT ARTILLERY.

| | | | |
|---|---|---|---|
| Hardy, H. T | H. Stew | Kaneville, Ill | Now M. D. |

### 1ST INFANTRY—(3 months.)

### 2D INFANTRY—Mustered out July 15, 1865.

| | | | |
|---|---|---|---|
| Ballou, Newton H | Surgeon | Mechanicsville, N. Y | To December, 1862. |
| Noyes, Luman A | Ass't S | Randolph, Vt. | To May, 1863. |
| Brush, Edwin R | " | Cambridge, Vt. | From November, 1863. |
| Carpenter, W. B | " | Burlington, Vt. | To 9th Inf. June, 1862. |
| Sherry, John W. | H. Stew | Albany, Vt. | Now M. D. |
| Atwood, A. A. | Ass't S. | Dead. | |
| Sawin, Wm J. | Surgeon | Dead. | |
| Hyde, Melvin J | " | Dead. | |

### 3D INFANTRY—Mustered out July 11, 1865.

| | | | |
|---|---|---|---|
| Meigs, John J. | Surgeon | Elko, Nevada | To July, 1865; also 1st H. Art. |
| Newell, Henry C | Ass't S. | St. Johnsbury, Vt. | To May, 1865. |
| Goodwin, David M | Surgeon | 300 Nicolet st., Minneapolis, Minn. | To July, 1864. |
| Janes, Henry | " | Brattleborough, Vt. | To Surg. U. S. Vols. May, 1863. |
| Smith Henry F | Ass't S. | Dead. | |

### 4TH INFANTRY—Mustered out July 13, 1865.

| | | | |
|---|---|---|---|
| Allen, Samuel J. | Surgeon | White River Junction, Vt. | To September, 1864. |
| Bixby, A. B | Ass't S. | South Londonderry, Vt. | To September, 1864. |
| Phillips, Edwin | " | Minneapolis, Minn | To 6th Inf. Nov., 1863. |
| Brook, Chas. S. | H. Stew | 110 Penn st., Williamsburgh, N. Y. | |
| Flesh, Marshall P. | " | Garden Park, Colo. | |
| Child, Willard A | Ass't S. | Dead | To 10th Inf. Aug., 1862. |
| Curtis, Edward M. | Surgeon | Dead | Also 6th Inf. |

VERMONT—Continued.

5TH INFANTRY—Mustered out June 29, 1865.

| | | | |
|---|---|---|---|
| Bradford, P. D | Surgeon | Northfield, Vt | To March, 1863. U. S. Ex. S. |
| Burdick, Arthur F | Ass't S | Underhill, Vt | To May, 1863. |
| Chesmore, Alwin H | Surgeon | Huntington, Vt | To September, 1864. |
| Allen, Cyrus H | " | Centreville, Cal | From Nov., 1864; also 8th Inf. |
| Russell, Edward P | H. Stew | Middlebury, Vt | Son of Surgeon Russell. |
| Atwood, Henry C | Ass't S | Salisbury, Vt | To June, 1863. |
| Russell, Wm. P | Surgeon | Dead. | |
| Colburn, Dan'l L. C | Ass't S | Dead. | |

6TH INFANTRY—Mustered out June 23, 1865.

| | | | |
|---|---|---|---|
| Woodward, R. C. M | Surgeon | Johnson, Vt | To October, 1861. |
| Chandler, Chas M | " | Montpelier, Vt | To October, 1863. U. S. Ex S. |
| Tuttle, Lyman M | Ass't S | Holyoke, Mass | To December, 1862. |
| Phillips, Edwin | Surgeon | Minneapolis, Minn | From Nov., 1863; also 4th Inf. |
| Cushman, A. J | H. Stew | Lincoln, Vt | 1861 to 1864. |
| Cushman, Elijah L | " | New Haven, Vt. | |
| Crandall, John B | " | Sterling, Ill | To Ass't Surg. 13th Inf., October, 1862. |
| Curtis, Edward M | Ass't S | Dead | Also 4th Inf. |

7TH INFANTRY—In service August 31, 1865.

| | | | |
|---|---|---|---|
| Blanchard, Enoch | Surgeon | Minonk, Ill | From September, 1862. |
| Trueworthy, E. W | Ass't S | Lowell, Mass | A. W. M. |
| Kelley, Francis W | Surgeon | Room 33 Central Block, Chicago, Ill. | To September, 1862. |
| Langdon, Henry H | Ass't S | Burlington, Vt | To March, 1863. |
| Tenney, Chas. H | " | Dead. | |
| Foster, Elihu S | " | Dead. | |

8TH INFANTRY—Mustered out June 28, 1865.

| | | | |
|---|---|---|---|
| Currier, Samuel H | Ass't S | Norwich, Vt | To October, 1862. |
| Gale, Geo. F | Surgeon | Brattleboro', Vt | To June, 1862. |
| Allen, Cyrus H | Ass't S | Centreville, Cal | To Surg. 5th Inf., Nov., 1864. |
| Gillett, Heman H | Surgeon | Post Mill Village, Vt | From July, 1862. |
| Ross, Oliver E | Ass't S | Rockport, Me | From Sept., 1863; also 12th Inf. |
| Ferrin, Chester M | H. Stew | Essex Junction, Vt. | |

9TH INFANTRY—In service August 31, 1865.

| | | | |
|---|---|---|---|
| Carpenter, Walter B | Surgeon | Burlington, Vt | To Nov., 1864; also 2d Inf. |
| Hall, Horace P | Ass't S | St. Albans, Vt | To March, 1863. |
| Goss, Story N | " | Chelsea, Vt | To Oct., 1863. U. S. Ex. S. |
| Vincent, Walter S | Surgeon | Burlington, Vt | To June, 1865. |
| Fairman, Erastus P | Ass't S | Woolcott, Vt | To June, 1865. |
| Belden, Henry D | H. Stew | Fairfield, Vt. | |

10TH INFANTRY—Part mustered out June 22, 1865, the rest transferred to the 5th Infantry.

| | | | |
|---|---|---|---|
| Rutherford, Jos. C | Ass't S | Newport, Vt | To 17th Inf. March, 1865. U. S. Ex. S. |
| Clark, Almon | " | Sheboygan, Wis | To 1st Cav. April, 1865. H. R. |
| Child, Willard A | Surgeon | Dead | Also 4th Inf. |

11TH INFANTRY—(See 1st Heavy Artillery.)

## VERMONT—Continued.

### 12TH INFANTRY—(9 months)—Mustered out July 14, 1863.

| Name | Rank | Residence | Remarks |
|---|---|---|---|
| Ketchum, Benj. F. | Surgeon | Cambridge, N. Y. | From October, 1862. |
| Conn, Granville P. | Ass't S. | Concord, N. H. | From October, 1862. |
| Ross, Oliver E. | " | Rockport, Me. | A. W. M. Also 8th Inf. |

### 13TH INFANTRY—(9 months)—Mustered out July 21, 1863

| Name | Rank | Residence | Remarks |
|---|---|---|---|
| Nichols, Geo. | Surgeon | Northfield, Vt | From Oct., 1864. Secretary of State. |
| Crandall, John B. | Ass't S. | Sterling, Ill. | From Oct., 1862; also Hos Steward 6th Inf. |
| Atherton, Chas. | Private Co. D. | Essex, Vt | Says he was nurse in 1863. |

### 14TH INFANTRY—(Militia, 9 months)—Mustered out July 30, 1863.

| Name | Rank | Residence | Remarks |
|---|---|---|---|
| *Woodward, A. T. | Surgeon | Brandon, Vt | A. W. M. |
| Ross, L. D. | Ass't S. | Poultney, Vt | From October, 1862. |
| Plant, Azro M. | " | St. Albans, Vt | A. W. M. |
| Jones, Frank | H. Stew | Alleged dead. | |
| Sprague, Edwin H. | Surgeon | | To December, 1862. |

### 15TH INFANTRY—(Militia, 9 months)—Mustered out August 5, 1863.

| Name | Rank | Residence | Remarks |
|---|---|---|---|
| Bullard, Gates B. | Surgeon | St. Johnsbury, Vt. | From May, 1863. U. S. Ex. S. |
| Frost, Carlton P. | " | Hanover, N. H. | To May, 1863. |

### 16TH INFANTRY—(9 months)—Mustered out August 10, 1863.

| Name | Rank | Residence | Remarks |
|---|---|---|---|
| Edson, P. O'M. | Surgeon | 109 Warren st., Roxbury, Mass. | Also 1st Cav. and 17th Inf. |
| Park, C. B., Jr. | " | Grand Junction, Iowa | From October, 1862; also 1st Heavy Artillery. |
| Spafford, Geo. | Ass't S. | Cavendish, Vt | From October, 1862. |
| Brooks, Nath'l G. | " | Charleston, N. H. | A. W. M. |

### 17TH INFANTRY—Mustered out July 14, 1865.

| Name | Rank | Residence | Remarks |
|---|---|---|---|
| Rutherford, Jos. C. | Surgeon | Newport, Vt. | From March, 1865; also 10th Inf. U. S. Ex. S. |
| Langdon, Seth W. | Ass't S. | Sheldon, Vt | From March, 1865. |
| Edson, P. O'Meara | Surgeon | 109 Warren st., Roxbury, Mass. | To February, 1865; also 1st Cav and 16th Inf. |
| Spohn, Henry | Ass't S. | Laredo, Tex | To November, 1864. |

## WASHINGTON TERRITORY.

### 1ST INFANTRY—Mustered out November 20 and December 11, 1865.

| Name | Rank | Residence | Remarks |
|---|---|---|---|
| Steinberger, C. M. | Surgeon | Walla Walla, W. T. | To September, 1865. |
| Whittemore, Sam'l | Ass't S | | To March, 1865. |

## WEST VIRGINIA.

### 1ST CAVALRY—Mustered out July 8, 1865.

| Name | Rank | Residence | Remarks |
|---|---|---|---|
| Gardner, Perin | Surgeon | Wilkesville, Ohio | From March, 1864; also 4th U. S. C. T. |
| Titus, Arthur | Ass't S. | Wheelersburgh or Portsmouth, Ohio. | To 3d Cav. March, 1865. |
| Enoch, Hiram D. | " | | To July, 1862. |
| White, Zach. A. | " | | From March, 1864. |

* Has list of killed and wounded at Gettysburgh for 14th Vermont.

## WEST VIRGINIA—Continued.

### 2D CAVALRY—Mustered out June 30, 1865.

Higgins, Daniel W ...H. Stew...Zaleski. Ohio.
Gilliam, Ed. L..........Ass't S ....Letart. W. Va.................From June, 1863. H. R. (probably.)
McEwen, Mathew....Surgeon...451 M st., Washington, D. C. From April, 1863, Bv't Lt. Col.
Nellis, Ozias............Ass't S....Commiskey, Ind ............To Nov., 1864; also 10th Inf.
Comstock, L. L........ " Charleston, W. Va.........To 7th Cav. Oct., 1862. Ex. S.
Neal, Thos. S...........Surgeon......................................To February, 1863.

### 3D CAVALRY—Mustered out June 30, 1865.

Davis, Aaron W.......Ass't S.....Murraysville, W. Va ......From February, 1865.
Pinnell, David S...... " Sycamore Dale, W. Va...To Dec , 1864; also 4th Cav.
Titus, Arthur...........Surgeon...Wheelersburgh or Portsmouth Ohio. From May, 1865; also 1st Cav.
McLane, Chas H.....H. Stew...Cassville, W. Va.
Parkinson, Benoni...Ass't S.....Washington or Ainsworth, Iowa. To 17th Inf. June, 1864.
Morton, Thos ..........Surgeon......................................To February, 1865.

### 4TH CAVALRY—Mustered out from March 6 to June 23, 1864.

Pinnell, David S ......Surgeon...Sycamore Dale. W. Va...From August, 1863; also 3d Cav.
Shaner, David .........Ass't S.....Allegheny, Pa ...............From November. 1863; also 6th and 7th Inf. Dead.

### 5TH CAVALRY—Transferred to the 6th Cavalry December 14, 1864.

Ford, Sample..........Ass't S.....Wheeling. W. Va...........To September, 1862.
Hazlett, R. W .. .....Surgeon...Wheeling, W. Va...........To March, 1863. U. S. Ex. S
Love, Eli, N............ " Waterford, Va ...............To August, 1864.
Millspaugh, T..........Ass't S.........................................To June, 1864.

### 6TH CAVALRY—(3d Virginia Volunteers)—Mustered out May 22, 1866.

Thayer, Abel H.......Surgeon .Grafton, W. Va...............From Oct., 1864. Ex. S.
Thomas, E. C.......... " Moundsville, W. Va........To August, 1864.
Dorsey, Dennis B.....Ass't S.........................................To August, 1862.

### 7TH CAVALRY—(Formerly 8th Infantry)—Mustered out August 1, 1865.

Comstock, L. L.........Surgeon...Charleston, W. Va.........From Oct., 1862; also 2d Cav. Ex. S.
Rouse, Jas H...........Ass't S.....469 E. Oak st.,Columbus, Ohio. From September, 1862.
Stanford, Lewis V.... " Chambersburgh, Mo.......From November 1862.
Barlow, Charles A....Surgeon...Fort Scott, Kan..............To April, 1862.
Putney, James......... " Alleged dead ...................To September, 1862.

### 1ST INFANTRY—Consolidated with the 4th Infantry to form the 2d Veterans December 21, 1864.

Gillespie, Jas. L.......Ass't S.....Sistersville, W. Va.........To 14th Inf. Nov., 1862; also 7th Vet. Vols.
Stidger, Sam'l B ...... " Cameron, W. Va............To July, 1862.
Kraft, A. W. D ........ " ...........................................To November, 1863.
English, John..........Surgeon...Clinton, W. Va...............From Dec , 1864; also 2d Vets.
Bagley, David.......... " ...........................................To November, 1864.

## WEST VIRGINIA—Continued.

1ST INFANTRY—(Veteran Infantry)—Mustered out July 21, 1865.

Hysell, Jas. H .........Surgeon...Pomeroy. Ohio ..............From Nov., 1864; also 9th Inf. U. S. Ex. S.
Meers, R. L ............Ass't S.........................................From March, 1865.

2D INFANTRY—(See 5th Cavalry.)

2D INFANTRY—(Veteran Infantry)—Mustered out July 16 and 18, 1865.

Waterman, H. C..... Ass't S.....Zanesville, Ohio ............From Jan., 1864; also 4th Inf.
English, John .........Surgeon...Clinton, W. Va..............From Dec., 1864; also 1st Inf.

3D INFANTRY—(See 6th Cavalry.)

4TH INFANTRY—Consolidated with the 1st Infantry to form 2d Veterans December 21, 1864.

Ackley, Geo. K........Surgeon...Pomeroy, Ohio ..............To March, 1863.
Philson, Jno. R........ " Racine. Ohio.....................To Oct., 1864. Dead.
Waterman, H. C......Ass't S.....Zanesville, Ohio............ To Oct., 1864; also 2d Vet Inf.
Barton, Thos. H ......H. Stew...Syracuse, Ohio.

5TH INFANTRY—Consolidated with 9th Infantry to form 1st Veterans November 9, 1864.

Mayer, Daniel......... Ass't S.....Charleston, W. Va.........From September, 1861.
Dally, Chas. D......... " Hannibal, Ohio...............To Surg. 13th Inf. Feb., 1864.
Randall, P. A.........Surgeon.........................................From September, 1861.

6TH INFANTRY—Mustered out July 10, 1865.

Wharton, J. T.........Surgeon...Credo, W. Va ..............From December, 1864.
Shanor, David.........Ass't S.....Allegheny, Pa ...............From April, 1864; also 4th Cav. and 7th Inf. Dead.
Safford, E D. .........Surgeon.........................................To July, 1864.
Wheeler, A. P......... " ..........................................Dismissed May, 1862.

7TH INFANTRY—Mustered out July 1, 1865.

Ross, Timothy W.....Ass't S.....Waynesburgh, Pa. ....... To August, 1863. Dead.
Scott, Isaac..............Surgeon...Parkersburgh, W. Va.....To Dec., 1864. U. S. Ex. S.
Shanor, David ......... " Allegheny, Pa.................From June, 1865; also 4th Cav. and 66th Inf.
Hicks, W. T ............Ass't S.........................................To January, 1865.

8TH INFANTRY—(See 7th Cavalry.)

9TH INFANTRY—Consolidated with 5th Infantry to form 1st Veterans November 9, 1864.

Hysell, Jas. H.........Ass't S.....Pomeroy, Ohio ..............From Feb., 1862; also 1st Vet. Inf U. S. Ex. S.
Morris, Jonathan .....Surgeon...Ironton. Ohio ..............From November, 1861.
Grant, Wm. L......... " Grafton. W. Va................To September, 1862.
Rouse, Jas. H. .........Act'g S....469 E. Oak street, Columbus, Ohio. Also 7th Cav.

10TH INFANTRY—Mustered out August 9, 1865.

Blair, Jonathan R....Surgeon...Buckhannon, W. Va......To June, 1865; also 16th U. S. C. T. Ex. S.
Nellis, Ozias............ " Commiskey. Ind............From July, 1865; also 2d Cav.
Bouse, Isaac W.. .....Ass't S.........................................To November, 1864.

## WEST VIRGINIA—Continued.

### 11th Infantry—Mustered out June 17, 1865.

| | | | |
|---|---|---|---|
| Bond, E. D. J | Surgeon | Davisville or Claysville, W. Va. | From January, 1865. |
| Hall, Benj. H | H. N'se | Wirt C. H., W. Va. | |
| Kindall, Jas. E | Ass't S. | Elizabeth, W. Va. | From February, 1864. |
| Voorhees, A. D | Surgeon | Dead | To October, 1864. |

### 12th Infantry—Mustered out June 16, 1865.

| | | | |
|---|---|---|---|
| Bryan, S P | Surgeon | Albia, Iowa | From July, 1863. |
| Neil, Alex | Ass't S. | Columbus, Ohio | From July, 1863. |
| Patton, F. H | " | West Newton, Pa. | From December, 1862. |
| Ruggles, Dwight | " | | To November, 1862. |
| Campbell, John C | Surgeon | | To March, 1863. |
| Frizzell, John | " | Wheeling, W. Va | To September, 1862. |
| Odbert, Chas. H | H. Stew | Wheeling, W. Va. | |

### 13th Infantry—Mustered out June 22, 1865.

| | | | |
|---|---|---|---|
| Lallance, Jacob | Ass't S. | Cottageville, W. Va. | From Feb., 1864. H. R. of Cedar Creek. |
| Shaw, Sam'l G | Surgeon | Point Pleasant, W. Va. | To September, 1863. |
| Dally, Chas. D | " | Hannibal, Ohio | From Feb., 1864; also 5th Inf. |
| Williams, A. D | Ass't S. | St. Louis, Mo | To January, 1865. |
| St. John, E. B | H. Stew | Point Pleasant, W. Va. | |

### 14th Infantry—Mustered out June 28, 1865.

| | | | |
|---|---|---|---|
| Brownfield, J. H | Ass't S. | Fairmont, W. Va. | From April, 1864. Ex. S. |
| Manown, Jas H | Surgeon | Kingwood, W. Va | From February, 1864. |
| Gillespie, Jas L | Ass't S. | Sistersville, W. Va | To March, 1864; also 1st Inf and 7th Vet. Vols. |
| Thacher, C. A | " | | To January, 1865 |
| Welch, Walter S | " | | To Surg. 15th Inf. April, 1863. |

### 15th Infantry—Mustered out June 14, 1865.

| | | | |
|---|---|---|---|
| Dovener, Robert G | Ass't S. | Newark, W. Va | To September, 1863. |
| Johnson, Jas, J | " | East Liverpool, Ohio | From March, 1864. |
| Howe, James F | " | Wetherford, Tex | To November, 1864. |
| Walsh, Walter S | Surgeon | | From May, 1863; also 14th Inf. |
| Starr, David L | " | | To March, 1863. |

### 16th Infantry—Mustered out June 10, 1863.

| | | | |
|---|---|---|---|
| Kilmer, Washington | Surgeon | | From November, 1862. |

### 17th Infantry—Mustered out June 30, 1865.

| | | | |
|---|---|---|---|
| Parkinson, Benoni | Surgeon | Washington, or Ainsworth, Iowa. | From Jan., 1865; also 3d Cav. |
| Ramsey, James R. | Ass't S. | Bridgewater, Pa | From September, 1864. |
| Stewart, Wm. H | " | Dead | From March, 1865. |

## WISCONSIN.

### 1st Cavalry—Mustered out July 19, 1865.

| | | | |
|---|---|---|---|
| Kramer, Ernest | Surgeon | Milwaukee, Wis. | To Feb., 1863; also 7th and 45th Inf. |
| Russell, Thos. P | Ass't S. | Oshkosh, Wis. | To November, 1862. |
| Robinson, N. S. | Surgeon | Neenah, Wis. | From July, 1865. H. R. |
| Winston, Egbert H. | Ass't S. | Evansville, Wis. | From May, 1863. |
| Young, Henry J. | " | Waseca, Minn. | To April, 1863. |
| Lord, C. H. | " | | To April, 1862. |
| Cansdell, H. W. | " | | To Surgeon 3d Battery. Not in A. G. R. |
| Turner, J. H. | " | | Not in A. G. R. |
| Persons, Horace T. | Surgeon | Alleged dead | To November, 1864. |
| Rudd, John C. | Ass't S. | | To November, 1864. |
| Read, J. A. | H. Stew | Tecumseh, Kans. | |

### 2d Cavalry—Mustered out November 15, 1865.

| | | | |
|---|---|---|---|
| Guernsey, A. H. | Ass't S. | Amherst, Wis. | To August, 1865. |
| Hanson, Moses P. | Surgeon | Milwaukee, Wis. | To November, 1865. |
| Kelso, J. Seaton | Ass't S. | Oakley, Iowa | From August, 1864. |
| McBean, Alex. | " | Chippewa Falls, Wis. | To Surgeon 4th U. S. C. H. A. Oct., 1363. |

### 3d Cavalry—Mustered out from September 8 to October 27, 1865.

| | | | |
|---|---|---|---|
| Lane, Joseph S. | Surgeon | 234 La Salle st., Chicago, Ill. | To August, 1865. |
| Reynolds, Benoni O. | " | Geneva Lake, Wis. | To February, 1865. |
| Warner, Wm. H. | Ass't S. | Girard or Ft. Scott, Kans. | To October, 1865. |

### 4th Cavalry—Mustered out May 28, 1866.

| | | | |
|---|---|---|---|
| Van Orstrand, A. H. | Surgeon | Green Bay, Wis. | To January, 1864. |
| Wilson, S. W. | " | Milwaukee, Wis. | Died Jan., 1880. Dead. |
| Roundy, D. C. | Ass't S. | Davenport, Iowa | To June, 1861. A. G. R. says Captain. |
| Harrison, W. H. | " | Texas | From April, 1864. |
| Page, J. L. | " | Racine, Wis. | To June, 1861. Not in A. G. R. |
| Smith, S Compton | " | | To October, 1861. |
| Horne, H. B. | " | | A. W. M. |

### 1st Heavy Artillery—Mustered out from June 26 to September 21, 1865.

| | | | |
|---|---|---|---|
| Borden, Wm. H. | Surgeon | Milton, Wis. | From October, 1864. |
| Waterhouse, Marvin | Ass't S. | Portage, Wis. | Died 1878. |
| Manley, Ira, Jr. | " | Portage City, or Markesan, Wis. | From November, 1864. |

### *Wisconsin Light Artillery.

| | | | |
|---|---|---|---|
| Halstead, L. C. | State S. | Wauzeka, Wis. | 7th Battery from May, 1862. G. |
| Marden, Alfred | H. Stew | Beaver Dam, Wis. | 5th Battery; acted as Surg. |
| †Lindsfeldt, A. F. St. Surg. | State S. | Sheboygan, Wis. | |
| Hobbins, William | Surgeon | Madison, Wis. | Also 8th Infantry. |
| Smith, Wm. H. | " | Albert Lea, Minn. | To Surgeon 28th Inf. |
| Cansdell, H. W. | " | | To Surgeon 22d Inf. |
| James, Robt. G. | " | | To Feb., 1864; also 10th Inf. |
| Riddell, Geo. | " | Chippewa, Wis. | |

* A. G. reports no Surgeons for Light Artillery.
† Was on duty with Battery up to December, 1863. Promoted to 15th Volunteers.

## WISCONSIN—Continued.

**1st Infantry**—Mustered out October 13, 1864; veterans and recruits transferred to the 21st Infantry.

| | | | |
|---|---|---|---|
| Corfe, Fred | Ass't S | Union, Iowa | From June, 1863. |
| Dixon, L. I | Surgeon | Milton, Vt | From October, 1861. |
| Devendorf, Dan'l B | Ass't S | Delavan, Wis | To 19th Inf. May, 1863. U. S. Ex. S. |
| McCullough, J. R | H. Stew | 98 Halsted st., Chicago, Ill. | M. D. |
| Crugon, James | Ass't S | Milwaukee, Wis | To March, 1863. |
| Green, Joseph | " | Hudson, Wis | Also 11th Infantry. Not in A. G. R. |

**2d Infantry**—Consolidated with 6th Infantry November 22, 1864

| | | | |
|---|---|---|---|
| Arndt, Peter S | Ass't S | 65 Randolph st., Chicago, Ill. or Kenosha, Wis. | To 31st Inf Dec., 1863. |
| Tucker, Samuel | " | Homer, Iowa | To December, 1862. |
| Ward, Andrew J | Surgeon | Madison, Wis | To July, 1864. Board Ex. S. |
| Babcock, Horace | Ass't S | Gowanda, N. Y | To September, 1863. |
| Fox, Philip | " | Madison, Wis | To July, 1864 |
| Lewis, J. M | Surgeon | Gunston, Va. or Oconomowoc, Wis. | To Col. 28th Inf. Oct., 1862. |
| Russell, T. P | Ass't S | Oshkosh, Wis | To July, 1861. |

**3d Infantry**—Mustered out July 18, 1865.

| | | | |
|---|---|---|---|
| Baxter, J. B. G | Ass't S | Pension Office | To Surg. U. S. V. Dec., 1861. |
| Conant, Geo. E | " | Neosho City, Mo | To November, 1862. |
| Conly, J. Griffin | Surgeon | Elk Point, Dak | From March, 1865. U. S. Ex. S. |
| Raymond, Don. A | " | Fond du Lac. Wis | To September, 1862. |
| Bartlett, O. F | " | Meridian. N. Y | To Jan., 1865; also 6th Inf. |
| Farr, E. J | Ass't S | Eau Claire, Wis | To July, 1862; also 30th Inf. Not in A. G. R |
| Kopff, Thos | Surgeon | Beaver Dam, Wis | From March to July, 1865. |
| Torrey, Wilson | " | Good Thunder, Minn | Dismissed July, 1863. Alleged dead. |
| King, Edward B | H. Stew | Green Bay, Wis | M. D. |
| Crane, H. O | Ass't S | Green Bay. Wis | To May, 1862. Alleged dead. |

**4th Infantry**—(See 4th Cavalry.)

**5th Infantry**—Mustered out July 11, 1865.

| | | | |
|---|---|---|---|
| Crane, Chas. E | Surgeon | Green Bay. Wis | To August, 1864. |
| Jones, Ambrose | Ass't S | Delton, Wis | From September, 1864. |
| Wilber, Geo D | Surgeon | Durango, Col | To July, '65; also 32d Inf. |
| Castleman, A. L | " | Alleged dead | To December, 1862. |
| Harwood, F. H | Ass't S | Milwaukee, Wis | To November, 1862 |
| Davis, J. W | " | | To August, 1864. |
| Allen, Wm. W | " | | From October, 1864. |
| Ewing. James S | " | | To August, 1864. |

**6th Infantry**—Mustered out July 14, 1865.

| | | | |
|---|---|---|---|
| Andrews, A. D | Ass't S | River Falls, Wis | To November, 1863. G. |
| Bartlett, Oscar F | " | Meridian. N. Y | To Oct., 1862; also 3d Inf. |
| Hall, John C | Surgeon | Monroe, Wis | From August, 1864. |
| Loy, Wm | Ass't S | Clifton or Annaton, Wis | From March, 1865. |
| Armstrong, L. G | " | Boscobel, Wis | To 48th Inf. March, 1865; also 8th Inf. |
| Chapman, C. B | Surgeon | | To Oct., '61; also 20th Inf. |
| Preston, A W | " | Olympia, Kan | To July, 1864. |
| McLoney, Jas. F | Ass't S | | A. W. M. |

WISCONSIN—Continued.

7TH INFANTRY—Mustered out July 3, 1865.

| | | | |
|---|---|---|---|
| Ayres, D. Cooper | Surgeon | Green Bay, Wis | From April, 1862. |
| Despins. Francis J | Ass't S. | Antigo, Wis | To March, 1865. |
| Kramer, Earnest | " | Milwaukee, Wis | To 1st Cav. June, 1862; also 45th Inf. |
| Palmer, Henry | Surgeon | Janesville, Wis | To April, 1862. |
| Brainard, L. B | Ass't S. | Waupaca. Wis. | To April, 1864. |
| Spaulding, E. F | " | East Boston, Mass | To July, 1865. |

8TH INFANTRY—Mustered out September 5, 1864

| | | | |
|---|---|---|---|
| Armstrong, L. G | Ass't S. | Boscobel, Wis. | To Nov., 1862; also 6th and 48th Inf. U. S. |
| Murta, Jos. E | Surgeon | La Grange, Tenn | From December, 1862. |
| Murdock, Henry M | Ass't S. | New Richmond, Wis | A. W. M. |
| Hobbins, Wm. | " | Madison. Wis | To January, 1862. |
| Jackson, Jas. A | " | Madison, Wis | A. W. M. Not in A. G. R. |
| Willson, Reuben | " | Mantorville, Minn | To August, 1864. |
| Thornhill, S. P | Surgeon | | Dissmissed Nov., 1862. |

9TH INFANTRY—Part mustered out December 3, 1864, the rest January 30, 1866.

| | | | |
|---|---|---|---|
| Nauman, Herrman | Surgeon | Milwaukee Wis. | To March, 1863. |
| Ottilie, Charles | " | La Crosse, Wis | From March, 1865. |
| Hasse, H. E | Ass't S. | Milwaukee, Wis | To Surg. 24th Inf. Not in A. G. R. |
| Haering, Theo | " | Bloomington, Ill | To December, 1864. |
| Loehr, Louis | Surgeon | Germany | To December, 1864. |

10TH INFANTRY—Mustered out November 3, 1864; veterans and recruits transferred to 21st Infantry.

| | | | |
|---|---|---|---|
| Marks, Solon | Surgeon | 136 Wisconsin st, Milwaukee, Wis. | From October, 1861. |
| Mitchell. Robert | Ass't S. | Merritt's Landing, Wis | To 27th Inf. Sept, 1863. |
| Reeve, Jas. T | " | Appleton, Wis | To Surg. 21st Inf. Not in A. G. R. |
| Benson, Harmon | " | Milwaukee, Wis | To S. 14th Inf. Mar, 1864. |
| Ballou, A. D | H. Stew | Delphos, Kan. | |
| Gordon. Wm. A | Ass't S. | | To February, 1863. |
| James Rob't G | " | Alleged dead | To November, 1864. |

11TH INFANTRY—Mustered out September 4, 1865.

| | | | |
|---|---|---|---|
| Green, Joseph | Ass't S. | Whitewater. Wis | To July, 1864. |
| Strong, Henry P | Surgeon | Beloit, Wis | To July, 1863. P. M. |
| Woodward, E. A | Ass't S. | Sun Prairie, Wis | Also 12th and 36th Inf. Not in A. G. R. |
| Wright. J. B | H. Stew | Merritt's Landing, Wis. | |
| Barnes, C. C | Ass't S. | | Not in A. G. R. |
| Boyce. H. W | Surgeon | Geneva, Wis | To June, 1863. |
| Everitt, Edward | Ass't S. | Alleged dead | From August, 1863. |
| Wilson, John T | " | Alleged dead | From September, 1864. |

12TH INFANTRY—Mustered out July 16, 1865.

| | | | |
|---|---|---|---|
| Marston, S L | Ass't S. | Campbellsport or New Cassel, Wis. | From July, 1863. |
| Seeley, S. E | " | Fulton, Ill | From July, 1864. G. |
| Lindsfeldt, A. F. St S | " | Sheboygan, Wis | State Surg. from Sept., 1861 to June, 1862. |
| Cary, Luther H | Surgeon | Fond du Lac, Wis | To June, 1863. |
| Rogers, Ezra M | " | Hartford, Wis. | From October. 1863. |
| Woodward, E. A | Ass't S. | Sun Prairie, Wis | To April, 1862; also 11th and 36th Inf. |
| Bennett, De W. C | " | | To January, 1863. |
| Cooper. J. B | " | | To Feb., 1863; also 27th Inf. Not in A. G. R. |
| Woodworth, L. P | H. Stew | Milford, Ill. | |

WISCONSIN—Continued.

13TH INFANTRY—Mustered out November 24, 1865.

| Name | Rank | Residence | Service |
|---|---|---|---|
| Cady, Selden | Surgeon | Kilbourn City, Wis., or Emmettsburgh, Iowa. | From April, 1865. |
| Coakley, Jas. E. | H. Stew | West Milton Junction, Wis. | From Oct., 1861, to Sept., 1863; also 22d Inf. |
| Evans, John M | Surgeon | Evansville. Wis | To March, 1865. |
| Horton, Elisha G | Ass't S. | Whitewater, Wis | To November, 1864. |
| Lord, Simon L | " | Evansville, Wis | To 32d Inf. April, 1863. |
| Smith, Chas. M | " | Evansville, Wis | To September, 1864. |
| Woodruff, C. D | " | Lima, N. Y | From June, 1865. |

14TH INFANTRY—Mustered out October 9, 1865.

| Name | Rank | Residence | Service |
|---|---|---|---|
| La Court, David | Surgeon | Chilton, Wis | To July, 1862. |
| Stangeland, E C | Ass't S. | Rock City, Ill. | To March, 1863. |
| Wiley, Wm. | " | Fond du Lac, Wis. | To November, 1861. |
| Walker, Wm. H | Surgeon | Fond du Lac Wis. | To April, 1862. Not in A. G. R. |
| Zielly, H. E | Ass't S. | Chilton, Wis | To Apr.,'62; also 48th Inf. |
| Benson, Harmon | Surgeon | Milwaukee, Wis. | To Feb.,'65; also 10th Inf. |
| Cameron, D. D | " | La Crosse Co., Wis | To August, 1862. |
| Fowler, H. T. | Ass't S. | | From June, 1865. |
| Talbert, G. E. | " | | To August, 1863. |
| McGuire, Francis | Surgeon | Blue Earth City, Minn | From March, 1865. |
| Howard, Edwin | H. Stew | La Crosse, Wis. | |

15TH INFANTRY—Mustered out from December 2, 1864, to February 13, 1865.

| Name | Rank | Residence | Service |
|---|---|---|---|
| Bell, Samuel | Ass't S. | Beloit, Wis | From September, 1864. |
| Heimoe, S. O. | Surgeon | Lawrence, Kans | To November, 1863. |
| Lindsfeldt, A. F. St S. | " | Sheboygan, Wis. | From December, 1863. G. |
| Trenkler, Oscar | Ass't S. | Albert Lea, Minn. | To June, 1863. |
| Hansen, S. J | " | | To October, 1862. |
| Newell, G. F | " | Watertown, Wis | To June, 1862. Not in A. G. R. |
| Whipple, A. H | " | | To November, 1862. |
| Wooster, D. P | " | | To March, 1863. |

16TH INFANTRY—Mustered out July 12, 1865.

| Name | Rank | Residence | Service |
|---|---|---|---|
| Eastman, Geo. W. | Surgeon | Platteville, Wis | To November, 1864. |
| Rogers, Jas. H | Ass't S. | New York city | To February, 1862. |
| McCallum, Jas | " | | A. W. M. Not in A. G. R. |
| Schermerhorn, W. S. | " | | From February, 1865. |
| Torey, Ira A | " | Dead | To 14th Inf. Oct., 1862 |
| Turner, Henry W. | Surgeon | Alleged dead | From March, 1865. |
| Hayes, Asa H. | Ass't S. | | Dismissed July, 1864. |

17TH INFANTRY—Mustered out July 14, 1865.

| Name | Rank | Residence | Service |
|---|---|---|---|
| McKennan, Henry | Surgeon | Sauk City or Baraboo, Wis. | To January, 1865. G. |
| Brett, Benj. C | " | Green Bay, Wis | A. W. M. Also 21st Inf. Not in A. G. R. |
| St. Sure, Geo | Surgeon | Sheboygan, Wis. | From April, 1865. |
| Davis, Chas. D | Ass't S. | Horicon, Wis | To Jan., 1865. Alleged dead |
| Jackson, Eben | " | Somerville, Mass | To July, 1863; also 25th and 30th U. S. C. T. |

18TH INFANTRY—Mustered out July 18, 1865.

| Name | Rank | Residence | Service |
|---|---|---|---|
| Buck, Erastus J. | Surgeon | Platteville, Wis. | From September, 1862. |
| Whitney, J. J. | Ass't S. | Emmettsburgh, Iowa | A. W. M. |
| Briggs, Geo. H. | " | Delevan, Wis. | To June, 1863. |
| Huntington, G F. | Surgeon | | To September, 1862. |
| Mead, Larkin G. | Ass't S. | | Revoked March, 1862. Not in A. G. R. |

## WISCONSIN—Continued.

### 19TH INFANTRY—Mustered out August 9, 1865.

Devendorf, D. B......Surgeon...Delavan, Wis.. ....... ......To April, 1865; also 1st Inf. U. S. Ex. S.
Dodge, E. F............Ass't S.....Fond du Lac, Wis.........From February, 1864.
Markham. H. C........ " Independence, Iowa ......To May, 1863. Ex. S.
Nichols, Lyndolf...... " Richland City, Wis.........To February, 1863.
Winter, Peter..........Surgeon.. 419 Warren ave., Chicago, Ill. To March, 1863.
Hitchcock. H. A ......Ass't S.......................................To July, 1863.
Chase, Philo W........ " .......................................To November, 1863
Hindman, D. R........H. Stew...Boone, Iowa.

### 20TH INFANTRY—Part mustered out July 14, 1865, the rest transferred to 35th Infantry.

Mosher, Mark A.......Ass't S.....Grand Rapids, or Berlin, Wis A. W. M.
Chapman, C. B........Surgeon...Olympia, Kans .............To Aug., 1864; also 6th Inf.
Munk, Emanuel.......Ass't S.....Milwaukee, Wis ............To January, 1863.
Peak, Orin...............Surgeon...Oak Park, Ill ................From September, 1864.

### 21ST INFANTRY—Part mustered out June 8, 1865, the rest transferred to 3d Infantry.

Brett, Benj. C .........Ass't S.....Green Bay, Wis.. ............To January, 1865.
Fuller, Sidney L...... " 88 Griswold st., Detroit, Mich. To 24th Ill. Inf. March, 1864.
Reeve, James T........Surgeon...Appleton, Wis...............From Nov., 1862. U. S. Ex. S.
Barnes, Henry L......Ass't S.....Ripon, Wis.........................From April, 1865
Hoyt, Wm. M. ........ " .......................................From April, 1865.

### 22D INFANTRY—Part mustered out June 12, 1865, the rest transferred to 3d Infantry

Blanchard, Caleb S...Ass't S....East Troy, Wis...............To July, 1863.
Burbank, Jerome..... " Waverly. Iowa...............To Sept., 1863; also 33d Inf.
Coakley, Jas. E........ " Milton Junction, Wis......To May, 1865; also 13th Inf.
Hatchard, Thos........Surgeon...Milwaukee. Wis.............From April, 1864.
Scofield, Proctor D...H. Stew...West Union. Iowa, or Janesville. Wis
Bicknell, Geo W.......Surgeon.......................................To February, 1863.
Cansdell, Henry W... " .......................................To March, 1864.

### 23D INFANTRY—Mustered out July 4, 1865.

Angell, J. W...........Surgeon...Sauk County, Wis., or Los Angeles, Cal. From July, 1863.
Irwin, E. Howard.....Ass't S.....Lodi, Wis.........................To April, 1863; also Capt. Co. H.
Prentice, Jas. D ......Surgeon...Portage, Wis .. ...............To February, 1863
Wood, Orestes H......Ass't S.....Brookfield, Mo..................Reported killed March, 1881.
Groening, John........Surgeon.......................................To June, 1863; also 35th Inf.

### 24TH INFANTRY—Part mustered out June 10, 1865, the rest transferred to 13th Infantry.

Hasse, Herman E.....Surgeon...Milwaukee. Wis..... ........From August, 1862.
Wheeler, J. P..........Ass't S.....Brighton, N. Y....... ......A. W. M.
Hoyt, Moses C......... " .......................................To May, 1863.

## WISCONSIN—Continued.

### 25TH INFANTRY—Mustered out June 7, 1865.

| Name | Rank | Residence | Remarks |
|---|---|---|---|
| Gott, Wm. A. | Surgeon | Viroqua, Wis. | From July, 1864. U. S. |
| Gage, Martin R. | " | Sparta, Wis. | To June, 1864. |
| Gunn, Samuel | H. Stew | Tomah, Wis. | |
| Dalgairns, Chas. A. | Ass't S. | | From November, 1864. |
| Young, A. | " | Prescott, Wis. | Revoked October 20, 1864. Not in A. G. R. |

### 26TH INFANTRY—Mustered out June 13, 1865.

| Name | Rank | Residence | Remarks |
|---|---|---|---|
| Huebschmann, F. | Surgeon | Milwaukee, Wis. | To September, 1864. |
| Vander Vaart, S. | " | Cedar Falls, Iowa | From November, 1864. |
| Fricke, Theo | Ass't S. | Cedarburgh, Wis. | To March, 1863. |
| Georgie, Carl | " | | To July, 1863. |

### 27TH INFANTRY—Mustered out August 29, 1865.

| Name | Rank | Residence | Remarks |
|---|---|---|---|
| Hutchinson, Geo | Ass't S. | Durand, Wis. | To December, 1863. |
| Mitchell, Robert | Surgeon | Douglas, Wis | From Oct., 1863; also 10th Inf. |
| Saltzman, J. C. | Ass't S. | Whitewater, Wis. | To June, 1864 |
| Cooper, Jas. B. | " | | From July, 1864. |
| Krack, Charles | Surgeon | Milwaukee, Wis. | To July, 1863. |

### 28TH INFANTRY—Mustered out August 23, 1865.

| Name | Rank | Residence | Remarks |
|---|---|---|---|
| Miller, D. McL. | Ass't S. | Oconomowoc, Wis. | From September, 1862. |
| Smith, Wm. H. | Surgeon | Albert Lea, Minn. | From Sept., 1862; also Lt. Art. |
| Frisbie, Chas. W. | Ass't S. | | To Aug., 1865. Not in A. G. R. |
| Hawes, Lewis K. | " | Alleged dead | To November, 1863. |

### 29TH INFANTRY—Mustered out June 22, 1865.

| Name | Rank | Residence | Remarks |
|---|---|---|---|
| Potter, Jacob L. | Surgeon | Menasha, Wis. | From Sept., 1864. Alleged dead. |
| Spalding, Wm. C. | " | Watertown, Wis. | To July, 1863. |
| Du Bois, Darwin | " | Lake Mills, Wis. | To July, 1864; also 46th Inf. Dead. |
| Hipolite, W. W. | Ass't S. | Devall's Bluff, Ark. | To 11th U. S. C. T. Mar., 1865; also 18th Ill. Inf. |
| Barber, Jos. H. | " | Davis City, Iowa | From April, 1865. |
| Addison, Robert | " | | To March, 1863. |
| McClure, J. F. | " | Beaver Dam, Wis | To Sept., 1862. Not in A. G. R. |
| Summerfeldt, W. B. | " | | To July, 1863. Not in A. G. R |
| Winch, Geo D. | " | | To August, 1863. |

### 30TH INFANTRY—Mustered out September 20, 1865.

| Name | Rank | Residence | Remarks |
|---|---|---|---|
| Baker, Edwin O. | Ass't S. | Menomonee, Wis. | From September, 1862. |
| Farr, Edwin J. | " | Eau Claire, Wis. | To July, 1865. |
| Hoyt, Otis | Surgeon | Hudson, Wis. | From September, 1862. |
| Jaggar, H. B. | Ass't S. | Hudson, Wis. | To Sept., 1865. Not in A. G. R. |

### 31ST INFANTRY—Cos. A to F, inclusive, mustered out June 20, 1865, the rest July 8, 1865.

| Name | Rank | Residence | Remarks |
|---|---|---|---|
| Arndt, Peter S. | Surgeon | 65 Randolph st. Chicago. | To Jan., 1865; also 2d Inf. |
| Bull, Jas. M | Ass't S. | Waterloo, Iowa | To July, 1864. |
| Mason, Darius | Surgeon | Milwaukee, Wis. | To Nov., 1863. H. R. |
| Wilber, Geo. D. | " | Mineral Point, Wis. | Also 5th and 32d Inf. Not in A. G. R. |
| Balcom, H. S | Ass't S. | Manitowoc, Wis. | From October, 1864. |
| Gailor, Jos. B. | " | | To November, 1863. |
| Thomas, Wm. M. | Surgeon | Darlington, Wis. | To June, 1865. |

WISCONSIN—Continued.

32D INFANTRY—Part mustered out June 12, 1865, the rest transferred to 16th Infantry.

| | | | |
|---|---|---|---|
| Fay, George W. | Ass't S. | Menasha, Wis. | To January, 1865. |
| Spalding, Wm. C. | Surgeon | Watertown, Wis. | To July, 1863 |
| Lord, Simon L. | " | Edgarton, Wis. | To September, 1864. |
| Sheppard, J. L. | Ass't S. | Sheboygan Falls, Wis. | From March, 1865. |
| Noyes, J. C. | Surgeon | Oshkosh, Wis. | From March, 1865. |
| Wilber, Geo. D. | " | Mineral Point, Wis. | To April, 1863; also 5th Inf. |
| La Dow, James | Ass't S. | | To January, 1863. |
| Dunn, S W | " | | From April, 1865. |
| Blood, Solomon | " | | To Nov. '63, also 39th Inf. |

33D INFANTRY—Mustered out August 9, 1865.

| | | | |
|---|---|---|---|
| Burbank, Jerome | Surgeon | Waverly, Iowa | From July, 1864; also 22d Inf. |
| Carley, D. W. | Ass't S. | Boscobel, Wis. | To January, 1864. |
| Whiting, Jos. B. | Surgeon | Janesville, Wis. | To June, 1864. |
| Blackall, C. R | Ass't S. | Chicago, Ill. | To February, 1864 |
| Berry, Edward E. | H. Stew | Platteville, Wis. | |
| Hanks, M. H. | Ass't S. | | From July, 1864. |

34TH INFANTRY—(9 months)—Mustered out September 8, 1863.

| | | | |
|---|---|---|---|
| Kopff, Theodore | Ass't S. | Beaver Dam, Wis. | From December, 1862. |
| Kelso, John S. | " | Ackley, Iowa | A. W. M. |
| Weinern, John E. | Surgeon | | To July, 1863. |

35TH INFANTRY—Mustered out March 15, 1866.

| | | | |
|---|---|---|---|
| Groening, John | Surgeon | | From Dec., 1863; also 23d Inf. |
| Garlick, Carmi P. | Ass't S. | | To February, 1865. |

36TH INFANTRY—Mustered out July 12, 1865.

| | | | |
|---|---|---|---|
| Woodward, E. A. | Surgeon | Sun Prairie, Wis. | To May, 1865. |
| Bunnell, L. H. | " | Winona Co., Minn. | From March, 1865. |
| Winch, George D. | Ass't S. | Alleged dead | To 42d Inf. Aug., 1864. |

37TH INFANTRY—Mustered out July 27, 1865.

| | | | |
|---|---|---|---|
| Roundy, Dan'l C. | Surgeon | 188 or 190 Clark st., Chicago, Ill., or Davenport, Iowa. | From April, 1864. |
| Calkins, Geo. H. | Ass't S. | Waupaca, Wis. | To March, 1864. |
| Sherman, Emery | " | Palmyra, Wis. | To June, 1865 |
| Orsick, John H. | " | Steven's Point, Wis. | From April, 1864. |

38TH INFANTRY—Companies G to K mustered out June 2, 1865, the rest July 26, 1865.

| | | | |
|---|---|---|---|
| Butterfield, H. L | Surgeon | Waupun, Wis. | From April, 1864. H. R. |
| Russell, Hugh | Ass't S. | Huron, Dak. Ter. | To July, 1865. |
| Pierson, C. B. | " | Spring Green, Wis | To November, 1864. |
| Tochterman, Chris. | " | Monroe, Wis. | From January, 1865. |

39TH INFANTRY—(100 days)—Mustered out September 22, 1864.

| | | | |
|---|---|---|---|
| Benedict, John H. | Ass't S. | | From June, 1864. |
| Clark, S. S. | " | Menomonee, Wis. | From May, 1864. |
| Blood, Solomon | Surgeon | | From May, 1864; also 32d Inf. |

WISCONSIN—Continued.

40TH INFANTRY—(100 days)—Mustered out September 20, 21, and 22, 1864.

| | | | |
|---|---|---|---|
| Jones, Amos S | Ass't S | Dayton, Ohio or Janesville, Wis. | From May, 1864. |
| Lamb, Geo. A | “ | Green Bay, Wis. | From June, 1864. |
| Blanchard, C. C | H. Stew | Delavan, Wis. | |
| Blanchard, O. W | Surgeon | Delevan, Wis | From May, 1864; also 49th Inf. |

41ST INFANTRY—(100 days)—Mustered out September 23 and 24, 1864.

| | | | |
|---|---|---|---|
| Wood, John D | Ass't S | Yankton, Dak. Ter. | From May, 1864. |
| Clarke, R. B | “ | | From June, 1864. |
| Smith, S. D | Surgeon | | From May, 1864. |

42D INFANTRY—(1 year)—Mustered out June 20, 1865.

| | | | |
|---|---|---|---|
| Winch, Geo. D | Surgeon | Alleged dead | To June, 1865; also 36th Inf. |
| Clement, John P | Ass't S | | From September, 1864. |
| Stevens, Oliver P | “ | Maxinkucku, Ind | A. W. M. |
| Goodrich, Harvey C. | Nurse | Geneva, Wis. | |

43D INFANTRY—(1 year)—Mustered out June 24, 1865.

| | | | |
|---|---|---|---|
| Ward, A. J | Surgeon | Madison, Wis. | To March, 1865. |
| Hayes, Chas. C | “ | Hyde Park, Mass | From March, 1865. H. R. |
| Ruger, H. H | Ass't S | | From April, 1865. |
| Searles, W. H | “ | Wausau, Wis. | A. W. M. Not in A. G. R. |

44TH INFANTRY—(1 year)—Mustered out August 28, 1865.

| | | | |
|---|---|---|---|
| Ball, Jas. M | Surgeon | Monroe, Wis | From Nov., 1864. H. R. |
| Harkins, Thos | Ass't S | Gotham, Wis. | A. W. M. |
| Ferrin, S. A | “ | Alleged dead | To May, 1865. |
| Best, Thos. E | “ | Alleged dead | To August, 1865. |

45TH INFANTRY—(1 year)—Mustered out July 17, 1865.

| | | | |
|---|---|---|---|
| Barndt, Allen S | Ass't S | Menominee Falls, Wis. | From December, 1864. |
| Dahm, Emil J | “ | Madison, Wis. | From December, 1864. |
| Kramer, Ernest | Surgeon | Milwaukee, Wis | From Dec., 1864; also 1st Cav. and 7th Inf. |

46TH INFANTRY—(1 year)—Mustered out September 27, 1865.

| | | | |
|---|---|---|---|
| Du Bois, Darwin | Surgeon | Lake Mills, Wis | From Feb., 1865; also 29th Inf. Dead. |
| Downs, D. L | Ass't S | Richland Centre, Wis. | To July, 1865. H. R. |
| Turner, G. R | “ | Mazo Manie, Wis. | From February, 1865. |

47TH INFANTRY—(1 year)—Mustered out September 4, 1865.

| | | | |
|---|---|---|---|
| Young, Henry J | Surgeon | Waseca, Minn. | From January, 1865. |
| Pelton, J. G | Ass't S | Spring Green, Wis | From January, 1865. |
| McIntosh, L. D | “ | Waseca, Minn. | From February, 1865. |

48TH INFANTRY—(1 year)—Mustered out from December 30, 1865, to March 24, 1866.

| | | | |
|---|---|---|---|
| Armstrong, L. G | Surgeon | Boscobel, Wis | From March, 1865; also 6th and 8th Inf. |
| Zielley, Henry E | Ass't S | Chilton, Wis | From March, 1865; also 14th Inf. |
| Squires, Jas. P | “ | | To October, 1865. |
| Pratt, Horace | “ | | Not in A. G. R. |

WISCONSIN—Continued.

49TH INFANTRY—(1 year)—Mustered out from November 1 to 8, 1865.

Gibbs, Jonathan ...... Ass't S..... Omro, Wis.. .................. From February, 1865.
Blanchard, P. W...... " Sharon, Wis ...................From February, 1865.
Blanchard, O. W......Surgeon..........................................From Feb., 1865; also 40th Inf.
Blanchard, C. C......H. Stew...Delavan, Wis.

50TH INFANTRY—(1 year)—Mustered out from April 19 to June 14, 1866.

Vivian, John H........Surgeon...Mineral Point, Wis.........From March, 1865.
Alexander, D. S......Ass't S......................................To June, 1865.
Fenn, Curtis T......... " ......................................From November, 1865.
Crosse, Chas. G....... " Sun Prairie, Wis............From October, 1865.

51ST INFANTRY—(1 year)—Mustered out from August 16 to 30, 1865.

Wood, Orestes H......Surgeon...Brookfield, Mo...............Also 23d Inf. Killed in 1881. Not in A. G. R.
Hall, Sam'l..............Ass't S.....Reedburgh, Wis.............To May, 1865. Not in A. G. R.
Jones, Erwin L........ " Oconomowoc, Wis .........From March, 1865; also 53d Inf.
Bennett, Rouse........ " Tomah, Wis.....................A. W. M.

52D INFANTRY—(1 year)—Mustered out July 28, 1865.

Dixon, Lewis J........Surgeon..........................................A. W. M. Not in A. G. R.
Wright, O. P. B.......Ass't S..........................................To July, 1865.
Teal, Cornelius....... " ..........................................To May, 1865.

53D INFANTRY—(1 year)—Consolidated with 51st Infantry June 30, 1865.

Jones, Erwin L........Ass't S.....Oconomowoc, Wis .........From March, 1865; also 51st Inf.
James, Robt G........Surgeon..........................................A. W. M. Also 10th Inf. Not in A. G. R.
Benson, L. M.. ........Ass't S.....Lowell, Wis.....................To May, 1865. Not in A. G. R.

## U. S. COLORED TROOPS.

1ST CAVALRY—Mustered out February, 4, 1866.

Manly, Bradford S...Surgeon...Potsdam, N. Y...............From Dec., 1863; also 3d N. Y. Light Artillery.
Gray, Wm. H..........Ass't S..........................................From December, 1863.

2D CAVALRY—Mustered out February 12, 1866.

Cisna, Wm. R .........Ass't S.....Shelby, Ohio.....................From October, 1865.
Manly, Marcus M.....Surgeon...737 Oxford st., Phila., Pa. To January, 1866.
Parker, M. G...........Ass't S.....Amo, Ind.........................To May, 1865.
Eakin, A. L ............A. A. S....3803 Chestnut st., Phila., Pa.
Pancoast, D. P......... " N. W. cor. 5th and Clinton sts., Camden, N. J.
Floyd, T. S.............. "

3D CAVALRY—Mustered out January 26, 1866.

Beadles, Wm. T.......Surgeon...Bushnell, Ill......................From Nov., 1863; also 4th Ill. Cav. U. S. Ex. S.
Keith, Price ............Ass't S..........................................From November, 1863.
French, Zeba D........ " Sumner, Ill.......................From August, 1865; also 11th Mo. Inf.

## U. S. COLORED TROOPS—Continued.

### 4TH CAVALRY—Mustered out March 20, 1866.

| | | | |
|---|---|---|---|
| Herrick, Lucius C. | Ass't S. | Woodstock, Ohio | From December, 1863. |
| Slawson, Daniel D. | Surgeon | | From March, 1864. |

### 5TH CAVALRY—Mustered out March 16, 1866.

| | | | |
|---|---|---|---|
| Bowen, Geo. W. | Surgeon | Toledo, Ohio | From October, 1864. |
| Smith, Herman J. | Ass't S. | 21 Central st., Lowell, Mass. | From October, 1864. |
| Swan, John | " | South Windham, Me | From November, 1864. |
| Carr, James A. | A. A. S. | Princeton, N. J. | |
| Peak, R. M. | " | New Haven, Ky. | |

### 6TH CAVALRY—Mustered out April 15, 1866.

| | | | |
|---|---|---|---|
| Ridgely, John | Surgeon | Lebanon, Ky | From July, 1865 |
| Riley, Chas. H. | Ass't S. | | From October, 1864. |
| Robbins, Wm. S. | " | | From December, 1864. |

### 1ST HEAVY ARTILLERY—Mustered out March 31, 1866.

| | | | |
|---|---|---|---|
| Cummings, Ralph W. | Surgeon | San Francisco, Cal | Died August, 1880 |
| Wight, E. M. | Ass't S. | Chattanooga, Tenn | From May, 1865. |
| Wyatt, Henry D. | " | Chattanooga, Tenn | From May, 1865. |

### 3D HEAVY ARTILLERY—(Formerly 2d)—Mustered out April 30, 1666.

| | | | |
|---|---|---|---|
| Binkerd, Adam D. | Ass't S. | Kern, Pa. | From August, 1865. |
| Bosley, Daniel | " | 244 Walnut st, Chicago, Ill. | From August, 1865. |
| Connell, J. J. | " | 507 E 119th st., N. Y. city | To July, 1865. |
| Hood, H. H. | Surgeon | Litchfield, Ill | From Sept., 1863; also 117th Ills. Inf. |
| Osborne, Francis M. | Ass't S. | Dead | Also 7th H. Art'y and 11th Inf. |

### 4TH HEAVY ARTILLERY—(Formerly 3d)—Mustered out February 25, 1666.

| | | | |
|---|---|---|---|
| Thompson, Jas. | Surgeon | Indianapolis, Ind. | To September, 1865 |
| Noyes, Hiram J. | Ass't S. | Meigsville, Ohio | From July, 1864. |
| Stockwell, Alanson | " | | From March, 1865. |
| McBean, Alexander | Surgeon | Chippewa Falls, Wis. | To Jan., 1864; also Wis. Cav. |
| Rice, Geo. L. | Ass't S. | | To May, 1864. |
| Raub, Abraham A. | " | | To March, 1864. |

### 5TH HEAVY ARTILLERY—(Formerly 4th)—Mustered out May 13, 1866

| | | | |
|---|---|---|---|
| Penniman, H. H. | Surgeon | | From Dec., 1863; also 17th Illinois Inf. |
| Greenleaf, Arthur W. | Ass't S. | | From Sept., 1865; also 34th Inf. |
| Wiggins, Aug. W. | " | | A. W. M. |

### 6TH HEAVY ARTILLERY—(Formerly 5th)—Mustered out May 13, 1866

| | | | |
|---|---|---|---|
| Peal, Geo. M. | Ass't S. | Metuchen, N. J. | From December, 1863. |
| Sargent, B. W. | Surgeon | Rochester, N. H. | From Oct., 1863; also 30th Mo. Inf. |
| Shafer, Geo. M. | Ass't S. | Bloom Centre, Ohio | From September, 1865. |
| Mitchell, Wm. S. | " | Brush Creek, Pa | To April, 1864. |
| Thomas, Simon | " | | Dismissed May, 1865. |
| Kendall, R. P. | A. A. S. | Beloit, Kan. | Also 11th U. S. C. T. |
| Henry, S. L. | " | 7th Dist., New Orleans, La. | |
| Ferris, F. W. | " | 33 Hathaway, st, Cincinnati, Ohio. | Also 13th U. S. C. H. Art. |

## U. S. COLORED TROOPS—Continued.

### 7TH HEAVY ARTILLERY—(See 11th Infantry.)

### 8TH HEAVY ARTILLERY—Mustered out February 10, 1866.

| Name | Rank | Address | Remarks |
|---|---|---|---|
| Traver, Richard D. | Ass't S. | | From August, 1864. |
| Price, Reuben W. | " | | From October, 1865. |
| De Wint, Fred'k | Surgeon | Dead | Dismissed October, 1865. |

### 9TH HEAVY ARTILLERY—Disbanded May 5, 1865.

| Name | Rank | Address | Remarks |
|---|---|---|---|
| Uterhart, Carl | Surgeon | | To Aug , 1865; also 119th N. Y. Inf. |

### 10TH HEAVY ARTILLERY—(Formerly 7th)—Mustered out February 22, 1867.

| Name | Rank | Address | Remarks |
|---|---|---|---|
| Landers, Thos. | Ass't S. | U. S. Pension Office | From September, 1865. |
| Fish, John | " | Auburn, Ohio | To Surg. 88th Inf. Jan., 1864. |
| Mather, Wm. H. | Surgeon | | From March, 1864. |
| Hurley, Jas. W. | Ass't S. | | From September, 1865. |

### 11TH HEAVY ARTILLERY—(Formerly 8th)—Mustered out October 2, 1865.

| Name | Rank | Address | Remarks |
|---|---|---|---|
| Draper, Jos. R. | Ass't S. | 672 E. Broadway, S. Boston, Mass. | From December, 1863. |
| Wilson, Wm. C | A. A. S. | 231 Canal st., New Orleans, La. | Not in A. G. R. |
| Carpenter, Benoni | Surgeon | Pawtucket, R. I. | Died 1878. |
| Mecorney, H | Ass't S. | Dead. | |

### 12TH HEAVY ARTILLERY—Mustered out April 24, 1866.

| Name | Rank | Address | Remarks |
|---|---|---|---|
| Westerling, Richard | Ass't S. | Elizabethtown, N. Mex. | From Feb., 1866; also 30th Inf. |
| Power, Lewis B. | Surgeon | | From July, 1864. |
| Evans, James L. | Ass't S. | | From November, 1864. |

### 13TH HEAVY ARTILLERY—Mustered out November 18, 1865.

| Name | Rank | Address | Remarks |
|---|---|---|---|
| Ferris, Frederick W. | Surgeon | 33 Hathaway st., Cincinnati, Ohio. | From Nov., 1864; also 6th U. S. C. H. A. |
| Piper, Wm. W. | Ass't A. | | From June, 1865. |
| Neal, Selden F. | " | | From June, 1865; also 72d Inf. |
| Abbot, Josiah | " | | To Surg. 119th Inf. April, 1865. |

### 14TH HEAVY ARTILLERY—Mustered out December 11, 1865.

| Name | Rank | Address | Remarks |
|---|---|---|---|
| Sitler, Isaac W. | Surgeon | | From November, 1864. |
| Hand, Chas. L. | Ass't S. | Stoney Brook, N. Y. | A. W. M. |

### 1ST INFANTRY—Mustered out September 29, 1865.

| Name | Rank | Address | Remarks |
|---|---|---|---|
| Bell, Sam'l A. | Ass't S. | 161 S. Sharp st., Baltimore, Md. | From June, 1865. |
| Crawford, Wm. H. | " | Nazareth, Pa. | Dismissed Aug., 1864. |
| Weist, Jacob R | Surgeon | Richmond, Ind | From Nov., 1863; also 4th Ohio Cav. U. S. Ex. S. |
| Willoughby, H. W. | Ass't S. | Hollis, N. H | To July, 1864. |

## U. S. COLORED TROOPS—Continued.

### 2D INFANTRY—Mustered out January 5, 1866.

| Name | Rank | Address | Remarks |
|---|---|---|---|
| McCulley, Wm. A | Surgeon | Independence, Kan | From Nov., 1863; also 65th Ohio Inf. |
| Wertz, J. M | Ass't S | Care P. Ft W. & C. R. R Co., Wooster, Ohio. | From October, 1861. |
| Eberhard, Chas | " | | From April, 1865. |
| Boothby, Alonzo | " | 60 Temple st., Boston, Mass. | To June, 1864. |
| Pettijohn, N. J | A. A. S | Las Vegas, N. M. | |
| Branch, Franklin | " | Tempa, Fla. | |
| Comick, W. T | " | Norfolk, Va | In U. S. A. |
| Eakin, A. L | " | 3803 Chestnut st., Philadelphia, Pa. | |
| Stocker, A. E | " | 2212 Fitzwater st., Philadelphia, Pa. | |
| Howard, J. C | " | Bronson, Fla. | |
| Tindall, D. W | " | Box 801 Quincy, Ill., or Taylor, Mo. | Also 3d and 11th Inf. |

### 3D INFANTRY—Mustered out October 31, 1865.

| Name | Rank | Address | Remarks |
|---|---|---|---|
| Barnes, Alonzo M | Surgeon | 3241 York Road, Phila., Pa. | From September, 1864. |
| Polk, Chas. G | Ass't S | 2219 Catharine st., Philadelphia, Pa. | To Jan., 1865; also 34th Inf. |
| Porter, Watson | " | Bridgeport, Conn | From April, 1864. |
| Farrington, Jas. B | " | | From August, 1865. |
| Lyman, John N | " | Columbus, Ohio | To December, 1863. |
| Tindall, D. W | A. A. S | Box 801 Quincy, Ill., or Taylor, Mo | Also 2d and 11th Inf. |
| Weeks, G. M | Surgeon | 4 W. 28th st., N. Y. city. | |
| Abbott, F. B | A. A. S | Elmira, N. Y. | |

### 4TH INFANTRY—Mustered out May 4, 1866.

| Name | Rank | Address | Remarks |
|---|---|---|---|
| Mitchell, John W | Surgeon | Palermo, Me | From Sept., 1863; also 21st Mass. Inf. |
| Odiorne, Geo. G | Ass't S | Jefferson, Iowa | From September, 1863. |
| Warry, Kenneth | " | Auburn, Kan | To August, 1865. Dead. |
| Gardner, Perrin | A. A. S | Wilksville, Ohio | Also 1st W. Va. Cav. |
| Heard, Lewis | " | Rochester, N. Y. | |
| Mackin, Charles | " | Milford, Mass. | |
| Potter, Z. H | " | U. S. Pension Office. | |

### 5TH INFANTRY—Mustered out September 20, 1865.

| Name | Rank | Address | Remarks |
|---|---|---|---|
| Eastman, J. A | Ass't S | Indianapolis, Ind | From August, 1865. |
| Gray, A. J | " | Care A. G. U. S. A | A. W. M. In U. S. A |
| Merrill, G. V. R | Surgeon | Monroeville, Ohio | From June, 1865; also 6th Inf. |
| Allen, Lyman | " | Sedalia, Mo | To April, 1865. |

### 6TH INFANTRY—Mustered out September 20, 1865.

| Name | Rank | Address | Remarks |
|---|---|---|---|
| Talbot, C. C | A. A. S | Lawrence, Mass. | |
| Barnes, Lemon | Surgeon | Manchester, Mich | From July, 1864. |
| Merrill, Geo. V. R | Ass't S | Monroeville, Ohio | To Surg. 5th Inf. June, 1865. |
| White, C. J | " | Dead | From June, 1865. |
| Ware, Edward H | " | Dead | A. W. M. Also 100th Infantry. |
| Ferris, Fred'k W | A. A. S | 33 Hathaway st., Cincinnati, Ohio. | Also 13th H. A. |

## U. S. COLORED TROOPS—Continued.

### 7TH INFANTRY—Mustered out October 13, 1866.

| | | | |
|---|---|---|---|
| Augusta, Alex. T | Surgeon | 1319 L st., Washington, D. C. | From October, 1863. |
| Morse, Joel | Ass't S | Dead | To Surg. 117th Inf. Mar., 1865. |
| Grange, Henry | “ | | To March, 1866. |
| Denuler, Z. P. | “ | | From June, 1865. |

### 8TH INFANTRY—Mustered out November 10, 1865.

| | | | |
|---|---|---|---|
| Breen, Michael | Ass't S | 158 Henry st., N. Y. city | From November, 1863. |
| Heichhold, C. P | Surgeon | Buffalo, N. Y | From September, 1863. |
| Miller, Christian | Ass't S | Dead | Dismissed Oct., 1864. |

### 9TH INFANTRY—Mustered out November 26, 1866.

| | | | |
|---|---|---|---|
| Newman, Thos | Ass't S | Philadelphia, Pa | From July, 1865. |
| Perry, Ira | “ | Nordhoff, Cal | From November, 1863. |
| Pease, E. M | Surgeon | Honolula, Sandwich I | From Dec., 1863; also 16th Con. Inf. |
| O'Donnell, John | Ass't S | | Dismissed Feb., 1864. |
| Matthews, J. Earl | A. A. S | 389 W. Fayette st., Baltimore, Md. | |

### 10TH INFANTRY—Mustered out May 17, 1866.

| | | | |
|---|---|---|---|
| Wevill, Richard H | Surgeon | 1014 S. 3d st., Phila., Pa | From November, 1863. |
| Moran, Thomas | Ass't S | Calvert, Texas | From March, 1865. |
| Clunie, William | “ | 149 Church st., Toronto, Canada. | From June, 1865. |
| Elderkin, John | “ | 84 Beekman st, N. Y. city. | To December, 1864. |
| Hair, B. W | A. A. S | Hamilton, Ohio | Also 100th U. S. C. T. |
| Vogel, Edward | “ | Addison, Ill. | |
| Farries, A. P | “ | Florida, N. Y. | |
| Bell, S. A. | “ | 161 S. Sharp st., Baltimore, Md. | |
| Draine, Wm | “ | Charleston, S. C. | |
| Noden, Wm | “ | Hampton, Canada, (old.) | |

### 11TH INFANTRY—(Old)—Consolidated with the 112th and 113th Infantry April 22, 1865.

| | | | |
|---|---|---|---|
| Hipolite, Wm. W | Surgeon | Devall's Bluff, Ark | From March, 1865; also 113th Inf. (new) & 29th Wis. Inf. |

### 11TH INFANTRY—(New)—Formerly 6th and 7th Heavy Artillery—Mustered out Janurry 12, 1866.

| | | | |
|---|---|---|---|
| Osborn, Francis M | Surgeon | Dead | To July, 1864. |
| Kendall, Reese P | “ | Beloit, Kan | To October, 1865; also 2d Ill. Cav. |
| Kempton, W. C | Ass't S | | To February, 1865. |
| Tindall, D. W | A. A. S | Box 801, Quincy, Ill. or Taylor, Mo. | Also 2d and 3d Inf. |

### 12TH INFANTRY—Mustered out January 16, 1866.

| | | | |
|---|---|---|---|
| Deal, W. G | Ass't S | Colfax, La | From September, 1865. |
| Russell, E. R | “ | Humboldt, Kan | To September, 1865. |
| Stegman, Gustavus | Surgeon | St. Louis, Mo | From Aug., 1863; also 2d Mo. Inf. |
| Anderson, David M | Ass't S | | To May, 1865. |

## U. S. COLORED TROOPS—Continued.

### 13TH INFANTRY—Mustered out January 10, 1866.

| | | | |
|---|---|---|---|
| Musgrave, P. D. | Ass't S. | Indianapolis, Ind | From October, 1863. |
| Bacon, Chas. H. | Surgeon | | To November, 1865. |
| Thomas, L. | Ass't S. | 11th street, above Race, Phila., Pa. | To October, 1864. |

### 14TH INFANTRY—Mustered out March 26, 1866.

| | | | |
|---|---|---|---|
| Green, W. H. | Ass't S. | Providence, R. I. | From August, 1865. |
| Ong, Jacob B. | " | Saint Leon, Ind. | To 18th Inf. May, 1865. |
| Ames, Fisher W. | Surgeon | 137 Plumb st., Cincinnati, Ohio | From Nov., 1863; also 6th Ohio Inf. |
| Block, Marx | Ass't S. | Chattanooga, Tenn | From August, 1865. |
| Oleson, Chas. W. | " | | To May, 1865. |

### 15TH INFANTRY—Mustered out April 7, 1866.

| | | | |
|---|---|---|---|
| Gregory, John | Surgeon | Farmington, Ill. | A. W. M. Dead. |
| Gratigny, L. H. | Ass't S. | 202 W. 4th st., Cincinnati, Ohio | To Surg. 109th Inf. June, 1864. |
| Johnson, J. J. | A. A. S. | East Liverpool, Ohio. | |
| York, Wm. H. | Ass't S. | | Cashiered Feb., 1866. |
| Ream, J. B. | " | | From April, 1865. |

### 16TH INFANTRY—Mustered out April 31, 1866.

| | | | |
|---|---|---|---|
| Gillman, O. L. | Ass't S. | Chattanooga, Tenn. | From February, 1864. |
| Welch, John | Surgeon | Mt. Vernon, Ohio | From August, 1864. |
| Blair, John R. | A. A. S. | Buckhannon, W. Va. | Also 10th W. Va. Inf. Ex. S. |
| Achenbach, A. H. | Ass't S. | | To October, 1864. |

### 17TH INFANTRY—Mustered out April 25, 1866.

| | | | |
|---|---|---|---|
| Clemons, P. H. | Surgeon | U. S. Pension Office | From Nov., 1863; also 99th Ohio Inf. |
| Merrill, Sam'l L. | Ass't S. | | From May, 1865. |
| Baker, Loyd W. | " | | To May, 1864. |

### 18TH INFANTRY—Mustered out February 21, 1866.

| | | | |
|---|---|---|---|
| Dods, Wm. B. | Surgeon | Tooele, Utah Ter. | From July, 1865. |
| Ong, Jacob B. | " | St. Leon, Ind. | From May, 1865; also 14th Inf. |

### 19TH INFANTRY—Mustered out January 15, 1867.

| | | | |
|---|---|---|---|
| Carter, Mills O. | Surgeon | Lowell, Mass. | From October, 1864. |
| Topliff, Chas. C. | Ass't S. | Fisherville, N. H. | Died April, 1881. |
| Wachter, C. | H. Stew | Ft. Davis, Tex. | A. G. R. says 2d Lieut. |
| McPherson, J. B. | Surgeon | | To August, 1864. |
| Ransom, John | Ass't S. | | From February, 1865. |

### 20TH INFANTRY—Mustered out October 7, 1865.

| | | | |
|---|---|---|---|
| Cushing, Thos. | Surgeon | Barre Centre, N. Y. | From December, 1863. |
| Dow, F. E. | Ass't S. | West Concord, N. H. | To June, 1865. |
| Stevens, David | " | New Brunswick, N. J. | From Jan., 1864; also 65th Inf. |
| Johnson, John D. | " | | From September, 1865. |

### 21ST INFANTRY—Mustered out April 25, 1866.

| | | | |
|---|---|---|---|
| Hawks, John M. | Surgeon | New Smyrna, Fla. | To Nov., 1865; also 33d Inf. |
| Roberts, N. S. | Ass't S. | | From July, 1863. |
| Burdette, Jas. F. | " | | From September, 1865. |

## U. S. COLORED TROOPS—Continued.

### 22D INFANTRY—Mustered out October 16, 1865.

| Name | Rank | Residence | Remarks |
|---|---|---|---|
| Merrill, C. G. G. | Surgeon | New Haven, Conn | From January, 1864. |
| Moore, Jas. O | Ass't S. | | From January, 1864. |
| Cooper, Stewart | " | | From July, 1865. |
| Phillips, Martin | " | | Dismissed March, 1865. |

### 23D INFANTRY—Mustered out November 30, 1865.

| Name | Rank | Residence | Remarks |
|---|---|---|---|
| Hall, Henry M | Ass't S. | Philadelphia, Pa | To Surg 41st Inf. Sept, 1864. |
| French, John O. | " | Hanover, Mass | From May, 1865. |
| Bethel, B. N | " | 632 N. 18th st., Phila., Pa. | From May, 1865. |
| Saxton, N. S | " | City Island, N. Y. | To December, 1864. |
| Potts, Geo. J | Surgeon | Quincy, Ill. (Old) | Cashiered October, 1865. |
| Sloan, Robt. J | A. A. S | Natchez, Miss. (Old) | From Aug. to Oct., 1865. |
| Copeland, Horatio F. | " | South Abingdon, Mass | In February, 1865. |

### 24TH INFANTRY—Mustered out September 30 and October 1, 1865.

| Name | Rank | Residence | Remarks |
|---|---|---|---|
| Hoffman, E. H | Surgeon | 909 North 25th st., St. Louis, Mo. | From Sept., 1865; also 11th Mo. Inf. |
| McCabe, E. R | " | Leighton, Iowa | To August, 1865. |
| Patte, Emile | Ass't S. | | From June, 1865. |

### 25TH INFANTRY—Mustered out December 6, 1865.

| Name | Rank | Residence | Remarks |
|---|---|---|---|
| Howley, Thos | Surgeon | St Johns, New Foundland. | From January, 1864. |
| Angeor, J. I. M | Ass't S. | | From February, 1864. |
| Adams, Carlos J | " | 253 W. Madison street, Chicago, Ill. | From March, 1864. |
| Jackson, Eben | " | Somerville, Mass | To Surg. 30th Inf. Feb., 1864; also 17th Wis. Inf. |

### 26TH INFANTRY—Mustered out August 28, 1865.

| Name | Rank | Residence | Remarks |
|---|---|---|---|
| Fox, E. C | Ass't S. | Galveston, Tex | From July, 1865; also 128th Inf. |
| Taulman, D. D | " | Cor. 6th and G sts., N. W., Wash., D. C. | From May, 1864. |
| Whitaker, J. L | Surgeon | Unionville, N. Y. | From June, 1865. |

### 27TH INFANTRY—Mustered out September 21, 1865.

| Name | Rank | Residence | Remarks |
|---|---|---|---|
| Niedermyer, H | Ass't S. | River Road, Cincinnati, Ohio. | From Jan., 1864; also 107th Ohio Inf. |
| Weld, Francis M | " | 11 E. 13th street, N. Y. city. | From May, 1864. |

### 28TH INFANTRY—Mustered out November 8, 1865.

| Name | Rank | Residence | Remarks |
|---|---|---|---|
| House, Peter R | Ass't S. | Avoca, N. Y | From August, 1864. |
| Blickhahn, G. H | Surgeon | | From July, 1864. |
| Pierucci, Celso | Ass't S. | 32 Market st., Springfield, Ohio. | From May, 1865; also 83d (old) Infantry. |

### 29TH INFANTRY—Mustered out November 6, 1865.

| Name | Rank | Residence | Remarks |
|---|---|---|---|
| Ewen, Clarence | Ass't S. | Care A. G. U. S. A | From November, 1864. |
| Evans, David J | " | San Bernardino, Cal | From June, 1865. |
| Fee, John | A. A. S | Kansas City, Mo | Not in A. G. R. |
| McKay, David | Surgeon | Dallas, Tex. | From June, 1864; also 79th N. Y. Inf. |

## U. S. COLORED TROOPS—Continued.

30TH INFANTRY—Mustered out December 10, 1865.

Westerling, R .........Ass't S.....Elizabethtown, N. M......From May, 1865; also 12th Heavy Artillery.
Farries, A. P .......... " ........................................From August, 1865.
Jackson, Eben.........Surgeon...Somerville, Mass............To March, 1865; also 25th Inf. and 17th Wis Inf.
Peoble, A. M.......... " Auburn or Augusta, Me. To June, 1865.
McComb, J. J .........Ass't S..........................................To December, 1864.

31ST INFANTRY—Mustered out November 7, 1865.

Barrett, P. G..........Surgeon...Hood's River, Oregon.....From Oct., 1864; also 7th Ohio Cav.
Tremaine, Wm. S.... " Care A. G. U. S. A........To Sept., 1864; also 24th Mass. Inf.
Martin, W. H..........Ass't S.....Died in 1875
Canhell, Clark......... " ........................................From July, 1865.
White, Frank.......... " ........................................Dismissed March, 1865.

32D INFANTRY—Mustered out August 22, 1865.

Wight, Chas. M.......Surgeon...Deceased ..........................From February, 1864.
Mason, Corodon......Ass't S.....Rushford, N. Y..............From March, 1864.
Green, Adolphus...... " 715 Lafayette steeet, St. Louis, Mo. To October, 1864.
Parks, N. O'D.........A. A. S....New Bowery, N. Y........From Dec., 1864, to May, 1865.
Dunn, Sam'l W........ " Maysville, Mo................From January to April, 1865.

33D INFANTRY—Mustered out January 31, 1866.

Minor, T. T.............Ass't S.....Port Townsend, Wash. Ter. To November, 1864.
Stewart, E. S........... " Covington, Ky.................From September, 1865.
Hawks, John M........ " New Smyrna, Fla...........To Surg. 21st Inf. Oct., 1863.
Crandall, Wm. B......Surgeon........................................From June, 1864; also 29th Conn.
Rogers, Seth............ " ........................................To December, 1863.

34TH INFANTRY—Mustered out February 28, 1866.

Hanson, D. D..........Surgeon...New York city.................From July, 1863.
Polk, Chas. G .........Ass't S.....2219 Catharine st., Philadelphia, Pa. From Aug., 1865; also 3d Inf.
Clements, T. R........ " ........................................From October, 1865.
Greenleaf, A. W......Ass't S..........................................To Oct., 1864; also 5th H. A.

35TH INFANTRY—Mustered out July 1, 1866.

Long, John R..........Ass't S.....Cain, W. Va...................To September, 1865.
Mann, Daniel.......... " 1114 Callowhill st., Philadelphia, Pa. To July, 1864.
Marcy, Henry O ......Surgeon...116 Boylston st., Boston, Mass. To May, 1865; also 43d Mass. Inf.
De Grasse, John......Ass't S.....Dead.
Eldridge, Wm. H.....Surgeon.........................................From July, 1865.
Haven, Alfred J ......Ass't S..........................................From September, 1865.

36TH INFANTRY—Mustered out October 28, 1866.

Lampson, M............Ass't S.....334 Communipaw ave., Jersey City, N. J. To March, 1865.
Stockton, J. C.........Surgeon...527 N. 43d st., Phila., Pa. From July, 1864.
Wild, Theodore........Ass't S..........................................From July, 1865.
Arthur, J. P............ " ........................................From July, 1865.
Mitchell, H. H..........Surgeon.........................................To June, 1864.

## U. S. COLORED TROOPS—Continued.

### 37TH INFANTRY—Mustered out February 11, 1867.

| | | | |
|---|---|---|---|
| Cowdrey, A. H | Surgeon | Stoneham, Mass | To June, 1865; also 7th Mass. Inf. |
| Hardy, D. W | " | Sandy Point, Me | From August, 1865. |
| Craig, Wm | Ass't S | Durango, Colo | From July, 1865. |
| Jones, John P | " | | From November, 1865. |

### 38TH INFANTRY—Mustered out January 25, 1867.

| | | | |
|---|---|---|---|
| Brown, Peter B | Ass't S | Somerset, N. Y | From October, 1865. |
| Crouse, Wm | " | 90 1st st., N. Y. city | Dismissed Sept., 1864 |
| Santoire, Sam'l | " | 37 La Fayette avenue, Brooklyn, N. Y. | From October, 1865. |
| Hall, Davis | Surgeon | Dead. | |

### 39TH INFANTRY—Mustered out December 4, 1865.

| | | | |
|---|---|---|---|
| Buckland, Frank | Ass't S | Cold Water, Mich | From May, 1864. Alleged dead. |
| La Barte, John N | " | Kingsville, Ohio | To February, 1865 Alleged dead. |
| Tucker, Maurice | Surgeon | Dead. | |

### 40TH INFANTRY—Mustered out April 25, 1866.

| | | | |
|---|---|---|---|
| Kaull, Wm. M | Surgeon | | From June, 1864. |
| Lee, Alfred H., Jr | Ass't S | | From August, 1865. |
| Draper, Edgar S | " | | From September, 1865. |

### 41ST INFANTRY—Mustered out December 10, 1865.

| | | | |
|---|---|---|---|
| Achim, Anselm | Ass't S | 302 St. Joseph st., Montreal, Canada. | To September, 1865. |
| Hall, Henry M | Surgeon | Philadelphia, Pa | To October, 1864; also 23d Inf. |
| Hemenway, Stacy | " | Fort Klamath, Oregon | From Dec., 1864; also 9th Ill. Cav., now A. Surg. U. S. A. |
| Lambert, Wm. P | Ass't S | | From July, 1865. |

### 42D INFANTRY—Mustered out January 31, 1866.

| | | | |
|---|---|---|---|
| Perry, Jos. J | Ass't S | Richmond, Ind | Dead. |
| Darby, John E | Surgeon | | From May, 1864; also 125th Ohio Inf. |

### 43D INFANTRY—Mustered out October 20, 1865.

| | | | |
|---|---|---|---|
| Lowe, Alexander | Ass't S | San Francisco, Cal | From March, 1864. |
| Waterhouse, Ai | Surgeon | Jamestown, N. Y | From March, 1864; also 7th Maine Inf Ex. S. |
| Chipman, Jas. L | Ass't S | Rehoboth, Mass | From June, 1865. |

### 44TH INFANTRY—Mustered out April 30, 1866.

| | | | |
|---|---|---|---|
| Strong, J. T | Surgeon | Plainville, Ind | From April, 1864. |
| Eastman, Jos. A | Ass't S | | From January, 1866. |

### 45TH INFANTRY—Mustered out November 4, 1865.

| | | | |
|---|---|---|---|
| Folsom, Norton | Surgeon | 19 Berkley st, Cambridge, Mass. | From April, 1864. |
| Hamilton, Rufus S | Ass't S | Montgomery, Vt | From March, 1865. |
| Morris, Henry A | " | Washington, D. C | From July, 1865. |

## U. S. COLORED TROOPS—Continued.

### 46TH INFANTRY—Mustered out January 30, 1866.

| Name | Rank | Residence | Remarks |
|---|---|---|---|
| Paterson, John J | Surgeon | Rockport, Ind | A. W. M. Also 1st Ind. Cav. Dead. |
| Bennett, Jas. H | Ass't S. | | From April, 1863. |
| Martin, Jas. A | " | | To January, 1865. |

### 47TH INFANTRY—Mustered out January 5, 1866.

| Name | Rank | Residence | Remarks |
|---|---|---|---|
| Fitch, Luther P | Ass't S. | Charles City, Iowa | From June, 1863. |
| Alexander, John | " | | To March, 1864. |
| Horton, N. N | Surgeon | Kansas City, Mo | From May, 1863. |
| Scofield, Darius | Ass't S. | | From April, 1864. |

### 48TH INFANTRY—Mustered out January 4, 1866.

| Name | Rank | Residence | Remarks |
|---|---|---|---|
| Bowen, Julius C. | Surgeon | 20 Savannah street, Rochester, N. Y. | To December, 1863. |
| Davis, A. C | " | Greenfield, Mo | To February, 1865 |
| McConaughy, J. B | " | | From May, 1865. |
| Ahern, Robert | Ass't S. | | From August, 1865. |
| Pegg, Chas. H | " | | From September, 1865. |
| Paterson, Arthur | " | | To June, 1864. |
| Hughes, John W | " | | Dismissed October, 1864. |

### 49TH INFANTRY—Mustered out March 22, 1866.

| Name | Rank | Residence | Remarks |
|---|---|---|---|
| Easton, Orsamus | Surgeon | New England, Ohio | To March, 1864. Dead. |
| Glenny, Wm. M | " | Albia, Iowa | From July, 1864. |
| Laning, Sylvester | " | North Liberty, Ind., or Kingman, Kans. | To Nov., 1863; also 48th Ind. Inf. |
| Luhring, Frederick | Ass't S. | Vicksburg, Miss | From September, 1864 |
| Patterson, Thos | H. Stew. | Rochelle, Ill. | |

### 50TH INFANTRY—Mustered out March 20, 1866.

| Name | Rank | Residence | Remarks |
|---|---|---|---|
| Huntsman, H. C | Surgeon | Oskaloosa, Iowa | From Aug., 1863; also 5th Iowa Inf. |
| Fisher, Wm. F | Ass't S. | | From September, 1864. |
| Dean, Dexter V | " | | From August, 1865. |
| Redkey, Geo. W | " | | To May, 1864. |

### 51ST INFANTRY—Mustered out June 16, 1866.

| Name | Rank | Residence | Remarks |
|---|---|---|---|
| Osborne, Henry | Surgeon | Dead | From March, 1864. |
| Arnold, Wm. M | Ass't S. | | From October, 1863. |

### 52D INFANTRY—Mustered out May 5, 1866.

| Name | Rank | Residence | Remarks |
|---|---|---|---|
| Osborn, Harris B | Ass't S. | Kalamazoo, Mich | From September, 1863. |
| Bailey, Wm. N | Surgeon | Plymouth, Ind | From Dec., 1863; also 113th Ill. Inf. |
| Powell, John S | Ass't S. | Hooperston, Ill | From October, 1864. |

### 53D INFANTRY—Mustered out March 8, 1866.

| Name | Rank | Residence | Remarks |
|---|---|---|---|
| Chase, Byron S | Surgeon | Akron, Ohio | From May, 1863; also 16th Ohio Inf. Dead. |
| Key, David | Ass't S. | | From July, 1864. |
| Wilkins, H. H | " | | Dismissed March, 1864. |

### 54TH INFANTRY—Mustered out from August 8 to December 31, 1866.

| Name | Rank | Residence | Remarks |
|---|---|---|---|
| Pyle, Elliott | Surgeon | Burlington, Iowa or Butler, Mo. | From Oct., 1863, to Aug., 1866; also 2d Iowa Inf. |
| Wilson, G. W | Ass't S. | Wolf Island, Mo | To October, 1866. |
| Smith, Lindsy D | " | | To December, 1863. |

## U. S. COLORED TROOPS—Continued.

### 55TH INFANTRY—Mustered out December 31, 1865.

| | | | |
|---|---|---|---|
| Clutter, Wm. H | Ass't S | Frankfort, Kan | To July, 1865. |
| Eaton, John M | " | Milford, Mass | To October, 1864. |
| Hall, Wm. C | " | West Minot, Me | From December. 1864. |
| Humphrey, Wesley | Surgeon | Moberly, Mo | From May, 1863; also 52d Ill. Inf. Ex. S. |
| Kugler, Jos | Ass't S | | From September, 1865. |

### 56TH INFANTRY—Mustered out September 15, 1866.

| | | | |
|---|---|---|---|
| La Force, D. A | Surgeon | Agency City or Ashland, Iowa. | From August, 1864. |
| Sykes, Jas | Ass't S | Beverly, Ill | From April, 1865. |
| Sholz, Geo | " | | To June, 1864. |
| Childs, Henry J | " | | To January, 1864. |

### 57TH INFANTRY—Mustered out October 18 and December 13, 1866.

| | | | |
|---|---|---|---|
| Dice, T. R | Surgeon | Utica, Mo | To December, 1865. G. |
| *Bridges, V. R | " | Mattoon, Ill | U. S. Examining Surg. |
| Wright, Chas. B | " | | From March, 1866. |

### 58TH INFANTRY—Mustered out April 30, 1866.

| | | | |
|---|---|---|---|
| Coats, Noyce | Surgeon | | From September, 1864. |
| Gray, Elias W | Ass't S | Bloomington, Ill | From October, 1863. |
| Bidlock, Wm. W | " | | From September, 1865. |
| Sloan, Robert J | Surgeon | | To April, 1864; also 30th Missouri Inf. |

### 59TH INFANTRY—Mustered out January 31, 1866.

| | | | |
|---|---|---|---|
| Bristol, B. J | Surgeon | Webster, Mo | From August, 1865. |
| Farrington, J. H | H. Stew | Rochester, N. H. | |
| Ingalls John | Ass't S | Memphis, Tenn | From Aug., 1863. Dead. |
| Rush, John | Surgeon | | To June, 1865. |

### 60TH INFANTRY—Mustered out October 15, 1865.

| | | | |
|---|---|---|---|
| Patton, Andrew | Surgeon | Nevada, Iowa | From September, 1864. |
| Knowles, Freeman | " | Keokuk, Iowa | To June, 1864. |
| Rayburn, Cyrus E | Ass't S | Brooklyn, Iowa | From Oct., 1864. Dead. |
| Richardson S. D | A. A. S. | Long Grove, Iowa | From March to May, 1864. |
| Baman, C. F | " | Boston, Mass | In June and July, 1864. |

### 61ST INFANTRY—Mustered out December 30, 1865.

| | | | |
|---|---|---|---|
| Quimby, S. J | Surgeon | Memphis, Tenn | From September, 1863. |
| Hazlewood, A | Ass't S | | From September, 1863. |
| Watts. Henry R | " | | Deserted Sept , 1863. |
| Dennis, Warden B | H. Stew | Effingham, Ill. | |

### 62D INFANTRY—Mustered out March 31, 1866.

| | | | |
|---|---|---|---|
| Cordan, Allen | Surgeon | Eldon, Iowa | From January, 1864. |
| Gordon, O. W | Ass't S | Fairfield, Iowa | To December, 1864 |
| Winslow, Chas | " | | From October, 1865. |

### 63D INFANTRY—Mustered out January 9, 1866.

| | | | |
|---|---|---|---|
| McCord, D. O | Surgeon | St. Joseph, Mo | From October, 1863 |
| Miles, Wm. H | Ass't S | | From November, 1863. |

* Was Surgeon of the 126th Illinois and attended members of this regiment at Devall's Bluff, Ark., from December, 1863, to February, 1864.

## U. S. COLORED TROOPS—Continued.

### 64TH INFANTRY—Mustered out March 13, 1866.

| Name | Rank | Residence | Remarks |
|---|---|---|---|
| Wright, T. J | Surgeon | | A. W. M. |
| Yost, John M. | Ass't S. | Mt. Zion, Iowa | From July, 1865. |

### 65TH INFANTRY—Mustered out January 8, 1867.

| Name | Rank | Residence | Remarks |
|---|---|---|---|
| Stevens, David | Ass't S. | New Brunswick, N. J. | From Nov., 1865; also 20th Inf. |
| Jordan, Josiah | Surgeon | Dead | Also 67th Infantry. |
| Fish, John | " | Auburn, Ohio | From August, 1865. |
| Leffingwell, H. S. | " | | To October, 1864. |

### 66TH INFANTRY—Mustered out March 20, 1866.

| Name | Rank | Residence | Remarks |
|---|---|---|---|
| Jay, Joseph R | Surgeon | | From January, 1864. |
| Brown, Jas. | Ass't S. | | From January, 1864. |

### 67TH INFANTRY—Consolidated with 65th Infantry July 12, 1865.

| Name | Rank | Residence | Remarks |
|---|---|---|---|
| Jordan, Josiah | Surgeon | Dead | Also 65th Inf. |
| Halleck, Richard S. | Ass't S. | | To September, 1864. |

### 68TH INFANTRY—Mustered out February 5, 1866.

| Name | Rank | Residence | Remarks |
|---|---|---|---|
| Lyford, B. F. | Ass't S. | Lock-box 1222, San Francisco, Cal. | From July, 1864. |
| Andrews, E. E. | Surgeon | | From March, 1864. |

### 69TH INFANTRY—Failed to complete.

### 70TH INFANTRY—Mustered out March 7, 1866.

| Name | Rank | Residence | Remarks |
|---|---|---|---|
| Reynolds, Oliver K. | Surgeon | Kane, Ill. | From April, 1864; also 71st Inf. |
| Whitaker, Jas. M. | Ass't S. | Windham, N. H. (?) | A. W. M. |
| Orr, Samuel L. | Surgeon | | To November, 1864. |

### 71ST INFANTRY—Consolidated with 70th Infantry November 8, 1864.

| Name | Rank | Residence | Remarks |
|---|---|---|---|
| Reynolds, Oliver K. | Surgeon | Kane, Ill. | From April, 1864; also 70th Inf. |

### 72D INFANTRY—Discontinued May 3, 1865.

| Name | Rank | Residence | Remarks |
|---|---|---|---|
| Twitchell, R. W. | Surgeon | Chatfield, Minn. | From July, 1864; also 119th Inf. and 9th Minn. Inf. Ex. S. |
| Bushnell, John H. | A. A. S. | 1212 10th street, N. W., Washington, D. C. | |
| Carter, Frank | Ass't S. | | To May, 1865. |
| Neal, Selden F. | " | | To 13th Inf. June, 1865. |

### 73D INFANTRY—Consolidated with 96th Infantry September 27, 1865.

| Name | Rank | Residence | Remarks |
|---|---|---|---|
| Huntington, R. M. | Ass't S. | Boone, Iowa | To May, 1865. |
| Payne, J. T | Surgeon | 242 Esplanade street, New Orleans, La | From September, 1862; also 96th Inf. |

### 74TH INFANTRY—Mustered out October 11, 1865.

| Name | Rank | Residence | Remarks |
|---|---|---|---|
| Willis, Lemuel M. | Surgeon | Boston, Mass. | To June, 1865; also 26th Mass. Inf. |
| Gihon, John H | " | | From September, 1865. |

### 75TH INFANTRY—Mustered out November 25, 1865.

| Name | Rank | Residence | Remarks |
|---|---|---|---|
| Howe, Alex. T. | Surgeon | | From November, 1862. |
| Wilkins, Clarence L. | Ass't S. | | From December, 1863. |

## U. S. COLORED TROOPS—Continued.

### 76TH INFANTRY—Mustered out December 31, 1865.

| | | | |
|---|---|---|---|
| Coad, Mathias | Ass't S | Williamstown, Mich | From July, 1863. |
| Brown, Henry W | Surgeon | Dead. | |
| Russell, Edward | " | | Dismissed April, 1862. |

### 77TH INFANTRY—Consolidated with 10th Heavy Artillery October 1, 1865.

| | | | |
|---|---|---|---|
| Poindexter, John | Surgeon | | From January, 1864; also 87th Ill. Inf. |
| Hurley, Jas. M | Ass't S | | From September, 1865. |
| Warner, John T | " | | To February, 1865; also 83d Inf. (old). |

### 78TH INFANTRY—Mustered out January 6, 1866.

| | | | |
|---|---|---|---|
| Lathrop, Moses C | Surgeon | | From October, 1863. |
| Ansell, Aaron | Ass't S | | From August, 1863. |
| David, Wm. G | Surgeon | | To August, 1865. |
| Osborn, Nehemiah | Ass't S | | Dismissed March, 1865. |

### 79TH INFANTRY—(Old)—Discontinued July 28, 1864.

| | | | |
|---|---|---|---|
| Fisher, Chas. L | Surgeon | Troy, N. Y | From March, 1863; also 84th and 123d Inf. |
| Hershay, David | Ass't S | New York city | From March, 1863; also 84th Inf. |
| Alleman, Levi J | " | Boone, Iowa | Transferred to 81st Inf April, 1863. |
| Baird, John H | " | | To December, 1864; also 82d Inf. |

### 79TH INFANTRY—(New)—Mustered out October 1, 1865.

| | | | |
|---|---|---|---|
| Ensor, J. Fulton | Surgeon | Columbia, S. C | From November, 1864 |
| Macy, E G | Ass't S | Clinton, Kan | To June, 1864. |
| Burr, C. S | " | Dead. | |
| Harrington, S C | Surgeon | Dead. | |
| Tenney, A. D | Ass't S | Dead. | |

### 80TH INFANTRY—Mustered out March 1, 1867.

| | | | |
|---|---|---|---|
| Scoon, Jas. H | Surgeon | Amsterdam, N. Y | A. W. M. |
| Mills, Lucius | Ass't S | | From July, 1865. |
| Failing, Walter | " | Evansville, Ind | A. W. M. |
| Percival, Geo. G | " | | To March, 1864. |

### 81ST INFANTRY—Mustered out November 30, 1866.

| | | | |
|---|---|---|---|
| Alleman, Levi J | Ass't S | Boone, Iowa | To August, 1863; also 79th Inf. (old.) |
| Blackwood, S. W | Surgeon | | From September, 1865. |
| Bogardus, John C | Ass't S | Kingston, N. Y | From September, 1865. |
| Johnson, John D | " | | From January, 1866. |
| Magee, John P | " | | To March, 1864. |
| Palmer, Daniel E | Surgeon | | To November, 1864 |
| Pilgrim, S. V | " | 108 Columbia st., New York city. | To April, 1864; also 145th Pa. Inf. |

### 82D INFANTRY—Mustered out September 10, 1866.

| | | | |
|---|---|---|---|
| Pierce, Chas M | Surgeon | Dead | From December, 1863. |
| Baird, John H | Ass't S | Dead | From April, 1865; also 79th Inf. (old.) |
| Ransom, John | " | | To January, 1864. |
| Hibbler, Rand. W | " | | To February, 1864. |

## U. S. COLORED TROOPS—Continued.

### 83D INFANTRY—(Old)—Discontinued July 28, 1864.

Warner, John T ......Ass't S.......................................Transferred to 77th Inf. August, 1864.
Pierucci, Celso.........Surgeon...32 Market st., Springfield. Ohio..To Feb., 1864, also 28th Inf.

### 83D INFANTRY—(New)—Mustered out October 9, 1865.

Wood, Jesse D.........Ass't S....Waveland, Kans..............A. W. M.
Walgamott, Geo. W..Surgeon.......................................To April, 1864; also 3d Kansas Inf.
Morse, D. A.............. " .......................................To July, 1865.
Thomas, Francis P...Ass't S.......................................To June, 1865.

### 84TH INFANTRY—Mustered out March 14, 1866.

Fisher, Charles L.....Surgeon...Troy, N. Y.....................Also 79th and 123d Inf.
Murray, H. A..........Ass't S.....New York city..............Dismissed March, 1866; also 87th Inf.
Cottrell, Geo. H ......H. Stew...Kalamazoo, Mich.
Hershay, David.......Surgeon...New York city..............To Dec., 1865; also 79th Inf.

### 85TH INFANTRY—Consolidated with the 77th Infantry May 24, 1864.

Spencer, Jas. E........Surgeon.......................................To November, 1864.

### 86TH INFANTRY—Mustered out April 10, 1866.

*Piquette, Francis E..Surgeon...Opelousas, La................To March, 1866.
Griswold, Wait R.....Ass't S.......................................To June, 1865.

### 87TH INFANTRY—(Old)—Consolidated with 95th Infantry November 26, 1864, to form 87th Infantry (new).

Sands, Sylvanus ......Ass't S.......................................From September, 1863.

### 87TH INFANTRY—(New)—Consolidated with 84th Infantry August 14, 1865.

Webster, Wm. S......Surgeon.......................................From April, 1864.
Murray, Henry A.....Ass't S.....New York city................From March, 1865; transferred to 8th Inf.
Pease, Byron W....... " Thomaston, Conn..........To January, 1865.

### 88TH INFANTRY—(Old)—Disbanded July 28, 1864

Fish, John ...............Surgeon...Auburn, Ohio.................To July, 1865; also 10th Heavy Art.
Reynolds, Albert .....Ass't S.....Independence, Iowa ......To January, 1864.

### 88TH INFANTRY—(New)—Consolidated with 3d Heavy Artillery December 16, 1865.

Manson, Chas. A......Ass't S.....177 State st., Springfield, Mass. From Sept., 1865, to Jan., 1866.
Simon, Wm...............Surgeon.......................................From May, 1865.

### 89TH INFANTRY—Disbanded July 28, 1864

Dean, Chas. A...... .Surgeon...Baton Rouge, La ..........To March, 1864; also 2d La. Inf.

### 90TH INFANTRY—Disbanded July 28, 1864.

Warren, Chas. E......Surgeon.......................................From Sept., 1863; transferred to 97th Inf. Aug. 1864.

*Had charge of Corps d'Afrique Hospital, New Orleans.

## U. S. COLORED TROOPS—Continued.

91ST INFANTRY—Consolidated with 74th Infantry July 7, 1874.

Green, J. Dunham...Surgeon..........................From October, 1863; also 1st Louisiana Inf.

92D INFANTRY—Mustered out December 31, 1865.

Murphy, John .........Surgeon..........................A. W. M. Also 37th Ill. Inf.
Miller, Wm. M ........Ass't S..........................To March, 1865.

93D INFANTRY—Disbanded June 23, 1865, and men transferred to the 81st and 82d Infantry. Officers (with three exceptions mustered) out on account of incompetency.

Wilkins, David ........Surgeon..........................To July, 1865.

94TH INFANTRY—Failed to complete.

95TH INFANTRY—Consolidated with 87th Infantry November 26, 1864.

Webster, W. S.........Surgeon..........................From April, 1864; transferred to 87th Infantry, (new.)
Pease, B. W ..........Ass't S..........................From May, 1864; transferred to 87th Infantry, (new.)
Warren, Chas. E...... " ..........................To Surg. 90th Inf. Sept., 1863.
Chubbuck, John ......Surgeon..........................To March, 1864.

96TH INFANTRY—Mustered out January 29, 1866.

Day, Alfred ............A. A. S....Mechanicsburgh, Pa ......April, 1865; not in A. G.'s Report
Fisher, Chas. H.........Surgeon...North Scituate, R. I ......From November, 1865.
Payne, J. T. ........... " 242 Esplanade st., New Orleans, La. To Nov., 1865; also 73d Inf.
Lewis, Geo. F..........A. A. S.. .Bridgeport, Conn.
Willson, John B........Surgeon..........................To January, 1865.
Martin, James.........Ass't S..........................To May, 1865.

97TH INFANTRY—Mustered out April 6, 1866.

Lester, Elias.............Surgeon...Seneca Falls, N. Y..... ...To July, 1864.
Warren, Chas. E...... " ..........................From September, 1863.
Bauer, Herman........Ass't S..........................From December, 1864.

98TH INFANTRY—Consolidated with 78th Infantry August, 26, 1865.

Lathrop, Moses C.....Surgeon..........................From Oct., 1863; also 19th Iowa Inf.

99TH INFANTRY—Mustered out April 23, 1866.

Gregory, Jas. R. ......Ass't S.....Westminster, Cal..........To June, 1864.
Huberich, H.............Surgeon...Dead.
Bacon, H. M............Ass't S..........................To December, 1863.

100TH INFANTRY—Mustered out December 26, 1865.

Elliott, Justin C......Surgeon...Titusville, Pa.................From June, 1864; also 18th Kentucky Inf.
Lescher, Sam'l B.....Ass't S.....Oakland City, Ind..........Dismissed May, 1865.
Ware, E. H............. " Dead..........................Also 6th Infantry.
Hair, B. W...............A. A. S....Hamilton, Ohio................Also 10th Infantry.

## U. S. COLORED TROOPS—Continued.

### 101st Infantry—Mustered out January, 21, 1866.

| | | | |
|---|---|---|---|
| Ford, Edward J | Surgeon | | From January, 1865. |
| Tuttle, F. A | Ass't S | | From October, 1865. |

### 102d Infantry—Mustered out September 30, 1865.

| | | | |
|---|---|---|---|
| Spiers, Wm. W | Ass't S | Chase, Kans | From June, 1864. Ex. S. |
| Vincent, Wesley | Surgeon | 181 W. Madison street, Chicago, Ill. | From February, 1864. |
| Curtis, —— | H. Stew | Flint, Mich. | |
| Jennings, E. P | Ass't S | | To October, 1864. |

### 103d Infantry—Mustered out from April 15 to 20, 1866.

| | | | |
|---|---|---|---|
| Babbitt, W. M | Surgeon | | To April, 1866; also 54th Mass. Inf. |
| Boice, Jas. S | Ass't S | | To April, 1866. |
| Wiser, Wm. H | " | | To April, 1866. |

### 104th Infantry—Mustered out February 5, 1866.

| | | | |
|---|---|---|---|
| Radzinsky, L. D | Surgeon | McKeesport, Pa | From June, 1865; also 36th N. Y. Inf. |
| Paine, A. Elliott | Ass't S | | From August, 1865. |

### 106th Infantry—Consolidated with 140th Infantry November 7, 1865.

### 107th Infantry—Mustered out November 22, 1866.

| | | | |
|---|---|---|---|
| Chalfant, C. M | Surgeon | 326 Pearl street, Cleveland, Ohio. | From August, 1864; also 111th Ohio Inf. |
| Mooar, Jacob W | A. A. S | 939 Elm st., Manchester, N. H. | Not in A. G. R. |
| Codman, Wm. S | Ass't S | Dead. | |
| North, Jas. W | " | | To May, 1865. |

### 108th Infantry—Mustered out March 21, 1866.

| | | | |
|---|---|---|---|
| Martin, Pearl | Surgeon | Medford, Mass | To August, 1865. |
| Ellis, Daniel F | " | | From December, 1865. |
| Woodman, J. W | Ass't S | | From October, 1864. |

### 109th Infantry—Mustered out February 6, 1866.

| | | | |
|---|---|---|---|
| Gratigny, L. H | Surgeon | 202 W. 4th street, Cincinnati, Ohio. | From June, 1864; also 15th Inf. |
| Kinne, T. Y | Ass't S | 82 Broadway, Paterson, N. J. | From October, 1865. |
| Wells, D. E | " | Dead. | |
| Graves, Milan | " | | To February, 1865. |

### 110th Infantry—Mustered out February 6, 1866.

| | | | |
|---|---|---|---|
| Donohue, T | Surgeon | St. Louis, Mo | From January, 1864. |
| Little, Jehu | Ass't S | Bloomington, Ill | From Sept., 1865; also 24th Missouri Inf. and Hosp't Stew. U. S. A. |

| | | | |
|---|---|---|---|
| Miner, Selden | Surgeon | Hancock, Wis | From December, 1865. |
| Thombs, P. R | Ass't S | Pueblo, Colo | From January, 1866. |
| Dickson, John | Surgeon | | To October, 1865. |

### 112 Infantry—Consolidated with 11th (old) and 113th (old) to form 113th Infantry (new) April 1, 1865.

### 113th Infantry—(Old)—Consolidated with the 11th (old) and 112th to form 113th Infantry (new) April 1, 1865.

## U. S. COLORED TROOPS—Continued.

### 113TH INFANTRY—(New)—Mustered out April 9, 1866.

Hipolite, Wm. W......Surgeon...Devall's Bluff, Ark.........From Mar., '65; also 11th Inf. & 29th Wis. Inf.
Wheelock, Jas. W....Ass't S.........................................From April, 1865.

### 114TH INFANTRY—Mustered out April 2, 1867.

Horr, Oren A...... ....Ass't S....Lewiston, Me..................To October, 1865.
Radmore, Chas. C...Surgeon...Lincoln, Neb...............From July, 1864; also 44th and 107th Ill. Inf.
Norris Albert L......Ass't S.........................................From October, 1866.
Perry, Orville H...... " .........................................To August, 1865.

### 115TH INFANTRY—Mustered out February 10, 1866.

Ham, John R..........Surgeon...Dover, N. H.................From October, 1865.
Walker, Robert C.....Ass't S.....Burlington, Iowa...........From November, 1864.

### 116TH INFANTRY—Mustered out January 17, 1867.

Egle, W. H...............Surgeon...Harrisburgh, Pa...........To November, 1865.
* Roberts, John H....H. Stew...Grand Rapids, Mich.
Merrill, Alfred W.....Ass't S.........................................From August, 1865.
Trask, Peleg B........ " .........................................To December, 1864.

### 117TH INFANTRY—Mustered out August 10, 1867.

Butcher, H. B. .........A. A. S....842 N. 19th st., Philadelphia, Pa. In September, 1866. Not in A. G. R.
Elliott, Chas. A.......Ass't S.....Somersworth, N. H........To March, 1865.
Rogers, Orville F..... " Dorchester, Mass............From November, 1864.
Spohn, Henry.........A. A. S...Laredo, Tex.....................In July and August, 1867. Not in A. G. R.
Harter, Peter C.......Ass't S.....Alleged dead.................Missing since Jan., 1866.
Putnam, Thos.........Surgeon.........................................Cashiered March, 1865.

### 118TH INFANTRY—Mustered out February 6, 1866.

Tevis, Joel T............Ass't S.....St. Paul or Rushville, Ind. From October, 1864.
Winn, Alex. M......... " Dead.
Adams, Russell D.....Surgeon.........................................From July, 1864.

### 119TH INFANTRY—Mustered out April 27, 1866.

Estabrook, Geo. C....Ass't S.....North Haven, Me...........From January, 1865.
Twitchell, R. W ......Surgeon...Chatfield, Minn...............From Sept., 1865; also 72d Inf. and 9th Minn. Inf. Ex. S.
Neal, Selden F.........Ass't S.........................................From November, 1865.
Hobbs, Benj ........... " Dead...................................To January, 1865; also 116th Inf.
Abbott, Josiah.........Surgeon.........................................To Sept., 1865; also 13th Heavy Artillery.

### 120TH INFANTRY—Disbanded June 21, 1865.

### 121ST INFANTRY—Disbanded June 30, 1865.

Jackson, J. B..........Surgeon.........................................To September, 1865.

### 122D INFANTRY—Mustered out February 8, 1866.

Willis, Chas. B.........Surgeon.........................................From October, 1864.
Creaghe, J. O. D......Ass't S.........................................From August, 1865.

* Was in Regular Army with regiment from February 18 to August 19, 1865, also in February, 1866.

## U. S. COLORED TROOPS—Continued.

### 123D INFANTRY—Mustered out October 16, 1865.

Fisher, Chas. L........Surgeon...Troy, N. Y.....................From January, 1865; also 79th and 84th Inf.
Sweet, Rich'd..........Ass't S....Saxonsburg, Pa...............From December, 1864.

### 124TH INFANTRY—Mustered out October 24, 1865.

House, Wm. W........Surgeon...Lincoln, Ill.........................From May, 1865.

### 125TH INFANTRY—Part mustered out October 31; the rest December 20, 1867.

Day, Wm. T...........Surgeon.............................................From April, 1865.

### 127TH INFANTRY—Mustered out October 20, 1865.

Chapman, E. A........Ass't S.....Belleville, N. Y...............From November, 1864.
Chase, John W .......H. Stew...Dedham, Mass.
Powell, Wm. C........Surgeon...Bristleton, Pa...................From September, 1864.

### 128TH INFANTRY—Mustered out October 10, 1866.

Fox, Edward C.......Ass't S.....Galveston, Tex................To October, 1866; also 26th Inf.
Durrant, Henry K...Surgeon.............................................To July, 1866.

### 135TH INFANTRY—Mustered out October 23, 1865.

Parks, Hinton F......Surgeon.............................................From March, 1865.
Shoales, Geo. A.......Ass't S...............................................From August, 1865.

### 136TH INFANTRY—Mustered out January 4, 1866.

Ranney, Geo. E......Surgeon.............................................From July, 1865.
Baker, Edward F.....Ass't S...............................................From September, 1865.

### 137TH INFANTRY—Mustered out January 15, 1866.

Briggs, C. F. H........Surgeon...Grand Haven, Mich........From April, 1865.
Stannard, W. D.......Ass't S...............................................From July, 1865.

### 138TH INFANTRY—Mustered out January 6, 1866.

Maxwell, Thos. J.....Surgeon...Briggsville, Ill...................From July, 1865; also 3d Iowa Cav.
Sweazey, Caleb.......Ass't S...............................................From July, 1865.

## U. S. SHARPSHOOTERS.

(Names and addresses as reported by the Surgeon-General U. S. A.)

1ST SHARPSHOOTERS—The veterans and recruits from Michigan were transferred to the 5th Michigan Infantry; the rest to the 2d U. S. Sharpshooters December 31, 1864.

Brennan, John W....Surgeon...143 Lexington ave., New York city. To November, 1863.
Brennan, Geo. M..... " 148 E. 30th street, New York city. To Nov., 1864. Dead.
Snelling, F. G.........Ass't S.....227 Lexington ave., New York city. To Surg. U. S. V. April, 1862.
Thompson, W. C......Surgeon...Indianapolis, Ind..............January and February, 1862.
Noyes, J. H.............Ass't S.....Ogden, Iowa.....................January and February, 1863.
Tripler, C. S............Surgeon...Dead.....................................December, 1861.
Hale, Chas. F..........Ass't S...............................................To 2d U. S. S. October, 1861.

2D SHARPSHOOTERS—The members of this regiment were transferred February, 1865, as follows: Company A to 5th Michigan Infantry; Company C to 105th Pennsylvania Infantry; Company D to 17th Maine Infantry; Companies E and H to 4th Vermont Infantry; and Companies F and G to 5th New Hampshire Infantry.

| Name | Rank | Address | Service |
|---|---|---|---|
| *Hawks, H. T | Ass't S | 45 E. 30th street, New York city. | From January to March 25, 1863. |
| Thompson, W. C | Surgeon | Indianapolis, Ind | February, 1862. |
| Reynolds, W. B | " | Lynn, Mass | To Jan., 1865. Dead. |
| Hale, C. F | " | | Dropped Nov., 1862. |
| Williams, A. A. C | " | Dead | To August, 1863. |
| Palmer, Oscar | Ass't S | | To October, 1864. |

## UNITED STATES VETERAN VOLUNTEERS.

(Names and addresses as reported by the Surgeon-General U. S A.)

1ST VETERAN VOLUNTEERS—(Engineers)—Mustered out in June, 1865, and September 26, 1865.

| Name | Rank | Address | Service |
|---|---|---|---|
| Farrow, W. H | A. A. S | Snow Hill, Md | September and October, 1865. |
| Haise, Geo A | Ass't S | Ridgeley, Mo | From February, 1865. |
| Brown, Albert G | " | Alexandria Mo | From March, 1865. |
| Sherwood, W. P | A. A. S | Millbrook, Ill | November, 1864. |
| Edelin, Alfred | Surgeon | Dead | From February, 1865. |

1ST VETERAN VOLUNTEERS—(Infantry)—Mustered out at different dates from January 10 to July 21, 1866.

| Name | Rank | Address | Service |
|---|---|---|---|
| Sheldon, J. J | Ass't S | Beattie, Kan | From February, 1865, to February, 1866. |
| Dean, Henry M | " | Muscatine, Iowa | From February, 1865, to January, 1866. |
| Stanton, J. O | A. A. S | Washington, D. C | January and February, 1865. U. S. Ex. S. |
| Betton, Thos F | Surgeon | Dead | From March, 1865, to March, 1866 |

2D VETERAN VOLUNTEERS—(Infantry)—Mustered out at different dates from February 3 to August 1, 1866.

| Name | Rank | Address | Service |
|---|---|---|---|
| Reynolds, Frank | Surgeon | Retired. Care A. G. U. S. A. | From March, 1865, to March, 1866; also 88th N. Y. Inf. |
| Mulford, Wm. C | Ass't S | Wilcox Wharf, Charles City County, Va. | From September, 1865, to March, 1866. |
| Trautman, Chas. T | " | Dead | From March, 1865, to March, 1866. |

3D VETERAN VOLUNTEERS—(Infantry)—Mustered out at different dates from March 6 to 20, 1866.

| Name | Rank | Address | Service |
|---|---|---|---|
| Wonsetler, Gideon | Surgeon | Hicksville, Ohio | From March, 1865, to May, 1866. |
| Forrest, John M | Ass't S | Oakland, Cal | From June, 1865, to March, 1866. |
| Cummings, Geo. W | " | | From March, 1865, to April, 1866. |

*Belonged to the 30th New York Volunteers.

## U. S. VETERAN VOLUNTEERS—Continued.

4TH VETERAN VOLUNTEERS—(Infantry)—Mustered out at different dates from March 1 to August 6, 1866.

Merritt, David.........Surgeon...2124 Fitzwater street, Philadelphia, Pa. From March, 1865, to April, 1866.
Paine, R. E...............Ass't S.....Camden, Maine..............From March, 1865, to March, 1866.
Matthews, Wash'n...A. A. S.....Now Ass't Surg. U. S. A..From September to December, 1865.
Miller, Geo. W.........Ass't S.....Dead..........................Dropped October, 1865.

5TH VETERAN VOLUNTEERS—(Infantry)—Mustered out from February 16 to July 20, 1866.

Miller, Wm. H.........Ass't S.....Luray, Va......................From May, 1865, to Mar., 1866; also 6th and 9th Vet. Vols.
Stevens, Joseph.......A. A. S....Towanda, Pa...............August and November, 1865.
Hunt, Sylvester H...Ass't S.........................................From May, 1865, to February, 1866.
Volk, Wm. W.........Surgeon...Dead..........................To October, 1865.
Shakerly, J. F.........A. A. S....Dead..........................November, 1865, to February, 1866.
Rizer, Martin..........Surgeon...Dead..........................From February, 1865, to March, 1866.

6TH VETERAN VOLUNTEERS—(Infantry)—Mustered out from March 15 to July 27, 1866.

Upton, Geo..............Ass't S.....Lagrangeville, N. Y......To March, 1866.
Stevens, Joseph.......A. A. S ...Towanda, Pa...................From Nov., 1865; also 5th and 9th Vet. Vols.
McDowell, A. W......Surgeon...Dead..........................To April, 1866.
Lloyd, David C.......Ass't S....Dead..........................To April, 1866.

7TH VETERAN VOLUNTEERS—(Infantry)—Mustered out from February 9 to July 23, 1866.

Gillespie, Jas. L......Surgeon...Sistersville, W. Va.........To April 1866; also 1st and 14th W. Va. Inf.
Wilson, Arthur H.....Ass't S.....504 E. Broadway, Boston, Mass To April, 1866.
Butler, J. W............A. A. S....Burnt Cabins, Pa............January, 1866.
Stayman, A. F.........Ass't S.....Dead..........................To February, 1866.

8TH VETERAN VOLUNTEERS—(Infantry)—Mustered out from February 15 to July 28, 1866.

McMillen, Geo W....Surgeon...Osage Mission, Kan.......To April, 1866.
Hines, C. M............Ass't S....Washington, D. C..........To February, 1866. Dead.
Transue, Abs ......... " Washington, D. C..........To May, 1866.

9TH VETERAN VOLUNTEERS—(Infantry)—Mustered out from February 26 to July 1, 1866.

Greely, Geo. P.........Surgeon...Nashua, N. H...............To May, 1866.
——, Samuel W.......Ass't S....St. Martin's New Brunswick. To March, 1866.
Marsh, Francis E.... " Quincy, Mich...............To March, 1866.
Stevens, Jos............A. A. S....Towanda, Pa...............May to June, 1865; also 5th and 6th Vet. Vols.

## UNITED STATES VOLUNTEER INFANTRY.

(Names and addresses as reported by the Surgeon General U. S. A.)

### 1st Infantry—Part mustered out November 27, 1865; the rest May 10 and 21, 1866.

| Name | Rank | Address | Service |
|---|---|---|---|
| Crapper, H. N | A. A. S. | Webster City, Iowa | July, 1865. |
| Matthews, Wash'ton | " | Care Adjutant General | Assistant Surgeon U. S. A. July, 1865. |
| Bradley, W. H | " | 181 W. Madison st., Chicago, Ill. | October, 1865. |
| Peters, DeWitt C | Ass't S. | Dead. | |
| Herrick, Geo. H. W. | Surgeon | Dead | To November, 1865. |

### 2d Infantry—(1 year)—Mustered out November 7, 1865.

| Name | Rank | Address | Service |
|---|---|---|---|
| Seymour, Fred | Surgeon | Van Buren and Halstead sts, Chicago, Ill. | To August, 1865. |
| McNeil, Daniel C | Ass't S. | Osceola, Mo | From February, 1865. |
| Williams, John F. | " | 411 Centre st., Chicago | From March, 1865. |
| *De Lamater, J. J | Surgeon | 811 11th st., N.W., Washington, D. C. | From October to December, 1864. |
| Crowley, Jas. W | A. A. S. | Salina, Kan | April and May, 1865. |
| Bunkley, J. Thos | " | | January, 1865. |
| Smith, Robert K | Surgeon | Dead | October, 1864 |

### 3d Infantry—(1 year)—Mustered out November 29, 1865.

| Name | Rank | Address | Service |
|---|---|---|---|
| Becker, Chas | Ass't S. | Carlinville, Ill | From April, 1865. |
| Yates, C. P | A. A. S. | Jacksonville, Mo | May, 1865. |
| Bennett, John C | Surgeon | | To June, 1865. |
| Harstig, Chas | Ass't S. | Dead | From April, 1865. |

### 4th Infantry—Mustered out June 18, 19, and July 2, 1866.

| Name | Rank | Address | Service |
|---|---|---|---|
| Russell, Leonard F. | Surgeon | Anoka, Me | From November, 1864 |
| Crapper, H. N | A. A. S. | Webster City, Iowa | August, 1865. |
| Glatfelder, N. M | Ass't S. | St. Louis, Mo | From September, 1865, to April, 1866. |
| Town, F. L | " | Care A. G. U. S. A. | January, 1866. Surgeon U. S. A. |

### 5th Infantry—Mustered out from October 11 to November 13, 1866.

| Name | Rank | Address | Service |
|---|---|---|---|
| Finlaw, Wm. C. | Surgeon | Santa Rosa, Cal | From April, 1865. |
| Smith, Henry J. | Ass't S. | 129 Geary st., San Francisco, Cal. | From April, 1865. |
| Riddler, John J. | " | Jefferson City, Mo | From May, 1865. |
| Campfield, R. B | A. A. S. | Belmont, Kan | April, 1866. |

### 6th Infantry—Mustered out from October 10 to November 3, 1866.

| Name | Rank | Address | Service |
|---|---|---|---|
| Lester, Gilbert B | Surgeon | Oswego, Ill | From May, 1865. |
| Silliman, H. R | Ass't S. | 1623 Pine st., Philadelphia, Pa. | From Sept. to Nov., '65. Retired, U. S. A. |
| Silliman, C. B | A. A. S. | Columbus, Neb | April, 1866. |
| Yates, C. P. | " | Jacksonville, Mo | June and July, 1865. |
| Wenz, Julius | Ass't S. | | From May, 1865. |

* Surgeon in charge of Fort Ripley, Minn., from 1871 to summer of 1874.

## HOSPITALS, ETC.

### BATON ROUGE, LA.

Green, F. C., Easthampton, Mass. } In 1863.
Dolson, Joseph S., Bath, N. Y. }
Mather, William H., (Surgeon 173d New York,) Suffield or Hartford, Conn.

### BRATTLEBOROUGH, VT.

Phelps, Edward E., Windsor, Vt. In 1864.
Goss, Story N., (Ex-Surgeon.) Chelsea, Vt. June to September, 1864.

### BEAUFORT, S. C.

Boynton, H., Woodstock, Vt. In 1862.

### CLIFFBURN, D. C.

Dearing, T. H., Braintree, Mass. In 1864.

### CORRY. AUGUSTA, ME.

Bradbury, O. N.. Norway, Me. From June 1, 1864, to September, 1865, and from January to July, 1866.

### CAMP LANDER, WENHAM, MASS.

Hurd, Y. G., (Surgeon 48th Massachusetts Infantry,) Ipswich, Mass. In 1862.

### DALE, WORCESTER, MASS.

Cutler, John H. In 1865.
Chamberlin, C. N., Lawrence, Mass. In 1865.
Lyon, E. B., New Britain, Conn. In 1865.

### DOUGLAS, WASHINGTON, D. C.

Sutton, G. L., East Fishkill, N. Y. From June, 1862, to April, 1863.

### EASTERN POINT FORT, GLOUCESTER, MASS.

Hildreth, Charles H.. (A. A. Surgeon,) Gloucester, Mass. In 1865.

### EAST NEW YORK, L. I.

Bricket, George E., 3d and 21st Maine Infantry, (Ex. Surgeon,) Augusta, Me. In 1863.

### EMERY, WASHINGTON, D. C.

Moseley, N. R., No. 53 West 36th street. New York City. In 1863-'64-'65.

### FREDERICK CITY, MD.

Lewis, J. B., Hartford, Conn. June, 1862, to —, —.

### FORT HAMILTON, N. Y.

Studley, W. H.. No. 160 E. 83d st., New York city. From August, 1862, to January, 1864.

### FOSTER, NEW BERNE, N. C.

Galioupe, I F., (Ex. Surgeon) Lynn. Mass. From June to August, 1863.
Cowgill, Clayton, ——, Del. In charge.

### FORT CONSTITUTION, PORTSMOUTH, N. H.

Smart, Wm. H., Clermont, N. Y. From 1863-'68.

### FORT RENO, D. C.

Whitney, W. W., Union, N. Y. In 1864-'65.

### FORTS PICKERING AND LEE, MASS.

Haddock, Charles, (Surgeon 8th Massachusetts Infantry.) Beverly, Mass. From May 4 to October 13, 1865.

### FORT FOOTE, MD.

Potter, Z. H., Ithaca. N. Y In 1864.

### FORT LYONS, VA.

Kirk, L R., Rising Sun. Md.

### FILBERT STREET, PHILADELPHIA, PA.

Dunglison, Richard J., Philadelphia, Pa. In 1864.

### GENERAL HOSPITAL, MADISON IND.

Sheets, William H., Jeffersonville, Ind. From 1863 to 1865.

HOSPITALS, ETC—Continued.

HAREWOOD, D. C.

Bontecou, R. B., (Ex. Surgeon,) Troy, N. Y. In 1863–'64.

JUDICIARY SQUARE, D. C.

Adams, J. F. A., Pittsfield, Mass. In 1863.

KNIGHT, NEW HAVEN, CONN.

Abernethy, A. H., Bridgeport, Conn. In 1862–'63.
Jewett, P. A., New Haven, Conn. Surgeon in charge.

LOWELL, PORTSMOUTH GROVE, R. I

Thurston, W. T., Woonsocket, R. I. In 1863.
Cushing, Jos. W., 29 Worcester street, Boston, Mass. In 1864.
Knowles, H. B., Calais, Me.

MOWER, PHILADELPHIA, PA.

Moon, William P., 44th and Haverford street, Philadelphia, Pa. In 1863–'64.

McKIM. BALTIMORE, MD.

Hartman, Andrew, Baltimore, Md. In 1864.

POST CAMP GILMORE, CONCORD, N. H.

Crosby, A. H., Concord, N. H.

SOLDIERS' AND SAILORS' HOME. NEW YORK.

Herrick, Everett, 126 Madison avenue, New York city.
Russell, Mrs. E. L., (Matron,) Grand Union Hotel, Saratoga, N. Y.

SLOAN, MONTPELIER, VT.

Crandall, H. A., Burlington, Vt. From July, 1863, to August, 1864–'65.

WHITE HOUSE LANDING, VA.

Millett, Asa, East-Bridgewater, Mass. In June, 1862.

3D BRIGADE, 22D A. C., NEAR FORT BAKER, D. C.

Russell, Allen S., Marion, N. Y. Records, 1864–'65.

## MISCELLANEOUS.

GEO. B. MILLS, Acting Assistant Surgeon U. S. Vols., Hospital No. 3, *Lookout Mountain, Tenn.* P. O., Pleasantville, Ohio.

W. V. RUTLEDGE, Acting Staff Surgeon U. S. A., was on duty at *Blind School Hospital, Macon, Ga.*, in 1865. P. O., 709 N. 9th st., Saint Louis, Mo.

A. P. WILLIAMS, Assistant Surgeon in charge of *Depot Camp, V. R. C., Washington, D. C.* P. O., Rutherford N. J.

JOHN H. W. FRANK, in charge of *Joe Holt General Hospital, Jeffersonville, Ind.*, from August 10, 1864, to December 17, 1864, and from March 13, 1865, to May 13, 1865. In charge of *Wilson General Hospital, Nashville, Tenn.*, from December 18, 1864, to March 31, 1865. P. O. address, Hardinsburgh, Ky.

DR. HENRY CUSHMAN, in charge of *Eruptive Hospital, Louisville, Ky.*, in 1863. P. O. Brighton, Iowa.

A. C. SWARTZWELDER, Surgeon U. S. V., was at same hospital. P. O. Waco, Texas.

NAZARETH PAQUETT served as nurse in 1st Division, 9th Army Corps Hospital. P. O., Petersburgh, Mich.

N. F. LITCHFIELD, Acting Assistant Surgeon A. S. A., in charge of Post Hospital, *Fort Sumner, Mich.*, 1863 and 1864. P. O., North Newbury, Mich.

WM. H. HIRE was a Contract Surgeon at *Saint James Hospital, New Orleans, La.*, from December 3, 1862, to July, 1863. Prior to the above he was at Marine Hospital, and Surgeon of the first board of enrollment of volunteers, at New Orleans. P. O address, New Orleans, La.

EDWARD J DARKEN was Assistant Surgeon from April, 1863, to April, 1868 On duty at Hospital No. 4, *Nashville, Tenn.*, and with 18th U. S. Infantry and with 3d Cavalry at *Fort Smith, Ark.*; then at *Fort Hamilton, N. Y.*; then at *Vicksburg* as Chief Medical Officer of Mississippi. P. O. address, No. 244 E. 25th st., New York city.

A. H. ROBINSON, of Concord, N. H., was an acting Assistant Surgeon in charge of Depot Hospital, at that place, from 1861 to 1864.

*Highest number of organizations from each State and Territory in the military service of the United States since April* 15, 1861.

| STATES, &C. | Infantry. | Cavalry. | Artillery. | Batteries. |
|---|---|---|---|---|
| Alabama | 4 | 1 | 1 | ...... |
| Arkansas | 4 | 4 | ...... | 1 |
| California | 8 | 2 | ...... | ...... |
| Colorado | 3 | 3 | ...... | 1 |
| Connecticut | 30 | 1 | 2 | 3 |
| Dakota | ...... | 1 | ...... | ...... |
| Delaware | 9 | 1 | 1 co. | 1 |
| District of Columbia | 2 | 1 | 1 co. | ...... |
| Florida | ...... | 2 | ...... | ...... |
| Illinois | 156 | 17 | 2 | 9 |
| Indiana | 156 | 13 | 1 | 26 |
| Indian Territory | 3 | ...... | ...... | ...... |
| Iowa | 48 | 9 | ...... | 4 |
| Kansas | 13 | 19 | ...... | 3 |
| Kentucky | 55 | 17 | 2 | 1 |
| Louisiana | 12 | 2 | 1 | 3 |
| Maine | 32 | 2 | 1 | ...... |
| Maryland | 13 | 3 | ...... | *4 |
| Massachusetts | 62 | 5 | 4 | 16 |
| Michigan | 30 | 11 | 1 | 14 |
| Minnesota | 11 | 2 | 1 | 3 |
| Mississippi | 6 | 1 | 2 | ...... |
| Missouri | 51 | 16 | 2 | ...... |
| Nebraska | 2 cos. | 2 | ...... | ...... |
| Nevada | 1 | 1 | ...... | ...... |
| New Hampshire | 18 | 2 | 1 | 1 |
| New Jersey | 40 | 3 | ...... | 5 |
| New Mexico | 5 | 1 | ...... | ...... |
| New York | 194 | 26 | 16 | 34 |
| North Carolina | 3 | ...... | 1 | ...... |
| Ohio | 198 | 13 | 2 | 26 |
| Oregon | 1 | 1 | ...... | ...... |
| Pennsylvania | 215 | 22 | 6 | *9 |
| Rhode Island | 12 | 3 | 14 | 1 |
| South Carolina | 4 | ...... | ...... | ...... |
| Tennessee | 10 | 14 | 2 | ...... |
| Texas | ...... | 2 | ...... | ...... |
| Vermont | 17 | 1 | 1 | 3 |
| Virginia | 1 co. | 1 | ...... | ...... |
| Washington Territory | 1 | ...... | ...... | ...... |
| West Virginia | 17 | 7 | ...... | *8 |
| Wisconsin | 53 | 4 | 1 | 13 |
| United States Army | 45 | 10 | 5 | ...... |
| United States Volunteers | 6 | ...... | ...... | ...... |
| United States Veteran Volunteers | 9 | ...... | ...... | ...... |
| United States Sharpshooters | 2 | ...... | ...... | ...... |
| United States Colored Troops | 138 | 6 | 14 | 1 |
| Corps d'Afrique | 25 | 1 | 1 | ...... |
| United States Veteran Reserve Corps | 24 reg'ts and 246 cos. in 1st Battalion. 174 companies in 2d Battalion. | | | |

* Batteries lettered, not numbered.

# PENSION AGENCY DISTRICTS.

CORRECTED TO APRIL 1, 1883.

---

AUGUSTA, ME—SELDEN CONNOR.
The State of Maine.

*BOSTON, MASS—D. W. GOOCH.
The States of Massachusetts, Connecticut, and Rhode Island.

*CHICAGO, ILL—ADA C. SWEET.
The State of Illinois.

COLUMBUS, OHIO—A. T. WIKOFF.
The State of Ohio.

CONCORD, N. H—E. L. WHITFORD.
The States of New Hampshire and Vermont

DES MOINES, IOWA—JACOB RICH.
The States of Iowa and Nebraska.

DETROIT, MICH—SAMUEL POST.
The State of Michigan.

INDIANAPOLIS, IND—FRED. KNEFLER.
The State of Indiana.

*KNOXVILLE, TENN—D T. BOYNTON.
The States of Virginia. West Virginia. North Carolina, Tennessee, South Carolina, Georgia, Florida, Alabama, Mississippi, Louisiana, Texas, and Arkansas.

LOUISVILLE, KY—R. M. KELLY.
The State of Kentucky.

MILWAUKEE, WIS—E. FERGUSON.
The States of Wisconsin and Minnesota, and the Territories of Dakota, Montana, and Wyoming.

*NEW YORK CITY, N. Y—CHAS. R. COSTER.
The Counties of Albany, Clinton, Columbia, Delaware, Dutchess, Essex, Greene, Kings, Queens New York, Orange, Putnam, Richmond, Rensselaer, Rockland, Saratoga, Schenectady, Sullivan, Suffolk, Ulster, Warren, Washington, and Westchester.

*PHILADELPHIA, PA—H. G. SICKEL.
The Counties of Berks, Bradford, Bucks, Carbon, Chester, Columbia, Dauphin, Delaware, Lackawanna, Lancaster, Lebanon, Lehigh, Luzerne, Monroe, Montgomery, Montour, Northampton, Northumberland, Philadelphia, Pike, Schuylkill, Sullivan, Susquehanna, Wayne, Wyoming, and York.

PITTSBURGH, PA—RUSSELL ERRETT.
The remaining Counties of the State.

*SAN FRANCISCO, CAL—HENRY COX.
The States of California, Nevada, and Oregon, and the Territories of Idaho, Washington, Arizona, and Utah, (Alaska.)

SYRACUSE, N. Y—T. L. POOLE.
Counties of the State not in New York City District.

TOPEKA, KANS—NATHANIEL A. ADAMS.
The States of Missouri, Kansas, and Colorado, the Territory of New Mexico, and the Indian Territory.

*WASHINGTON, D. C—THEOPHILUS GAINES.
The States of New Jersey, Delaware, Maryland, the District of Columbia, and all the National Home and foreign pensioners.

---

* Pays Navy Pensions.

# ERRATA.

## ALABAMA.

1st Cavalry—Stuart Absalom B., Surgeon, Santa Rosa, Cal. Also 10th Missouri Infantry. (Pages 70, 173.)

McDavitt, Virgil, Assistant Surgeon, Quincy, Ill. (Page 72.)

## COLORADO.

2d Cavalry—Vance, D. M., Assistant Surgeon. (Page 72.)

Thompson, S. B., Assistant Surgeon. (Page 72.)

King, Dean W., Assistant Surgeon, Boulder, Col. (Page 72.)

## KENTUCKY.

5th Cavalry—Alexander, R. M., Assistant Surgeon, Burksville, Ky. Alleged dead. (Page 128.)

6th Cavalry—Peters, Preston, Acting Assistant Surgeon, Louisville, Ky. (Page 128.)

7th Cavalry—Burnham, A. T., Assistant Surgeon. (Page 129.)

14th Cavalry—Daniels, John M., Con't Surgeon, Proctor or Pleasant Hill, Ky. Alleged dead by P. M. (Page 129.)

17th Cavalry—Wright, Alex., private. Was Acting Hospital Steward from May, 1865. (Page 129.)

1st Infantry—Menzies, S. G., Surgeon, 137 W. 6th street, Cincinnati, Ohio. Alleged dead. (Page 130.)

5th Infantry—Miller, S. J. F., Assistant Surgeon, National Military Home, Milwaukee, Wis. (Page 130.)

12th Infantry—Mullins, W. H., Surgeon, Richmond, Ky. (Page 131.)

14th Infantry—Miller A. C., Surgeon, Cleveland, Ohio. Dead. (Page 132.)

17th Infantry—Hubbard, Stewart, Assistant Surgeon, Woodlawn, Neb. (Page 132.)

39th Infantry—Hereford, J. H., Surgeon, Prestonburg, Ky. (Page 134.)

Sweatman, H. S., Acting Assistant Surgeon, Louisa, Ky. (Page 134.)

55th Infantry—Palmer, E. R., Assistant Surgeon, Louisville, Ky. (Page 135.)

## LOUISIANA.

1st New Orleans Infantry—Paine, J. T., Surgeon, 242 Esplanade, New Orleans, La (Page 136.)

## MARYLAND.

2d and 4th Infantry, E. S.—Owings, H. W., Surgeon, 274 Madison avenue, Baltimore, Md. (Page 143.)

7th Infantry—Buhrman, Harvey, Assistant Surgeon, Foxville, Md.; also 11th Infantry. (Page 144.)

## MISSOURI.

1st Battalion S. M. Cavalry—Bruere, John, Assistant Surgeon, St. Charles. Mo. (Page 166.)

2d Cavalry—Dickinson, E. C., Surgeon, Kansas City, Mo.; also 11th and 14th S. M. Cavalry. Dead. (Page 167.)

6th Cavalry—Bluder, O. C., Acting Assistant Surgeon, Hiattville, Kan. (Page 167.)

7th Cavalry—Foster, Wm. D., Assistant Surgeon, Hannibal. Mo. (Page 168.)

6th Infantry—Mathews, N. C., Acting Assistant Surgeon, Jakes Prairie, Mo. (Page 172.)

30th Infantry—Sargent, B. W. To 6th U. S. Col. H. Art. November 1863. Dead. (Page 175.)

43d Infantry—Dill, Ed. W., Assistant Surgeon, Westport, Mo. Dead. (Page 176.)

Egleston, John Q., Surgeon, Olathe, Kan.; also 25th Infantry. (Page 176.)

## TENNESSEE.

4th Cavalry—Brown, John G., Surgeon. Dead. (Page 285.)

7th Cavalry—Arbuckle, Edward, Surgeon, Elm Tree, Tenn. (Page 285.)

# INDEX TO LIST OF BATTLES, ETC.



# INDEX TO ROSTER OF SURGEONS.

# EXPLANATIONS.

"G."—Good.
"I."—Intemperate.
"R."—Records.
"U. M."—Unsound mind.
"H. R."—Has records, or private memoranda.
"A. G. R."—Adjutant General's Report.
"A. W. M."—Appointed and waiting muster into the U. S. service.
"Dism."—Dismissed.
"U. S. Ex. S." or "Ex. S."—U. S. Examining Surgeon for Pension Office.

"To Jan'y, '64," in column of remarks, means the time at which the Surgeon left the organization, either by resignation, discharge, or transfer.

"From Feb'y, '62," means the time that Surgeon was commissioned to the rank that appears opposite his name. A Surgeon may have been commissioned in January, 1862, as Assistant Surgeon, and promoted to Surgeon in March, 1864; the last-named date would appear opposite his name as Surgeon from "March, 1864," whereas he may have been serving in the same organization as Assistant Surgeon for two years or more prior to that date.

OFFICE OF "THE UNION VOLUNTEER,"
604 13TH STREET,
WASHINGTON, D. C., *April*, 1883.

## TO THE PUBLIC.

Mr. Newton A. Strait, the compiler of this work, has been indefatigable in his efforts, and his labors have made this index as correct as possible to date; and the soldiers of the country owe him a debt of gratitude for his labors in their behalf.

The Adjutant and Surgeon Generals' reports were not always correct, in which case he consulted other authorities, thus making a book invaluable to every soldier in the land.

We have found it necessary to place a second edition of 10,000 copies on the market, and from the demand, believe 100,000 will be needed. Any changes of address, the fact of *death*, or unavoidable omission, will be gladly received, and such notice by postal or otherwise will be appreciated.

Mr. Strait has made this work so necessary to soldiers having claims for pensions pending, as well as to Surgeons and Grand Army Posts, that we expect each one will eventually possess himself of a copy.

Respectfully,
G. M. VAN BUREN,
*Publisher.*

# Index

The *Roster* in several instances lists the same person with either a variation or a misspelling of either the first or the last name. In these cases we have indicated the variation by putting it in parentheses following the initial entry. An asterisk (*) indicates that two listings are more than likely the same person. A number sign (#) indicates that two listings may or may not be the same person.

Norman Publishing is a division of Jeremy Norman & Company, Inc., leading international dealers in rare books and manuscripts in the history of medicine and science.

The following people collaborated on the production of the *List of Battles and Roster of Regimental Surgeons*.

Steven Hiatt, Copy Editor
Jill Rotenberg, Project Manager
Martha Steele, Editorial Assistant
Seventeenth Street Studios, Designer

The layout was done by Donna Kelley at Zetatype Desktop Publishers of San Francisco, using Ventura Publisher. The type is Bodoni, a Postscript font from Adobe Systems.

Linotronic output by Pinnacle Type, San Francisco.

Printed and bound by Braun-Brumfield, Inc., Ann Arbor.

With its geometrical framework, the Norman Publishing logo resembles the constructed letters of the Renaissance, but there the resemblance ends. The logo incorporates the capital letter N within an arc of the logarithmic spiral, one of the most beautiful mathematical curves appearing in nature. It links together the graphic arts and the sciences, reflecting the dual commitments of Norman Publishing.

NORMAN
PUBLISHING TM